UK Ambulance Services
Clinical Practice
Guidelines 2013

Disclaimer

The Association of Ambulance Chief Executives and the Joint Royal Colleges Ambulance Liaison Committee have made every effort to ensure that the information, tables, drawings and diagrams contained in these guidelines are accurate at the time of publication. However, the 2013 guidelines are advisory and have been developed to assist healthcare professionals, and patients, to make decisions about the management of the patient's health, including treatments. This advice is intended to support the decision making process and is not a substitute for sound clinical judgement. The guidelines cannot always contain all the information necessary for determining appropriate care and cannot address all individual situations; therefore, individuals using these guidelines must ensure they have the appropriate knowledge and skills to enable suitable interpretation.

The Association of Ambulance Chief Executives does not guarantee, and accepts no legal liability of whatever nature arising from or connected to, the accuracy, reliability, currency or completeness of the content of these guidelines.

Users of these guidelines must always be aware that such innovations or alterations after the date of publication may not be incorporated in the content. As part of its commitment to defining national standards, the association will periodically issue updates to the content and users should ensure that they are using the most up-to-date version of the guidelines. These updates can be found on www.2013guidelines.com, www.AACE.org.uk or www.warwick.ac.uk/go/jrcalcguidelines. Please note however that the Association of Ambulance Chief Executives assumes no responsibility whatsoever for the content of external resources.

Although some modification of the guidelines may be required by individual ambulance services, and approved by the relevant local clinical committees, to ensure they respond to the health requirements of the local community, the majority of the guidance is universally applicable to NHS ambulance services. Modification of the guidelines may also occur when undertaking research sanctioned by a research ethics committee.

Whilst these guidelines cover the full range of paramedic treatments available across the UK they will also provide a valuable tool for ambulance technicians and other pre-hospital providers. Many of the assessment skills and general principles will remain the same. Those not qualified to paramedic level must practise within their level of training and competence.

UK Ambulance Services
Clinical Practice
Guidelines 2013

Edited for JRCALC by

Joanne D Fisher, Simon N Brown, Matthew Cooke

and for NASMeD by

Alison Walker, Fionna Moore, Pam Crispin

With thanks to:

Mark Millins, Kevin Webb, Bartholomew Wood, David Whitmore,
Stephen Hines, Mark Whitbread and Andy Swinburn

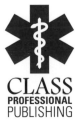

CLASS
PROFESSIONAL
PUBLISHING

© Association of Ambulance Chief Executives (AACE) 2013

Printing history
First edition published 2000, second edition 2004, third edition 2006
This edition 2013

The authors and publisher welcome feedback from the users of this book.
Please contact the publisher:
Class Professional Publishing Ltd,
The Exchange, Express Park, Bristol Road, Bridgwater TA6 4RR
Telephone: 01278 427843
Email: post@class.co.uk
Website: www.classprofessional.co.uk

Class Professional Publishing is an imprint of Class Publishing Ltd

A CIP catalogue record for this book is available from the British Library
ISBN 978 1 85959 363 9

Designed and typeset by Typematter

Line illustrations by David Woodroffe

Printed in Slovenia by arrangement with KINT Ljubljana

Contents

Foreword

Dr Anthony C Marsh SBStJ DSci (Hon) MBA MSc FASI

Chairman of the Association of Ambulance Chief Executives

I am delighted to acknowledge at the very start of these 2013 guidelines the tremendous amount of hard work that has gone into their publication. I wish to express my thanks to the contributors at JRCALC, especially the clinical guideline committee chaired by Dr Simon Brown and also the team at Warwick University who have worked so hard to collate this 2013 edition.

I am also very proud of the contribution made by so many Paramedics, whether researching evidence, writing sections or editing copy. It is a great testament to the profession that they now play such a significant part in influencing their own clinical practice.

The Association of Ambulance Chief Executives would also like to thank the National Ambulance Service Medical Directors group chaired by Dr Alison Walker for their invaluable expertise. We will all wish to ensure updates to this edition are produced when required. Future editions will be produced in a timely manner and in formats that best support clinical practice on the front line. This will enable us to provide the very best clinical care and to achieve the best outcomes for patients.

Dr Simon N Brown

Chairman of the Guideline Development Group, Joint Royal Colleges Liaison Committee

The 2013 Clinical Practice Guidelines provide guidance for NHS paramedics; although the principles are applicable to the work of all pre-hospital clinicians. The guidelines are an important part of clinical risk management and ensure uniformity in the delivery of high quality patient care. As such, they form the basis for UK paramedic training and education.

Significant revisions have been made to this edition including the introduction of new guidelines for major pelvic trauma, airway and breathing management, intravascular fluid therapy (page-for-age), obstetrics and gynaecological emergencies overview, management of the newborn, and the assessment and management of incapacitating agents, clopidogrel, dexamethasone, patient's own midazolam, misoprostol, ondansetron and tranexamic acid. In addition, there is a new section for use at the scene of chemical, biological, radiological, nuclear and explosive incidents, which includes drug guidelines for atropine, ciprofloxacin, dicobalt, doxycycline, obidoxime, potassium iodate, and pralidoxime mesylate.

There is also new guidance on the management of minor illness in children, to help identify those that can be safely left at home; this is in recognition of the increase in calls to children with minor illness and acknowledging that paramedics receive less training in the management of children with minor illness and injury. Guidelines include an overview of minor illness, febrile illness, respiratory illnesses and gastroenteritis.

An important change is the move to **<C>ABC** from **ABC** for all trauma guidelines, to indicate the importance of identifying and managing catastrophic haemorrhage. These guidelines also contain the latest guidance for cardiopulmonary resuscitation.

Professor Matthew W Cooke

Guideline Academic Director and Professor of Emergency Medicine, Warwick Medical School

The UK Ambulance Service Clinical Practice Guidelines have evolved from locally-derived guidance, mainly developed using non-systematic approaches, to systematically-developed evidence based national clinical practice guidelines. The guidelines utilise rigorous national standards for guideline development.

The multidisciplinary approach involving all UK ambulance services and many other stakeholders in the development has provided a wealth of experience and expertise. This has also enhanced ownership and will lead to improved clinical outcomes, when combined with appropriate service delivery systems.

Any clinical guidelines are designed to support the clinical decision making of the professional. These guidelines have been developed to work in the rapidly evolving world of the autonomous clinical practitioner delivering personalised care, whilst also appreciating the importance of utilising best evidence.

We are indebted to those who have helped in producing guidelines, or have allowed their work to be reproduced, for this edition.

Consent Statement

Consent in Pre-hospital Care

The laws and guidance that relate to consent to assessment, treatment, care and other interventions are different in the countries and/or jurisdictions that constitute the United Kingdom.

Therefore, these guidelines do not offer guidance on obtaining consent beyond the general advice in this statement. The Joint Royal Colleges Ambulance Liaison Committee (JRCALC) advises strongly that readers should seek specific guidance on consent from their Ambulance Services or Trusts or other relevant employers.

JRCALC advises that obtaining consent in ways that are lawful in the jurisdiction in which each reader works is fundamental to meeting patients' legal and ethical rights in determining what happens to them and to their own bodies. Therefore, it is important to ensure that you have legally valid consent to conduct assessments, treatments and other interventions, and provide care. Consent must be obtained from each patient or their legally valid representative (defined according to the law in the relevant country or jurisdiction) prior to conducting examinations, treatment, or providing care.

In pre-hospital situations, it is not uncommon for patients to refuse assessment, care or treatment. Although patients may refuse, there may be, depending on the circumstances, continuing moral duties and legal responsibilities for ambulance clinicians to provide further intervention, particularly if life-threatening risk is involved. Again, ambulance clinicians are advised to obtain advice from their employers about circumstances of this nature so the actions they take are appropriate to the legal jurisdiction in which they are working.

Further guidance can be obtained from:

- The Department of Health for England: http://www.dh.gov.uk/en/index.htm
- The Scottish Government: http://www.scotland.gov.uk/Topics/Health
- The Welsh Assembly Government: http://wales.gov.uk/?lang=en
- The Department of Health, Social Services and Public Safety in Northern Ireland: http://www.dhsspsni.gov.uk/

Guideline Developers and Contributors

Guideline Contributors	Organisation/Affiliation
Simon Brown (Chairman)	South Central Ambulance Service
Andy Collen	South East Coast Ambulance Service NHS Trust/College of Paramedics
Carl Keeble	East Midlands Ambulance Service
Caroline Leech	University Hospitals Coventry and Warwickshire NHS Trust
Cathryn James	Yorkshire Ambulance Service
Charles Deakin	South Central Ambulance Service
Chris Evans	Welsh Ambulance Service
Darren Walter	North West Ambulance Service
Dhushy Surendra Kumar	Royal College of Anaesthetists
Fiona Jewkes	The Royal College of Paediatrics and Child Health
Fionna Moore	London Ambulance Service
Helen Simpson	Royal College of Obstetrics and Gynaecology
Henry Guly	Plymouth Hospitals NHS Trust
Ian Mursell	Coventry University/West Midlands Ambulance Service
Jane Worthington	London Ambulance Service
John Black	South Central Ambulance Service
John Stephenson	East Midlands Ambulance Service
Jonathan Dermott	East of England Ambulance Service
Jonathan Ellis	East Midlands Ambulance Service
Julian Mark	Yorkshire Ambulance Service
Julian Sandell	The Royal College of Paediatrics and Child Health
Kevin Webb	Welsh Ambulance Service
Kim Hinshaw	Royal College of Obstetrics and Gynaecology
Malcolm Woollard	College of Paramedics
Mark Bloch	Aberdeen Royal Infirmary
Mark Whitbread	London Ambulance Service NHS Trust/College of Paramedics
Martin Lewis	South East Coast Ambulance Service
Matthew Cooke	The University of Warwick
Matthew O'Meara	The University of Warwick
Mike Jenkins	Welsh Ambulance Service
Mike Smyth	West Midlands Ambulance Service NHS Trust/College of Paramedics
Nicky Fothergill	East Midlands Ambulance Service
Paul Cassford	Isle of Wight Ambulance Service
Paul Grant	South Central Ambulance Service
Paul Johnson	London Ambulance Service
Phil Hallam	West Midlands Ambulance Service
Quen Mok	The Royal College of Paediatrics and Child Health
Ravi Chauhan	The University of Warwick
Richard Steyn	Heart of England NHS Foundation Trust
Richard Whitfield	Welsh Ambulance Service NHS Trust/College of Paramedics
Richard Williams	Royal College of Psychiatrists
Rob Russell	Royal Centre for Defence Medicine
Robin Beal	Isle of Wight Ambulance Service
Robin Lawrenson	Scottish Ambulance Service/College of Paramedics
Rodger Gregson	Yorkshire Ambulance Service
Sarah Black	South Western Ambulance Service
Stef Cormack	West Midlands Ambulance Service
Stephen Hines	London Ambulance Service
Steve Mortley	East of England Ambulance Service
Tim Hodgetts	College of Emergency Medicine
Tom Clarke	North East Ambulance Service
Tom Mallinson	The University of Warwick
Tom Quinn	The University of Surrey
Tony Bleetman	Great Western Ambulance Service
Tullie Yeghen	Lewisham Healthcare NHS Trust
Vicky O'Leary	Great Western Ambulance Service
Adam Zenkner	The University of Warwick
Adrian Castle	London Ambulance Service

Guideline Developers and Contributors

Guideline Developers	Organisation/Affiliation
Alan Dobson	Royal College of Nursing
Alex Knight	The University of Warwick
Alison Walker	Yorkshire Ambulance Service
Andrew Downes	East of England Ambulance NHS Trust/College of Paramedics
Professor Andy Newton	South East Coast Ambulance NHS Trust/College of Paramedics
Andy Rosser	West Midlands Ambulance Service
Bill Mason	Scottish Ambulance Service
Bob Fellows	London Ambulance Service/College of Paramedics
Chris Horswell	The University of Warwick
Christopher Jones	University of Teeside/College of Paramedics
Colin Cessford	North East Ambulance Service
Dan Staines	West Midlands Ambulance Service
David McManus	Northern Ireland Ambulance Service
David Wilmot	Great Western Ambulance Service
David Halliwell	South Western Ambulance Service
Dominic Tolley	West Midlands Ambulance Service
Donal O'Donaghue	Surviving Sepsis Campaign
Elizabeth Kershaw	East Midlands Ambulance Service
Emma Hines	Medical Negligence Solicitor
Fizz Thompson	South Central Ambulance Service
Gary Strong	Great Western Ambulance Service
Gavin Perkins	The UK Resuscitation Council
Geraint Farr	Welsh Ambulance Service
Gillian Bryce	South Western Ambulance Service
Graeme Mattison	The University of Warwick
Iain McNeil	Royal College of General Practitioners
James Coe	The University of Warwick
James Gray	East Midlands Ambulance Service
James Webster	The University of Warwick
Jeremy Mayhew	South East Coast Ambulance Service
Katie Hawkins	The University of Warwick
Keith Porter	Faculty of Pre-hospital Care
Kyee Han	North East Ambulance Service
Lee Styles	East of England Ambulance Service
Lesley Altoft	Great Western Ambulance Service
Mark Ainsworth-Smith	South Central Ambulance Service
Matthew Wyse	West Midlands Ambulance Service
Mick Colquhoun	The UK Resuscitation Council
Mike Ward	Joint Royal Colleges Ambulance Liaison Committee
Niro Siriwardena	East Midlands Ambulance Service
Pam Hardy	East Midlands Ambulance Service
Paul Fell	North East Ambulance Service
Rachel Ryan	British National Formulary
Rodger Gadsby	The University of Warwick
Ron Daniels	Surviving Sepsis Campaign
Rose Jarvis	The University of Warwick
Russell Thornhill	Isle of Man Ambulance Service
Sam Oestreicher	Staff Side Ambulance Council
Sean Mitchell	South East Coast Ambulance Service
Shaun Carter	Isle of Wight Ambulance Service
Simon Stockley	Royal College of General Practitioners
Steven Rawstorne	Great Western Ambulance Service
Stuart Cooper	East of England Ambulance Service
Victoria Leeson	Great Western Ambulance Service
Wim Blancke	Royal College of Anaesthetists
Yenushka Llangakoon	The University of Warwick

Update Analysis

Significant revisions have been made to this edition. The layout of the guidelines has a standard approach for presenting information, and where possible, sections on incidence, severity and outcome and pathophysiology are included. The assessment and management sections have also been standardised and are now presented in table format. References to stand-alone guidance for fluid therapy, oxygen therapy and airway and breathing management are made to reduce repetition of information in each guideline. The administration and dosages tables for drugs have been re-formatted and now include column headings for age, initial dose, repeat dose, dose interval, concentration, volume and maximum dose. Assessment and management algorithms have been created for all conditions where appropriate and included in the pocket guide.

There is new guidance for the management of major pelvic trauma, airway and breathing management, obstetrics and gynaecological emergencies overview, management of the newborn, and the assessment and management of incapacitating agents. In addition guidance for intravascular therapy has been developed and includes algorithms for quick reference. An important change is the move to **<C>ABC** from **ABC** for all trauma guidelines to indicate the importance of identifying and managing catastrophic haemorrhage; a definition of catastrophic haemorrhage and guidance for its management, including the use of haemostatic agents, is also provided. There is also new guidance on the management of minor illness in children, to help identify those that can be safely left at home; this is in recognition of the increase in calls to children with minor illness and acknowledging that paramedics receive less training in the management of children with minor illness and injury. Guidelines include an overview of minor illness, febrile illness, respiratory illnesses and gastroenteritis.

New drug guidelines for administration of clopidogrel, dexamethasone, patient's own midazolam, misoprostol, ondansetron and tranexamic acid have been added. A new section for use at the scene of chemical biological, radiological, nuclear and explosive incidents has been added and includes new drug guidelines for the administration of ciprofloxacin, dicobalt, doxycycline, obidoxime, potassium iodate, and pralidoxime mesylate that may be required for these incidents.

These guidelines contain the latest guidance for cardiopulmonary resuscitation http://www.resus.org.uk.

The following table indicates where key changes have been made and is a signpost to changes within the guidelines, but is not a substitute for reading and assimilating the new guidelines.

Update Analysis

Section 1

General guidance	Addition/update of guidance and rationale
Consent Statement	The laws and guidance that relate to consent to assessment, treatment, care and other interventions are different in the countries and/or jurisdictions that constitute the United Kingdom. Therefore, these guidelines do not offer guidance on obtaining consent beyond the general advice contained in this statement. The Joint Royal Colleges Ambulance Liaison Committee (JRCALC) advises strongly that readers should seek specific guidance on consent from their Ambulance Services or Trusts or other relevant employers. JRCALC advises that obtaining consent in ways that are lawful in the jurisdiction in which each reader works is fundamental to meeting patients' legal and ethical rights in determining what happens to them and to their own bodies. Therefore, it is important to ensure that you have legally valid consent to conduct assessments, treatments and other interventions, and provide care. Consent must be obtained from each patient or his or her legally valid representative (defined according to the law in the relevant country or jurisdiction) prior to conducting examinations, treatment, or providing care. In pre-hospital situations, it is not uncommon for patients to refuse assessment, care or treatment. Although patients may refuse, there may be, depending on the circumstances, continuing moral duties and legal responsibilities for ambulance clinicians to provide further intervention, particularly if life-threatening risk is involved. Again, ambulance clinicians are advised to obtain advice from their employers about circumstances of this nature so the actions they take are appropriate to the legal jurisdiction in which they are working. Further guidance can be obtained from: ● **The Department of Health for England (DH)**: http://www.dh.gov.uk/en/index.htm ● **The Scottish Government**: http://www.scotland.gov.uk/Topics/Health ● **The Welsh Assembly Government**: http://wales.gov.uk/?lang=en ● **The Department of Health, Social Services and Public Safety in Northern Ireland**: http://www.dhsspsni.gov.uk/
Patient Confidentiality	● The importance of recording accurate information about patients is further emphasised. ● Guidance is included on what action to take if personal data has been lost or disclosed to unauthorised persons. ● The section on requests by the media has been expanded to include guidance on managing personal media criticism.
Pain Management	● An emphasis on a more balanced approach to pain management by treating the cause, introducing more than one agent i.e. psychological, physical and pharmacological methods, and administering analgesia incrementally, except in cases where it is clear that a stronger analgesic is required. ● A change to the assessment of pain with the inclusion of the SOCRATES mnemonic and an emphasis on administering analgesia as soon as clinically possible after arriving on scene. ● The inclusion of intravenous paracetamol. ● The need to adhere to strict Service guidelines on the use of the intra-osseous route for pain relief which is not routinely recommended. ● The routine use of metoclopramide for nausea induced by morphine administration is also no longer recommended. ● A section is included on ketamine which is being used by some Service and local protocols should be adhered to on this.

Update Analysis

General guidance	Addition/update of guidance and rationale
Pain Management in Children	• As with adults there is an emphasis on a more balanced approach to pain management by treating the cause, introducing more than one agent i.e. psychological, physical and pharmacological methods, and administering analgesia incrementally, except in cases where it is clear that a stronger analgesic is required. • The use of the Wong-Baker faces is recommended for the assessment of children in pain, and for pre-verbal children the FLACC scale (table 1.8) is now recommended. • An emphasis on administering analgesia as soon as clinically possible after arriving on scene. • The inclusion of intravenous paracetamol. • Paramedics should note that the section on regional anaesthesia in children is currently for specialist pre-hospital Doctors only.
Safeguarding Children	• There is increased emphasis that the first priority is the health and safety of the child by the inclusion of the ABCDE and <C>ABCDE assessment paradigms. • Definitions of harm have been updated (Working Together to Safeguard Children, 2010). • The generic safeguarding report form has been removed and ambulance clinicians should use forms provide by their Service.
Sexual Assault	• Further information on different types of sexual assault. • An expansion of section on forensic examination.
Vulnerable Adults	• There is increased emphasis that the first priority is the health and safety of the patient by the inclusion of the ABCDE and <C>ABCDE assessment paradigms. • The generic safeguarding report form has been removed and ambulance clinicians should use forms provided by their Service.
Death of a Child (Including Sudden Unexpected Death in Infancy)	• The title of this guideline has changed to "Death of a child, including sudden unexpected deaths in infancy, children and adolescents (SUDICA)". • Emphasises inter-agency communication and working and describes the conditions unequivocally associated with death in children aged <18 years. • An example of a local child death procedure is provided for information.

Section 2

Resuscitation	Addition/update of guidance and rationale
Resuscitation	<ul><li>Overall:<ul><li>– All resuscitation and related guidance now reflects the 2010 European Resuscitation Council Guidelines .</li><li>– The endotracheal route is no longer recommended for drug administration.</li></ul></li></ul>
Airway and Breathing Management	<ul><li>A new guideline providing stepwise guidance on airway and breathing management.</li><li>Reduced emphasis on tracheal intubation which needs to be undertaken only by highly skilled individuals.</li><li>Emphasis on the use of capnography with both tracheal intubation and SGAs to provide feedback on CPR.</li><li>A reference table with airway sizes by type is provided.</li></ul>
Traumatic Cardiac Arrest	<ul><li>A distinction is made between blunt and penetrating traumatic cardiac arrest.</li><li>Penetrating trauma resulting in a cardiac arrest should be rapidly transferred to hospital with full ALS support. In blunt trauma full ALS should be performed for 20 minutes in the absence of non-survivable injuries before termination of resuscitation attempts.</li><li><C>ABC has replaced ABC to reflect the importance of assessing and managing catastrophic haemorrhage i.e. extreme bleeding likely to cause death in minutes.</li></ul>
ROLE	<ul><li>Conditions unequivocally associated with death have been amended and are:<ul><li>– Massive cranial and cerebral destruction</li><li>– Hemicorporectomy or similar massive injury</li><li>– Decomposition putrefaction</li><li>– Incineration</li><li>– Hypostasis</li><li>– Rigor mortis</li><li>– Fetal maceration.</li></ul></li><li>The 15 minute time limit for not commencing CPR has been clarified to 15 minutes since the onset of cardiac arrest.</li></ul>
Basic Life Support (Adults)	<ul><li>Ambulance clinicians should look for signs of life and if they are confident in the technique, they may add a pulse check for diagnosing cardiac arrest and decide whether they should begin compressions or not. This decision must be made within 10 seconds.</li><li>A strong emphasis on delivering high quality, uninterrupted chest compressions remains essential. Compress the chest to a depth of 5–6cm at a rate of 100–120 compressions min^{-1}, allowing full chest recoil, and minimising interruptions to chest compressions.</li><li>In the event of ROSC following BLS the recovery position is no longer recommended.</li></ul>

Resuscitation	Addition/update of guidance and rationale
Advanced Life Support	• The use of capnography during ALS will provide feedback on the quality of CPR and is encouraged. • Good quality CPR should be given while a defibrillator is retrieved, applied and charged. • Routine delivery of a pre-specified period of CPR prior to the first shock is no longer recommended. • Immediate resumption of chest compressions following defibrillation is emphasised; in combination with continuation of compressions with continuation of compressions during defibrillator charging. The delivery of defibrillation should be achievable with an interruption in chest compressions of < 5 seconds. • Drugs should not be administered via the tracheal tube, if IV access cannot be achieved then the intra-osseous route should be used. • When treating VF/VT adrenaline 1 mg 1:10,000 IV/IO is given after the 3rd and 5th shock. Amiodarone 300 mg IV/IO is given after the 3rd shock and an additional 150mg amiodarone IV/IO is given after the 5th shock. • Atropine is no longer recommended for routine use in asytole or PEA. • Reduced emphasis on tracheal intubation unless it can be achieved by a highly skilled individual with minimal interruption to chest compressions. • Increased emphasis on the use of capnography to confirm quality of CPR, provide early indication of ROSC. It can also confirm tracheal tube placement, where performed, and can be used with an SGA. • Recognition of the potential harm of hyperoxaemia after ROSC is achieved: Titrate inspired oxygen to achieve a SpO_2 of 98%.
ROSC	• An emphasis on conveying the patient to an appropriate PPCI centre if the cause of the arrest was non-traumatic in origin. • The use of active cooling in non-traumatic cases. Note that this is a specialist technique requiring appropriate equipment and Service guidelines should be adhered to.
Foreign Body Airway Obstruction	• No significant changes.
Maternal Resuscitation	• Further emphasis on undertaking a time critical transfer for pregnant mothers as soon as ventilation is achieved and CPR commenced; continuing CPR en-route to minimise delay on scene.
Basic Life Support (Children)	• Updated in line with 2010 European Resuscitation Council Guidelines. • Ambulance clinicians should look for signs of life and, if they are confident in the technique, they may add a pulse check for diagnosing cardiac arrest and decide whether they should begin compressions or not. This decision must be made within 10 seconds. • A ratio of 15 compressions to 2 ventilations should be used; however, if the clinician is working alone a ratio of 30:2 is acceptable. • Compress the chest to at least ⅓ of the anterior-posterior chest diameter in all children i.e. ≈ 4cm in infants and ≈ 5cm in children. • For both infants and children the compression rate should be 100 – 120 min⁻¹. • There are no changes to the use of AEDs in children. Attenuating pads should be used where possible in children aged 1–8 if available. In children < 1 year it is acceptable to use an AED (preferably with attenuating pads).

Update Analysis

Resuscitation	Addition/update of guidance and rationale
Newborn Life Support	<ul><li>For term infants air should be used for resuscitation at birth. If, despite effective ventilation, oxygenation (ideally guided by oximetry) remains unacceptable, use of higher concentration of oxygen should be considered.</li><li>For babies < 32 weeks gestation use an oxygen air mix.</li><li>The compression ratio for CPR remains 3:1.</li><li>If adrenaline is given then the IV route is recommended at a dose of 10–30 micrograms kg^{-1}.</li></ul>
Advanced Life Support Support (Children)	<ul><li>In children the practice of tracheal intubation should be avoided in most circumstances.</li><li>The use of capnography with a SGA will help assess the quality of CPR.</li><li>A single shock strategy with a non-escalating dose of 4 j kg^{-1} is recommended for children.</li><li>Once spontaneous circulation is restored, inspired oxygen should be titrated to avoid the risk of hyperoxaemia.</li><li>Amiodarone is given after the 3rd shock and a second dose after the 5th shock in VF/pulseless VT arrests and dosages should be adjusted according to age.</li></ul>
Foreign Body Airway Obstruction (Children)	<ul><li>No significant change.</li></ul>

Section 3a

Medical emergencies – undifferentiated complaints	Addition/update of guidance and rationale
Abdominal Pain	• A reference table with details of conditions, characteristics of pain and associated symptoms has been included. • Reinforcement of the use of the mnemonic SOCRATES for the assessment of pain. • A reminder to consider abdominal aortic aneurysm in patients over 50 years of age with renal colic type pain, sudden abdominal pain or backache. • All children less than one year of age with bile stained vomit should be admitted. • Emphasis on providing adequate analgesia to patients with abdominal pain.
Cardiac Rhythm Disturbance	• Greater emphasis on the assessment of the patient which should follow the ABCDE approach. Key elements of this process include assessing for adverse signs, obtaining IV access and establishing monitoring (ECG, BP and SpO_2). • A 12 lead ECG should be recorded whenever possible as this can help to determine the precise rhythm, either before treatment or retrospectively.
Decreased Level of Consciousness	• This section has been renamed Altered Level of Consciousness to reflect the differences between a transient loss of consciousness, a decreased level of consciousness and coma. • There is now emphasis on the recognitions of conditions that require urgent treatment and require transfer to hospital and those which are transient and can be referred to a GP at a later stage. • Transient loss of consciousness reflects advice from the National Institute for Health and Clinical Excellence (NICE) guideline.
Dyspnoea	• The reference table for differential diagnoses has been expanded to include acute coronary syndrome, anaphylaxis, chronic obstructive pulmonary disease, foreign body airway obstruction, acute heart failure and pneumothorax. • The causes of dyspnoea have been tabulated for ease of reference.
Headache	• Emphasis on the importance of taking a detailed history using the mnemonic SOCRATES. • Clearer guidance on excluding mimics, such as stroke, head injury/trauma and glycaemic problems. • Definition of primary and secondary headaches. • Clear list of red flags. • Guidance to convey the first presentation of severe headaches to the ED. • Avoidance of morphine in the pain management of headaches. • Bundling all the time critical features into the same area of the guideline and supporting red flags. • Importance of referring patients to primary care if appropriate and not leaving patients without a care plan.
Mental Disorder	• No significant change.

Update Analysis

Medical emergencies – undifferentiated complaints	Addition/update of guidance and rationale
Medical Emergencies Overview (Adults)	• A reference table of time critical feature/conditions has been included. • Guidance for patients with suspected sepsis is emphasised with signs and symptoms listed and a reminder that patients with sepsis will benefit from early fluid therapy, and an alert/information message. • Adrenal crisis has replaced the term Addisonian crisis as it is a more inclusive term.
Non-Traumatic Chest Pain/Discomfort	• A note has been added that symptoms should not be assessed any differently in men/women or in different ethnic groups. • A revised list of accompanying features.
Medical Emergencies Overview (Children)	• A change to the assessment of capillary refill so that now it is only assessed on the sternum or the forehead. • Emphasis on the management of A and B problems on scene and C problems en route to the ED. • Adrenal crisis has replaced the term Addisonian crisis as it is a more inclusive term. • 0.9% sodium chloride is now the fluid of choice.
Minor Illness Overview (Children)	• This is a new guideline for the assessment and management of children with less serious illness that the ambulance service may be called to. • The guideline provides an overview with directions to other related illnesses including fever, gastroenteritis and respiratory illness.
Febrile Illness (Children)	• This is a new guideline for the assessment and management of fever in children, based on the clinical practice guideline "Feverish illness in children" issued by NICE. • The guideline uses the traffic light system to assess and group children into risk categories which guides management. • There is guidance on the interpretation of vital signs and information on specific febrile illnesses. • Guidance on non-conveyance of children with fever is provided.
Respiratory Illness (Children)	• This is a new guideline for the assessment and management of respiratory illness including bronchiolitis, croup, upper respiratory tract infections and pneumonia. • Guidance on non-conveyance is provided.

Section 3b

Medical emergencies – specific conditions	Addition/update of guidance and rationale
Heat Related Illness	• The updated guideline for heat related illness replaces the previous guidance for heat exhaustion and heat stroke. In addition, classic heat stroke is now referred to as non-exertional heat stroke throughout the guideline. • Heat related illnesses are now considered in terms of a continuum of conditions ranging from heat stress to heat stroke causing multi-organ dysfunction. Heat stress can be recognised in symptomatic patients with normal or mildly elevated temperature; heat exhaustion is recognised in symptomatic patients with a core temperature of >37°C and <40°C, while heat stroke is seen in symptomatic patients with a core temperature ≥40°C. Further diagnostic features of each condition have also been added to assist with assessment and management. • The new guideline highlights the potential time critical nature of heat related illnesses in general. The need for urgent cooling is emphasised, as is the need for a time critical transfer to hospital, in cases of haemodynamic compromise or an altered level of consciousness. The use of cold or iced water or ice packs is now advocated.
Hyperventilation Syndrome	• An emphasis on the fact that hyperventilation should be a diagnosis of exclusion. • A reference table of signs and symptoms has been added. • Guidance on the non-conveyance of patients is included.
Hypothermia	• The core body temperature categories for moderate (32–28°C) and severe hypothermia (<28°C) have changed. • In severe hypothermia it is acknowledged that the fastest way to re-warm patients is by extracorporeal warming, however this is not available in every hospital so local guidelines should be followed. • Recognition that mixed forms of hypothermia can occur, e.g. the exhausted walker who collapses and falls into a stream.
Sickle Cell Crisis	• This guideline was first published in April 2009. • The term sickle cell disease has replaced sickle cell anaemia throughout the guideline as it was felt to be an all-embracing term for the variants of the condition, so replaces the term anaemia, which only refers to HbSS. • A more comprehensive explanation of the sickling process has been included. • The causes which may precipitate crisis have been extended to include surgery and mental stress. • The signs and symptoms have been extended to include long bones, pyrexia, headache and priapism. • 12-lead ECG should be undertaken for patients with chest pain. • The term ACS, previously incorrectly recorded as 'Acute Coronary Syndrome' has been replaced with Acute Chest Syndrome, with an explanation of this condition inserted as a footnote. • The importance of early analgesia is again stressed; however the importance of using the oral or subcutaneous rather than the intravenous route is highlighted, as is the need to follow an individualised care plan where this is available. • A note that until a reliable SpO_2 measurement is available it is safer to over-oxygenate.

Update Analysis

Medical emergencies – specific conditions	Addition/update of guidance and rationale
	• Increased emphasis on pain management with a preference for oral or subcutaneous administration. • Entonox use has proved contentious in this group of patients as prolonged exposure is potentially dangerous. Limited use is stressed, though it remains a valuable analgesic for these patients.
Meningococcal Septicaemia	• Amendments to the clinical findings list. • Emphasis on the importance of a TIME CRITICAL transfer for all patients where meningococcal disease is suspected. • Emphasis on the fact that a rash may be absent.
Acute Coronary Syndrome	• New guidance on the management of patients presenting with a history suggestive of acute myocardial ischaemia. • Emphasis on PPCI when available and appropriate. • A reminder that patients with non-ST-segment-elevation myocardial infarction are at high risk and should be treated as a medical emergency.
Allergic Reactions including Anaphylaxis (Adults)	• This algorithm has been updated to reflect the RCUK guidance and as such the order of drug administration has been changed to the following: • Oxygen • Adrenaline • Fluid challenge • Chlorphenamine • Hydrocortisone • The use of salbutamol is still recommended as an addition to the RCUK guidance.
Asthma (Adults)	• There is an emphasis on the use of inhalers, rather than nebulisers, in non-oxygen dependent acute asthma and mild asthma attacks. • In patients with life threatening asthma, the stipulation that the transfer time to hospital must be over 30 minutes before steroids can be administered has been removed, as the evidence suggests that steroids should be given sooner rather than later. The decision as to which steroid to administer is dependent upon local policy. • A new algorithm has been developed with clear indications for transferring patients to further care based on the patient's severity and response to treatment. • The addition of a reference table with features of severity for near-fatal, life-threatening, severe and moderate asthma. • The addition of a reference table of risk factors for developing near-fatal asthma.
Chronic Obstructive Pulmonary Disease	• Reference tables with features of an acute exacerbation, conditions with similar features to an acute exacerbation and causes of an acute exacerbation have been included. • An indication to ask if the patient has an individualised treatment plan.
Convulsions (Adults)	• Emphasises the administration of the patient's own midazolam or intravenous diazepam for the management of convulsions.

Update Analysis

Medical emergencies – specific conditions	Addition/update of guidance and rationale
	• A caution has been added when inserting an oropharyngeal airway in patients with suspected basal skull fracture or facial injury. • Dislocated shoulder has been added to the list of injuries that can occur in patients suffering a convulsion. • Extended guidance on non-conveyance is provided including information and advice for carers and referral options.
Gastrointestinal Bleeds	• An note to exclude PV bleeding in females has been added.
Glycaemic Emergencies (Adults)	• It is recommended that patients taking the oral sulphonylurea hypoglycaemic agent glibenclamide are transferred to further care. • Extended guidance on non-conveyance is provided including information and advice for carers and referral options. • Reference tables for risk factors and signs and symptoms included.
Heart Failure	• The title of the guideline has changed from pulmonary oedema. • It is now recommended that Continuous Positive Airway Pressure (CPAP) should be used wherever available. • It is emphasised that morphine should not be used to reduce preload, but should be administered to manage pain when present. • The clinical significance of third heart sound and elevated jugular venous pressure has been included in the assessment and management of patients.
Implantable Cardioverter Defibrillator	• The distance from the implanted cardioverter defibrillator that the defibrillator electrode can be placed has been increased from 5 to 8 centimetres.
Overdose/Poisoning (Adults)	• An expanded list of common poisons. • Opiates has been added to the Illegal drugs table. • Leave at home guidance added for some circumstances.
Pulmonary Embolism	• No significant changes.

Stroke/Transient Ischaemic Attack	• The stroke and transient ischaemic attack guideline has been updated to take account of the recent update of the 'diagnosis and initial management of acute stroke and transient ischaemic attack' guideline by the National Institute for Health and Clinical Excellence and the Department of Health's National Stroke Strategy.
	• Although there are no significant changes to the assessment and management of patients suffering a stroke or transient ischaemic attack, there are changes in tone to reflect the importance of this topic nationally and recognition of the need to reduce unnecessary delay including:
	  – Upgrading the FAST test to the 'time critical features' section.
	  – De-emphasising some non-essential interventions such as the 12 lead ECG and intravenous access, which should be considered en-route if indicated.

Update Analysis

Medical emergencies – specific conditions	Addition/update of guidance and rationale
Allergic Reactions including anaphylaxis (Children)	• This algorithm has been updated to reflect the RCUK guidance and as such the order of drug administration has been changed to the following – • Oxygen • Adrenaline • Fluid challenge • Chlorphenamine • Hydrocortisone • The use of salbutamol is still recommended as an addition to the RCUK guidance. • The doses of adrenaline and hydrocortisone have also been changed.
Asthma (Children)	• Hydrocortisone has been introduced for the management of life threatening asthma, because anaphylaxis can also cause severe wheezing and mimic (or be misdiagnosed as) life threatening asthma. • The use of inhalers, rather than nebulisers, in non-oxygen dependent acute asthma attacks is emphasised. • The caution to exclude the presence of a pneumothorax has been removed. • A new algorithm has been developed with clear indications for transferring patients to further care based on the patient's severity and response to treatment.
Convulsions (Children)	• Intravenous diazepam is recommended rather than further doses of rectal diazepam in prolonged seizures that fail to respond to initial rectal/buccal medications.
Gastroenteritis (Children)	• This is a new guideline for the assessment and management of gastroenteritis in children. • The guidance includes a reference table of the signs and symptoms associated with clinical dehydration and shock. • Guidance on non-conveyance is provided including information and advice for parents and carers.
Glycaemic Emergencies (Children)	• The dosage of IV 10% glucose for children has been changed to 2 ml kg^{-1} to reflect national guidance. • Emphasises the risks of cerebral oedema and the importance of a time critical transfer of children with diabetic ketoacidosis. • The introduction of reference tables for risk factors and signs and symptoms included.
Overdose/Poisoning (Children)	• An expanded list of common poisons. • Opiates have been added to the illegal drugs table. • Leave at home guidance added for some circumstances.

Section 4

Trauma	Addition/update of guidance and rationale
Overall	• <C>ABC has replaced **ABC** in all the trauma guidelines in order to emphasise the importance of identifying and managing catastrophic haemorrhage. • **A definition of** catastrophic haemorrhage has been provided; '**extreme bleeding likely to cause death in minutes**'.
Trauma Emergencies Overview (Adults)	• The primary survey has been updated to reflect current guidance. • To support the move to **<C>ABC** from **ABC** new guidance for identifying and managing catastrophic haemorrhage is provided, including the use of haemostatic agents; algorithms have been developed for quick reference. • Indications for the administration of tranexamic acid are included. • The NHS Clinical Advisory Group on Trauma Pre-hospital Major Trauma Triage Tool >12 years is provided as an appendix. • Undertaking a dynamic risk assessment is re-emphasised. • A SCENE assessment tool is provided to assist in the initial management of a traumatic incident. • The use of the ATMIST tool is recommended for hand-over. • Emphasis on a maximum on scene time of 10 minutes unless the patient is trapped.
Trauma Emergencies Overview (Children)	• To support the move to **<C>ABC** from **ABC** new guidance for identifying and managing catastrophic haemorrhage is provided, including the use of haemostatic agents; algorithms have been developed for quick reference. • A SCENE assessment tool is provided to assist in the initial management of a traumatic incident. • Indications for the administration of tranexamic acid in children are included.
Abdominal Trauma	• Information on the effects and nature of blast injuries has been included.
Head Trauma	• The caution about not assuming that alcohol is the cause for depressed level of consciousness has been extended to include the effects of drugs. • Neurological assessment is to be re-assessed every 15 minutes. • A pedestrian or cyclist struck by a motor vehicle and an occupant ejected from a motor vehicle have been added to the list for mechanism of injury for intracranial head injury. • A reminder to consider and report any suspicions of non-accidental injury. • Additional indicators of head injury have been added: • Amnesia for events before/after injury. • Persistent headache following injury. • Convulsion following injury. • Vomiting following injury. • Indications for spinal immobilisation have been specified: GCS <15 on initial assessment, neck and back tenderness, focal neurological deficit, paraesthesia in the extremities or other clinical suspicions of cervical spine injury. • A note to consider whether the patient is on anticoagulant therapy or has a bleeding/clotting disorder has been added. • An algorithm for significant head trauma has been developed.
Limb Trauma	• Information on degloving injuries has been included. • Relocation of a dislocated patella is now included.

Trauma	Addition/update of guidance and rationale
Neck and Back Trauma	• A reminder has been added that some patients can sustain thoracic or lumbar injuries, in addition to, or in isolation from cervical spine injuries, therefore, if thoracic or lumbar injuries are suspected, even if the cervical spine has been cleared, then full spinal immobilisation should be undertaken if possible.
	• To improve the flow on the immobilisation algorithm the questions have been slightly amended so that '**YES**' answers now point to immobilisation and '**NO**' answers to immobilisation not required.
	• A reminder that older patients can sustain significant neck and back injuries from relatively minor trauma e.g. a fall from standing height.
	• A caution has been added in the case of older patients, especially those with cervical spine abnormalities such as ankylosing spondylitis, that when immobilised and positioned absolutely flat or fitted with a collar they may not be able to breathe adequately, therefore, a "best possible" approach should be adopted which may include manual in-line immobilisation.
	• The scoop stretcher is now advocated as the preferred method of immobilisation. Once a patient is on a scoop they can be transported on it unless there is a protracted journey time (>45 mins) when they should be ideally transferred to a vacuum mattress.
	• A long board should be used only as an extrication device and log rolling should be avoided where possible
Major Pelvic Trauma	• This is a new guideline first issued in April 2009 subsequent to publication of the 2006 UK ambulance service clinical practice guidelines; the main changes are:
	– Pelvic fracture should be considered based upon mechanism of injury.
	– The majority of pelvic fractures are stable pubic ramus or acetablar fractures.
	– Any patient with hypotension and potentially relevant mechanism of injury MUST be considered to have a **TIME CRITICAL** pelvic injury.
	– 'Springing' or distraction of the pelvis must not be undertaken.
	– Pelvic stabilisation should be implemented as soon as is practicable whilst still on scene.
	– Consider appropriate pain management.
Thoracic Trauma	• The stabilisation of a flail chest is no longer recommended as the underlying pulmonary contusion is the priority.
	• Specific reference to police wearing protection vests has been removed as other occupations also wear them.
	• Specific reference to ballistic protection vests has been removed as other types of vest are available e.g. stab vests.
	• Open chest wound has been added to the list of conditions to consider in the brief secondary survey for **NON-TIME CRITICAL** patients.
	• A reminder to look for asymmetrical chest movement when measuring the respiratory rate has been added.
	• A caution has been added regarding needle thoracocentesis which may not always decompress pneumothoraces in large patients; in such cases, a thoracostomy with or without a chest drain may need to be performed by an appropriately skilled practitioner.
	• Additional guidance on the management of children is included.
	• Additional guidance on the management of blast injury and air embolism.

Trauma	Addition/update of guidance and rationale
Trauma in Pregnancy	• This guideline has been moved to the trauma section. • The term 'found in cardiac arrest' has replaced 'dead' in the text.
Burns and Scalds (Adults)	The signs and increased risk of airway burns has been expanded to include: • Loss of consciousness. • Fires/blasts in enclosed spaces. • The calculation of burn area for the palm is 0.7–0.9% Total Body Surface Area (TBSA) this has been rounded to 1% for ease of estimation. • A note that large breast(s)/obesity will alter TBSA estimates has been added. • Serial halving is now not recommended. • The duration of irrigation of burns with water has changed to 20–30 minutes; irrigation can be undertaken up to three hours post injury. • A caution regarding the avoidance of ice or iced water has been added. • The duration of irrigation with water for the treatment of chemical burns is now a minimum 15 minutes and ideally until arrival at definitive care. • Water gel dressings are advocated in absence of water for irrigation. • Revised guidance for fluid administration
Electrical Injuries	• The title of the guideline has changed from electrocution to electrical injuries. • An assessment and management algorithm has been included.
Immersion and Drowning	• The title of the guideline has changed from the immersion incident to immersion and drowning. • A reminder that in **TIME CRITICAL** conditions speed of removal from the water takes precedent over preferred position i.e. horizontal. • The guideline emphasises the importance of a firm surface when undertaking chest compressions. • References to secondary drowning have been removed.

Update Analysis

Section 5

Obstetrics and gynaecology	Addition/update of guidance and rationale
Overall changes	<ul><li>The guideline has been formatted in a different order to reflect practice.</li><li>The assessment paradigm is now ABCED**F or <C>** ABCED**F** where F is for assessment of the fundus.</li><li>The preferred destination for patient transfer to further care is indicated for each condition/illness and may have changed in some instances.</li><li>Definitions and signs and symptoms have been placed prominently.</li><li>Large bore cannulae are emphasised for intravascular fluid administration.</li></ul>
Obstetrics and Gynaecology Emergencies Overview	<ul><li>A new guideline providing an overview for the care of patients with obstetrics and gynaecology conditions, including information on the physiological and anatomical changes that occur during pregnancy that affect patient care. General information of this type that was contained within the specific and in-text references are made within the specific guidelines.</li></ul>
Birth Imminent: Normal Delivery and Complications	<ul><li>This guideline focuses on birth imminent and delivery complications and therefore guidance starts at the second stage of labour when the cervix is fully dilated to 10 cm.</li><li>A separate table for each complication is provided so information can be accessed quickly.</li><li>**Prolapsed umbilical cord** – it is recommended that only ONE attempt is made to replace the cord in order to prevent cord spasm.</li><li>**Placental abruption** – a note has been added to consider in the presence of severe continuous pain.</li><li>**Shoulder dystocia** – given the TIME CRITICAL nature of this complication the guidance has been expanded to include further details of the McRobert's manoeuvre and the all-fours position with supporting diagrams. In addition details of the suprapubic and intermittent pressure have been included.</li><li>Insertion of large bore cannula if the patient has not delivered the placenta within 20 minutes.</li><li>Diagrams for the neutral position and cutting the cord have been included.</li></ul>
Care of the Newborn	<ul><li>A new guideline designed for the care of the newborn in the pre-hospital environment. This guideline covers the differences in physiology of the newborn baby, which is changing within the first few hours after birth and guidance on the management of premature babies.</li></ul>
Haemorrhage in Pregnancy	<ul><li>Early and late haemorrhage is now defined by the period of gestation. Haemorrhage in early pregnancy is defined as 22 weeks or less gestation and haemorrhage in late pregnancy is defined as more than 22 weeks gestation.</li><li>Guidance for the administration of misoprostol is provided.</li></ul>
Pregnancy Induced Hypertension	<ul><li>The guideline has been divided into two sections. Section one provides guidance for the care of patients with pregnancy-induced hypertension and severe pre-eclampsia and section two provides guidance for the care of patients with ecalmpsia.</li><li>The definitions and signs and symptoms are given above the assessment and management tables.</li></ul>

Update Analysis

Obstetrics and gynaecology	Addition/update of guidance and rationale
Vaginal Bleeding: Gynaecological Causes	• A ten day time period has been added to indicate when bleeding may occur post operatively. • The term 'cervical shock' has been replaced with the more widely recognised term 'vagal stimulation'.

Section 6

Drugs	Addition/update of guidance and rationale
Generic changes	• Thirteen new drug guidelines have been developed including: iprofloxacin, clopidogrel, dexamethasone, dicobalt, doxycycline, patient's own midazolam, misoprostol, obidoxime, ondansetron, potassium iodate, pralidoxime mesylate and tranexamic acid.
	• Where a Prescription-Only Medicines (POMs) exemption exists the MHRA has agreed a Patient Group Direction (PGD) is no longer required for paramedics to administer drugs, where a JRCALC drug protocol is issued. Currently POMs exemptions have not been issued for intravenous paracetamol, ondansetron, and tranexamic acid, therefore a PGD is required. A POMs exemption is not required for dexamethasone as the intravenous preparation is administered orally.
	• The dosage and administration tables have been re-designed and now include column headings for initial dose, repeat dose, dose interval, concentration, volume and maximum dose for each drug where appropriate.
	• The children's drug doses have been updated following publication of new UK Child Growth Standards. Drug doses have been rounded for practical purposes. Although some doses may differ from the exact dose calculated using dose per/kg formulae, these differences are not clinically significant and will not compromise patient care.
Drug Overview	• A table listing possible drug routes for each of the drug guidelines has been included.
	• **Table 6.4** lists the drugs and their possible routes of administration. In cases of parenteral administration, where at all possible, intravenous (IV) cannulation should be attempted, except for children in cardiac arrest where intra-osseous cannulation is the preferred method. **NB** If a vein cannot be found it is not necessary to attempt IV cannulation.
Adrenaline	• Cardiac arrest: – A dose for birth has been introduced. – There are changes in the administration schedule to: – **Shockable rhythms:** administer adrenaline after the 3rd shock and then after alternate shocks i.e. 5th, 7th etc. • **Non-shockable rhythms:** administer adrenaline immediately IV access is achieved then alternate loops.
Amiodarone	• A second dose of amiodarone is now given in a shockable rhythm following the 5th shock and dose is dependent on age.
	• The following *'acts to stabilise and reduce electrical irritability of cardiac muscle'* replaces **significant sodium channel blocking activity** to clarify the action of amiodarone.
Aspirin	• No significant changes.
Atropine	• The indication for cardiac arrest in asystole or PEA has been removed.
	• It is further emphasised that 'hypoxia is the most common cause of bradycardia in children, therefore interventions to support ABC and oxygen therapy should be the first-line therapy'.
	• Information and dosages for organophosphate poisoning is contained in a separate guideline in the CBRNE section.

Trauma	Addition/update of guidance and rationale
	• The adult dose for bradycardia has changed to 600 micrograms to reflect current supply of 600 microgram ampoules. However, it can be given in aliquots of either 500 or 600 micrograms to a maximum of 3 milligrams if supply changes.
Benzylpenicillin	• No significant changes.
Chlorphenamine (Chorpheniramine, Piriton)	• Two additional preparations, tablets and oral solution, have been included. • Prostatic disease has been included as a caution.
Clopidogrel	• The clopidogrel guideline was first issued in August 2008 subsequent to publication of the 2006 clinical practice guidelines. • Two major trials have reported their results, both of which support the extension of the use of clopidogrel to the STEMI end of the acute coronary syndrome spectrum. The 2007 update of the American College of Cardiology/American Heart Association STEMI guidelines, and the guidance on acute coronary syndromes published by the Scottish Intercollegiate Guidelines Network (SIGN) last year also recommend clopidogrel (although the SIGN guideline remit is restricted to in-hospital, rather than pre-hospital care). • Many cardiac networks are now recommending addition of clopidogrel to the pre-hospital treatment of STEMI patients, and the Joint Royal Colleges Ambulance Liaison Committee Cardiac Sub-Committee also recommended that clopidogrel be added to the prehospital treatment to bring ambulance practice in line with hospital practice (clopidogrel is increasingly being given on arrival in the emergency department). A small number of ambulance services are providing clopidogrel with the agreement of local Cardiac Networks. The clopidogrel drug protocol is now finalised. Based on current best evidence and expert consensus, the Joint Royal Colleges Ambulance Liaison Committee Guideline Development Group are recommending for patients with ST segment elevation myocardial infarction aged **75 years or less**: • 300 mg of clopidogrel orally for patients who are receiving, or where it is anticipated that patents will receive, thrombolysis • 600 mg of clopidogrel orally where it is anticipated that patients will undergo primary percutaneous coronary intervention.
Dexamethasone	• Dexamethasone is a new addition for children age one month to six years with moderate to severe croup. • It is recommended that the IV preparation is administered orally.
Diazepam	• The typographical error published in the 2006 UK Ambulance Service Clinical Practice Guidelines has been amended. The rectal tubes for administration are now specified by milligrams not millilitres. • The larger dosage table emphasises that the maximum dose for under 2's is 5 milligrams.
Entonox/Nitronox	• No significant changes.
Furosemide	• The ages for contra-indication of administering furosemide has been increased from 16 to 18 years.

Trauma	Addition/update of guidance and rationale
Glucagon	• Hypotension has been added as a side effect.
Glucose 10%	• The paediatric dose has been changed to 2 ml/kg^{-1} to reflect national advice. • A caution has been added to emphasise that glucose 10% should be administered via a large bore cannula to minimise the risk of irritation, especially extravasations.
Glucose 40% Oral Gel	• Change in the presentation section to 10 grams of glucose in a 25 gram tube of gel.
Glyceryl Trinitrate	• No significant changes.
Heparin	• The three drugs that comprised the thrombolytics guideline – heparin, reteplase, tenecteplase – have become separate guidelines.
Hydrocortisone	• The term adrenal crisis has been added as it encompasses a group of conditions which included Addisonian crisis.
Ibuprofen	• An emphasis on a balanced approach to pain management. • Hypovolaemia has been added as a contra-indication. • The dose for a one month infant is no longer recommended.

Intravascular Fluid Therapy (Adults)	• A new guideline providing guidance on intravascular fluid therapy in children and including an algorithm for quick reference.
	• Pathophysiologic considerations in intravascular fluid therapy.
	• Indications for intravascular fluid therapy in haemorrhagic emergencies.
	• Indications for intravascular fluid therapy in non-haemorrhagic emergencies.
	• Indications for intravascular fluid therapy in special circumstances:
	  – Crush injury
	  – Obstetric emergencies
	  – Sepsis
	  – Burns.
	• The indication for intravascular fluid for burns now recommends that if the burn surface area is:
	  – <15% do not administer fluid.
	  – ≥15 – <25% and time to hospital is greater than 30 minutes then administer 1 litre sodium chloride 0.9%
	  – ≥25% administer 1 litre sodium chloride 0.9%

Intravascular Fluid Therapy (Children)	• A new guideline providing guidance on intravascular fluid therapy in children and including an algorithm for quick reference. • Indications for intravascular fluid therapy in special circumstances: • Diabetic ketoacidosis • Haemorrhage • Burns. • The indication for intravascular fluid for burns now recommends that if the burn surface area is: – <10% do not administer fluid.

Trauma	Addition/update of guidance and rationale
	– ≥10 – <20% and time to hospital is greater than 30 minutes then administer sodium chloride 0.9% 10ml/kg over an hour. – ≥20% administer sodium chloride 0.9% 10ml/kg over an hour.
Ipratropium Bromide	● A caution has been added that If COPD is a possibility nebulisation should be limited to six minutes.
Lidocaine	● Removed from the JRCALC guidelines because lidocaine is no longer recommended.
Metoclopramide	● There are no significant changes to this guideline. ● However, with the introduction of ondansetron, a more effective anti-emetic with fewer side effects, it is envisaged that metoclopramide will eventually be removed.
Misoprostol	● A new guideline for the control of postpartum haemorrhage if syntometrine or other oxytocics are unavailable, contra-indicated, or if they have been ineffective at reducing haemorrhage after 15 minutes (Syntometrine and misoprostol reduce bleeding through different pathways; therefore if one drug has not been effective after 15 minutes, the other may be administered in addition). ● Misoprostol was chosen because it does not require refrigeration and therefore it has a longer shelf life. Currently there is no rectal preparation of misoprostol therefore the same tablets can be administered orally or rectally.
Morphine Sulphate	● The parenteral and oral preparations of morphine have been combined into one guideline. ● Dosages for intramuscular and subcutaneous administration of morphine are presented for patients with major trauma, shock, or cardiac conditions when the intravascular or intra-osseous routes are not available. ● An emphasis on a balanced approach to pain management.
Naloxone Hydrochloride	● In cases where naloxone is administered via the intravascular or intra-osseous route, the repeat dose is equal to the initial dose and is administered every three minutes up to the maximum dose until an effect is noted.
Ondansetron	● Ondansetron is a new guideline for 2011; it is an anti-emetic which is effective in the prevention and treatment of opiate-induced nausea and vomiting, the treatment of nausea and/or vomiting in adults and the treatment of travel associated nausea or vomiting in children. ● At the time of going to print a PGD is required.
Oxygen	● An update of the JRCALC oxygen clinical practice guideline was first issued in 2009 based on O'Driscoll BR, Howard LS, Davison AG, on behalf of the British Thoracic Society. BTS guideline for emergency oxygen use in adult patients. Thorax 2008;63(Suppl_6):vi1-68. ● http://www.brit-thoracic.org.uk/guidelines/emergency-oxygen-use-in-adult-patients.aspx ● This update includes significant changes in practice for some conditions in ADULTS e.g. stroke or myocardial infarction. ● Administration of supplemental oxygen is based on target saturation range.

Trauma	Addition/update of guidance and rationale
	• Initial dosage i.e. flow rate is determined by condition. • Conditions are grouped together into four main categories of illness and or injury: critical illness, serious illness, and COPD and other conditions requiring controlled or low-dose oxygen and conditions requiring no supplemental oxygen unless patients are hypoxaemic. • Target saturations for each of the four categories are set out in four tables together with other relevant guidance including the initial dose and method of administration. • In some instances there is a choice of administrative device e.g. simple face mask to nasal cannulae to allow for maximum flexibility. • An algorithm has been developed to support implementation of this guidance.

Paracetamol	• The range of preparations has increased to include:
	  – two oral preparations, **infant paracetamol** for ages 3 months to 5 years and **paracetamol six plus** for ages 6 to 11 years
	  – **intravenous paracetamol** for ages 6 months to adult are now included
	  – **paracetamol tablets** for ages 12 years – adult.
	• An emphasis on a balanced approach to pain management.
	• At the time of going to print a PGD is required for intravenous administration.

Patient's Own Midazolam	• A new guideline written to provide information on buccal administration of the patient's own prescribed midazolam when a grand-mal convulsion continues ten minutes after a carer has administered a first dose of midazolam. The current management options, if patients are still convulsing ten minutes after the carer has administered midazolam, are either to cannulate and administer intravenous diazepam or to administer rectal diazepam; both options involve time delays and it would be preferable to administer a second dose of midazolam. A recent amendment to the Misuse of Drugs Act now permits paramedics to be in possession of midazolam under a PGD, although while these are developed it is permissible for a paramedic or technician to administer a patient's own prescribed medication, if they are competent to administer medication via the buccal route and are familiar with the indications, actions and side effects of the medication.
Reteplase	• The three drugs that comprised the thrombolytics guideline reteplase, tenecteplase and heparin have become separate guidelines. • The thrombolysis checklist now follows the indications issued by the European Society of Cardiology. • An emphasis on undertaking primary percutaneous coronary intervention where available as this is now the dominant reperfusion treatment.
Salbutamol	• A caution has been added that If COPD is a possibility nebulisation should be limited to six minutes. • Muscle cramps and rash have been included as side effects.
0.9% Sodium Chloride	• 0.9% sodium chloride is now recommended as the intravascular fluid of choice.

Trauma	Addition/update of guidance and rationale
Sodium Lactate	● The administration of sodium lactate has been de-emphasised and 0.9% sodium chloride is the intravascular fluid of choice.
Syntometrine	● The indications for the administration of Syntometrine have been extended to include miscarriage with life-threatening bleeding and a confirmed diagnosis e.g. where a patient has gone home with medical management and starts to bleed. ● Additional information has been provided indicating that the action pathways for Syntometrine and misoprostol are different and therefore if one drug has not been effective after 15mins, the other may be administered in addition.
Tenecteplase	● The three drugs that comprised the thrombolytics guideline tenecteplase, reteplase, and heparin have become separate guidelines. ● The thrombolysis checklist now follows the indications issued by the European Society of Cardiology. ● An emphasis on undertaking primary percutaneous coronary intervention where available as this is now the dominant reperfusion treatment.
Tetracaine	● No significant changes.
Tranexamic Acid	● Tranexamic acid is a new guideline for patients who require intravascular fluid. Tranexamic acid is an anti-fibrinolytic which reduces the breakdown of blood clot. ● At the time of going to print a PGD is required.
Page-for-Age (Children)	● The guideline has expanded to include information and dosages for chlorphenamine, dexamethasone, ibuprofen, and ondansetron. ● Sizes of i-gel airways are now provided in the table. ● Drug routes are specified for all drugs in the drug route column; including when a drug is not appropriate for a specific age. ● The guideline has changed its name from 'age per page' to 'page per age'.

Section 7

Special Situations	Addition/update of guidance and rationale
Overall	• A special situations section has been created that brings together the guidance on the assessment and management of chemical, biological, radiological, nuclear and explosive incidents together with related drugs. • Six new drug guidelines are included: ciprofloxacin, dicobalt, doxycycline, obidoxime, potassium iodate, and pralidoxime mesylate; see below for details.
Major Incident	• The METHANE tool has been added to this section to specifically deal with major incidents.
Chemical, Biological, Radiological, Nuclear and Explosive (CBRNE) Incidents	• The guidance for chemical, biological, radiological, nuclear incidents guideline has been extended to include guidance on the assessment and management of patients following explosive incidents. • The guidance emphasises the role of the Hazardous Area Response Teams (HART)/Fire Services in the management of incidents. • More guidance is provided on the signs and symptoms of CBRNE incidents.
Atropine (CBRNE)	• A separate guideline has been created to provide guidance specially related to organophosphate poisoning. • Additional information on administration. • The inclusion of two further preparations: • An auto-injector containing 2 milligrams of atropine sulphate in 0.7 ml. • Nerve Agent Antidote Kit (NAAK) containing 2 milligrams of atropine sulphate.
Ciprofloxacin (CBRNE)	• This is a new guideline for 2013 and is only to be dispensed on the instruction of the Health Protection Agency or Medical Director. • Ciprofloxacin is for patients who have been exposed to a known or suspected biological agent such as anthrax, plague, tularaemia, or other biological agent.
Dicobalt (CBRNE)	• This is a new guideline for 2013 and is only to be dispensed on the instruction of the Health Protection Agency or Medical Director. • Dicobalt is for patients with a clinical diagnosis of severe poisoning with hydrogen cyanide, or cyanide salts; in the presence of respiratory depression, and impaired consciousness e.g. glasgow coma score <8.
Doxycycline (CBRNE)	• Doxycycline is a new guideline for 2013 and is for patients who have been exposed to anthrax, plague, tularaemia or other biological agent.
Obidoxime (CBRNE)	• This is a new guideline for 2013 and is only to be dispensed on the instruction of the Health Protection Agency or Medical Director. • Obidoxime is administered as an adjunct to atropine in the treatment of organophosphorus (OP) poisoning by nerve agents.
Potassium Iodate (CBRNE)	• This is a new guideline for 2013 and is only to be dispensed on the instruction of the Health Protection Agency or Medical Director.

Update Analysis

Special Situations	Addition/update of guidance and rationale
	● Potassium iodate is for patients with a known, expected or suspected exposure to radioactive iodine, at or above a level judged appropriate by a Director of Public Health (or delegate).
Pralidoxime Pralidoxime Mesylate	● Pralidoxime mesylate is for patients with a clinical diagnosis of poisoning by organophosphorus (OP) nerve agents, as an adjunct to maintenance of oxygenation and atropine administration.
Incapacitating Agents	● New guidance on the assessment and management of patients for conditions and injuries following the deployment of incapacitating agents including conducted electrical weapons, incapacitant sprays, projectiles and batons.

Glossary of Terms

The glossary of terms listed below is designed to assist reading ease and is **NOT** provided as a list of short-hand terms. The Joint Royal Colleges Ambulance Liaison Committee reminds the user that abbreviations are not to be used in any clinical documentation.

Term

AAA	Abdominal Aortic Aneurysm
ACPO(TAM)	Association of Chief Police Officers (Terrorism and Allied Matters)
ACS	Acute Coronary Syndrome
AED	Automated External Defibrillation
AHTPS	Alder Hey Triage Pain Score
ALS	Advanced Life Support
AMHP	Approved Mental Health Professional
APGAR	**A** – Airway **P** – Pulse **G** – Grimace **A** – Appearance **R** – Respiration
ARDS	Acute Respiratory Distress Syndrome
ASHICE	**A** – Age **S** – Sex **H** – History **I** – Injuries or illnesses **C** – Current condition **E** – Estimated time/mode of arrival
ASW	Approved Social Worker
ATLS	Advanced Trauma Life Support
ATO	Ammunition Technical Officer
ATP	Anti-Tachycardia Pacing
AVPU	**A** – Alert **V** – Responds to voice **P** – Responds to pain **U** – Unresponsive
AWE	Atomic Weapons Establishment
bd	Twice daily
BLS	Basic Life Support
BM	Stick Measures blood sugar
BP	Blood Pressure
BR	Breech
BSA	Body Surface Area
BVM	Bag-Valve-Mask
CABG	Coronary Artery Bypass Grafting
CAC	Central Ambulance Control
CALD	Chronic Airflow Limitation Disease

(CB)IED	(Chemical or Biological) Improvised Explosive Device
CBRNE	Chemical, Biological, Radiological, Nuclear, Explosive
CBRT	(Capillary bed refill time)
CCC	Civil Contingencies Committee
CCCG	Chief Constable's Co-Ordinating Group
CD	Controlled Drug
CHD	Coronary Heart Disease
CMLO	Consequence Management Liaison Officer
CNS	Central Nervous System
CO	Carbon monoxide
CO$_2$	Carbon dioxide
COPD	Chronic Obstructive Pulmonary Disease
COBR	Cabinet Office Briefing Room
CPAP	Continuous Positive Airway Pressure
CPP	Cerebral Perfusion Pressure
CPR	Cardiopulmonary Resuscitation
CRT	Capillary Refill Test
CRT	Cardiac Resynchronisation Therapy
CSF	Cerebrospinal Fluid
CT	Computerised Tomography
CVA	Cerebo Vascular Accident
DIC	Disseminated Intravascular Coagulation
DKA	Diabetic Ketoacidosis
DM	Diabetes Mellitus
DNA	Deoxyribonucleic Acid
DNAR	Do Not Attempt Resuscitation Order
DST	Defence, Science and Technology Laboratory
DVT	Deep Vein Thrombosis
E	Ecstasy
EC	Enteric Coated
ECG	Electrocardiograph
ED	Emergency Department
EDD	Estimated Date of Delivery

EHO	Environmental Health Officer	**MAOI**	Monoamine Oxidase Inhibitor antidepressant
EMS	Emergency Medical Services	**MAP**	Mean Arterial Pressure
EOD	Explosives Ordnance Disposal	**MCD**	Maximum Cumulative Dose
ET	Endotracheal	**mcg**	Microgram
ETA	Expected Time of Arrival	**MDMA**	Methylene Dioxymethamphetamine
FCP	Forward Control Point	**mg**	Milligram
FMC	Forward Military Commander	**MI**	Myocardial Infarction
FSC	Forward Scientific Controller	**MIMMS**	Major Incident Medical Management and Support
g	Grams	**ml**	Millilitre
GCS	Glasgow Coma Scale	**mmHG**	Millimetres of Mercury
GI	Gastrointestinal	**mmol**	Millimoles
GLO	Government Liaison Officer	**mmol/l**	Millimoles per Litre
GLT	Government Liaison Team	**MOI**	Mechanisms of Injury
GP	General Practitioner	**MR**	Modified Release
GSW	Gunshot Wounds	**MSC**	**M** – Motor
GTN	Glyceryl Trinitrate		**S** – Sensation
HazMat	Hazardous Material		**C** – Circulation
HIV	Human Immunodeficiency Virus	**NARO**	Nuclear Accident Response Organisation
HONK	Hyperosmolar Non-Ketotic Syndrome	**Neb**	Nebulisation
IBS	Irritable Bowel Syndrome	**NP**	Nasopharyngeal
ICD	Implantable Cardioverter Defibrillator	**NSAID**	Non-Steroidal Anti-inflammatory Drug
ICP	Intracranial Pressure	**NSAP**	Non-Specific Abdominal Pain
IHD	Ischemic Heart Disease	**O$_2$**	Oxygen
IM	Intramuscular	**OP**	Oropharyngeal
IO	Intraosseous	**P**	Parity
IPE	Individual Protective Equipment	**PCO$_2$**	Measure of the Partial Pressure of Carbon dioxide
IPPV	Intermittent Positive Pressure Ventilation	**PE**	Pulmonary Embolism
IV	Intravenous	**PEA**	Pulseless Electrical Activity
JHAC	Joint Health Advisory Cell	**PEF**	Peak Expiratory Flow
JIG	Joint Intelligence Group	**PHTLS**	Pre-hospital Trauma Life Support
JMC	Joint Military Commander	**PIC**	Police Incident Commander
JVP	Jugular Vein Pressure	**PID**	Pelvic Inflammatory Disease
KED	Kendrick Extraction Device	**PIH**	Pregnancy Induced Hypertension
kg	Kilogram	**PMBS**	Police Main Base Station
LA	Left Atrium	**PO**	Pulmonary Oedema
LMA	Laryngeal Mask Airway	**POLSA**	Police Search Adviser
LMP	Last Menstrual Period	**POM**	Prescription Only Medicine
LMW	Low Molecular Weight	**PPCI**	Primary Percutaneous Coronary Intervention
LOC	Level of Consciousness	**PPE**	Personal Protective Equipment
LSD	Lysergic Acid Diethylamide	**pr**	Per Rectum
LVF	Left Ventricular Failure		

prn	When required	**SO13**	Metropolitan Police Anti-Terrorist Squad
qds	Four times a day	**SpO$_2$**	Oxygen Saturation Measured With Pulse Oximeter
Rh+ve	Rhesus positive		
Rh-ve	Rhesus negative	**SSA**	Senior Scientific Authority
ROLE	Recognition Of Life Extinct	**SSRIs**	Selective Serotonin Re-Uptake Inhibitors
RSI	Rapid Sequence Intubation	**STEMI**	ST Segment Elevation Myocardial Infarction
RTC	Road Traffic Collision		
RVP	Rendezvous Point(s)	**STEP**	Safety Triggers For Emergency Personnel
SaO$_2$	Oxygen Saturation Of Arterial Blood	**SVT**	Supraventricular Tachycardia
SAS	Special Air Squadron	**TBSA**	Total Body Surface Area
SBP	Systolic Blood Pressure	**tds**	Three times a day
SBS	Special Boat Squadron	**TIA**	Transient Ischaemic Attack
SC	Subcutaneous	**UTI**	Urinary Tract Infection
SCI	Spinal Cord Injury	**VAS**	Visual Analogue Scale
SF	Special Forces	**VF**	Ventricular Fibrillation
SIO	Senior Investigating Officer	**VT**	Ventricular Tachycardia
SMC	Senior Military Commander	**VTE**	Venous Thromboembolism

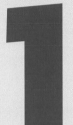

General Guidance

General Guidance

Patient Confidentiality

1. Introduction [1–7]

Health professionals have a duty of confidentiality regarding patient information. They also have a priority, which is to ensure that all relevant information about their patients, their assessments, examinations and advice is recorded clearly and accurately, and passed to other staff whenever it is necessary for provision of ongoing care.

Sometimes, aspects of legislation relating to these issues appear to conflict with each other. This guideline provides a brief overview of the relevant legislation under the following headings:

- Patient Identifiable Information.
- Data Protection Act 1998 (DPA).
- NHS Policy.
- Protecting Patient Information.
- Patients' Rights of Access to Personal Health Records.
- Disclosure to Other Bodies and Organisations.
- Research.
- Consent.

2. Patient Identifiable Information [1, 2, 7–11]

Patient Identifiable Information is any information that may be used to identify a patient directly or indirectly. It may include:

- Patient's name, address, postcode or date of birth.
- Any image or audiotape of the patient.
- Any other data or information that has the potential, however remote, to identify a patient (e.g. rare diseases, drug regimes, statistical analysis of small groups).
- Patients' record numbers.
- Combinations of any of the items here that may increase the risk of a breach of confidentiality, that include all verbal, written and electronic disclosure, whether formal or incidental.

3. Data Protection Act [1, 12–14]

The main principles of the (DPA) should be read in conjunction with this guideline. This Act describes processes for obtaining, recording, holding, using and sharing information:

- Patients must be informed and give consent to any sharing of their personal information. Exceptions to this general rule may exist (see sections on Disclosure and Consent).
- Only the minimum amount of data should be collected and used to achieve the agreed purpose.
- Information can only be retained for as long as it is needed to achieve its purpose.
- Strict rules apply to sharing information and with whom it may be shared.

4. NHS Policy [1–4]

All NHS employees must be aware of, and respect a patient's right to confidentiality. A disciplinary offence may have been committed for any behaviour contrary to their organisation's policy or the *NHS Code of Practice: Confidentiality (in Scotland, the NHS COP on Protecting Patient Confidentiality)*. Ambulance clinicians should be aware of how to gain access to training, support or information, which they may need and be able to show that they are making every reasonable effort to comply with the relevant standards.

5. Protecting Patient Information [6, 15]

There are five essential steps that all ambulance clinicians should take to ensure that they comply with the relevant standards of confidentiality. They are listed below:

5.1 Record information given by, and about patients concisely and accurately. [1, 2]

- Inaccurate clinical records about patients may contain false information that has been created by, for example, omissions, errors, unfounded comments or speculation. This breaches DPA standards. It also brings the professional integrity of ambulance clinicians and their employing organisations into question. Any comments and opinions, whether verbal, written or electronic, must be justifiable and accurate.

5.2 Keep patient information physically secure. [7, 13, 16]

- Ambulance services have particular difficulties in ensuring that information is not shared accidentally with the public. Not only must patients be treated confidentially, but the information gained must not be disclosed to anyone else unless to do so genuinely promotes patient care. (Comments to the public must be guarded). Information given to other clinicians when handing over patients' care should not be overheard or shared with people who are not directly involved in each patient's care. Patients' records, either electronic or written, must be protected against unwarranted viewing: thus, patients' clinical records must be shielded from the view of other people, stored securely after case closure, and only handed over to staff who are entrusted with ongoing care of particular patients or other authorised personnel who have legitimate reasons for possessing the information. Personal health data must be destroyed in an approved manner and according to each organisation's policies when they have served their function. Discussions of each patient must not disclose personal information unless there is genuine and provable health benefit.

- Leaders of healthcare and health information systems believe that electronic health information systems, which include computer-based patient records, can improve healthcare. Achieving this goal, requires systems to be in place that: protect the privacy of individual persons and data about patients; provide appropriate access; and use data security measures that are adequate. Sound policies and practices relating to handling confidential information must be in place prior to deploying health information systems. Strong and enforceable policies on privacy and security of confidential and patient identifiable information must shape the development and implementation of these systems.

5.3 Follow guidance before disclosing any patient information [3, 4]

- It is not sufficient for ambulance clinicians to understand the basic principles of confidentiality alone. They must also understand and comply with their employing organisations' requirements for information-sharing. Similarly, it is the responsibility of each service to ensure that policies for data-sharing are produced, communicated, monitored, updated and reviewed. There must be a Data Protection Officer, Information Governance Manager, and/or a Caldicott Guardian available to advise ambulance clinicians if they have any doubts about sharing information.

5.4 Conform to best practice [1, 14–16]

- All grades of ambulance clinicians come into contact with the public and other NHS clinicians. Any temptation for ambulance clinicians to share information unnecessarily with other people who are known to them must be avoided, and the responsibility lies firmly with the holder of the data, both personally and in respect of employing organisations. Commitment to best practice should be applied to all information in any form about patients (e.g. patients' records, electronic data, surface mail, email, faxes, telephone calls, conversations that may be overheard, and private comments to friends or colleagues).

- If, for any reason, ambulance staff discover that personal data has been lost or has the potential for being viewed by anyone not authorised to view it, they have a duty to immediately:

  – take every action possible to recover the data and/or protect them, and

  – to inform immediately an officer in their employing organisation who has responsibility for data (or their immediate supervisor) that such an event has occurred

  – record the event.

5.5 Anonymise information where possible [3, 5]

- Information about patients is said to be anonymised when items such as those listed in section 2 are removed. It means that patients cannot be identified by any receiver of the information and any possibility of recognition is extremely small.

- Ambulance clinicians are advised to anonymise confidential data about patients wherever possible and reasonable. If information is recorded, retained or transmitted in any way, it should be anonymised unless to do so would frustrate any genuine reasons for its collection/storage that create identifiable benefits to patients' health.

6. Patients' rights of access to their personal health records [2 ,11]

Patients have a right to see, and obtain a copy of personal health information held about them. This

right in law includes any legally appointed representative and those persons who have parental responsibility for children who are patients. Children also have this right provided they have the capability to understand the information. Services have the right to charge for this information; and there are guidelines on the processes that are to be followed.

- There are exceptions to the rights of patients to see their personal health information. The information is subject to legal restrictions if it could identify someone else and if that information cannot be removed from the record. Also, a request can be refused if there is substantial opinion that access to the information could cause serious harm to a particular patient or to someone else's physical or mental well-being. These instances are extremely rare in ambulance service operations. If there were to be doubt about whether exceptions such as these do exist, staff should consult the Caldicott Guardian, Information Governance Manager or Data Protection Officer and agreement should be reached with each patient's lead-clinician.

- Notwithstanding the exceptions noted here, clinicians should make every effort to support each patient's right to gain access to their personal health information. It is a requirement that this information should be received by a patient who requests it within 40 days of their request. Services should have clear written procedures in place to deal with these requests.

7. Disclosure of information to other bodies and organisations [2, 3, 14, 16, 17]

7.1 Police

- The police have the right of access to personal information (name, address, etc.) in their investigation, detection and prevention of any crime. They also have the right of access to confidential health information (type of illness or injury, etc) in their investigation, detection or prevention of a serious crime (e.g. rape, arson, terrorism, murder, etc.).

- They have no right to expect to receive information when criminality, crew safety or public safety are not involved. Generalised information regarding attendance at an incident may be passed to the police through locally agreed procedures, when details of the location of an incident and what is involved **may** be disclosed – but passage of personal or confidential health data **may not**.

7.2 Local Authorities

- A local authority officer may require any person holding health, financial or other records relating to a person whom the officer knows or believes to be an adult at risk to give the records, or copies of them, to the officer, for the purposes of enabling or assisting the authority to decide whether it needs to do anything in order to protect an adult at risk from harm.

7.3 Secretary of State (by proxy)

- The Secretary of State's *'security management functions'* in relation to the health service mean that his powers to take action for the purpose of protecting and improving the security of health service providers (and persons employed by them) includes releasing documents for the purpose of preventing, detecting or investigating fraud, corruption or other unlawful activities.

7.4 Fire Service and other emergency services

There is no right of access for emergency service personnel other than the police to patients' personal health information. Situations may occur in which ambulance clinicians feel that such disclosure would be in the best interests of a particular patient, or that, by not disclosing it, other emergency workers could be put at risk. Ambulance clinicians should be fully aware of their obligations towards their patients' confidentiality. Avoidable breaches of confidentiality occur when colleagues and authorities (such as the police and persons in a judicial context) ask for information. On these occasions ambulance clinicians should follow the best practice advice given in the relevant section of the NHS Code of Practice on Protecting Patient Confidentiality; otherwise, access to information should be governed by formal documented requests and consideration by the Data Protection Officer, Information Governance Manager and/or the Caldicott Guardian.

7.5 The media

- There is no basis for disclosure of confidential or patient identifiable information to the media. Services may receive requests for information in special circumstances (e.g. requests for updates on celebrity patients or following large incidents and when responding to press statements – public interest exemption). In instances such as these the explicit consent of the persons about whom information is sought should be gained and recorded prior to any disclosure. Occasionally, services or ambulance clinicians can be criticised in the press by patients or by someone else with whom a patient has a relationship. Criticism of this nature may contain inaccurate or misleading detail of behaviour, diagnosis, or treatment. Services or ambulance clinicians should always seek advice from professional bodies on how to respond (if at all) to press criticism and about any legal redress that may be available. Although these instances may cause frustration or distress, they do not relieve anyone of their duty to respect the confidentiality of any patient.

7.6 For commercial purposes

- Ambulance services are not registered to use information for primarily commercial purposes. If such use was permitted, each patient would have to give explicit consent for information given by, or about them to be used within the express commercial setting and each patient should be given an opt-out facility. This includes all intended purposes of all parties to the agreement and lists of all persons/groups who would have access to the data. Due to the nature of commercial enterprise, this consent must be explicit (expressly and actively given) as opposed to implied (acceptance without voicing an objection).

8. Research [3]

All data for research should be anonymised wherever possible. If anonymisation would be contrary to the aims of the research, prior consent must be gained. Formal research guidelines exist for the use of health-related data and they must be adhered to.

9. Consent [2, 18, 19]

Consent and patients' confidentiality are inextricably linked. In essence, each patient is said to be the owner of their own personal, non-anonymised patient information and/or data. Therefore, each patient should give approval before information provided by, or about them is used by other people. There are exceptions to this general rule:

- There may be legal requirements to disclose data without consent (e.g. due to persons having **notifiable diseases**). Even then, however, each patient must be informed that this situation has arisen.

- When there is a risk to a patient's well-being by not informing other professionals without consent (e.g. where a child or vulnerable adult, an adult without capacity, or a patient who is being treated using powers given by the Mental Health Act, may be in need of protection) and informing the relevant authorities would appear to be to the patient's wider benefit.

- Inability to consent (e.g. some children, adults who lack capacity or patients who are seriously ill or injured and who could reasonably be expected to give consent if it were otherwise possible to do so). Even in circumstances such as these, information must be used cautiously and anonymised when possible. A proxy, guardian or parent should be consulted if such a person is available.

- Use of personal information without consent may be justified if it is in the **public interest** to do so. This may occur to prevent or detect a serious crime, for example.

In all of the instances that are described here, the advice of the service's Caldicott Guardian, Information Governance Manager and/or Data Protection Officer should be sought prior to using or releasing any personal health information or data. Each service must advise their own ambulance clinicians in relation to consent, and this advice must be studied by ambulance clinicians.

KEY POINTS

Patient Confidentiality

- Health professionals have a duty of confidentiality regarding information about or that may identify patients. They also have a priority to ensure that all relevant information is recorded clearly and accurately, and passed to others when this is necessary for providing ongoing care.

- Inaccurate clinical records may contain false information about patients, which is created by, for example, omissions, errors, unfounded comments or speculation. Any comments or opinions, whether verbal, written or electronic, must be justifiable and accurate.

- Data Protection Officers, Information Governance Managers and Caldicott Guardians are available to advise and assist ambulance clinicians of the ambulance services.

- Consent and confidentiality of information that is held about patients are inextricably linked. In essence, patients are the owners of personal, non-anonymised information that is provided by, or about them, and they, therefore, are required to give approval before it is used by other people.

- Ensure you are aware of the rules in your service regarding patients' confidentiality and follow them – but remember that ongoing care of patients should never be compromised in their application.

Further Reading

The principles within the following documents have significant impact on patient confidentiality issues, and should be considered essential reading.

1. Health and Care Professions Council. Standards of conduct, performance and ethics: Your duties as a registrant.

2. Confidentiality: NHS Code of Practice (NHS Scotland Code of Practice on Protecting Patient Confidentiality).

3. Data Protection Act 1998.

Methodolgy

For details of the methodology used in the development of this guideline refer to the guideline webpage.

Pain Management in Adults

1. Introduction

Pain is one of the commonest symptoms in patients presenting to ambulance services.

Control of pain is important not only for humanitarian reasons but also because it may prevent deterioration of the patient and allow better assessment. Analgesia should be administered as soon as clinically possible after arriving on scene although this can be done en-route so as not to delay time-critical patients.

There is no reason to delay relief of pain because of uncertainty with the definitive diagnosis. It does not affect later diagnostic efficacy.

Many studies have demonstrated the inadequacy of pre-hospital pain relief and that time to pain relief is reduced by prehospital administration of analgesia.

Pain is a multi-dimensional construct (see below).

Pain consists of several elements:
- Treatment of the underlying condition.
- Non-pharmacological methods including:
  - psychological support and explanation
  - physical methods e.g. splinting.
- Pharmacological treatment.

Pain relief will depend on:
- Cause, site, severity and nature of the pain.
- Age of the patient.
- Experience/knowledge of the clinician.
- Distance from receiving unit.
- Available resources.

---

2. Assessment

An assessment should be made of the requirements of the individual. Pain is a complex experience that is shaped by gender, cultural, environmental and social factors, as well as prior pain experience. Thus the experience of pain, including assessment and tolerance levels, is unique to the individual.

It is important to remember that the pain a patient experiences cannot be objectively validated in the same way as other vital signs. Attempts to estimate the patient's pain should be resisted, as this may lead to an underestimation of the patient's experience. Several studies have shown that there is a poor correlation between the patient's pain rating and that of the healthcare professional, with the latter often underestimating the patient's pain.

Instead, ambulance clinicians need to seek and accept the patient's self-report of their pain. This is reinforced by a popular and useful definition of pain: 'pain is whatever the experiencing person says it is, existing whenever he/she says it does.'

Pain scoring

All patients in pain should have their pain assessed using the mnemonic **SOCRATES** for its:
- site
- onset
- character
- radiates
- associated symptoms
- time/duration
- exacerbating or relieving factors
- severity.

All patients with pain should have a pain severity score undertaken. It has been recognised that pain scoring increases awareness of pain, reveals previously unrecognised pain and improves analgesic administration.

There are a variety of methods of scoring pain using numerical (analogue) rating scales and simple scoring systems. JRCALC recommend that a simple 0-10 point verbal scale (0 = 'no pain' and 10 = 'the worst pain imaginable') will be the most suitable method in most prehospital situations.

This should be undertaken on all patients who are in pain and should be repeated after each intervention (the timing of the repeat score depends on the expected time for the analgesic to have an effect). The absolute value is used in combination with the patient assessment to determine the type of analgesia and route of administration that is most appropriate. The trend in the scores is more important than the absolute value in assessing efficacy of treatment. Scoring will not be possible in all circumstances (e.g. cognitively impaired individuals, communication difficulties, altered level of consciousness) and in these circumstances behavioural cues will be more important in assessing pain.

3. Management

Analgesia should normally be introduced in an incremental way, considering timeliness, effectiveness and potential adverse events and titrating to effect. However, it may be apparent from the assessment that it is appropriate to start with stronger analgesia e.g. in apparent myocardial infarction or fractured long bones. Entonox should be supplied until the other drugs have had time to take effect and if the patient is still in pain, other analgesics administered. Administering analgesia in this step-wise, incremental, titratable manner, utilising a balanced analgesic approach, minimises the amount of potent analgesia that is required whilst still obtaining good analgesic effect with fewer side effects.

Any pain relief must be accompanied by careful explanation of the patient's condition and the pain relief methods being used.

Patients with chronic pain, including those receiving palliative care, may experience breakthrough pain despite their usual drug regime. They may require large doses of analgesics to have significant effect. If possible, contact should be made with the team caring for the patient.

4. Treating the Cause

Many conditions produce pain and it is vital to treat the cause of the pain, including underlying conditions. This will also help relieve the pain in many situations e.g. giving GTN in cardiac pain or oxygen in sickle cell crisis.

Pain Management in Adults

NOTE: Most commonly, a patient requires a combination of pharmacological and non-pharmacological methods of pain relief (refer to Tables 1.1–1.3 and Figure 1.1). For example: entonox, morphine or ketamine may be required to enable a splint to be applied.

Table 1.1 – NON-PHARMACOLOGICAL METHODS OF PAIN RELIEF

Psychological
Fear and anxiety worsen pain; reassurance and explanation can go a long way towards alleviation of pain.

Distraction is a potent analgesic, commonly used in children, but may also apply to adults; simple conversation is the simplest form of distraction. It is important to keep the patient as comfortable as possible e.g. warm.

Dressings
Burns dressings that may cool, such as those specifically designed for the task or cling film, can alleviate the pain. Burns should not be cooled for more than 20 minutes total time and care should be taken with large burns to prevent the development of hypothermia. However, analgesia should also be provided at the earliest opportunity.

Splintage
Simple splintage of fractures provides pain relief as well as minimising ongoing tissue damage, bleeding and other complications.

Table 1.2 – PHARMACOLOGICAL METHODS OF PAIN RELIEF (refer to specific drug protocols)

Inhalational analgesia
Entonox (50% Nitrous oxide 50% Oxygen) is a good analgesic for adults who are able to self-administer and who can rapidly be taught to operate the demand valve. It is rapidly acting but has a very short half-life, so the analgesic effect wears off rapidly when inhalation is stopped. It can be used as the first analgesic whilst other pain relief is instituted. It can also be used as part of a balanced analgesic approach (several agents working at different sites to enable effective analgesia with fewer side effects), particularly during painful procedures such as splint application and patient movement.

Oral analgesia
Paracetamol and ibuprofen may be used in isolation or together for the management of mild to moderate pain when used in appropriate dosages. It is important to assess the presence of contra-indications to all drugs including simple analgesics. Non-steroidal anti-inflammatory drugs are responsible for large numbers of adverse events, because of their gastro-intestinal and renal side effects and their effects on asthmatics. Some ambulance services may also choose to add a paracetamol/codeine combination and/or other opioid based oral analgesics e.g. tramadol to their formulary.

Parenteral and enteral analgesia
Morphine is approved for administration by paramedics. However, opioids are not as effective (especially when used in isolation) for the management of musculoskeletal type pain and may well lead to significant side effects before achieving adequate analgesia for skin and musculoskeletal pain and therefore other agents such as IV paracetamol should be considered (see medication sheets). As with other opioids morphine is reversed by naloxone. When administering opioids, facilities for maintaining airway, breathing, circulation and naloxone **MUST** be available. If clinically significant sedation or respiratory depression occurs following the administration of opioids the patient's ventilations should be assisted. Decisions to reverse the opioid's effect using an opioid antagonist such as naloxone should be made cautiously as this will return the patient to their pre-opioid pain level and may lead to even more sympathetic stimulation with associated cardio-vascular and endocrine detrimental effects e.g. hyperglycaemia.

The intravenous route has the advantage of rapid onset and the dose can be easily titrated against analgesic effect. In certain patients the intramuscular/subcutaneous routes may be used effectively and may be most appropriate for certain patient specific protocols for certain groups of patients such as end of life and sickle cell disease. Intra-osseous pain relief should only be considered in very specific circumstances and local Trust guidelines should be followed.

Oral morphine is useful for less severe pain but has the disadvantage of delayed onset, some unpredictability of absorption and having to be given in a set dose. It has the advantage of avoiding the need for intravenous access. It is widely used for patients with mild/moderate pain from injuries such as forearm fractures and hip fractures. Those with severe pain are best treated with an intravenous preparation, augmented with entonox and other agents if required. In the event of break-through pain with palliative care, advice should be sought from the patient's care team whenever possible. Opioids are often required in sickle cell disease (a review is underway to look at the optimal analgesic treatment in sickle cell disease). There is limited evidence to suggest that metoclopramide is effective in relieving the nausea induced by opioids in hospital situations but this has not been evaluated in the prehospital environment where motion sickness may also contribute, however, other anti-emetic agents should be utilised when required and available e.g. ondansetron.

Intranasal opioids (morphine, diamorphine and fentanyl)
Intranasal opioids are not currently approved for administration by paramedics. Although it has been suggested that they may be useful in the prehospital environment and are sometimes used by doctors, legal restrictions on the administration of opioids by paramedics have to be addressed before this will be possible. Intranasal opioid analgesia is becoming used more frequently in hospital and has the advantage of potent, rapid action without needing parenteral administration; however it may be logistically more difficult in the prehospital context.

Topical analgesia
In vulnerable adults or needle phobic adults, where venepuncture may be required in a non-urgent situation, tetracaine 4% gel/amethocaine can be applied to the skin overlying a suitable vein and the area covered with an occlusive dressing. Such an application takes about 30–40 minutes to work.

Methods of Pain Management which Require Appropriately Trained Prehospital Practitioners

These methods are included because it is necessary to know what can be done to reduce pain before hospital, if time and logistics allow. An appropriately trained practitioner should be called early to the scene if it is thought that such assistance may be necessary. Hospital personnel may not all have these skills.

Table 1.3 – METHODS THAT REQUIRE APPROPRIATELY TRAINED PRACTITIONERS

Ketamine analgesia/anaesthesia

Ketamine is particularly useful in entrapments where a person can be extricated with combined analgesic and sedative effects.

Ketamine is a parenteral analgesic, with a relatively small opioid action, that at higher doses is a general anaesthetic agent. It is particularly useful in serious trauma because it is less likely to significantly depress blood pressure, or respiration compared to other agents. Adults may experience unpleasant emergence phenomena if used in moderate to higher analgesic or anaesthetic dosages. Ketamine produces salivation so careful airway management is important, although unnecessary interference should be avoided as laryngospasm may occasionally occur. Atropine may be used with care concurrently to minimise hypersalivation.

Regional anaesthesia

There is limited room for regional nerve blocks because of the environment and the need to transport the patient to hospital in a timely manner. However, they can be effective in certain circumstances of severe pain and do not induce drowsiness or disorientation. Femoral nerve blocks may be useful and provide good analgesia for a lower limb injury such as a fractured femur. Clinicians undertaking regional anaesthesia must be suitably trained, prepared and experienced including the management of local anaesthetic toxicity.

KEY POINTS

Management of Pain in Adults

- Pain should be treated as early as possible in all patients unless there is an exceptional specific reason not to.
- Pain relief does not affect later diagnosis.
- A balanced analgesic approach to pain management consists of treating the cause wherever possible, and analgesia involving psychological, physical and pharmacological interventions (more than one agent, when possible, in smaller and titrated doses to achieve better analgesia with fewer side effects by acting at different areas involving the pain pathways).
- Balanced analgesia remains the objective and should be tailored according to both patient and practitioner variables.
- All patients should have a pain score before and after each intervention.

Methodology

For details of the methodology used in the development of this guideline refer to the guideline webpage.

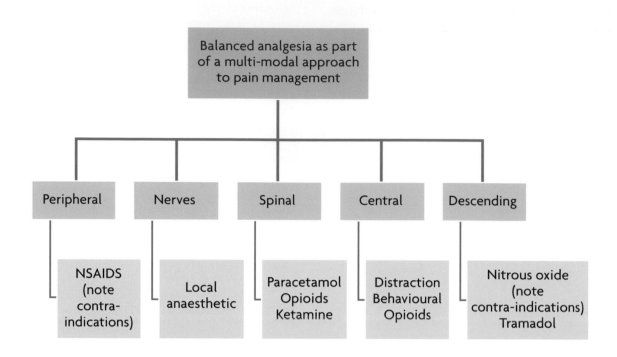

Figure 1.1 – Balanced approach to analgesia.

Pain Management in Children [20]

1. Introduction

All children in pain need analgesia, regardless of age or situation and when appropriate, analgesia should be administered as soon as clinically possible after arriving on scene although this can be done en-route so as not to delay time-critical patients. There is no reason to delay relief of pain because of uncertainty with the definitive diagnosis.

Pain is one of the commonest symptoms in patients presenting to ambulance services.

Control of pain is important not only for humanitarian reasons but also because it may prevent deterioration of the child and allow better assessment.

There is no excuse for leaving a child in pain because of lack of necessary skills in the clinician. If necessary, suitable expertise should be sought to provide pain relief.

Pain is a multi-dimensional construct (see below).

Pain consists of several elements:

- Treatment of the underlying condition.
- Non-pharmacological methods including:
  - psychological support and explanation
  - physical methods e.g. splinting
- Pharmacological treatment.

Pain relief will depend on:

- Cause, site, severity and nature of the pain.
- Age of child.
- Experience/knowledge of the clinician.
- Distance from receiving unit.
- Available resources.

---

2. Assessment

An assessment should be made of the requirements of the child. Pain is a complex experience that is shaped by gender, cultural, environmental, social and personal factors, as well as prior pain experience. Thus the experience of pain is unique to the individual.

It is important to remember that the pain a child experiences cannot be objectively validated in the same way as other vital signs. Attempts to estimate the child's pain should be resisted, as this may lead to an underestimation of the child's experience. Several studies have shown that there is a poor correlation between the patient's pain rating and that of the health professional's, with the latter often underestimating the patient's pain.

Instead, ambulance clinicians need to seek and accept the child's self-report of their pain. This is reinforced by a popular and useful definition of pain: 'pain is whatever the experiencing person says it is, existing whenever they says it does'.

All children in pain should have their pain assessed for its location, nature, severity and duration. Any factors related to, or that, exacerbate or improve the pain should also be assessed.

Pain scoring

There is no validated method of pain scoring for children in the prehospital environment. It is suggested that, pending this, a method that has been validated in the paediatric emergency department (ED) setting is used. The Wong and Baker 'faces' (scoring 0 = no hurt, 1–2 = hurts little bit, 3–4 = hurts little more, 5–6 = hurts even more, 7–8 = hurts whole lot, 9–10 = hurts worst) (**refer to Appendix 1**) are useful for younger children. The FLACC scale is useful for preverbal children and may also be used for older children if needed (**refer to Appendix 2**).

The trend in the scores is more important than the absolute value in assessing efficacy of treatment. Scoring will not be possible in all circumstances (e.g. cognitively impaired individuals, and those with communication difficulties or altered level of consciousness) and in these circumstances behavioural cues will be more important in assessing pain.

3. Management

Analgesia should normally be introduced in an incremental way with each agent being titrated to effect, considering timeliness, effectiveness and potential adverse events. Utilising a balanced analgesic approach will often allow improved efficacy with reduced side-effects. Generally this should always include the non-pharmacological methods of treatment as a starting point and background to all pharmacological therapy (refer to Tables 1.4–1.7).

However, it may be apparent from the assessment that it is appropriate to start with stronger analgesia because of the child's condition; for example, a child with bilateral fractured femurs is likely to require vascular access to provide circulatory replacement and will be in severe pain. It would, therefore, be inappropriate to only try paracetamol and ibuprofen and wait for them to work. Other agents including inhaled (entonox) and intravenous/transmucosal agents as part of a balanced analgesic approach would be indicated at an early stage (this may include paracetamol, opioids and ketamine when appropriate). This along with non pharmacological methods of pain control would provide the best possible analgesia with a lower risk of side effects. However, in a child with a small superficial burn one might try paracetamol with or without ibuprofen and along with non-pharmacological methods, this may be adequate. The child will still require regular re-assessment and a change of approach if needed.

Entonox should be given using an appropriate technique until the other drugs have had time to take effect, and if the child is still in pain. Administering analgesia in this step-wise, incremental way minimises the amount of potent analgesia that is required while still achieving adequate analgesia with fewer side effects.

Any pain relief must be accompanied by careful explanation, involving the child, where possible, and the carer. Include details of the child's condition, the pain relief methods being used, and any possible side effects.

Pain Management in Children

Table 1.4 – NON-PHARMACOLOGICAL METHODS OF PAIN RELIEF

Psychological

Fear and anxiety worsen pain and a child-friendly environment (for example removing equipment which may cause fear and having toys or child-friendly pictures around) may go a long way towards alleviation of pain as may keeping the patient comfortable e.g. warm.

The presence of a parent has been shown to reduce the unpleasantness of hospital emergency procedures more than any other single factor and there is no reason why this should not be true in the prehospital setting.

Distraction (toys, stories, games etc.) is a potent analgesic – whatever is to hand may be used, but there is no substitute for forward planning.

Dressings

Burns dressings that may cool, such as those specifically designed for the task or cling film, can alleviate the pain in the burnt or scalded child. Burns should not be cooled for more than 20 minutes total time and care should be taken with large burns to prevent the development of hypothermia.

Splintage

Simple splintage of fractures provides pain relief as well as minimising ongoing tissue trauma, bleeding and other complications.

NOTE: These should be part of all other methods of pain relief.

Table 1.5 – PHARMACOLOGICAL METHODS OF PAIN RELIEF (refer to specific drug protocols)

Topical analgesia

It is no longer acceptable to consider the prehospital portion of the child's treatment in isolation although the prehospital context must be taken into account with regards to prioritising of care, skill-sets and time-line. The child is on a pathway of care, from the prehospital scene to the most appropriate setting within definitive care. Care that can be improved by one sector (prehospital) to enhance the quality of another (e.g. hospital cannulation) should be provided. Local anaesthetic agents such as **tetracaine gel 4%/amethocaine** can be applied to the skin overlying a suitable vein and the area covered with an occlusive dressing if it is thought likely that the child will require venepuncture on arrival in hospital. Such an application may take about 30–40 minutes to work.

Oral analgesia

Paracetamol and **ibuprofen** may be used in isolation or together for the management of mild to moderate pain as long as appropriate dosages of both are utilised.

Oral morphine solution may also prove very effective in the child with moderate to severe pain such as a fractured forearm (although in isolation is not the ideal class of drug for musculoskeletal pain), but has the disadvantage of delayed onset, some unpredictability of absorption and having to be given in a set dose. It has the advantage of avoiding the need for intravenous access. Those with severe pain are best treated with an intravenous preparation, augmented with entonox if required.

Inhalational analgesia

Entonox (50% Nitrous oxide, 50% Oxygen) is a good analgesic for children who are able to self-administer and who can rapidly be taught to operate the demand valve. It is rapid acting but has a very short half-life, so the analgesic effect wears off rapidly when inhalation is stopped. It can be used as the first analgesic whilst other pain relief is instituted. It can also be used in conjunction with morphine, particularly during painful procedures such as splint application and patient movement. Quite young children, providing they can be taught to operate the demand valve, and the child's fear of the noise of the gas flow and the mask can be overcome, can use the system. Flavoured (e.g. bubblegum) clear masks may help the child overcome the fear.

Parenteral and enteral analgesia

Morphine remains an important component for balanced analgesia and can be administered intravenously, intra-osseously, and orally (**refer to morphine drug guidelines**). Opioid analgesics should be given intravenously rather than intramuscularly to avoid erratic absorption when possible. When used in isolation for musculoskeletal pain, there may be an increased risk of side effects before achieving adequate analgesia, emphasising the need for a balanced analgesic approach. Therefore other agents such as IV paracetamol should be considered (see medication sheets).

As with the other opioids, morphine is reversed by naloxone. When administering opioids to children, ability to maintain airway/breathing/circulation and naloxone **MUST** be available and the required dose calculated in case urgent reversal is necessary. If clinically significant sedation or respiratory depression occurs following the administration of opioids, the child's ventilation should be assisted. Decisions to reverse the opioid effects using an opioid antagonist such as naloxone should be made cautiously as this may return the child to their pre-opioid pain level depending on dosage of naloxone given, which should therefore be titrated to desired effect.

Intranasal opioids (morphine, diamorphine and fentanyl) are not currently approved for paramedic administration. Intranasal opioid analgesia is becoming used more frequently in hospital and has the advantage of potent, rapid action without needing parenteral administration. However, it is fairly difficult to prepare the appropriate dose and concentration in the pre-hospital context.

In certain patients the subcutaneous routes may be used effectively and may be most appropriate for certain patient specific protocols for certain groups of patients such as end of life and sickle cell disease. In the event of break-through pain with palliative care, advice should be sought from the patient's care team whenever possible.

There is no evidence that metoclopramide is effective in relieving nausea induced by opioids. Children have a significant risk of dystonic reactions with metoclopramide and therefore it is not advised in these circumstances.

Other anti-emetics (e.g. Ondansetron) can be used for opioid induces nausea and vomiting.

4. Pain Relief which Requires Appropriately Trained Practitioners

These methods are included because it is necessary to know what can be done to reduce pain in children before hospital, if time and logistics allow. A suitably licensed and trained prehospital practitioner should be called early to the scene if it is thought that such assistance may be necessary. Hospital personnel may not all have these skills.

Table 1.6 – PAIN RELIEF WHICH REQUIRES APPROPRIATELY TRAINED PRACTITIONERS

Ketamine analgesia/anaesthesia

Ketamine is particularly useful in entrapments where a child can be extricated with combined analgesic and sedative effects. At present only doctors and suitably trained and authorised paramedics may carry ketamine.

Ketamine has a predominantly non-opioid mechanism of action. At higher doses it can be used as a general anaesthetic agent. It is particularly useful in serious trauma because it may not significantly depress blood pressure or respiration depending on the particular patient (acute and chronic comorbidity) and the time since injury.

Older children in particular may experience unpleasant emergence phenomena but these tend to be less common in the young especially if appropriate analgesic doses are utilised and titrated to effect. Ketamine in higher doses (not often a problem with appropriate analgesic doses titrated to effect)

produces salivation so careful airway management is important, although unnecessary interference should be avoided as laryngospasm may occasionally occur. Atropine may be used with care concurrently to minimise hypersalivation.

Regional anaesthesia

There is very limited room for regional nerve blocks because of the environment and the need to transport the child to hospital in a timely manner. However, they can be effective in certain circumstances of severe pain and do not induce drowsiness or disorientation. Femoral nerve blocks may be useful and provide good analgesia for a fractured femur. Clinicians undertaking regional anaesthesia must be suitably trained, prepared and experienced and fully understand and have the mechanism to treat local anaesthetic toxicity in the prehospital environment.

Pain Management in Children

Table 1.7 – PREHOSPITAL ANALGESIC DRUGS USED IN CHILDREN

Drug	Route	Pain Severity	Advantages	Disadvantages
Tetracaine 4% gel	Topical	N/A	Reduces pain of venepuncture.	Takes about 30–40 minutes to work.
Paracetamol	Oral (the rectal route is no longer recommended for analgesia).	Mild-moderate (may be opioid sparing when used for more severe pain as better efficacy for musculoskeletal pain than opioids alone).	Readily accessible and well tolerated orally. Well accepted antipyretic.	Slow action when given orally. Inadequate and unpredictable plasma levels if given rectally.
Ibuprofen	Oral (other IV NSAIDS are available but currently not available for paramedic use).	Mild-moderate (may be opioid sparing when used for more severe pain as better efficacy for musculoskeletal pain than opioids alone).	Moderately good analgesic, antipyretic and anti-inflammatory.	Slow action. May cause bronchospasm in asthmatics. Caution in trauma and patients with regards platelet and renal function.
Entonox	Inhaled	Mild-moderate (may be opioid sparing when used for more severe pain as better efficacy for musculoskeletal pain than opioids alone).	Quick, dose self-regulating. Relative contra-indications are important.	Fear of mask. Understanding, coordination and cooperation required. (Demand valves for younger children becoming more available. Cannot use free-flow if not scavenging in confined space e.g. ambulance.)
Oral morphine	Oral	Moderate	Good analgesic for minor/moderate pain particularly of a visceral nature.	May need to adjust dose of IV morphine if given subsequently. Reduced oral bioavailability. Slow action.
Morphine	Intravenous Intra-osseous	Severe	Rapid onset. Reversed with Naloxone (although requires care). Some euphoria.	Not ideal as solo agent when used for musculoskeletal pain. Need access. Respiratory depression, vomiting. Controlled drug.
Diamorphine[a]	Intranasal Intravenous Intra-osseous	Moderate to severe pain particularly of visceral nature.	Intranasal – quick and effective although logistically difficult in prehospital practice. Best efficacy if used with other agents e.g. paracetamol.	As for morphine if given IV. More euphoria. Intranasal not currently approved for paramedics.
Ketamine[a]	Intravenous Intramuscular Oral	Severe pain from either musculoskeletal or visceral aetiologies (excluding acute coronary syndromes).	Can be increased to general anaesthesia in experienced hands. Less respiratory and cardiovascular depression than other strong analgesic/anaesthetic drugs. Concerns re raised ICP less clinically relevant than previously thought.	Emergence phenomena, salivation, occasional laryngospasm (usually with higher doses, therefore small doses 0.1 mg/kg/dose for analgesia and titrate to effect). Comes in three different concentrations which may lead to confusion.

[a] Currently not approved for general paramedic administration; doctor and suitably trained and authorised paramedic administration only.

Pain Management in Children

KEY POINTS

Management of Pain in Children

- All children in pain need analgesia.
- The method of pain relief used will depend on the cause, site, severity, nature of the pain and age of child.
- Analgesia should be introduced incrementally and titrated to effect.
- Pain scoring faces and the FLACC scale are useful for use with young children.
- A balanced analgesic approach to pain management consists of treating the cause wherever possible, and analgesia involving psychological, physical and pharmacological interventions (more than one agent, when possible, in smaller and titrated doses to achieve better analgesia with fewer side effects by acting at different areas involving the pain pathways).
- Balanced analgesia remains the objective and should be tailored according to both patient and practitioner variables.

APPENDIX 1 – The Wong-Baker FACES Pain Rating Scale

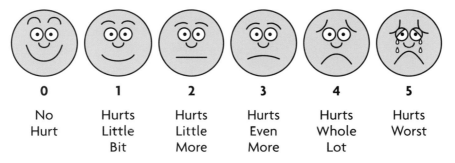

0	1	2	3	4	5
No Hurt	Hurts Little Bit	Hurts Little More	Hurts Even More	Hurts Whole Lot	Hurts Worst

This rating scale is recommended for persons aged 3 years and older.

Instructions: Point to each face using the words to describe the pain intensity. Ask the child to choose face that best describes own pain and record the appropriate number.

Explain to the person that each face is for a person who feels happy because he has no pain (hurt) or sad because he has some or a lot of pain.

Face 0 is very happy because he doesn't hurt at all.
Face 1 hurts just a little bit.
Face 2 hurts a little more.
Face 3 hurts even more.
Face 4 hurts a whole lot.
Face 5 hurts as much as you can imagine, although you don't have to be crying to feel this bad.

Ask the person to choose the face that best describes how they are feeling.

From Hockenberry MJ, Wilson D, Winkelstein ML: Wong's Essentials of Pediatric Nursing, ed. 7, St. Louis, 2005, p. 1259. Used with permission. Copyright, Mosby.

APPENDIX 2 – The FLACC Scale

The **Face, Legs, Activity, Cry, Consolability scale** or **FLACC scale** is a measurement used to assess pain for children up to the age of 7 years or individuals who are unable to communicate their pain. The scale is scored on a range of 0–10 with 0 representing no pain. The scale has five criteria which are each assigned a score of 0, 1 or 2.

Methodology

For details of the methodology used in the development of this guideline, refer to the guideline webpage.

Table 1.8 – THE FLACC SCALE

Criteria	Score - 0	Score - 1	Score - 2
Face	No particular expression or smile	Occasional grimace or frown, withdrawn, uninterested	Frequent to constant quivering chin, clenched jaw
Legs	Normal position or relaxed	Uneasy, restless, tense	Kicking, or legs drawn up
Activity	Lying quietly, normal position, moves easily	Squirming, shifting back and forth, tense	Arched, rigid or jerking
Cry	No cry (awake or asleep)	Moans or whimpers, occasional complaint	Crying steadily, screams or sobs, frequent complaints
Consolability	Content, relaxed	Reassured by occasional touching, hugging or being talked to, distractible	Difficult to console or comfort

1. Introduction

- Safeguarding, promoting welfare and protecting children from significant harm is reliant on effective joint working between agencies and professionals.

- **Duty of care** – as a healthcare worker who may come into contact with children, you have a duty to report concerns about abuse. If you do not report the abuse you may be putting the victim at greater risk. You may also discourage them from disclosing again, as they may feel they were not believed. This may put other people at risk.

- All partners who work with children including local authorities, police, health service, courts, professionals, the voluntary sector and individual members of local communities share the responsibility for safeguarding and promoting the welfare of children and young people. It is vital that all partners are aware of, and appreciate, the role that each of them plays in this area – for further information on the roles and responsibilities of each partner refer to *Working Together to Safeguard Children 2010*.

- Social services and the police have statutory authority and a responsibility to investigate allegations or suspicions about child abuse.

- Ambulance clinicians are often the first professionals on scene and therefore may identify initial concerns regarding a child's welfare and be able to alert social care, the police, the GP, or other appropriate health professional, in line with locally agreed procedures. Accurate recording of events/actions may be crucial to subsequent enquiries.

- The role of the Ambulance Service is not to investigate suspicions but to ensure that any suspicion is passed to the appropriate agency, e.g. social care or the police. Ambulance clinicians need to be aware of child abuse issues and the aim of this guideline is to:

- Ensure all staff are aware of, and can recognise, cases of suspected child abuse, or children at risk of significant harm and provide guidance enabling operational and control staff to assess and report cases of suspected child abuse.

- Ensure that all staff involved in a case of suspected abuse are aware of the possible outcome and of any subsequent actions.

- Further information on local procedures can be obtained from the named professional for safeguarding within individual Ambulance Trusts. The contact details for the named professional for safeguarding can be obtained from ambulance control.

2. Significant Harm

All children have the right:

- To be protected from significant harm/ill-treatment.[a]

- To be protected from impairment of their health[b] and development.[c]

- To grow up in circumstances consistent with the provision of safe and effective care.

The maltreatment of children, physically, emotionally, sexually or through neglect can have a major impact on their health, well-being and development.

There are no absolute criteria on which to rely when judging what constitutes significant harm. In some cases a single traumatic event may constitute significant harm, but more generally it is a compilation of significant events, both acute and long-standing, which interrupt, change, or damage the child's physical and psychological development. Considerations include:

- The degree and extent of physical harm.

- The duration and frequency of abuse and neglect.

- The extent of premeditation.

- The degree of threat, coercion, sadism, and bizarre or unusual elements.

- In order to understand and identify significant harm, consider:
  - the nature of harm, in terms of maltreatment or failure to provide adequate care
  - the impact on the child's health and development
  - the child's development within the context of the family and wider environment
  - any special needs, such as a medical condition, communication impairment or disability, that may affect the child's development and care within the family and the capacity of parents to meet adequately the child's needs.

- Abuse and neglect are forms of maltreatment and children may suffer as a result of a deliberate act, or failure on the part of a parent or carer to act to prevent harm – descriptions of abuse and neglect are detailed in Table 1.10.

- Children may be abused in a family or in an institutional or community setting, by those known to them or, more rarely, by a stranger.

- Children in a care setting can be subject to exploitation, e.g. for prostitution.

Children in need

- Children are defined as being 'in need' when:
  - they are unlikely to reach or maintain a satisfactory level of health or development
  - their health and development will be significantly impaired, without the provision of services (section 17 (10) of the Children Act 1989)
  - they have a disability.

- Local Authorities have a duty to safeguard and promote the welfare of children in need.

---

[a] Harm means ill-treatment or the impairment of health or development, including, for example, impairment suffered from seeing or hearing the ill-treatment of another. Ill-treatment includes sexual abuse and forms of ill-treatment which are not physical.

[b] Health means physical or mental health.

[c] Development means physical, intellectual, emotional, social or behavioural development.

3. Recognition of Abuse

Ambulance clinicians may receive information or make observations which suggest that a child has been abused or is at risk of harm, for example:

- The nature of the illness/injury.
- The account given for the illness/injury may be inconsistent with what is observed.
- Observation of hazards in the home.
- Child(ren) have been locked in a room.
- Signs of distress shown by other children in the home.
- Observations regarding the condition of other children or adults in the household e.g. an environment where domestic violence has taken place. In the case of domestic dispute between adults, the presence of children in the household creates a need to notify even if the child(ren) was not injured.
- Parents or carers who seek medical care from a number of sources.

Non-accidental injury

- When assessing an injury in any child, you should be aware of the possibility of the injury being non-accidental and you should consider this possibility in every case, even if you promptly dismiss the idea.
- For an injury to be accidental it should have a clear, credible and acceptable history and the findings should be consistent with the history and with the development and abilities of the child.

Suspicions of abuse should be raised by:

- Any injury in a non-mobile baby.
- Accidents/injuries in unusual places, e.g. the buttocks, trunk, inner thighs.
- Extensive injuries or signs of both recent and old injuries.
- Small deep burns in unusual places.
- Repeated burns and scalds.
- 'Glove and stocking' burns.
- Poor state of clothing, cleanliness and/or nutrition.
- Delayed reporting of the injury.
- Inappropriate sexual knowledge for the child's age.
- Overt sexual approaches to other children or adults.
- Fear of particular people or situations, e.g. bath time or bedtime.
- Drug and alcohol abuse.
- Suicide attempts and self-injury.
- Running away and fire-setting.
- Environmental factors and family situations (e.g. domestic violence, drug or alcohol abuse, learning disabilities).

The following symptoms should give cause for concern and further assessment:

- Soreness, discharge or unexplained bleeding in the genital area.
- Chronic vaginal infections.
- Bruising, grazes or bites to the genital or breast area.
- Sexually transmitted diseases.
- Pregnancy especially when the identity of the father is vague.

When assessing an injured child, you should use your clinical knowledge regarding what level of accidental injury would be appropriate for their stage of development. Although stages of development vary (e.g. children may crawl or walk at different ages), injuries can broadly be divided between mobile and non-mobile children.

Non-mobile babies

- Any injury in a non-mobile baby must be considered carefully and have a credible explanation if it is to be considered accidental.
- Healthy babies do not bruise or break their bones easily. They do not bruise themselves with their fists or toys, bruise themselves by lying against the bars of a cot, or acquire bruises on the legs when they are held for a nappy change.
- Bruising on the ears, face, neck, trunk and buttocks is particularly suspicious. A torn frenulum (behind the upper lip) is rarely accidental in babies, and bleeding from the mouth of a baby should always be regarded as suspicious.

Fractures

- Fractures may not be obvious on observation and the baby may present only with crying on handling. Often a fracture will not be diagnosed until an X-ray is performed. Fractures in babies are seldom caused by 'rough handling' or putting their legs through the bars of the cot. Babies rarely fracture their skull after a fall from a bed or a chair. Fractures in non-mobile infants should be assessed by an experienced paediatrician to exclude non-accidental injury (refer to Table 1.9 for types of fractures).

Table 1.9 – TYPES OF BONE FRACTURES

Greenstick
The bones bend rather than break. This is a very common accidental injury in children.

Transverse
The break goes across the bone and occurs when there is a direct blow or a direct force on the end of the bone, e.g. a fall on the hand may break the forearm bones or the distal humerus.

Spiral or oblique
A fracture line which goes right around the bone or obliquely across it is due to a twisting force, which may be a feature in non-accidental injuries.

Metaphyseal
Occur at the extreme ends of the bone and are usually only confirmed radiologically. These are caused by a strong twisting force.

Table 1.9 – TYPES OF BONE FRACTURES *continued*

Skull
These must be consistent with the history and explanation given. Complex (branched), depressed or fractures at the back of the skull are suspect.

Rib
These do not occur accidentally, except in a severe crushing injury. Any other cause is highly suspicious of non-accidental injury.

Shaking injuries

- When small babies are shaken violently their head and limb movements cannot be controlled, causing brain damage and haemorrhage within the skull.

- Finger bruising on the chest may indicate that a baby has been held tightly and shaken. These babies usually present with collapse or respiratory problems and the diagnosis is only made on further detailed assessment.

Burns and scalds

- See below.

Mobile Babies and Toddlers

Bruising

- It is normal for toddlers to have accidental bruises on the shins, elbows and forehead. Bruises in unusual areas such as the back, upper arms and abdomen do not tend to occur accidentally.

- Bruising caused by a hand slap leaves a characteristic pattern of 'stripes' representing the imprint of fingers. Forceful gripping leaves small round bruises corresponding to the position of the fingertips. 'Tramline' bruising is caused by a belt or stick and shows as lines of bruising with a white patch in-between. Bites result in small bruises forming part or all of a circle.

Burns and scalds

- Burns are caused by the application to the skin of dry heat and the depth of the burn will depend on the temperature of the object and the length of time it is in contact with the skin.

- Abusive burns are frequently small and deep, and may show the outline of the object (e.g. the soleplate of an iron) whereas accidental burns rarely do so because the child will pull away in response to pain.

- Cigarette burns are not common. They are round, deep and have a red flare around a flat brown crust. These burns usually leave a scar.

- Scalds are caused by steam or hot liquids. Accidental scalds may be extensive but show splash marks unlike the sharp edges of damage done when the child is dunked in hot water (although splash marks may also feature in a non-accidental burn indicating that the child had tried to escape hot water). The glove and stocking pattern of burns on the arms and legs is typical of non-accidental injury. The head, face, neck, shoulders and front of the chest are the areas affected when a child pulls over a kettle accidentally.

Fractures

- Children's bones tend to bend rather than break and require considerable force to damage them. There are various kinds of fractures (refer to Table 1.9), depending on the direction and strength of the force which caused them.

- Unless there is an obvious bony deformity, bony injuries may not be apparent on initial clinical assessment. A clear history and appreciation of the mechanism of injury are crucial parts of the initial assessment and must be clearly documented.

Deliberate poisoning and attempted suffocation

- These are very difficult to assess and may need a period of close observation in hospital. Deliberate poisoning, such as might be found in a child in whom illness is fabricated or induced by carers with parenting responsibilities (factitious or induced illness), may be suspected when a child has repeated puzzling illnesses, usually of sudden onset. The signs include unusual drowsiness, apnoeic attacks, vomiting, diarrhoea and fits.

Older Children and Adolescents

- If the injury is accidental, older children will give a very clear and detailed account of how it happened. The detail will be missing if they have been told what to say.

- Overdosing and other self-harm injuries must be taken seriously in this age group, as they may indicate sexual or other abuse (such as exploitation).

Who is Vulnerable to Abuse?

Although any child can potentially be a victim of abuse, there are some groups of children who may be particularly vulnerable. Factors which may put a child at increased risk of harm include both child and parental factors (adapted from Child Protection Companion, RCPCH 2006).

Child factors:

- Prematurity.
- Feeding difficulties.
- Disability (including learning difficulties).
- Severe physical illnesses or sensory impairments.
- Children with special needs, for example, those who are deaf or autistic. These children may demonstrate challenging behaviour, which may or may not be as a result of abuse.
- Chronic illness.
- Children who are looked after.

Parental factors:

- Parental unavailability for whatever reason increases the risk to the child of all forms of abuse, especially

Safeguarding Children

neglect and emotional abuse. Specific consideration of the effects of the parent's problem on the children must be made, whatever the circumstances of presentation. Sources of stress within families may have a negative impact on a child's health, development or well-being, either directly or because they affect the capacity of parents to respond to their child's needs. Sources of stress may include social exclusion, domestic violence, unstable mental illness of a parent or carer, or drug and alcohol misuse. Parents who appear overanxious about their child when there is no sign of illness or injury may be signalling their inability to cope.

- Parental factors which might have a negative impact on parenting capacity include:
  - learning difficulties
  - mental health problems
  - substance abuse
  - domestic violence
  - chronic ill health
  - physical disability
  - unemployment or poverty
  - homelessness/frequent moves
  - social isolation
  - young, unsupported parents
  - parents with poor role models of their own.

4. Special Circumstances

Individuals who pose a risk to children

- Once an individual has been sentenced and identified as presenting a risk of harm to children, agencies have a responsibility to work collaboratively to monitor and manage the risk of harm to others.

- Where an offender is given a community sentence, Offender Managers or Youth Offending Team workers will monitor the individual's risk of harm to others and their behaviour, and liaise with partner agencies as appropriate.

- Multi-Agency Public Protection Arrangements (MAPPA) should be in place to enable agencies to work together within a statutory framework for managing risk of harm to the public.

Disabled children

- Abuse may be difficult to separate from symptoms of disability e.g. increase in seizures in a child with epilepsy if anticonvulsants are withheld. Induced and fabricated illness may be even more difficult to recognise because the child may have coexistent diagnoses. Important points to remember about abuse of disabled children are:
  - it may be more common than abuse of non-disabled children but evidence for this is poor
  - it may be under reported
  - children may have difficulty communicating their abuse
  - abuse may compound pre-existing disability, or be the cause of the disability
  - all forms of abuse are seen including neglect and sexual abuse

  - it is easy to fail to recognise abuse in disabled children by making too many allowances for the disability as a cause of problems
  - be aware that professionals can be drawn into collusion with families.

- These children are at risk of achieving poor outcomes. Ambulance clinicians need to be aware of the role they can play in recognition of these children, identifying their particular needs and preventing significant harm. In the current multicultural society of the United Kingdom, it is important to recognise that there may be children and families in need of skilled interpreters. You should also recognise the differences that may exist in child-rearing practices in minority groups.

- Special circumstances you should consider are:
  - **Children and young people living away from home** – it has been estimated that 4% of foster carers/placements are abusive to children. Many looked-after children and young people that live independently have been abused or neglected prior to going into care. This is a particular group where assessment may be made more difficult, because of pre-existing symptoms and behaviour. There should be a low threshold in seeking advice from experienced professionals in these circumstances (e.g. designated/named professional).
  - **Asylum-seeking children or refugees**, **both with families and unaccompanied** – the importance of having skilled interpreters in assessment of these children cannot be over-emphasised. The children's behaviour on entering the country may already have been influenced by previous experience. It is important to remember their general health needs and the families will need help in accessing services.
  - **Children with troubled parent/s** (see also **Parental factors** above) These include children of substance misusing parents, children living with domestic violence, children whose parents have chronic mental or physical health problems, children whose parents have a learning disability, children with a parent in prison. Effects on the child are profound and include fearfulness, withdrawal, anxious behaviour, lack of self-confidence and social skills, difficulties in forming relationships, sleep disturbance, non-attendance at school, aggression, bullying, post-traumatic stress disorder, behaviour suggestive of ADHD.

The following children may also have unmet health needs – low immunisation levels, poor dental health and non-attendance at clinic appointments.

  - **Children in the Armed Forces** – extra strains are placed upon the families engendered by frequent moves, frequent changes of school, separation of parents by the nature of the job and separation from immediate support from family and friends.
  - **Children of travelling families** – are subjected to the same problems because of frequent moves. They may also suffer from poor health, poor access to primary health care and vaccinations, in addition to poor living conditions.

Safeguarding Children

- **Runaway children and prostitution** – many runaway children may already have been the subject of abuse and are at risk of exploitation and prostitution. Children of troubled families are more likely to be involved in prostitution than other groups. They also are at risk of child trafficking for sexual exploitation.
- **Children as young carers** – neglect and emotional abuse may be part and parcel of the difficulties of taking on parental responsibilities and a caring role at a young age. Young carers lose out on normal childhood experiences (e.g. school attendance, peer groups).

5. Procedure

If physical, sexual, or emotional abuse or neglect is suspected, follow local procedures; information can be obtained from the named professional for safeguarding within individual Ambulance Trusts. Ambulance clinicians may obtain contact information from ambulance control.

5.1 If the child is the patient

- The first priority is the health and safety of the child. Ambulance clinicians should follow the usual **ABCDE** and **<C>ABCDE** assessment (**refer to medical and trauma overview guidelines**). Children with significant injury should be transferred to further care without delay.
- Where a child is thought to be at immediate risk, they should be referred to the police as an emergency by contacting ambulance control for a 999 response.

In all circumstances:

- Limit questions to those of routine history taking, asking questions only in relation to the injury or for clarification of what is being said. It is important to stop questioning when your suspicions are clarified. Unnecessary questioning or probing may affect the credibility of subsequent evidence.
- Accept the explanations given and do not make any suggestions to the child as to how an injury or incident may have happened.
- Care must be taken not to directly accuse parents or carers of abuse as this may result in a refusal to transfer to further care and place the child at further risk. However, you should always work in partnership with parents as far as possible, and inform them of your concerns and the need to share these with the statutory agencies, unless to do so would put the child or others at greater risk of harm. Professional judgement is crucial as to what information should be shared with parents.
- Any allegation of abuse by a child is an important indicator and should always be taken seriously – it is important to listen to the 'voice of the child' and what they are saying. Do not ask probing questions.
- Adult responses can influence how able a child feels to reveal the full extent of the abuse. Listen and react appropriately to instil confidence. It is important to note that children may only tell a small part of their experience initially.

- It is important to make an accurate record of events and actions. Write down exactly what you have been told. The child's first language may not be English and care must be taken not to use family members or carers as interpreters in cases of suspected abuse. Take note of any inconsistency in history and any delay in calling for assistance.
- On arrival inform the receiving staff and the most senior member of nursing staff on duty of your concerns or suspicions. When reporting suspected abuse, the emphasis must be on shared professional responsibility and immediate communication.
- Complete safeguarding documentation/report as per local procedures; complete in private if possible. Follow local/Trust protocols/guidelines.
- Ambulance clinicians must report suspected child abuse to the relevant statutory bodies e.g. social care and the police, but they do not have a statutory duty to investigate it.
- Where a practitioner feels that their concerns have not been taken up, they have a duty to escalate their concerns to a higher level by discussing this with their line manager, a more experienced colleague or named/designated doctor or nurse.

5.2 If the child is not the patient

- If the circumstances are suspicious, the ambulance clinician(s) should consider the implications of leaving the child.
- If the child is accompanying another person (e.g. a parent/carer) who is being conveyed, the ambulance clinician(s) should inform ED staff of their concerns.
- If no one is transferred to hospital, follow local/Trust protocols/guidelines and inform them of the incident/concerns at the earliest opportunity.
- Complete safeguarding documentation/report as per local procedures; complete in private if possible.
- Follow local/Trust protocols/guidelines of the circumstances.

5.3 Allegations against ambulance staff

- An allegation made by a child against a member of ambulance staff is no different to an allegation made against any other healthcare professional and the appropriate procedures should be followed i.e. a referral to social care or the police. In other words, a child protection inquiry must follow such allegations.
- The member of staff who is alleged to have abused the child will have to report the allegation to his line manager who should follow employment procedures – i.e. suspend the member of staff while investigations are conducted. There should be close liaison between the police doing the investigation and the line manager who should be guided by the police as to how much information about the inquiry should be relayed to the member of staff. There will also need to be a support system in place for the member of staff.

Table 1.10 – EXAMPLES OF TYPES OF ABUSE AND NEGLECT

Emotional abuse

The persistent emotional maltreatment of a child so as to cause severe and persistent adverse effects on the child's emotional development. It may:

● Involve conveying to children that they are worthless or unloved, inadequate, or valued only insofar as they meet the needs of another person.

● Involve not giving the child opportunities to express their views, deliberately silencing them or 'making fun' of what they say or how they communicate.

● Feature age or developmentally inappropriate expectations being imposed on children, e.g. interactions that are beyond the child's developmental capability, as well as overprotection and limitation of exploration and learning, or preventing the child participating in normal social interaction.

● Involve seeing or hearing the ill-treatment of another.

● Involve serious bullying (including cyberbullying), causing children frequently to feel frightened or in danger, or the exploitation or corruption of children. Some level of emotional abuse is involved in all types of maltreatment of a child, though it may occur alone.

Emotional abuse alone can be difficult to recognise as the child may be physically well cared-for and the home in good condition. Some factors which may indicate emotional abuse are:

● If the child is constantly denigrated before others.

● If the child is constantly given the impression that the parents are disappointed in them.

● If the child is blamed for things that go wrong or is told they may be unloved/sent away.

● If the parent does not offer any love or attention, e.g. leaves them alone for a long time.

● If the parent is obsessive about cleanliness, tidiness etc.

● If the parent has unrealistic expectations of the child, e.g. educational achievement/toilet training.

● If the child is either bullying others or being bullied themselves.

● If there is an atmosphere of domestic violence, adults with mental health problems or a history of drug or alcohol abuse.

Sexual abuse

Sexual abuse involves forcing or enticing a child or young person to take part in sexual activities, not necessarily involving a high level of violence, whether or not the child is aware of what is happening.

Both girls and boys of all age groups are at risk. The sexual abuse of a child is often planned and chronic. A large proportion of sexually abused children have no physical signs, and it is therefore necessary to be alert to behavioural and emotional factors that may indicate abuse. Although some children are abused by strangers, most are abused by someone known to them. Some are abused by other children, including siblings, who may also be at risk of abuse. The majority of abusers are male, although occasionally women abuse children sexually or cooperate with men in the abusing behaviour.

The activities may involve physical contact, including assault by penetration e.g. rape or oral sex or non-penetrative acts such as masturbation, kissing, rubbing and touching outside of clothing. They may include non-contact activities, such as involving children in looking at, or in the production of, sexual images, watching sexual activities, encouraging children to behave in sexually inappropriate ways, or grooming a child in preparation for abuse (including via the internet).

Physical abuse

Physical abuse may involve hitting, shaking, throwing, poisoning, burning or scalding, suffocating, or otherwise causing physical harm. Physical harm may also be caused when a parent or carer fabricates the symptoms of, or deliberately induces ill-health; this situation is commonly described using terms such as 'factitious or induced illness'.

Neglect

Neglect is more difficult to recognise and define than physical abuse, but its effects can be life-long. Impairment of growth, intelligence, physical ability and life expectancy are only a few of the effects of neglect in childhood.

The persistent failure to meet a child's basic physical and/or psychological needs is likely to result in the serious impairment of the child's health or development.

A neglected or abused infant may show signs of poor attachment. They may lack the sense of security to explore, and appear unhappy and whining. There may be little sign of attachment behaviour, and the child may move aimlessly round a room or creep quietly into corners.

Neglect may occur during pregnancy as a result of maternal substance abuse. Once a child is born, neglect may involve a parent or carer failing to:

● Provide adequate food, clothing and shelter (including exclusion from home or abandonment).

● Protect a child from physical and emotional harm or danger.

● Ensure adequate supervision (including the use of inadequate care-givers).

● Ensure access to appropriate medical care or treatment.

● Respond to the child's basic emotional needs.

In pre-school and school-age children, indicators of neglect may include poor attention span, aggressive behaviour and poor co-operative play. Indiscriminate friendly behaviour to unknown adults is often a feature of children who are deprived of emotional affection. Other signs include repetitive rocking or other self-stimulating behaviour. Personal hygiene may be poor because of physical neglect, and this may lead to rejection by peers.

Safeguarding Children

KEY POINTS

Safeguarding children

- The safety and welfare of the child is paramount.
- There is a duty to report concerns. Staff should not investigate suspicions themselves.
- Be aware of the special circumstances that the child is in which may increase the risk of abuse.
- Police should be involved where there may be an immediate risk to the child.
- Staff should document the circumstances giving rise to their concern as soon as possible.

Further reading

The National Service Framework for Children, Young People and Maternity Services, which sets out a ten-year plan to stimulate long-term and sustained improvement in children's health and well-being.

There are many other documents which are important to inform strategy and delivery of services. These are referenced on the Government's website http://www.dcsf.gov.uk/everychildmatters/

Methodology

For details of the methodology used in the development of this guideline, refer to the guideline webpage.

Sexual Assault [30–39]

1. Introduction

- Sexual assault is extremely distressing; managing such cases demands sensitive, non-judgemental medical and emotional care and an awareness of the forensic requirements.

- Patients are likely to be very distressed about the events surrounding sexual assault. They may not want to involve anybody else, and may not consent to disclosure of information to other parties such as the police. Do not judge, or give the appearance of judging the patient. Be kind and considerate, and allow the patient space, and as much choice about options for their treatment as possible. They may feel worthless, guilty and humiliated; dominant and controlling behaviour will intensify these feelings.

- Alcohol and drugs such as Rohypnol may also be involved.

- It may be appropriate for the patient to be accompanied by another person. The patient may be anxious when left alone with a person of the same sex as the assailant. On the other hand, they may be reassured by the presence of a professional person. The wishes of the patient must be considered and attempts made to reassure them and make them feel safe.

- **Further care** – it is important to encourage all victims of sexual assault to attend a specialised unit for forensic examination, and inform the police. Both will be able to provide physical, medical and emotional support.

- In cases of sexual assault in vulnerable adults and children **refer to suspected abuse of vulnerable adults and recognition of abuse and safeguarding children**.

2. Incidence

- Sexual assault affects approximately 23% of women, 3% of men, 21% of girls and 11% of boys. Rape affects 5% of women and 0.4% of men. In 2009/10 there were approximately 20,000 sexual assaults and 14,000 rapes against women, reported to the police In England and Wales. However, many assaults go unreported.

- One-fifth of all rapes reported to the police involved children under the age of 16 years. Child sexual abuse is more likely in missing children, looked-after children, children with a disability and those whose family experience domestic violence.

3. Severity and Outcome

The severity of the assault can vary from sexual touching to sustaining life-threatening injuries. The outcome of the assault can lead to long-term psychological and physical effects.

4. Pathophysiology

- **Sexual assault** is touching another person in a sexual way without consent.

- **Serious sexual assault** is penetration of the vagina or anus with a part of the body or anything else without consent.

- **Rape** is penetration of the vagina, anus or mouth with a penis without consent.

5. Assessment and Management

For the assessment and management of sexual assault refer to Table 1.11.

Methodology

For details of the methodology used in the development of this guideline refer to the guideline webpage.

KEY POINTS

Sexual Assault
- **Sexual assault may be concurrent with other injuries which will need treating.**
- **Treatment should avoid disturbing evidence where possible.**
- **Leave the investigation to the police.**
- **Accommodate patient wishes where possible.**
- **Police may have special facilities for managing patients.**

Sexual Assault

Table 1.11 – ASSESSMENT and MANAGEMENT of:

Sexual Assault

ASSESSMENT	MANAGEMENT
● Assess ABCD	If any of the following **TIME CRITICAL** features present **major ABCD problems**: ● Start correcting **A** and **B** problems. ● Undertake a **TIME CRITICAL** transfer to nearest receiving hospital. ● Continue patient management en-route. ● Provide an alert/information call.
● Assess	● Limit questions to those identifying the need for medical treatment, but allow the patient to talk and document what is said – it is not appropriate to probe for details of the assault and could affect the outcome of criminal investigations. ● Manage according to condition. ● Acute injury – **refer to trauma emergencies overview**. ● Acute illness – **refer to medical emergencies overview**. ● It may be appropriate to delay assessment for non-urgent injuries until transfer to specialised unit for forensic examination to avoid further distress and disturbing the evidence.
● Approach	● Sensitive and respectful manner. ● Call police promptly – so the scene may be secured. ● If possible ensure privacy. ● Consider cultural/religious issues. ● Where possible accommodate patient's requests. ● Where possible avoid disturbing the scene. ● Where possible avoid being alone with the patient.
● Forensic examination	Forensic examination will focus specifically on the areas affected, including wounds, mouth, anus and vagina and other areas where the patient has been kissed, licked or bitten, as these areas may well be contaminated with the assailant's DNA; therefore patients should not: ● Wash (shower/bathe) or brush their teeth. ● Change clothes, throw away or destroy clothes. ● Urinate. The police will want to collect early evidence samples including a urine sample to screen for the presence of drugs as some drugs have a very short half-life. ● A mouth swab and mouth wash may also be requested by the police. ● Defecate. ● Smoke. ● Drink/eat. ● If a blanket is required for modesty or warmth a single-use blanket should be used and kept with the patient – the blanket needs to be retained in order to analyse cross-contamination. ● If the patient is not wrapped in a single-use blanket, place a sterile sheet or single-use blanket under the patient where they sit or lie and retain for forensic examination. ● Avoid cleaning any wounds unless clinically absolutely necessary – if possible keep 'washings'. ● If required, lightly apply dry dressings – retain any used dressing and swabs for forensic examination; also keep the sterile packets they were contained in order to examine cross-contamination. NB All of these recommendations are vital to conserve evidence for a successful prosecution of the offender; **BUT** the need for this approach must be conveyed with great sensitivity to the patient who may well want to wash and change.
● Transfer[a]	● Encourage all patients to attend further care and to inform the police. ● Transfer patients to further care according to local guideline. ● Many services no longer employ 'courtesy calls'. Follow local procedures around information provided prior to arrival / shared with triage nurse. ● Hand over to an appropriate member of staff and not in a public area. ● Where a patient is competent and refuses hospital treatment, advise them to seek further medical attention. They may need post-exposure prophylaxis, vaccination, and/or contraception, all of which can be provided confidentially.
● Documentation	Complete the clinical record in great detail contemporaneously: ● Document only facts not personal opinion. ● Document what the patient says. ● Clinical findings with relevant timings. ● Ambulance identification number. ● A police statement may be required later.

[a] In some areas arrangements exist for patients to be examined and interviewed in police or other facilities.

1. Introduction

- All vulnerable adults have the right to be protected from harm. Safeguarding vulnerable adults from significant harm is reliant on effective joint working and communication between responsible agencies and professionals.

- This guidance is for the management of people aged 18 years or over; for those under the age of 18 years **refer to the safeguarding children guideline**.

- **Duty of care** – as a healthcare worker who may come into contact with vulnerable adults, there is a duty to report concerns about abuse. Not reporting abuse may put the person at greater risk. It may also discourage people from disclosing again, as they may feel they were not believed and this may put others at risk.

- Ambulance clinicians are often the first professionals on scene and therefore may identify initial concerns regarding abuse. The role of the Ambulance Service is not to investigate suspicions but to ensure that any suspicion is passed to the appropriate agency, e.g. social care or the police in line with locally agreed procedures.

- Ambulance clinicians need to be aware of issues and local policies and procedures related to the abuse of vulnerable adults. The aim of this guideline is to assist ambulance clinicians to recognise and report cases of suspected abuse of a vulnerable adult.

- The principles of adult protection differ from those of child protection, in that adults have the right to take risks and may choose to live at risk if they have the capacity to make such a decision. Their wishes should not be overruled without full consideration. For example, older people are not 'confused'; similarly, people with learning disabilities or mental health problems may have the capacity to make some decisions about their lives, but not others.

- All Local Authorities should have Inter-Agency Adult Protection Procedures which comply with the 'No Secrets' guidance and many authorities will also have an Inter-agency Adult Protection Committee / Safeguarding Adults Board. In addition, the Care Quality Commission is responsible for the standard of care provided in nursing homes, residential care homes and by domiciliary care agencies.

2. Incidence

The National Adult Social Care Intelligence Service survey of councils in England with responsibility for adult social services found the majority of referrals were:

- In the 18–64 age group.
- For women.
- For people with physical disabilities.
- Regarding physical abuse.
- Undertaken in the person's own home.
- Perpetrated by social care staff.

However, not all councils reported data; in those that did, some data were incomplete. Also it is likely that abuse of vulnerable adults is underreported.

3. Assessment

- Abuse can be perpetrated by a range of people (Table 1.12) and take a number of forms (Table 1.13). Abuse can be a single or repeated act that can result in significant harm.

- A vulnerable adult is defined as a person *'who is or may be in need of community care services by reason of mental or other disability, age or illness; and who is or may be unable to take care of him or herself, or unable to protect him or herself against significant harm or exploitation.'*

- Abuse is the *'violation of an individual's human and civil rights by any other person or persons.'*

When assessing the seriousness of abuse consider the:

- **Vulnerability** of the individual.
- **Nature and extent** of the abuse.
- **Length of time** it has been occurring.
- **Impact** on the individual.
- Risk of **repeated or increasingly serious** acts involving this or other vulnerable adults.

Table 1.12 – POTENTIAL SOURCES OF ABUSE

- Spouse, relatives and family members
- Professional staff
- Paid care workers
- Volunteers
- Other service users
- Neighbours
- Friends and associates
- People who deliberately exploit vulnerable people
- Strangers

Table 1.13 – TYPES OF ABUSE

Physical
- Hitting
- Slapping
- Pushing
- Kicking
- Misuse of medication
- Restraint or inappropriate sanctions

Sexual
- Rape
- Sexual assault
- Sexual acts to which the vulnerable adult has not consented or could not consent or was pressured into consenting

Psychological
- Emotional abuse
- Threats of harm or abandonment
- Deprivation of contact
- Humiliation

Table 1.13 – TYPES OF ABUSE *continued*

Psychological *continued*
- Blaming
- Controlling
- Intimidation
- Coercion
- Harassment
- Verbal abuse
- Isolation
- Withdrawal from services or supportive networks

Financial/material
- Theft
- Fraud
- Exploitation
- Pressure in connection with wills, property, inheritance or financial transactions
- Misuse or misappropriation of property, possessions or benefits

Neglect
- Ignoring medical or physical care needs
- Failure to provide access to appropriate health, social care or educational services
- Withholding of the necessities of life, such as medication, adequate nutrition and heating

Discriminatory
- Racist
- Sexist
- Based on a person's disability
- Harassment
- Slurs or similar treatment

4. Management

- The first priority is the health and safety of the patient. Ambulance clinicians should follow the usual **ABCDE** and **<C>ABCDE** assessment – **refer to medical and trauma overview guidelines**.

- If the ambulance clinicians are concerned that the abuser may be present, the ambulance clinicians should not let the person(s) know they are suspicious, as this may result in a refusal to attend hospital or a situation where a vulnerable adult may be placed at further risk.

- Any inconsistency in history and any delay in calling for assistance should be noted. A patient who is frightened may be reluctant to say what may be the cause of their injury/condition, especially if the person responsible for the abuse is present.

- If necessary, ask appropriate questions of those present to clarify the situation, but avoid unnecessary questioning or probing, as this may affect the credibility of subsequent evidence.

- Accurate recording of events/actions/information may be crucial to subsequent inquiries. It may be helpful to make a note of the person's body language.

- It is important to ascertain the wishes of the patient and to take into account whether or not they want to be conveyed to hospital. However, the decision not to convey a patient to hospital is one that must be fully considered. In some cases the ambulance clinician may consider that the patient clearly does not have the capacity to make a judgement with respect to their need for medical care, and may decide to act under the Doctrine of Necessity (if there is risk to life or limb), or make alternative arrangements for the patient if their condition requires less immediate treatment (e.g. a general practitioner visit the following day).

- If the patient needs to be transferred to further care, and another person tries to prevent this, crews may need to consider whether to involve the police; inform ambulance control about the situation.

- Report concerns to the appropriate agency i.e. local social services and/or police.

- If the patient is transferred to further care inform a senior member of the receiving staff of the concerns regarding possible abuse. Be careful not to alert the alleged abuser or place the vulnerable adult at risk of further abuse or intimidation.

- If the patient is not transferred to further care or if the ambulance clinicians have concerns about someone else in the household or on the premises, they should contact ambulance control and inform them of their concerns.

- Inform the appropriate clinical manager as per local /Trust guidelines.

- Complete documentation/report as per local procedures; complete in private if possible.

NB The patient may not be the person at risk of harm; it may be a person in the household or someone accompanying the patient.

Further information – on local procedures can be obtained from the named professional for safeguarding within individual Ambulance Trusts. The contact details can be obtained from ambulance control.

Methodology

For details of the methodology used in the development of this guideline refer to the guideline webpage.

KEY POINTS

Safeguarding Vulnerable Adults
- **Vulnerable adults have a right to be protected.**
- **Abuse can take a number of forms.**
- **Concerns of suspected abuse must be reported to the appropriate agency i.e. local social services and/or police.**
- **Ambulance clinicians must document the circumstances giving rise to concern as soon as possible.**
- **The wishes of the patient should be taken into account where possible.**
- **Ambulance clinicians should not investigate allegations.**

1. Introduction

- Being called to a death of an infant, child or adolescent is one of the most difficult experiences that an ambulance clinician will encounter. They are usually the first professionals to arrive at the scene, and, at the same time as making difficult judgements about resuscitation, they have to deal with the devastating initial shock of the parents/carers.

- Despite the recent fall in incidence,[a] sudden unexpected death in infancy (SUDI) remains the largest single cause of death in infants aged one month to one year. SUDI can also occasionally occur in children older than 1 year of age.

- In 50% of SUDI a specific cause for the death is found, either from a careful investigation of the circumstances or from post-mortem findings.

- The vast majority of SUDI occur from natural causes. 10% of SUDI are thought to arise from some form of maltreatment by their parents/carers and so a joint paediatric and police investigation is required for **all** SUDIs. When informed of a SUDI, ambulance control should notify the police Child Abuse Investigation Team to initiate this process.

- This document draws on national experiences and is in accord with the recommendations of the Kennedy Report.

2. Multi-agency Approach

The Kennedy Report requires a multi-agency approach to the management of SUDI, in which all the professionals involved keep each other informed and collaborate.

Objectives

The main objectives for ambulance clinicians when called to a child death are:

- Resuscitation (**refer to Paediatric Basic (BLS) and Advanced Life Support (ALS) guidelines**) should be attempted in all cases, unless there is a condition unequivocally associated with death or a valid advance directive (**refer to Recognition of Life Extinct (ROLE) guideline**).

- Detecting a pulse in a sick infant can be extremely difficult so the absence of peripheral pulses is not a reliable indication of death. Similarly, a sick infant may have marked peripheral cyanosis and cold extremities (**refer to paediatric medical and trauma emergencies guidelines**).

- It is better for parents/carers to know that resuscitation was attempted but failed, than to be left feeling that something that might have saved their infant was not done.

- Once resuscitation has been initiated, the infant should be transported at once to the nearest suitable emergency department, with resuscitation continuing en-route.

Care of the family

- The initial response of professionals (and you will probably be the first on the scene) will affect the family profoundly.

- Having experienced this hugely distressing event, parents/carers exhibit a variety of reactions e.g. overwhelming grief, anger, confusion, disbelief or guilt. Be prepared to deal with any of these feelings with sympathy and sensitivity, remembering some reactions may be directed at you as a manifestation of their distress.

- Think before you speak. Chance remarks may cause offence and may be remembered indefinitely e.g. 'I'm sorry he looks so awful'.

- Avoid any criticism of the parents/carers, either direct or implied.

- Ask the child's name and use it when referring to them (do not refer to the child as 'it').

- If possible, do not put children in body bags. It is known that relatives do not perceive very traumatic events in the way that unrelated onlookers might and it is important they are allowed to see, touch and hold their loved one.

- Explain what you are doing at every stage.

- Allow the parents/carers to hold the child if they so wish (unless there are obvious indications of trauma), as long as it does not interfere with clinical care.

- The parents/carers will need to accompany you when you take the infant to hospital. If appropriate, offer to take one or both in the ambulance. Alternatively ensure that they have other means of transport, and that they know where to go.

- If they have no telephone, offer to help in contacting a relative or friend who can give immediate support, such as looking after other children or making sure the premises are secure.

Document

- Time arrived on scene.

- The situation in which you find the infant e.g. position in cot, bedding, proximity to others, room temperature, etc.

- A brief description from the parents/carers of the events that led up to them finding the dead child e.g. when last seen alive, health at that time, position when found, etc. The police and community paediatrician will go through these events in greater detail, but the parent/carer's initial statement to you may be particularly valuable in the investigation.

- Write all this information down as soon as you have the opportunity, giving times and other details as precisely as possible.

Communication with other agencies

- After you have arrived at the house and confirmed that the infant is dead or moribund, the police child abuse investigation team must be informed (see your locally agreed procedure – Figure 1.2 shows South Central's Child Death Procedures flowchart, as an example).

- In unexpected child deaths, advise the parents/carers that the death will be reported to the Coroner, and that they will be interviewed by the Coroner's Officer and the police in due course.

---

[a] The national 'Reduce the Risk' campaign of 1991 advocating infants sleep on their backs produced a dramatic reduction (70%) in sudden infant deaths.

- Share the information you have collected with the police and with relevant health professionals.

Transferring the infant

- The infant should be taken to the nearest appropriate emergency department, not direct to a mortuary. This should apply even when the infant has clearly been dead for some time and a doctor has certified death at home (it will on occasions be necessary to remind a doctor that taking the infant to a hospital is now the preferred procedure, as recommended by Kennedy).

- The main reasons for taking the infant to the hospital rather than the mortuary are that at hospital an immediate examination can be made by a paediatrician, early samples can be taken for laboratory tests, parents/carers can talk with the paediatricians and other local support services can be contacted.

- Pre-alert the emergency department of your arrival, asking them to be ready to take over resuscitation if this is ongoing.

Support for ambulance clinicians

- The death of a child is very distressing for all those involved, and opportunities for debriefing or counselling should be available for ambulance clinicians.

- Follow local procedures for post critical incident debriefing local guidelines/processes.

- Some clinicians will feel ongoing distress. This is normal but should be recognised and other forms of therapy, from informal support from colleagues, to formal counselling, may be required.

- As part of the ambulance service safeguarding processes information from local paeditricians and ambulance service safeguarding leads will be available if required for further discussion

- Unsuccessful resuscitation attempts on children weigh heavily on many people's shoulders and it is very important to remember that the vast majority of children who arrest outside hospital will die, whoever is there, or whatever is done – less than 10% of paediatric out-of-hospital cardiac arrests survive. Such outcomes are almost never the fault of those attempting resuscitation who will have done everything possible to help that child.

Conclusion

- Findings from the Foundation for the Study of Infant Deaths have show that parents/carers regard the actions and attitudes of ambulance clinicians to them as really important and speak very highly of the way both they and their child were treated.

- Your role is not only essential for immediate practical reasons but also has a great influence on how the family deals with the death long after the initial crisis is over.

Additional Reading

http://www.dcsf.gov.uk/everychildmatters/. A guide to inter-agency working to safeguard and promote the welfare of children.

Children Act 2004.

Methodology

For details of the methodology used in the update of this guideline refer to the guideline webpage.

KEY POINTS

Death of a Child (including Sudden Unexpected Death in Infancy)

- **A child death is one of the most emotionally traumatic and challenging events that an ambulance clinician will encounter.**
- **Resuscitation should always be attempted unless there is a condition unequivocally associated with death or a valid advance directive.**
- **Communication and empathy are essential, and the family must be treated with compassion and sensitivity throughout.**
- **Ensure the family is aware of where you are taking their infant/child.**
- **Collect information pertaining to the situation in which you find the child, a history of events and any significant past medical history.**
- **Follow agreed protocols with regards to inter-agency communication and informing the police.**
- **In unexpected deaths, when appropriate explain to the family that the death will be reported to the Coroner and that they will be interviewed by the Coroner's Officer and the police in due course.**

Death of a Child, including Sudden Unexpected Death in Infancy, children and adolescents (SUDICA)

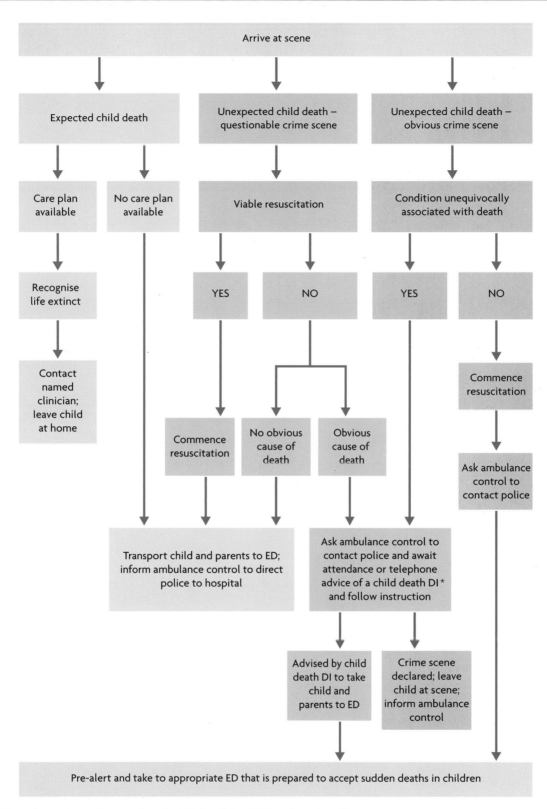

SECTION 1 General Guidance

Arrive at scene

- Expected child death
  - Care plan available
    - Recognise life extinct
      - Contact named clinician; leave child at home
  - No care plan available
- Unexpected child death – questionable crime scene
  - Viable resuscitation
    - YES
      - Commence resuscitation
    - NO
      - No obvious cause of death
      - Obvious cause of death
- Unexpected child death – obvious crime scene
  - Condition unequivocally associated with death
    - YES
    - NO
      - Commence resuscitation
        - Ask ambulance control to contact police

Transport child and parents to ED; inform ambulance control to direct police to hospital

Ask ambulance control to contact police and await attendance or telephone advice of a child death DI* and follow instruction

- Advised by child death DI to take child and parents to ED
- Crime scene declared; leave child at scene; inform ambulance control

Pre-alert and take to appropriate ED that is prepared to accept sudden deaths in children

Conditions unequivocally associated with death in children less than 18 years:
1. Massive cranial and cerebral destruction
2. Hemicorporectomy or similar massive injury
3. Decomposition/putrefaction
4. Incineration

NB Hypostasis and rigor mortis are not to be considered in children – these should all be conveyed.

Child Death Detective Inspector* – A Detective Inspector who is trained in the management of child death incidents to ensure the multi-agency investigation is commenced and evidence gathered to ascertain the full facts of the child's death.

Figure 1.2 – Example of a local child death procedure from South Central Ambulance Service – reproduced with kind permission.

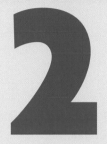

Resuscitation

Resuscitation

Airway and Breathing Management [47, 48, 58–60]

1. Introduction

- Airway obstruction is life-threatening and needs rapid intervention.
- Most patients can be managed using simple techniques.
- Spinal immobilisation must be started at the same time as airway control (but does not take priority over airway control). **Refer to neck and trauma guideline**.

- The size of airway differs between patients; Table 2.1 provides a guide for airway sizes in children and adults.
- Assessment of breathing includes both airway and respiratory effort (refer to Figure 2.1 and 2.2).

Table 2.1 – AIRWAY SIZES BY TYPE

Age	Oropharyngeal	Endotracheal	Laryngeal	I-gel
		Airway Size by Tube Type		
Birth	000	Diameter: 3.0 mm Length: 10 cm	1.0	1.0
1 month	00	Diameter: 3.0 mm Length: 10 cm	1.0	1.0
3 months	00	Diameter: 3.5 mm Length: 11 cm	1.5	1.5
6 months	00	Diameter: 4 mm Length: 12 cm	1.5	1.5
9 months	00	Diameter: 4 mm Length: 12 cm	1.5	1.5
12 months	00 OR 0	Diameter: 4.5 mm Length: 13 cm	1.5	1.5 OR 2.0
18 months	00 OR 0	Diameter: 4.5 mm Length: 13 cm	2.0	1.5 OR 2.0
2 years	0 OR 1	Diameter: 5 mm Length: 14 cm	2.0	1.5 OR 2.0
3 years	1	Diameter: 5 mm Length: 14 cm	2.0	2.0
4 years	1	Diameter: 5 mm Length: 15 cm	2.0	2.0
5 years	1	Diameter: 5.5 mm Length: 15 cm	2.0	2.0
6 years	1	Diameter: 6 mm Length: 16 cm	2.5	2.0
7 years	1 OR 2	Diameter: 6 mm Length: 16 cm	2.5	2.0
8 years	1 OR 2	Diameter: 6.5 mm Length: 17 cm	2.5	2.5
9 years	1 OR 2	Diameter: 6.5 mm Length: 17 cm	2.5	2.5
10 years	2 OR 3	Diameter: 7.0 mm Length: 18 cm	3.0	2.5 OR 3.0
11 years	2 OR 3	Diameter: 7.0 mm Length: 18 cm	3.0	2.5 OR 3.0
Adult >70kg	4 OR 5	Female diameter: 7.0–8.0 mm length: 22–24 cm Male diameter: 8.0–9.0 mm length: 23–25 cm	4 OR 5	4 OR 5

This table is an indicative guide only. Individual manufacturer's sizes may vary.

Airway and Breathing Management

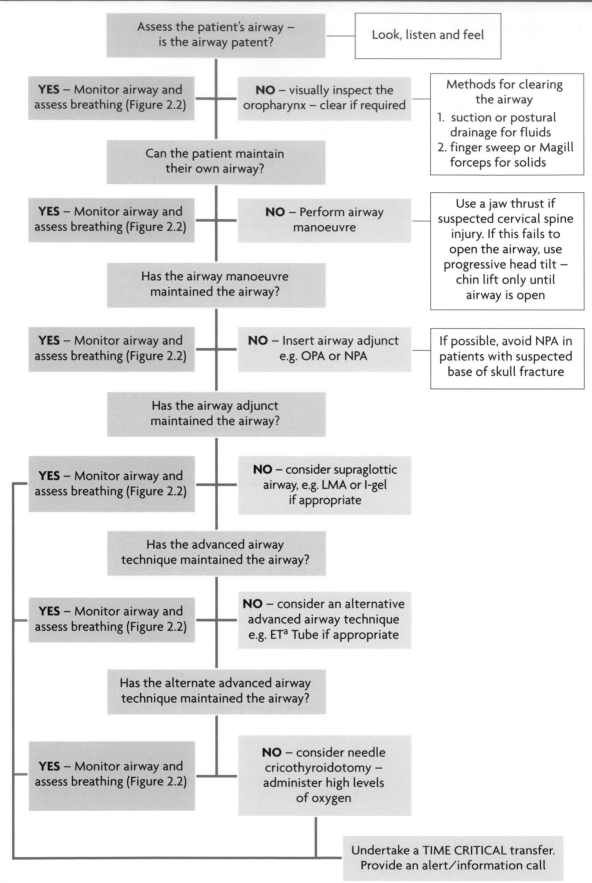

Assess the patient's airway – is the airway patent?

Look, listen and feel

YES – Monitor airway and assess breathing (Figure 2.2)

NO – visually inspect the oropharynx – clear if required

Methods for clearing the airway
1. suction or postural drainage for fluids
2. finger sweep or Magill forceps for solids

Can the patient maintain their own airway?

YES – Monitor airway and assess breathing (Figure 2.2)

NO – Perform airway manoeuvre

Use a jaw thrust if suspected cervical spine injury. If this fails to open the airway, use progressive head tilt – chin lift only until airway is open

Has the airway manoeuvre maintained the airway?

YES – Monitor airway and assess breathing (Figure 2.2)

NO – Insert airway adjunct e.g. OPA or NPA

If possible, avoid NPA in patients with suspected base of skull fracture

Has the airway adjunct maintained the airway?

YES – Monitor airway and assess breathing (Figure 2.2)

NO – consider supraglottic airway, e.g. LMA or I-gel if appropriate

Has the advanced airway technique maintained the airway?

YES – Monitor airway and assess breathing (Figure 2.2)

NO – consider an alternative advanced airway technique e.g. ET[a] Tube if appropriate

Has the alternate advanced airway technique maintained the airway?

YES – Monitor airway and assess breathing (Figure 2.2)

NO – consider needle cricothyroidotomy – administer high levels of oxygen

Undertake a TIME CRITICAL transfer. Provide an alert/information call

Figure 2.1 – Airway assessment and management overview.

[a] **Capnography** assists in confirmation and continuous monitoring of tracheal tube placement, provides feedback on the quality of CPR and provides an early indication of return of spontaneous circulation. It has been shown to have 100% sensitivity and 100% specificity in identifying correct tracheal tube placement. Although it should be used in conjunction with visualisation of the tracheal tube entering the cords and auscultation, its use when undertaking tracheal intubation is strongly recommended. In the absence of a waveform capnograph it may be preferable to use a supraglottic airway device when advanced airway management is indicated. ET CO_2 can be monitored with an SGA and is useful in providing positive feedback on quality of CPR.

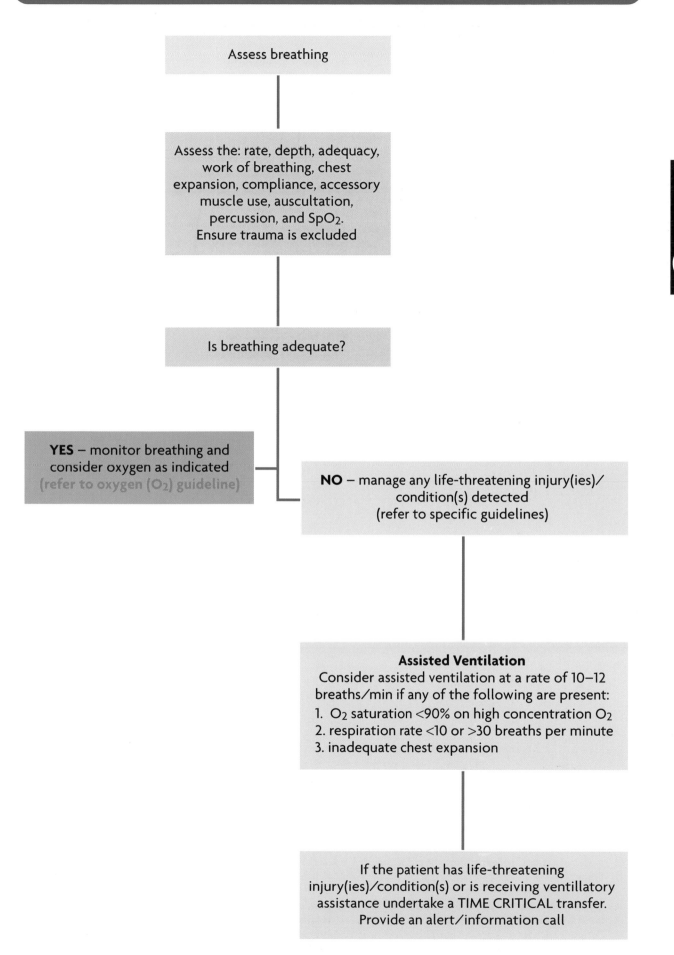

Assess breathing

Assess the: rate, depth, adequacy, work of breathing, chest expansion, compliance, accessory muscle use, auscultation, percussion, and SpO_2. Ensure trauma is excluded

Is breathing adequate?

YES – monitor breathing and consider oxygen as indicated (refer to oxygen (O_2) guideline)

NO – manage any life-threatening injury(ies)/ condition(s) detected (refer to specific guidelines)

Assisted Ventilation
Consider assisted ventilation at a rate of 10–12 breaths/min if any of the following are present:
1. O_2 saturation <90% on high concentration O_2
2. respiration rate <10 or >30 breaths per minute
3. inadequate chest expansion

If the patient has life-threatening injury(ies)/condition(s) or is receiving ventillatory assistance undertake a TIME CRITICAL transfer. Provide an alert/information call

Figure 2.2 – Breathing assessment and management overview.

Traumatic Cardiac Arrest [47, 58–60]

1. Introduction

- Traumatic cardiac arrest is a very different condition from the more usual cardiac arrest which is often related to ischaemic heart disease.
- Management of traumatic cardiac arrest must be directed towards identifying and treating the underlying cause of the arrest or resuscitation is unlikely to be successful.
- Traumatic cardiac arrest may develop as a result of:
  i. Hypoxia caused by manageable issues such as obstruction of the airway (e.g. facial injury or decreased level of consciousness) or breathing problems (e.g. pneumo/haemothorax).
  ii. Hypoperfusion caused by compromise of the heart (e.g. stab wound causing cardiac tamponade) or hypovolaemia (either occult or revealed haemorrhage).

2. Assessment and Management

For the assessment and management of traumatic cardiac arrest refer to Table 2.2.

Methodology

For details of the methodology used in the update of this guideline refer to the guideline webpage.

[Further related reading includes 61, 63, 64, 66, 67]

Table 2.2 – ASSESSMENT and MANAGEMENT of:

Traumatic Cardiac Arrest

ASSESSMENT	MANAGEMENT
● Assess potential cause(s)	Manage by applying standard trauma management principles (**refer to trauma emergencies guideline**). Any problem should be dealt with adequately before moving on to the next: **<C>** Control any **CATASTROPHIC HAEMORRHAGE** (extreme bleeding likely to cause death in minutes) – assess for the presence **LIFE-THREATENING EXTERNAL BLEEDING** – **refer to trauma emergencies overview guideline**. **A** – Airway obstruction; ensure the airway is open and clear. **B** – Impaired breathing; search for and manage a sucking chest wound or a tension pneumothorax (**refer to thoracic trauma guideline**). If not absolutely certain, then needle thoracocentesis should be performed on both sides. Support and assist ventilation (**refer to airway and breathing management guideline**). **C** – Hypovolaemia as a result of major blood loss; apply external haemorrhage control and obtain vascular access while transferring without delay to definitive treatment. **D** – Major head injury (**refer to head trauma guideline**) or spinal cord injury (**refer to neck and back trauma guideline**) impairing ventilation through CNS depression or loss of neuromuscular function.
● Commencing CPR	● Resuscitation should be commenced in all patients, irrespective of whether the arrest was witnessed, unless the patient is clearly beyond help (non-survivable injury, rigor mortis, decomposition etc.). Once resuscitation is commenced, full ALS-based resuscitation (**refer to advanced life support guidelines**) should be attempted for an appropriate duration (see below). ● In paediatric traumatic cardiac arrest, CPR should always be commenced unless the child has unsurvivable injuries and ROLE is appropriate (**refer to ROLE guideline**). ● In penetrating traumatic cardiac arrest, patients must be transferred rapidly to hospital because surgical intervention is often needed to treat the cause of the arrest. In these patients, a 'scoop and run' policy is appropriate. Do not stay on scene to resuscitate a patient with penetrating injury. ● If a patient has not responded after 20 minutes of advanced life support (ALS) then resuscitation can be terminated (see below).
● Terminating CPR	● Termination of resuscitation in a patient who has suffered a traumatic cardiac arrest (blunt) should be considered if the patient has not responded (i.e. the patient is apnoeic, pulseless, without organised cardiac electrical activity and without pupillary light reflexes) to 20 minutes of ALS, providing all reversible causes have been treated. Patients in cardiac arrest due to penetrating trauma can only have all reversible causes treated in hospital and a **TIME CRITICAL** transfer of these patients should be undertaken. ● The only exceptions to this are pregnancy (when the patient should be rapidly transferred to hospital to deliver the infant), in the presence of hypothermia and with trauma involving children. In this latter case follow paediatric resuscitation guidelines and undertake a **TIME CRITICAL** transfer to a hospital Emergency Department with ongoing resuscitation. ● After stopping resuscitation, the Recognition of Life Extinct by Ambulance Clinicians (ROLE) procedure should be followed (**refer to ROLE guideline**) and the police informed.

KEY POINTS

Traumatic Cardiac Arrest

- **Traumatic cardiac arrest is different from cardiac arrest due to primary cardiac disease.**
- **Assessment and management should follow the trauma guideline, treating problems as they are found.**
- **Once a decision to start resuscitation is taken, full ALS-based resuscitation for at least 20 minutes should be performed.**
- **If there is no response to resuscitation after 20 minutes of ALS and all potentially reversible causes have been treated, further effort is futile. However, resuscitation of children should be continued to hospital.**
- **Patients who have suffered cardiac arrest due to penetrating trauma should have full ALS based. resuscitation continued with a minimal on scene time and a time critical transfer to hospital undertaken.**
- **The ROLE procedure should be followed if resuscitation is terminated.**

Recognition of Life Extinct by Ambulance Clinicians [48, 59, 68, 69]

1. Introduction

In patients with cardio-pulmonary arrest, vigorous resuscitation attempts must be undertaken whenever there is a chance of survival.

Nevertheless, it is possible to identify patients in whom there is absolutely no chance of survival, and where resuscitation would be both futile and distressing for relatives, friends and healthcare personnel and where time and resources would be wasted undertaking such measures.

The views of an attending general practitioner (GP), ambulance doctor or relevant third party should be considered.

2. Conditions Unequivocally Associated with Death where Resuscitation should not be Attempted

All the conditions, listed below, are unequivocally associated with death in **ALL** age groups (see below for further details):
1. massive cranial and cerebral destruction
2. hemicorporectomy or similar massive injury
3. decomposition/putrefaction
4. incineration
5. hypostasis
6. rigor mortis.

In the newborn, fetal maceration is a contra-indication to attempted resuscitation.

Further Details

Decapitation: Self-evidently incompatible with life.

Massive cranial and cerebral destruction: Where the injuries are considered by the ambulance clinician to be incompatible with life.

Hemicorporectomy (or similar massive injury): Where the injuries are considered by the ambulance clinician to be incompatible with life.

Decomposition/putrefaction: Where tissue damage indicates that the patient has been dead for some hours, days or longer.

Incineration: The presence of full thickness burns with charring of greater than 95% of the body surface.

Hypostasis: The pooling of blood in congested vessels in the dependent part of the body in the position in which it lies after death (**See Guidance Note 1**).

Rigor mortis: The stiffness occurring after death from the post mortem breakdown of enzymes in the muscle fibres (**See Guidance Note 2**).

In all other cases resuscitation must be commenced and the facts pertaining to the arrest must be established.

Following arrival and the recognition of an absent pulse and apnoea (in the presence of a patent airway), chest compression and ventilations should be commenced whilst the facts of the collapse are ascertained.

3. In the Following Conditions, Resuscitation can be Discontinued

● The presence of a DNACPR (Do Not Attempt Cardio-pulmonary Resuscitation) order or an Advanced Decision (Living Will) that states the wish of the patient not to undergo attempted resuscitation (see 3b below).

● A patient in the final stages of a terminal illness where death is imminent and unavoidable and CPR would not be successful, but for whom no formal DNAR decision has been made.

● There would be no realistic chance that CPR would be successful if **ALL** the following exist together:
  – 15 minutes since the onset of cardiac arrest
  – no bystander CPR prior to arrival of the ambulance
  – the absence of any of the exclusion factors on the flowchart (Figure 2.3)
  – asystole for >30 seconds on the ECG monitor screen.

● Submersion for longer than 1.5 hours (NB submersion **NOT** immersion) (**See Guidance Note 3**).

Whenever possible a confirmatory ECG, demonstrating asystole, should be documented as evidence of death. In this situation a 3 or 4 electrode system using limbs alone will cause minimum disturbance to the deceased. If a paper ECG trace cannot be taken it is permissible to make a diagnosis of asystole from the screen alone (NB due caution must be applied in respect of electrode contact, gain and, where possible, using more than one ECG lead). The use of the flow chart shown in Figure 2.3 is recommended.

If there is a realistic chance that CPR could be successful then resuscitation must continue to establish the patient's response to Advanced Life Support interventions. If the patient does not respond despite full ALS intervention and remains asystolic for >20 minutes then the resuscitation attempt may be discontinued.

Removal of tracheal tubes and/or indwelling cannulae should be in accordance with local protocol.

4. Do not Attempt Resuscitation (DNAR)/Advanced Decision to Refuse Treatment (Living Will)

Ambulance clinicians should initiate resuscitation unless:

1. A formal DNAR order is in place, either written and handed to the ambulance clinician or verbally received and recorded by ambulance control from the patient's attendant requesting the ambulance providing that:
   a. the order is seen and corroborated by the ambulance clinician on arrival
   b. the decision to resuscitate relates to the condition for which the DNAR order is in force: resuscitation should not be withheld for coincidental conditions.

2. The patient is in the final stages of a terminal illness where death is imminent and unavoidable and CPR would not be successful, but for whom no formal DNAR decision has been made.

3. An Advanced Decision (Living Will) has been accepted by the treating physician (patient's GP or hospital consultant) as a DNAR order. This should be communicated to ambulance control and logged against the patient's address.

    a. Patients may have an Advanced Decision (Living Will) although it is not legally necessary for the refusal to be made in writing or formally witnessed. This specifies how they would like to be treated in the case of future incapacity. Case law is now clear that an advance refusal of treatment that is valid, and applicable to subsequent circumstances in which the patient lacks capacity, is legally binding. An advance refusal is valid if made voluntarily by an appropriately informed person with capacity. Staff should respect the wishes stated in such a document.

    b. In an out-of-hospital emergency environment, there may be situations where there is doubt about the validity of an advance refusal or DNAR order. If staff are **NOT** satisfied that the patient had made a prior and specific request to refuse treatment, they should continue to provide all clinical care in the normal way.

5. Action to be Taken after Death has been Established

For guidance on the actions to be taken following verification of death refer to Figure 2.4.

Complete documentation — including all decisions regarding do not attempt resuscitation (DNAR) / advanced decision to refuse treatment.

In light of the fact that earlier guidelines have been in use by a number of services for almost 10 years, we no longer believe that it is necessary for a medical practitioner to attend to confirm the fact of death. Moreover, the new GP Contract contains no obligation for a GP to do so when requested to attend by ambulance control.

Services should be encouraged, in conjunction with their coroner's service (or Procurator Fiscal in Scotland), to develop a local procedure for handling the body once death has been verified by ambulance personnel.

We further propose the adoption of a locally approved leaflet for handing to bereaved relatives.

GUIDANCE NOTE 1
Initially, hypostatic staining may appear as small round patches looking rather like bruises, but later these coalesce to merge as the familiar pattern. Above the hypostatic engorgement there is obvious pallor of the skin. The presence of hypostasis is diagnostic of death — the appearance is not present in a live patient. In extremely cold conditions hypostasis may be bright red in colour, and in carbon monoxide poisoning it is characteristically 'cherry red' in appearance.

GUIDANCE NOTE 2
Rigor mortis occurs first in the small muscles of the face, next in the arms, then in the legs (30 minutes to 3 hours). Children will show a more rapid onset of rigor because of their large surface area/body mass ratio. The recognition of rigor mortis can be made difficult where,

rarely, death has occurred from tetanus or strychnine poisoning.

In some, rigidity never develops (infants, cachectic individuals and the aged) whilst in others it may become apparent more rapidly (in conditions in which muscle glycogen is depleted): exertion (which includes struggling), strychnine poisoning, local heat (from a fire, hot room or direct sunlight).

Rigor should not be confused with cadaveric spasm (sometimes referred to as instant rigor mortis) which develops immediately after death without preceding flaccidity following intense physical and/or emotional activity. Examples include: death by drowning or a fall from a height. In contrast with true rigor mortis only one group of muscles is affected and **NOT** the whole body. Rigor mortis will develop subsequently.

GUIDANCE NOTE 3
Submersion victims
Attempting to predict criteria for commencing resuscitative efforts on victims found in water is fraught with danger because of many interacting factors that may contribute to extending accepted anoxic survival times.

Chief among these is the heat exchange that occurs in the lungs following aspiration of water.

Should the water temperature be very cold, it will rapidly cool the blood in the pulmonary circulation, which in turn selectively cools the brain for as long as a viable cardiac output continues. Should brain temperature be rapidly cooled to a degree where protection from hypoxia/anoxia is possible (circa 20°C) in the 70 seconds or thereabouts before cardiac failure occurs, then the chances of successful resuscitation are considerably enhanced even if cardio-respiratory arrest has been present for an hour or more. For this outcome to be likely, the water temperature has to be near freezing, and usually, but not necessarily, the body mass relatively small. Hence the majority of the accounts of successful resuscitation after submersion pertain to small children being rescued from 'ice water'.

It would seem prudent that resuscitative efforts **should** be made on:

1. Those with a witnessed submersion time of 1.5 hours or less, even though they appear to be dead on rescue.

2. All those where there is a possibility of their being able to breathe from a pocket of air while underwater.

3. Anyone showing any signs of life on initial rescue.

4. Those whose airway has been only intermittently submerged for the duration of their immersion, e.g. those wearing lifejackets but in whom the airway is being intermittently submerged, provided the body still has a reasonably fresh appearance.

5. Resuscitative efforts are unlikely to be successful in those submerged for periods exceeding 1.5 hours with the exception of those in categories 2–4 above.

Recognition of Life Extinct by Ambulance Clinicians

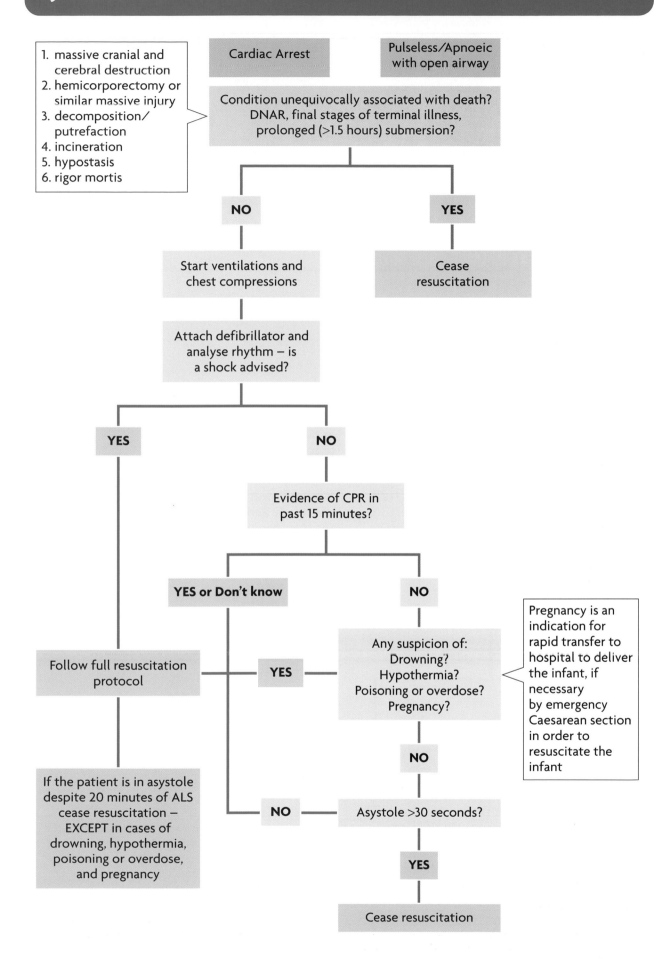

1. massive cranial and cerebral destruction
2. hemicorporectomy or similar massive injury
3. decomposition/ putrefaction
4. incineration
5. hypostasis
6. rigor mortis

Cardiac Arrest

Pulseless/Apnoeic with open airway

Condition unequivocally associated with death? DNAR, final stages of terminal illness, prolonged (>1.5 hours) submersion?

NO

YES

Start ventilations and chest compressions

Cease resuscitation

Attach defibrillator and analyse rhythm – is a shock advised?

YES

NO

Evidence of CPR in past 15 minutes?

YES or Don't know

NO

Follow full resuscitation protocol

YES

Any suspicion of: Drowning? Hypothermia? Poisoning or overdose? Pregnancy?

Pregnancy is an indication for rapid transfer to hospital to deliver the infant, if necessary by emergency Caesarean section in order to resuscitate the infant

NO

If the patient is in asystole despite 20 minutes of ALS cease resuscitation – EXCEPT in cases of drowning, hypothermia, poisoning or overdose, and pregnancy

NO

Asystole >30 seconds?

YES

Cease resuscitation

Figure 2.3 – Recognition of life extinct by ambulance clinicians algorithm.

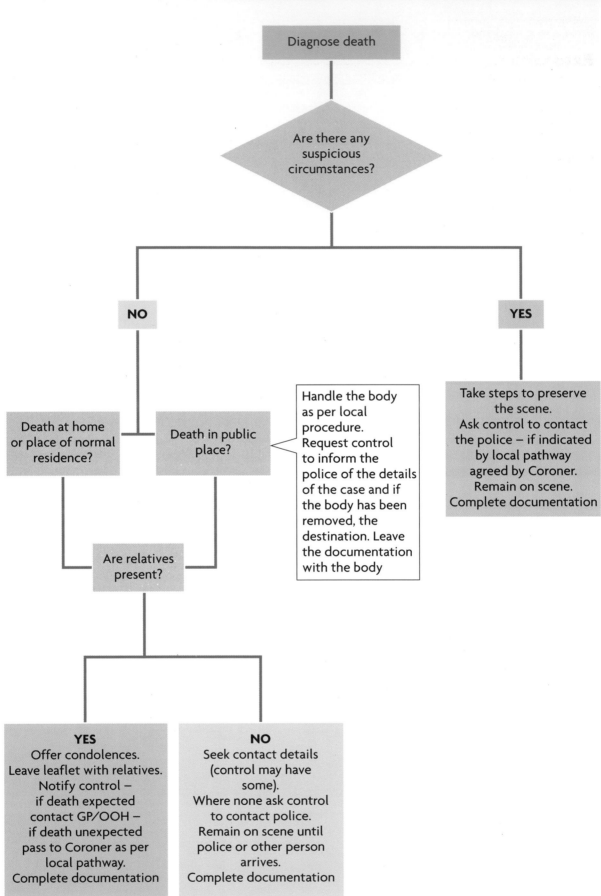

Figure 2.4 – Action to be taken after verification of fact of death.

Recognition of Life Extinct by Ambulance Clinicians

KEY POINTS

Recognition of Life Extinct by Ambulance Clinicians

- Ambulance clinicians are increasingly called upon to diagnose death and initiate the appropriate responses to death.
- In patients with cardio-pulmonary arrest, vigorous resuscitation efforts must be made whenever there is a chance of survival, however remote.
- Some conditions are incompatible with recovery and in these cases resuscitation need not be attempted.
- In some situations, once the facts of the patient/situation/etc. are known, resuscitation efforts can be discontinued.
- Patients can and do make anticipatory decisions NOT to be resuscitated. An Advanced Decision (Living Will), if verifiable, must be respected.
- These guidelines should be read in conjunction with local policies and procedures.

Methodology

For details of the methodology used in the development
of this guideline refer to the guideline webpage.

Basic Life Support (Adult) [59]

1. Introduction

● Basic life support (BLS) refers to maintaining airway patency, and supporting breathing and circulation without the use of equipment other than a protective device, usually a facemask or shield. In the prehospital environment, BLS includes the use of a bag-valve-mask and oropharyngeal airway.

● BLS is undertaken as a prelude to defibrillation, often with an automated external defibrillator (AED).

2. Assessment and Management

● For the assessment and management of adult basic life support refer to Table 2.3 and the adult basic life support sequence detailed in Figure 2.5.

Table 2.3 – ASSESSMENT and MANAGEMENT of:

Basic Life Support (Adult)

This sequence is for a single ambulance clinician, however, when more than one clinician is present, tasks can be shared and undertaken simultaneously.

ASSESSMENT	MANAGEMENT
● Assess safety	● Ensure that you, the patient and any bystanders are safe.
● Check responsiveness	● Gently shake the patient by the shoulders and ask loudly: '**Are you all right?**'
– The **responsive** patient	● Take history and make assessment of what is wrong, with further action determined accordingly.
– The **unresponsive** patient	● Obtain further resources if appropriate. ● Turn the patient onto their back and then open the airway using head tilt and chin lift. Look in the mouth. If a foreign body or debris is visible attempt to remove it with a finger sweep, forceps or suction as appropriate. ● When there is a risk of back or neck injury, establish a clear upper airway by using jaw thrust or chin lift in combination with manual in-line stabilisation of the head and neck by an assistant (if available). If life-threatening airway obstruction persists despite effective application of jaw thrust or chin lift, add head tilt a small amount at a time until the airway is open; establishing a patent airway takes priority over concerns about a potential back or neck injury.
● Keeping the airway open	● Look, listen and feel for normal breathing, taking no more than 10 seconds to determine if the patient is breathing normally. If you have any doubt whether breathing is normal, act as if it is **NOT** normal. ● Agonal breathing (occasional gasps, slow, laboured noisy breathing) is common in the early stages of cardiac arrest. It is a sign of cardiac arrest and should not be confused as a sign of life/circulation.
● If the patient is breathing normally:	● Turn into the recovery position. ● Undertake assessment, monitoring and transport accordingly. ● Re-assess regularly.
● If the patient is not breathing normally:	● It may be difficult to be certain that there is no pulse. ● If there are no signs of life (lack of movement, normal breathing, or coughing), or there is doubt, start chest compressions at a rate of 100–120 compressions per minute. ● Compression depth should be 5–6 cm. Allow the chest to recoil completely after each compression. Take approximately the same amount of time for each compression and relaxation. Minimise interruptions to chest compression. Do not rely on a palpable pulse (carotid, femoral, or radial) as a gauge of effective blood flow.
● Combine chest compression with rescue breaths	● After 30 compressions, open the airway again and provide two ventilations with the most appropriate equipment available, using an inspiratory time of one second with adequate volume to produce normal chest expansion. Each time compressions are resumed the ambulance clinician should place their hands without delay in the centre of the chest. ● Add supplemental oxygen as soon as possible. ● Continue chest compressions and ventilation in a ratio of 30:2. ● Stop to recheck only if the patient starts breathing normally; otherwise do not interrupt chest compressions and ventilation. ● Performing chest compressions is tiring; try to change the person doing chest compressions every two minutes; ensure the minimum of delay during the changeover. Once the airway is secure (for example after supraglottic airway insertion) continue chest compressions uninterrupted at a rate of 100–120 per minute (except for defibrillation or further assessment as indicated). ● Ventilate 8–10 times per minute. Avoid hyperventilation. ● If attempts at ventilation do not make the chest rise as in normal breathing, then before the next attempt at ventilation: – check the patient's mouth and remove any obstruction – recheck that the airway position is optimal with adequate head tilt/chin lift or jaw thrust – do not attempt more than two breaths each time before returning to chest compressions.

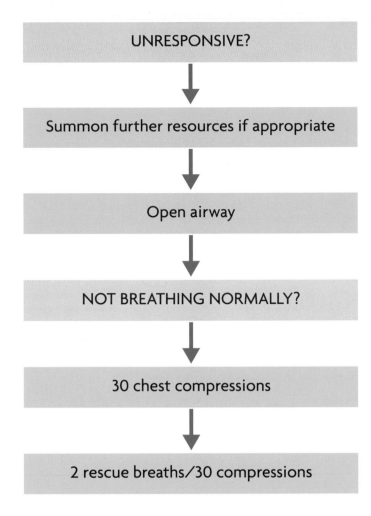

Figure 2.5 – Adult basic life support sequence – Modified from the Resuscitation Council (UK) Guidelines 2010 algorithm for the JRCALC Resuscitation Supplement 2010 (www.resus.org.uk).

3. Additional Information

CPR in confined spaces – Over-the-head CPR and straddle CPR may be considered for resuscitation in confined spaces.

Use of the Automated External Defibrillator (AED)

1. Make sure you, the patient and any bystanders are safe.

2. In the unlikely event that you do not have an AED with you, perform CPR until an AED arrives.

3. As soon as an AED is available:
   - switch on the defibrillator and attach the electrode pads. If more than one ambulance clinician is present, CPR should be continued whilst this is done
   - follow the spoken/visual directions
   - ensure nobody touches the patient whilst the AED is analysing the rhythm.

4a. If a shock is indicated continue compression as AED is charging if possible:
   - ensure nobody touches the patient
   - push the shock button as directed
   - continue as directed by the voice/visual prompts.

4b. If no shock is indicated:
   immediately resume CPR using a ratio of 30 compressions to 2 rescue breaths
   - continue as directed by voice/visual prompts.

5. Continue to follow AED prompts until:
   - the patient starts to breathe normally
   - ALS is started
   - you are exhausted.

Methodology

For details of the methodology used in the development of this guideline refer to the guideline webpage.

Basic Life Support (Adult)

KEY POINTS

Adult Basic Life Support

- Agonal breathing is common in the early stages of cardiac arrest and should not be confused as a sign of life/circulation.
- If there are no signs of life, start chest compressions at a rate of 100–120 per minute using a ratio of 30 compressions to 2 breaths.
- Once the airway is secure, chest compressions should be uninterrupted with ventilations 8–10 times per minute; avoid hyperventilation.
- As soon as an AED is available switch on the defibrillator and attach the electrode pads and follow voice/visual prompts.

Advanced Life Support (Adult) [58, 70, 74]

1. Introduction

The heart rhythms associated with cardiac arrest are divided into two groups:

1. **shockable rhythms** – ventricular fibrillation and pulseless ventricular tachycardia (VF/VT)
2. **non-shockable rhythms** – asystole and pulseless electrical activity (PEA).

- The principal difference in the management of these two groups is the need for attempted defibrillation in VF/VT. Subsequent actions including chest compressions, airway management and ventilation, venous access, administration of adrenaline and the management of reversible factors, are common to both groups.

- The interventions that unequivocally improve survival are early defibrillation and effective basic life support. Attention should focus therefore on early defibrillation and high quality, uninterrupted cardio-pulmonary resuscitation (CPR).

- A solo responder should not interrupt chest compressions for any reason other than to deliver two breaths or defibrillate the patient. Intravenous (IV) access, drug delivery and advanced airway management require two or more responders. While these procedures are performed, interruptions to chest compressions must be kept to an absolute minimum.

- High quality, uninterrupted chest compressions are crucial in achieving improved survival. Chest compressions at the correct rate (100–120/min) and depth (5–6 cm) with complete relaxation should commence immediately and continue while the defibrillator is charging; only pausing to assess the rhythm or deliver the shock (as appropriate) before recommencing the compressions.

- Intravenous access should be established as soon as an appropriately trained responder is able to do so. If IV access is not possible, intraosseous access should be considered.

2. Assessment and Management

For assessment and management of cardiac arrest refer to Table 2.4 and Figure 2.6. For the care of patients following Return Of Spontaneous Circulation (ROSC) refer to Table 2.5 and Figure 2.7.

Table 2.4 – ASSESSMENT and MANAGEMENT of:

Adult Advanced Life Support

ASSESSMENT	MANAGEMENT
Having confirmed cardiac arrest:	• Request further resources. • Start CPR beginning with chest compressions. Ventilate with high concentration oxygen. • As soon as the defibrillator arrives, diagnose the rhythm by applying self-adhesive pads to the chest and attempt defibrillation as appropriate.
1. SHOCKABLE RHYTHMS (VF/PULSELESS VT)	• Attempt defibrillation (one shock – 150–200 Joules biphasic or 360 Joules monophasic). • Immediately resume chest compressions (30:2) without re-assessing the rhythm or feeling for a pulse. • Continue CPR for 2 minutes, and then pause briefly to check the monitor.
If VF/VT persists:	• Give a further (2nd) shock (150–360 Joules biphasic or 360 Joules monophasic). • Resume CPR immediately and continue for 2 minutes. • Pause briefly to check the monitor. • If VF/VT persists, give a further (3rd) shock (150–360 Joules biphasic or 360 Joules monophasic). • As soon as CPR has resumed, give adrenaline 1mg 1:10,000 IV. Give 300 mg amiodarone IV while continuing CPR for a further 2 minutes. • Pause briefly to check the monitor. • If VF/VT persists, give a further (4th) shock (150–360 Joules biphasic or 360 Joules monophasic). • Resume CPR immediately and continue for 2 minutes. • Pause briefly to check the monitor. • If VF/VT persists give a further (5th) shock (150–360 Joules biphasic or 360 Joules monophasic). • Resume CPR immediately and give adrenaline 1 mg 1:10,000 IV and an additional 150 mg amiodarone IV while continuing CPR for a further 2 minutes. • Give adrenaline 1mg 1:10,000 IV immediately after alternate shocks (i.e. approximately every 3–5 minutes). • Give further shocks after each 2 minute period of CPR and after confirming that VF/VT persists.
If organised electrical activity is seen, check for a pulse	• If a pulse is present, start post-resuscitation care. • If no pulse is present, continue CPR and switch to the non-shockable algorithm.
If asystole is seen:	• Continue CPR and change to follow the non-shockable algorithm.

Table 2.4 – ASSESSMENT and MANAGEMENT of:

Adult Advanced Life Support *continued*

ASSESSMENT	MANAGEMENT
2. NON-SHOCKABLE RHYTHMS (ASYSTOLE AND PEA)	If these rhythms are identified: ● Start CPR 30:2 and give adrenaline 1 milligram as soon as intravascular access is achieved. ● If asystole is displayed, without stopping CPR, check the leads are attached correctly. ● Secure the airway as soon as possible to enable continuous chest compressions without pausing for ventilation. ● After two minutes CPR 30:2 recheck the rhythm. If asystole is present or there has been no change in ECG appearance, resume CPR immediately. ● If VF / VT present, change to the shockable rhythm algorithm. ● If an organised rhythm is present, attempt to palpate a central pulse. ● If a pulse is present, begin post-resuscitation care. ● If no pulse is present (or there is any doubt) continue CPR. Give adrenaline 1 milligram IV every 3–5 minutes (alternate loops). ● If signs of life return during CPR, check the rhythm and attempt to palpate a pulse.

| POTENTIALLY REVERSIBLE CAUSES
Potential causes or aggravating factors for which specific treatment exists must be considered during any cardiac arrest. For ease of memory these are presented | Assess the 4Hs and 4Ts according to their initial letter. Those amenable to treatment include:

1. **Hypoxia** – ensure adequate ventilation, adequate chest expansion and breath sounds. Verify tracheal tube placement, using capnography.[a]

2. **Hypovolaemia** – PEA caused by hypovolaemia is usually due to haemorrhage from trauma, gastrointestinal bleeding or rupture of an aortic aneurysm. Intravascular volume should be restored rapidly with IV fluid. Rapid transport to definitive surgical care is essential.

3. **Hypothermia – refer to hypothermia and immersion incident guidelines**.

4. **Hyperkalaemia** and other electrolyte disorders are unlikely to be apparent in the pre-hospital arena or respond to treatment. Consider early removal to hospital. | 1. **Tension Pneumothorax** – the diagnosis is made clinically; decompress as soon as possible by needle thoracocentesis.

2. **Cardiac Tamponade** is difficult to diagnose as the typical signs (high venous pressure, hypotension) disappear after cardiac arrest occurs. Cardiac arrest after penetrating chest trauma is highly suggestive of cardiac tamponade. These patients should be transported to hospital immediately without any delay on scene as pericardiocentesis or thoracotomy cannot routinely be performed outside hospital.

3. **Toxins** – only rarely will an antidote be available outside hospital, and in most cases supportive treatment will be the priority.

4. **Thromboembolism** – massive pulmonary embolism is the commonest cause but diagnosis in the field is difficult once arrest has occurred. Specific treatments (like thrombolytic drugs) are not available to ambulance personnel in the UK at present. |

| THE WITNESSED, MONITORED ARREST | **If a patient who is being monitored has a witnessed arrest:**
● Confirm cardiac arrest, request further resources if appropriate.
● If the rhythm is VF/VT and a defibrillator is not immediately available, consider a precordial thump.
● If the rhythm is VF/VT and a defibrillator is immediately available, give a shock first and immediately commence CPR; treat any recurrence of VF/pulseless VT following the shockable rhythm algorithm.
● Where the arrest is witnessed but unmonitored, using self-adhesive hands-free defibrillation pads will allow assessment of the rhythm more quickly than attaching ECG electrodes. |

[a] **Capnography** assists in confirmation and continuous monitoring of tracheal tube placement, provides feedback on the quality of CPR and provides an early indication of return of spontaneous circulation. It has been shown to have 100% sensitivity and 100% specificity in identifying correct tracheal tube placement. Although it should be used in conjunction with visualisation of the tracheal tube entering the cords and auscultation, its use when undertaking tracheal intubation is strongly recommended. In the absence of a waveform capnograph it may be preferable to use a supraglottic airway device when advanced airway management is indicated.

Advanced Life Support (Adult)

Table 2.5 – ASSESSMENT and MANAGEMENT of:

Return of Spontaneous Circulation (ROSC)

Return of spontaneous circulation (ROSC) is an important first step on the pathway to recovery from cardiac arrest. Following ROSC some patients may suffer post-cardiac-arrest syndrome, the severity of which will depend on the duration and cause of the cardiac arrest. Post-cardiac-arrest syndrome often complicates the post-resuscitation phase and comprises:

- **Brain injury:** coma, seizures, myoclonus, varying degrees of neurocognitive dysfunction and brain death; this may be exacerbated by microcirculatory failure, impaired autoregulation, hypercarbia, hyperoxia, pyrexia, hyperglycaemia and seizures.

- **Myocardial dysfunction:** this is common after cardiac arrest but usually improves in the following weeks.

- **The systemic ischaemia/reperfusion response:** the whole body ischaemia/reperfusion that occurs with resuscitation from cardiac arrest activates immunological and coagulation pathways contributing to an inflammatory response and multiple organ failure.

- **Persistence of the precipitating pathology.**

For the care of patients following ROSC see below.

ASSESSMENT	MANAGEMENT
- Return Of Spontaneous Circulation	- Transfer the patient directly to the nearest appropriate hospital in accordance with local protocols relating to PPCI. - Early recurrence of VF is common, so ensure continuous monitoring in order to deliver further shocks if appropriate. - Continue patient management en-route – see below. - Provide an alert/information call.
- Oxygen	- Measure oxygen saturation. - Maintain oxygen saturations of 94–98%.
- Ventilation	- Use of an automatic ventilator is preferable to manual ventilation. - Monitor ventilation rate and volume. - Monitor end-tidal CO_2 (NB Readings may be low because of reduced cardiac output rather than hyperventilation. Normal range = 3.5–5.0 kPa).
- ECG	- Undertake a 12-lead ECG.
- Blood glucose level	- Measure blood glucose level. - If the patient is hypoglycaemic (BM <4.0 mmol) **refer to glycaemic emergencies guideline.**
- Cooling	- In cases of non-traumatic cardiac arrest, in patients that have not regained consciousness, start active cooling in line with local protocols.

KEY POINTS

Advanced Life Support (Adult)

- **Begin good quality, uninterrupted chest compressions immediately. Attempt defibrillation as soon as a defibrillator is available.**
- **For shockable rhythms defibrillate and resume chest compressions (30:2) for 2 minutes without re-assessing the rhythm or feeling for a pulse; then check rhythm, if VF/VT persists follow ALS algorithm.**
- **Give adrenaline 1mg 1:10,000 and amiodarone 300 milligrams immediately after the 3rd shock.**
- **For non-shockable rhythms start CPR at a ratio of 30:2 and give adrenaline 1mg 1:10,000 as soon as intravascular access is achieved.**
- **Give adrenaline every second cycle (3–5 minutes).**
- **Always consider reversible features (4Hs and 4Ts) and correct if possible.**

Methodology

For details of the methodology used in the development of this guideline refer to the guideline webpage.

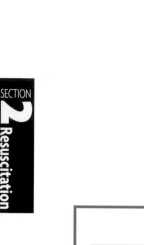
Advanced Life Support (Adult)

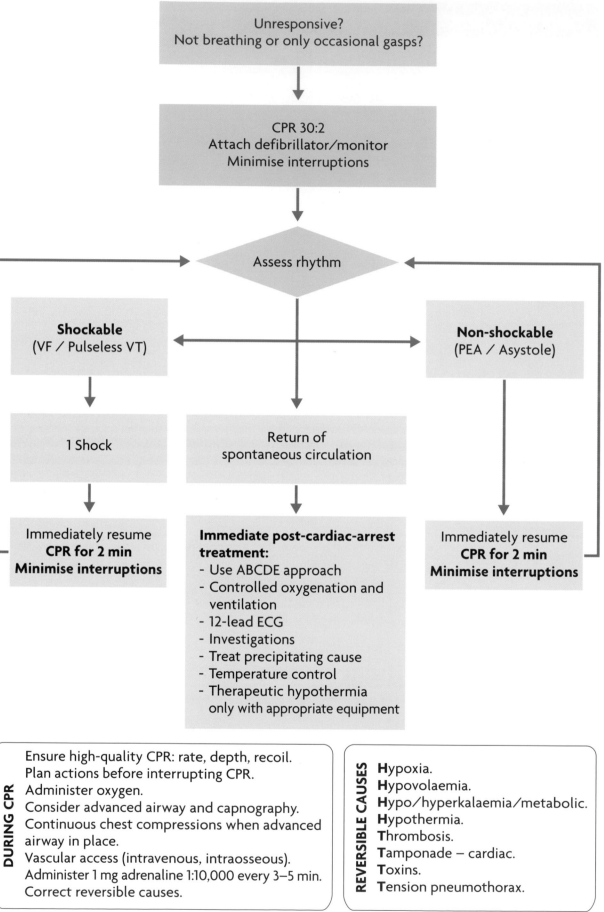

Unresponsive?
Not breathing or only occasional gasps?

↓

CPR 30:2
Attach defibrillator/monitor
Minimise interruptions

↓

Assess rhythm

Shockable
(VF / Pulseless VT)

Non-shockable
(PEA / Asystole)

1 Shock

Return of
spontaneous circulation

Immediately resume
CPR for 2 min
Minimise interruptions

Immediate post-cardiac-arrest treatment:
- Use ABCDE approach
- Controlled oxygenation and ventilation
- 12-lead ECG
- Investigations
- Treat precipitating cause
- Temperature control
- Therapeutic hypothermia only with appropriate equipment

Immediately resume
CPR for 2 min
Minimise interruptions

DURING CPR
Ensure high-quality CPR: rate, depth, recoil.
Plan actions before interrupting CPR.
Administer oxygen.
Consider advanced airway and capnography.
Continuous chest compressions when advanced airway in place.
Vascular access (intravenous, intraosseous).
Administer 1 mg adrenaline 1:10,000 every 3–5 min.
Correct reversible causes.

REVERSIBLE CAUSES
Hypoxia.
Hypovolaemia.
Hypo/hyperkalaemia/metabolic.
Hypothermia.
Thrombosis.
Tamponade – cardiac.
Toxins.
Tension pneumothorax.

Figure 2.6 – Advanced life support algorithm – modified from the Resuscitation Council (UK) Guidelines 2010 algorithm for the JRCALC Resuscitation Supplement 2010 (www.resus.org.uk).

Return of Spontaneous Circulation (ROSC)

Transfer
- Transfer the patient to the nearest appropriate hospital according to local protocols
- Early recurrence of VF is common so monitor continuously – further shocks may be indicated.
- Provide an alert / information call.
- Continue patient management en-route. Address 4 Hs and 4Ts, according to local guidelines. Keep the patient flat during removal to vehicle

Oxygen saturations
Monitor oxygen saturation.
Maintain oxygen saturations between 94–98%

Ventilation
Monitor ventilation rate and volume.
Monitor end-tidal CO_2.
(NB Readings may be low because of reduced cardiac output rather than hyperventilation – normal range = 3.5–5.0 kPa)

ECG
Undertake a 12-lead ECG

Blood glucose level
Measure blood glucose level – if patient is hypoglycaemic (BM<4.0 mmol)
refer to glycaemic emergencies guideline

Cooling
In unconscious, non-traumatic cardiac arrest patients, start active cooling as soon as possible, according to local guidelines
(only with appropriate equipment)

Figure 2.7 – Assessment and management of Return of Spontaneous Circulation (ROSC).

Foreign Body Airway Obstruction (Adult) [59, 62, 69]

1. Introduction

- Foreign body airway obstruction is an uncommon but potentially treatable cause of accidental death.
- In adults, food, usually fish, meat or poultry, is the commonest cause of obstruction.
- Most cases occur when eating and are therefore usually witnessed. The signs and symptoms vary, depending on the degree of airway obstruction (Table 2.6).

2. Assessment and Management

- For the assessment and management of adult foreign body airway obstruction refer to Table 2.7 and Figure 2.8.

Table 2.6 – GENERAL SIGNS OF FOREIGN BODY AIRWAY OBSTRUCTION

- **Attack usually occurs while eating**
- **Patient may clutch their neck**

Mild airway obstruction
- In response to question – '**Are you choking?**'
- The patient speaks and answers '**Yes**'.

Other signs – the patient is able to:
- speak
- cough
- breathe.

Severe airway obstruction
- In response to question – '**Are you choking**?'
- The patient is unable to speak and may respond by nodding.

Other signs:
- patient unable to breathe
- breathing sounds wheezy
- attempts at coughing are silent
- patient may be unconscious.

Table 2.7 – ASSESSMENT and MANAGEMENT of:

Foreign Body Airway Obstruction (Adult)

ASSESSMENT	MANAGEMENT
- Assess for severity of obstruction (Table 2.6)	
- Mild airway obstruction	- Encourage the patient to cough but do nothing else. - Monitor carefully. - Rapid transport to hospital.
- Severe airway obstruction – conscious patient	- Give up to five back blows – after each back blow check to see if the obstruction has been relieved. - If five back blows do not relieve the airway obstruction, give up to five abdominal thrusts. - If five abdominal thrusts do not relieve the obstruction, continue alternating five back blows with five abdominal thrusts.
- Severe airway obstruction – unconscious patient	- If the patient is unconscious or becomes unconscious, begin basic life support – **refer to adult BLS guidance**. - During CPR the patient's mouth should be quickly checked for any foreign body that has been partly expelled each time the airway is opened.
- If these measures fail and the airway remains obstructed:	- Attempt to visualise the vocal cords with a laryngoscope. - Remove any visible foreign material with forceps or suction. - If this fails or is not possible, and you are trained in the technique, perform needle cricothyroidotomy.
Additional information	- Chest thrusts/compressions generate a higher airway pressure than back blows. - Avoid blind finger sweeps. Manually remove solid material in the airway only if it can be seen. - Following successful treatment for FBAO, foreign material may remain in the upper or lower respiratory tract and cause complications later. Patients with a persistent cough, difficulty swallowing or the sensation of an object being stuck in the throat must be assessed further. - Abdominal thrusts can cause serious internal injuries and all patients so treated must be assessed for injury in hospital.

Foreign Body Airway Obstruction (Adult)

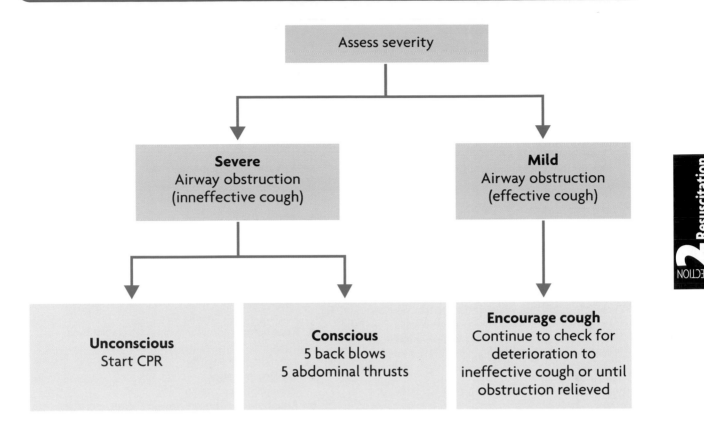

Figure 2.8 – Adult foreign body airway obstruction algorithm – modified from the Resuscitation Council (UK) Guidelines 2010 algorithm for the JRCALC Resuscitation Supplement 2010 (www.resus.org.uk).

Methodology

For details of the methodology used in the development of this guideline refer to the guideline website.

KEY POINTS

Foreign Body Airway Obstruction (FBAO) (Adult)

● Potentially treatable cause of death; often occurs whilst eating.

● Asking the patient 'Are you choking?' can aid diagnosis.

● Back blows and abdominal thrusts may relieve the obstruction; check after each manoeuvre to see if obstruction is relieved.

● Abdominal thrusts can cause internal injuries and patients should be assessed in hospital.

● Avoid blind finger sweeps; manually remove solid material in the airway ONLY if it can be seen.

General Introduction

- It is important to recognise that there are two patients.
- Effective resuscitation of the mother will provide effective resuscitation of the fetus.
- Resuscitation priority is the mother.

1. Cardiac Arrest

Undertake a TIME CRITICAL transfer as soon as ventilation is achieved and CPR commenced.

1.1 Introduction

- The approach to resuscitating an obstetric patient is the same as that of any adult in cardiac arrest; but in the third trimester additional measures must be undertaken to maximise the efficacy of resuscitation.
- Because fetuses can tolerate significant levels of hypoxia, resuscitation should be initiated immediately and **NOT** terminated in prehospital care, even in cases where the mother's condition is, or appears non-survivable or unequivocally associated with death, as this will maximise the chances of both maternal and fetal survival.

1.2 Risk factors

There is an increased risk of maternal mortality for patients who are:

- Socially disadvantaged.
- From poor communities.
- From minority ethnic groups.
- Late in booking for antenatal care or have poor attendance.
- Obese.
- The victims of domestic violence.
- Substance abusers.

1.3 Pathophysiology

- Cardiac arrest in pregnancy is very rarely due to a primary cardiac cause. Common causes of sudden maternal death include pulmonary or amniotic fluid embolus.
- There are a number of physiological and anatomical changes during pregnancy that may influence the management of the obstetric patient (**refer to obstetrics and gynaecology overview guideline**).

1.4 Assessment and management

For the assessment and management of cardiac arrest during pregnancy refer to Table 2.8.

2. Shock

2.1 Pathophysiology

The failure of perfusion of the tissues with oxygenated blood due to loss of circulating fluid volume may be due to:

- **Hypovolaemic shock** – loss of circulating fluid volume due to haemorrhage.
- **Septic shock** – movement of circulating fluid volume into the interstitial spaces due to increased capillary permeability.
- **Cardiogenic shock** – pump failure or obstruction in the circulatory system.
- **Anaphylactic shock** – severe allergic reaction.
- **Neurogenic shock in trauma** – loss of nervous control of blood vessels leading to relative hypovolaemia.

2.2 Risk factors

There are a number of associated risk factors including:

- Intercurrent heart disease (**cardiogenic shock**).
- Thromboembolism or amniotic fluid embolism (**cardiogenic shock**).

Table 2.8 – ASSESSMENT and MANAGEMENT of:

Cardiac Arrest

ASSESSMENT	MANAGEMENT
• Undertake a primary survey ABCDEF	• Manage as per standard advanced life support (**refer to ALS guideline**). • Assess and exclude treatable causes including hypovolaemia, sepsis and anaphylactic shock.
	• **Caution** – ventilation with a bag-valve-mask may lead to regurgitation and aspiration. Consider early tracheal intubation which reduces the risk of gastric aspiration and may make ventilation of the lungs easier. A supraglottic airway is a suitable alternative (**refer to airway and breathing management guideline**). • Undertake a **TIME CRITICAL** transfer to nearest suitable receiving hospital; provide an alert/information call – ask to have an **OBSTETRICIAN ON STANDBY IN THE EMERGENCY DEPARTMENT** for an emergency Caesarean section (in this situation delivering the fetus **MAY** facilitate maternal resuscitation).
	• Manually displace the uterus to the left or tilt the patient to the left (15–30 degrees) to remove compression of the inferior vena cava. NB The angle of tilt needs to allow good quality chest compressions (**refer to obstetrics and gynaecology overview**).
	• Aim to establish intravascular access using a **LARGE BORE** cannula without delay in transfer to hospital. • Attempt IO access if rapid IV cannulation is not possible.

Maternal Resuscitation

- Non-obstetric infections and genital tract sepsis (**septic shock**).
- Trauma (**hypovolaemic shock**).
- Obstetric haemorrhage (**hypovolaemic shock**).
- Inverted uterus (**hypovolaemic shock**).
- Ruptured ectopic pregnancy (**hypovolaemic shock**).
- Incomplete miscarriage (**hypovolaemic shock**).
- Opiate-induced histamine release or other drug allergy (**anaphylaxis**).

2.3 Pathophysiology
- The body's main mechanism for maintaining maternal circulation in the event of blood loss is to restrict blood flow to the uterus. This results in a reduction of placental perfusion and associated fetal hypoxia.

- There are a number of other physiological and anatomical changes during pregnancy that may influence the management of the obstetric patient (**refer to obstetrics and gynaecology overview guideline**).

2.4 Assessment and management
For the assessment and management of shock during pregnancy refer to Table 2.9.

Methodology
For details of the methodology used in the development of this guideline refer to the guideline webpage.

Table 2.9 – ASSESSMENT and MANAGEMENT of:

Shock

ASSESSMENT	MANAGEMENT
● Undertake a primary survey ABCDEF	
● Cardiogenic anaphylactic shock	**Refer to specific resuscitation guidelines.** **Refer to anaphylaxis/allergic reactions guideline.** ● Manually displace the uterus to the left or tilt the patient to the left (15–30 degrees) to remove compression of the inferior vena cava. NB The angle of tilt needs to allow good quality chest compressions (**refer to obstetrics and gynaecology overview**). ● Administer supplemental oxygen and aim for a saturation of 94–98% (refer to oxygen guideline). ● Undertake a **TIME CRITICAL** transfer to nearest suitable receiving hospital; provide an alert/information call. Ask to have an **OBSTETRICIAN ON STANDBY IN THE EMERGENCY DEPARTMENT** for an emergency Caesarean section if the mother has suffered cardiorespiratory collapse (in this situation delivering the fetus **MAY** facilitate maternal resuscitation). ● Monitor blood pressure, ECG, and blood glucose level. ● Treat the underlying condition. ● Insert at least one **LARGE BORE** IV cannulae – do not delay transfer. ● In hypovolaemia, septic shock, and anaphylactic shock administer IV sodium chloride 0.9% given in 250 ml aliquots to maintain a systolic blood pressure of 90 mmHg or if there is significant external haemorrhage >500 ml, altered mental status, or arrhythmias (refer to intravascular fluid therapy guidelines).
● Assess patient's level of pain	● Pain management (**refer to adult pain management guidelines**). ● Nil by mouth.

KEY POINTS

Maternal Resuscitation
- **Do not withhold or terminate maternal resuscitation.**
- **ALWAYS manage patients >22 weeks gestation with manual displacement of the uterus to the left or a left lateral tilt (15–30 degrees).**
- **Gastric regurgitation is more likely; be ready with suction (consider early intubation or supraglottic airway insertion) to reduce gastric insufflation.**
- **Insert at least one LARGE BORE IV cannulae.**
- **Cardiac arrest may be caused by pulmonary arrest or amniotic fluid embolism.**
- **Due to physiological changes of pregnancy, patients may initially compensate for hypovolaemia.**
- **If the patient is unstable, ask to have an OBSTETRICIAN ON STANDBY IN THE EMERGENCY DEPARTMENT.**

Basic Life Support (Child) [47]

1. Introduction

- The following sequence is that followed by those with a duty to respond to paediatric emergencies – refer to Table 2.10 and/or Figure 2.9.

Age definitions

- An infant is a child under one year old.
- A child is between one year and puberty.

These guidelines are not intended to apply to the resuscitation of the newborn (refer to neonatal resuscitation guideline).

Table 2.10 – ASSESSMENT and MANAGEMENT of:

Basic Life Support (Child)

The following sequence is that followed by those with a duty to respond to paediatric emergencies (also refer to Figure 2.9)

ASSESSMENT	MANAGEMENT
● Assess safety	● Ensure that you, the child and any bystanders are safe.
● Check responsiveness	● Gently stimulate the child and ask loudly 'Are you all right?' – **DO NOT** shake infants, or children with suspected cervical spinal injuries.
● If the child responds (by answering or moving):	● Leave the child in the position found (provided the child is not in further danger). ● Check the child's condition. ● Summon help if necessary. ● Re-assess the child regularly.

● If the child does not respond:	● Summon additional resources if required if necessary.
	
	● Open the child's airway by tilting the head and lifting the chin:
	  – with the child in the position found, place your hand on the forehead and gently tilt the head back
	  – at the same time, with your fingertip(s) under the point of the child's chin, lift the chin. Do not push on the soft tissues under the chin as this may block the airway
	  – if you still have difficulty in opening the airway, try the jaw thrust method: place the first two fingers of each hand behind each side of the child's mandible (jaw bone) and push the jaw forward. Both methods may be easier if the child is turned carefully onto their back.
	● When there is a risk of back or neck injury, establish a clear upper airway by using jaw thrust or chin lift alone in combination with manual in-line stabilisation of the head and neck by an assistant (if available).
	● If life-threatening airway obstruction persists despite effective application of jaw thrust or chin lift, add head tilt a small amount at a time until the airway is open; **establishing a patent airway takes priority over concerns about a potential back or neck injury**.

● Keeping the airway open	● Look, listen and feel for normal breathing by putting your face close to the child's face and looking along the chest:
	  – look for chest movements
	  – listen at the child's nose and mouth for breath sounds
	  – feel for air movement on your cheek.
	● Look, listen and feel for no more than 10 seconds before deciding that breathing is absent.

a. If the child **IS** breathing normally:	● Turn the child onto their side into the **RECOVERY POSITION** (see below) taking appropriate precautions if there is any possibility of injury to the spine. ● Check for continued breathing.
b. If the child is **NOT** breathing or is making agonal gasps (infrequent, irregular breaths):	● Carefully remove any obvious airway obstruction. ● Turn the child carefully on to their back taking appropriate precautions if there is any possibility of injury to the spine. ● Give 5 initial rescue breaths. ● While performing rescue breaths, note any gasp or cough response to your action. These responses (or their absence), will form part of your assessment of 'signs of life', which will be described later.

Table 2.10 – ASSESSMENT and MANAGEMENT of:

Basic Life Support (Child) *continued*

The following sequence is that followed by those with a duty to respond to paediatric emergencies (also refer to Figure 2.9)

ASSESSMENT	MANAGEMENT
	Rescue breaths for an INFANT: ● Ensure a neutral position of the head and apply chin lift. ● Use a bag-valve-mask device if available (with a mask appropriate to the size of the child) and inflate the chest steadily over 1–1½ seconds watching for chest rise. ● Maintaining head tilt and chin lift, watch the chest fall as air comes out. ● Repeat this sequence 5 times. ● Identify effectiveness by observing the child's chest rise and fall in a similar fashion to the movement produced by a normal breath. **Rescue breaths for a CHILD >1 year of age:** ● Ensure head tilt and chin lift. ● Use a bag-valve-mask device if available (with a mask appropriate to the size of the child) and inflate the chest steadily over 1–1½ seconds watching for chest rise. ● Maintaining head tilt and chin lift, watch the chest fall as air comes out. ● Repeat this sequence 5 times. ● Identify effectiveness by observing the child's chest rise and fall in a similar fashion to the movement produced by a normal breath.
	Rescue breaths for an INFANT if no bag-valve-mask is available: ● Ensure a neutral position of the head and apply chin lift. ● Take a breath and cover the mouth and nose of the infant with your mouth, making sure you have a good seal. ● In an older infant, if the mouth and nose cannot be covered, seal either the infant's nose or mouth with your mouth (if the nose is used, close the lips to prevent air escape). ● Blow steadily into the child's mouth and nose over 1–1½ seconds, sufficient to make the chest visibly rise. ● Maintain head tilt and chin lift, take your mouth away from the child and watch for the chest to fall as air comes out. ● Take another breath and repeat this sequence five times. ● Identify effectiveness by seeing that the child's chest has risen and fallen in a similar fashion to the movement produced by a normal breath. **Rescue breaths for a CHILD >1 year of age if no bag-valve-mask is available:** ● Ensure head tilt and chin lift. ● Pinch the soft part of the nose closed with the index finger and thumb, with the hand on the forehead. ● Open the mouth a little, but maintain chin lift. ● Take a breath and place your lips around the mouth, making sure that you have a good seal. ● Blow steadily into the mouth over 1–1½ seconds watching for chest rise. ● Maintain head tilt and chin lift, take your mouth away from the child and watch for the chest fall as air comes out. ● Take another breath and repeat this sequence five times. ● Identify effectiveness by seeing that the child's chest has risen and fallen in a similar fashion to the movement produced by a normal breath.
● If you have difficulty achieving an effective breath, the airway may be obstructed	● Open the child's mouth and remove any visible obstruction. ● **DO NOT** perform a blind finger sweep. ● Ensure that there is adequate head tilt and chin lift but also that the neck is not over extended. ● If head tilt and chin lift has not opened the airway, try the jaw thrust method. ● Make up to 5 attempts to achieve effective breaths. ● If still unsuccessful, move on to chest compressions.

● Assess the child's circulation	● Take no more than 10 seconds to look for signs of life. This includes any movement, coughing, or normal breathing (not agonal gasps – these are infrequent, irregular breaths).
	 ● Check the pulse but ensure you take no more than 10 seconds to do this:
	   – in a child over 1 year – feel for the carotid pulse in the neck
	   – in an infant – feel for the brachial pulse on the inner aspect of the upper arm
	   – If you are not sure if there is a pulse, **assume there is NO pulse**.

a. If you are confident that you can detect signs of a circulation within 10 seconds:	● Continue rescue breathing, until the child starts breathing effectively on their own. ● If the child remains unconscious, turn them on to their side (into the recovery position), taking appropriate precautions if there is any chance of injury to the neck or spine. ● Re-assess the child frequently.

Table 2.10 – ASSESSMENT and MANAGEMENT of:

Basic Life Support (Child) continued

The following sequence is that followed by those with a duty to respond to paediatric emergencies (also refer to Figure 2.9)

ASSESSMENT	MANAGEMENT
b. If there are: no signs of a circulation OR no pulse OR a slow pulse (less than 60/min with poor perfusion) OR you are not sure	● Start chest compressions. ● Combine rescue breathing and chest compressions.
For all children, compress the lower half of the sternum	● Avoid compressing the upper abdomen by locating the xiphisternum (i.e. find the angle where the lowest ribs join in the midline) and compressing the sternum one finger's breadth above this point. ● Compressions should be sufficient to depress the sternum by at least 1/3rd of the depth of the chest. ● Release the pressure, and then repeat at a rate of 100–120 per minute. ● After 15 compressions, tilt the head, lift the chin and give two effective breaths. ● Continue compressions and breaths in a ratio of 15:2. ● Lone rescuers may use a ratio of 30:2, particularly if they are having difficulty with the transition between compression and ventilation. ● Although the rate of compressions is 100–120 per minute, the actual number of compressions delivered will be less than 100 per minute because of pauses to give breaths. ● The best method for compression varies slightly between infants and children (see below).
● Chest compressions in infants	● The lone rescuer should compress the sternum with the tips of 2 fingers. ● If there are 2 or more rescuers, use the encircling technique: – place both thumbs flat side by side on the lower half of the sternum (as above) with the tips pointing towards the infant's head – spread the rest of both hands with the fingers together to encircle the lower part of the infant's rib cage with the tips of the fingers supporting the infant's back – press down on the lower sternum with the two thumbs to depress it at least one-third of the depth of the infant's chest.
● Chest compression in children >1 year of age	● Place the heel of one hand over the lower half of the sterum (as above). ● Lift the fingers to ensure that pressure is not applied over the child's ribs. ● Position yourself vertically above the child's chest and, with your arm straight, compress the sternum to depress it by at least one-third of the depth of the chest. ● In larger children or for small rescuers, this may be achieved most easily by using both hands with the fingers interlocked.
● Continue resuscitation until	● The child shows signs of life (spontaneous respiration, pulse, movement). ● You become exhausted.
	Additional Information **RECOVERY POSITION** An unconscious child with a clear airway that is breathing spontaneously should be turned on their side into the recovery position: ● The child should be placed in as near a true lateral position as possible with their mouth dependent to allow free drainage of fluid. ● A small pillow or a rolled-up blanket placed behind their back may be used to maintain an infant/small child in a stable position. ● It is important to avoid any pressure on the chest that impairs breathing. ● It should be possible to turn a child onto their side and to return them back easily and safely, taking into consideration the possibility of cervical spine injury. ● The airway should be accessible and easily observed. ● The adult recovery position is suitable for use in children.

Basic Life Support (Child)

Methodology

[Further related reading includes 61, 64]

For details of the methodology used in the development of this guideline refer to guideline webpage.

KEY POINTS

Paediatric Basic Life Support

- If the child is not breathing, carefully remove any obvious airway obstruction but DO NOT perform blind finger sweeps.
- Give 5 initial rescue breaths.
- Blow steadily into the mouth over 1–1½ seconds watching for chest rise.
- If there are:
  - no signs of life,
  - or no or a slow pulse (<60 bpm with poor perfusion)
  - or you are not sure, start chest compressions at a rate of 100–120 per minute.
- Continue alternating compressions and breaths in a ratio of 15:2.

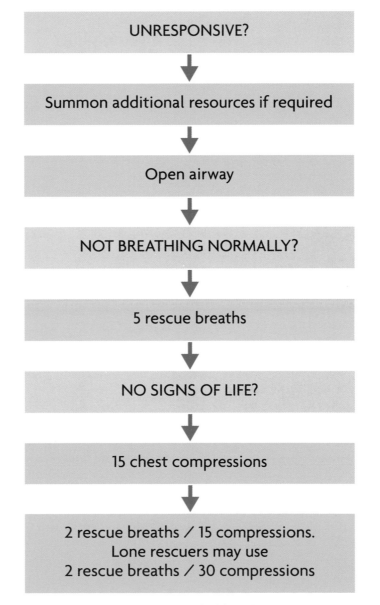

UNRESPONSIVE?

↓

Summon additional resources if required

↓

Open airway

↓

NOT BREATHING NORMALLY?

↓

5 rescue breaths

↓

NO SIGNS OF LIFE?

↓

15 chest compressions

↓

2 rescue breaths / 15 compressions.
Lone rescuers may use
2 rescue breaths / 30 compressions

Figure 2.9 – Child basic life support sequence algorithm – modified from the Resuscitation Council (UK) Guidelines 2010 algorithm for the JRCALC Resuscitation Supplement 2010 (www.resus.org.uk).

Newborn Life Support [48]

1. Introduction

- Passage through the birth canal is a hypoxic experience for the fetus since placental respiratory exchange is prevented for the 50–75 seconds duration of the average contraction. Most babies tolerate this well, but those few that do not may require help to establish normal breathing at delivery.

- The newborn life support guideline provides this help and comprises the following elements:
    1. drying and covering the baby to conserve heat
    2. assessing the need for any intervention
    3. opening the airway
    4. lung aeration
    5. rescue breathing
    6. chest compression.

2. Physiology

- In the face of in utero hypoxia, the breathing centres in the fetal brain become depressed and spontaneous breathing ceases. The fetus can maintain an effective circulation during periods of hypoxia, so the most urgent requirement for any asphyxiated baby at birth is aeration of the lungs. Then, provided the circulation has remained intact, oxygenated blood will be conveyed from the lungs to the heart and onwards to the brain. The centres responsible for breathing should recover and the baby will breathe spontaneously.

- Merely aerating the lungs is sufficient in the majority of cases. Where cardiac function has deteriorated to an extent that the circulation is inadequate, a brief period of chest compression may be needed.

- In a very small number of cases, lung aeration and chest compression will not be sufficient – the outlook in this group is poor.

3. Sequence of Actions (refer to Figure 2.10)

Keep the baby warm and assess

- Babies are small and born wet. They become cold very easily, particularly if they are allowed to remain wet and exposed.

- A healthy baby will be born blue but will have a good tone, will cry within a few seconds of delivery, will have a good heart rate (normally 120–150 per minute), and will become pink within the first 90 seconds or so.

- A less healthy baby will be blue, will have less good tone, may have a slow heart rate (less than 100 per minute) and may not establish adequate breathing by 90–120 seconds.

- An ill (very hypoxic) baby will be born pale and floppy, not breathing and with a very slow heart rate.

4. Assessment and Management

For the assessment of newborns and management of cardiorespiratory problems refer to Table 2.11 and Figure 2.10.

Methodology

For details of the methodology used in the development of this guideline refer to the guideline webpage.

KEY POINTS

Newborn Life Support

- **Passage through the birth canal is a hypoxic experience and some babies may require help to establish normal breathing at delivery.**
- **Babies become cold very easily; dry the baby, remove any wet towels and replace with dry ones. Once in the ambulance keep the compartment as warm as possible.**
- **Ensure the airway is open by placing the baby on their back with the head in a neutral position.**
  If the baby is very floppy it may be necessary to apply a chin lift or jaw thrust.
- **If the baby is not breathing adequately by about 90 seconds give 5 inflation breaths.**
- **If chest compressions are necessary compress the chest quickly and firmly at a ratio of 3:1 compressions to inflations.**
- **Use a two thumbs, encircling technique.**

Newborn Life Support

Table 2.11 – ASSESSMENT and MANAGEMENT of:

Newborn Life Support

ASSESSMENT	MANAGEMENT
● In all cases	● Ensure the ambient temperature is as high as possible. ● Clamp and cut the cord. ● Dry the baby. ● Remove wet towels and cover the baby with dry towels.
● Assess	● **Colour.** ● **Tone.** ● **Breathing rate.** ● **Heart rate:** – assess heart rate by listening with a stethoscope (feeling for a peripheral pulse is not reliable) – in noisy or very cold environments, palpating the pulse at the umbilical cord may be an alternative and may save unwrapping the baby (this is only reliable when the pulse is >100 bpm) – attach a pulse oximeter. NB Attaching to the wrist using an infant probe can give an accurate heart rate in approximately 90 seconds.
● Re-assess breathing and heart rate, every 30 seconds ● Decide whether help is required (and likely to be available) and whether rapid evacuation to hospital is indicated. If transferring to hospital follow pre-alert procedure	● An increase in heart rate is usually the first clinical sign of improvement. ● Once the baby is in the ambulance, the patient compartment should be kept as warm as possible (especially if pre-term) even if uncomfortable for the mother and attendant.
Airway	The airway must be open for a baby to breathe effectively: ● Place the baby on their back with the head in a neutral position i.e. neither flexed nor extended. ● If the baby is very floppy, a chin lift or jaw thrust may be necessary.
Breathing ● If the baby is not breathing adequately by approximately 90 seconds:	● Give 5 inflation breaths – use a 500 ml bag-valve-mask device. NB Until birth the baby's lungs have been filled with fluid; aeration of the lungs in these circumstances is likely to require sustained application of pressures of about 30 centimetres of water for 2–3 seconds. These are known as **inflation breaths**. Bag–valve-mask devices should incorporate a safety device that allows this pressure to be generated yet prevents higher pressures that might damage the lungs.
Heart Rate If the heart rate increases: ● If the heart rate increases but the baby does not start breathing: ● If the heart rate does not increase following inflation breaths:	● Assume that lung aeration has been successful. ● Continue to provide regular breaths (**ventilation breaths**) at a rate of about 30–40 per minute until the baby starts to breathe on their own. NB Ventilation breaths do not need as long an inspiratory time as inflation breaths (~ 1 second). Continue to monitor the heart rate. If the rate should drop <100 bpm it suggests insufficient ventilation. In this situation, increase the rate of inflation or use a longer inspiratory time. ● Either lung aeration has not been adequate or the baby requires more than lung aeration alone. It is most likely that you have not aerated the lungs effectively. If the heart rate does not increase and the chest does not move with each inflation, you have not aerated the lungs; in this situation consider: 1. Is the head in the neutral position? 2. Do you need jaw thrust? 3. Do you need a longer inflation time? 4. Do you need help with the airway from a second person? 5. Is there obstruction in the oropharynx (laryngoscope and suction)? 6. Do you need an oropharyngeal airway? ● Check the baby's head is in the neutral position; that breaths are at the correct pressure and applied for the correct time and the chest moves with each breath. ● If the chest still does not move, consider an obstruction in the oropharynx that may be removable under direct vision.

Table 2.11 – ASSESSMENT and MANAGEMENT of:

Newborn Life Support *continued*

ASSESSMENT	MANAGEMENT
• If after 5 inflation breaths the heart rate remains slow (<60 bpm), or the heart beat is absent despite good passive chest movements in response to inflations:	• Start chest compressions.
• If the baby is not vigorous at birth or does not respond very rapidly to bag-valve-mask ventilation:	• **TIME CRITICAL** transfer. • Provide an alert/information call.
• If the mother has received morphine or any other opiate within the previous four hours and the baby does not breathe adequately:	• Administer **naloxone** intramuscularly (**refer to naloxone drug guideline**) and provide respiratory support until it takes effect.
Circulation • If chest compressions are necessary:	• Ensure that the lungs have been successfully aerated. • In newborns, encircle the lower chest with both hands in such a way that the two thumbs can compress the lower third of the sternum, at a point just below an imaginary line joining the nipples, with the fingers over the spine at the back. • Compress the chest quickly and firmly in such a way as to reduce the antero-posterior diameter of the chest by a third. • **The ratio of compressions to inflations in newborn resuscitation is 3:1.**
Meconium	• Attempting to aspirate meconium from a baby's mouth and nose while their head is still on the perineum does not prevent meconium aspiration and is not recommended. • Attempts to aspirate meconium from a vigorous baby's airway after birth will not prevent meconium aspiration and is not recommended. • If a baby is born through thick meconium and is unresponsive at birth, the oropharynx should be inspected and cleared of meconium. The larynx and trachea should also be cleared if a suitable laryngoscope is available. This should not however unduly delay initial attempts to inflate the lungs.
	Additional Information There is no evidence to suggest that any one concentration of **oxygen** is better than another when starting resuscitation. Air has also been shown to be equally effective. Whenever possible, additional **oxygen** should be available if there is not a rapid improvement in the baby's condition.

[Further related reading includes 65]

SECTION 2 Resuscitation

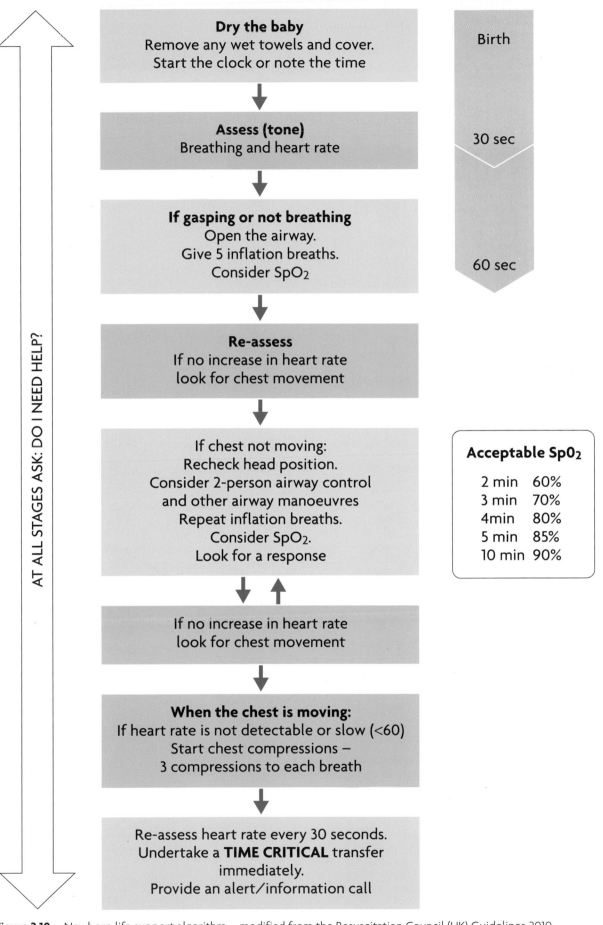

Dry the baby
Remove any wet towels and cover.
Start the clock or note the time

Assess (tone)
Breathing and heart rate

If gasping or not breathing
Open the airway.
Give 5 inflation breaths.
Consider SpO$_2$

Re-assess
If no increase in heart rate
look for chest movement

If chest not moving:
Recheck head position.
Consider 2-person airway control
and other airway manoeuvres
Repeat inflation breaths.
Consider SpO$_2$.
Look for a response

If no increase in heart rate
look for chest movement

When the chest is moving:
If heart rate is not detectable or slow (<60)
Start chest compressions –
3 compressions to each breath

Re-assess heart rate every 30 seconds.
Undertake a **TIME CRITICAL** transfer
immediately.
Provide an alert/information call

AT ALL STAGES ASK: DO I NEED HELP?

Birth

30 sec

60 sec

Acceptable SpO2

2 min	60%
3 min	70%
4min	80%
5 min	85%
10 min	90%

Figure 2.10 – Newborn life support algorithm – modified from the Resuscitation Council (UK) Guidelines 2010 algorithm for the JRCALC Resuscitation Supplement 2010 (www.resus.org.uk).

Advanced Life Support (Child) [47, 60]

1. Introduction

Paediatric resuscitation practices have been simplified to minimise the differences between the adult and paediatric protocols.

Age definitions:

● an infant is a child under one year old.

● a child is between one year and puberty.

These guidelines are not intended to apply to the resuscitation of newborn (**refer to neonatal resuscitation guideline**).

2. Assessment and Management

For children requiring advanced life support follow the assessment and management guidance in Table 2.12 and Figure 2.11.

Table 2.12 – ASSESSMENT and MANAGEMENT of:

Advanced Life Support (Child)

ASSESSMENT	MANAGEMENT
1. Establish basic life support 2. Oxygenate, ventilate, and start chest compressions	● **Refer to basic life support (child) guideline**. ● Ensure a patent airway by using an airway manoeuvre as described in the child basic life support guideline. An adjunct such as an oropharyngeal airway may be needed. ● Provide positive pressure ventilation delivering high flow oxygen. ● Provide ventilation, initially by bag and mask. ● Provide compressions and ventilations at a ratio of 15 compressions to 2 ventilations (the compression rate should be 100–120 per minute and the ventilation rate about 10 per minute). ● If bag-valve-mask ventilation is impossible or impractical, and if the clinician is trained, a laryngeal mask or possibly another supraglottic airway can be used. ● In most circumstances, tracheal intubation should be avoided in children. The technique is difficult and used only rarely as the skill is very difficult to acquire and maintain. ● Once airway has been secured then continuous compressions should be performed; take care to ensure that ventilations remain effective.
3. Attach a defibrillator or monitor	● Assess and monitor the cardiac rhythm. ● Place one defibrillator pad/paddle on the chest wall just below the right clavicle and the other in the left anterior axillary line. ● Use paediatric pads for children <1 year of age and adult pads ≥1 year of age. For infants, if there are only large pads or paddles available, then it may be more appropriate to apply them to both the front and back of the chest. ● Monitoring electrodes should be placed in the conventional positions.
4. Check for signs of circulation and assess rhythm	**Look for signs of life** e.g. moving, responsiveness, coughing, and normal breathing. **Assess the rhythm on the monitor:** ● Non-shockable (i.e. Asystole or Pulseless Electrical Activity (PEA)). ● Shockable (Ventricular Fibrillation (VF) or Pulseless Ventricular Tachycardia (VT)).
5. Non-shockable (Asystole, Pulseless Electrical Activity (PEA))	Asystole and PEA are the commonest paediatric cardiac arrest rhythms. Perform continuous CPR: ● Ventilate with high concentration **oxygen**. ● If ventilating with a bag-mask device, give 15 chest compressions to 2 ventilations for all ages. NOTE: Once there is return of spontaneous circulation (ROSC), ventilate gently at a rate of 12–20 per minute (as over inflation of the lungs can cause increased intrathoracic pressure, which has a detrimental effect on venous return and hence cardiac output).
● Administer adrenaline	● Obtain circulatory access. Insert a peripheral venous cannula. If venous access is not readily attainable, give early consideration to intraosseous access. ● Give **adrenaline** 10 micrograms/kg (0.1 ml/kg of 1 in 10,000 solution) IV/IO (**see adrenaline guideline**.)
● Continue CPR	
● Repeat the cycle	● Give 10 micrograms/kg of **adrenaline** (see adrenaline guideline) every 3–5 minutes. (10 micrograms/kg is the dose for all subsequent doses i.e. 'high-dose' **adrenaline** is no longer used). ● Continue effective chest compressions and ventilation without interruption, at a ventilatory rate of approximately 10 per minute and a compression rate of 100–120 per minute. ● Once airway has been secured then continuous compressions should be performed without pausing for ventilation. ● When circulation is restored, ventilate the child at a rate of 12–20 breaths per minute.

Table 2.12 – ASSESSMENT and MANAGEMENT of:

Advanced Life Support (Child) *continued*

ASSESSMENT	MANAGEMENT	
● Consider and correct reversible causes: **4Hs 4Ts**	1. Hypoxia 2. Hypovolaemia 3. Hyper/hypokalaemia 4. Hypothermia	1. Tension pneumothorax 2. Tamponade 3. Toxic/therapeutic disturbance 4. Thromboembolism

ASSESSMENT	MANAGEMENT
6. Shockable (VF/pulseless VT) These rhythms are less common in paediatric practice but more likely when there has been a witnessed and sudden collapse or in children with underlying cardiac disease	**Defibrillate the heart:** ● Give 1 shock of 4 Joules/kg if using a manual defibrillator, rounding the shock up as necessary to the machine settings (this energy level is appropriate for both biphasic and the older monophasic defibrillators). If using an AED in a child over the age of 8 years, use the adult shock energy – paediatric attenuation is not required. If using an AED in a child under the age of 8 years, use a machine with paediatric attenuation (according to the manufacturer's instructions) when available. An AED should not routinely be attached to infants unless they have a history of cardiac problems. Where an infant is found to have a shockable rhythm, use a manual defibrillator to administer 4 Joules/kg. (In infants, if a manual defibrillator is not available, a paediatric attenuated AED may be used.) If no paediatric attenuated AED is available, use the adult shock energy at all ages.
	● **Resume CPR:** without re-assessing the rhythm or feeling for a pulse, resume CPR immediately, starting with chest compressions. ● **Continue CPR for 2 minutes**.
● Then pause briefly to check the monitor	**If still VF/pulseless VT:** ● Give a 2nd shock at 4 Joules/kg **as for the 1st shock (see start of step 6)**. ● **Resume CPR immediately after the second shock.**
● Consider and correct reversible causes	● **4Hs 4Ts** (see above.) ● Continue CPR for 2 minutes.
● Pause briefly to check the monitor	**If still VF/pulseless VT:** ● Give a 3rd shock followed by **adrenaline** 10 micrograms/kg PLUS an intravenous or intraosseous bolus of **amiodarone** 5 milligrams/kg (refer to amiodarone guideline for further information). ● Resume CPR immediately and continue for another 2 minutes.
● Pause briefly to check the monitor	**If still VF/pulseless VT:** ● Give a 4th shock. ● Resume CPR, and continue giving shocks every 2 minutes, minimising the breaks in chest compressions as much as possible. ● Give **adrenaline** after every other shock (i.e. every 3–5 minutes) until ROSC.
● After each 2 minutes of uninterrupted CPR, pause briefly to assess the rhythm	**If still in VF/VT:** ● Continue CPR with the shockable rhythm (VF/VT) sequence. **If asystole:** ● Continue CPR and switch to the non-shockable (asystole/PEA) sequence as above.
● **If an organised rhythm appears at any time, check for a central pulse**	● If there is return of a spontaneous circulation (**ROSC**) begin post-resuscitation care. ● If there is **NO** pulse, and there are no other signs of life, or you are not sure, continue CPR as for the non-shockable sequence as above.

Methodology

For details of the methodology used in the development of this guideline refer to the guideline webpage.

[Further related reading includes 63, 75]

Advanced Life Support (Child)

KEY POINTS

Advanced Life Support (Child)

- Changes in guidelines have been made for simplification and to minimise the difference between the paediatric and adult protocols.
- One defibrillating shock rather than three stacked shocks should be used.
- Intubation is rarely indicated and should only be undertaken by those with appropriate skills.

Automated External Defibrillators (AEDs)

- If using an AED in a child <8 years, paediatric attenuation should be used whenever possible.
- An unmodified AED may be used in children older than one year.
- If an infant is known to have a shockable rhythm or underlying cardiac problem, a paediatric attenuated AED may be used.
- If an unmodified AED is the only machine available, it may be used at all ages or the child/infant will die.

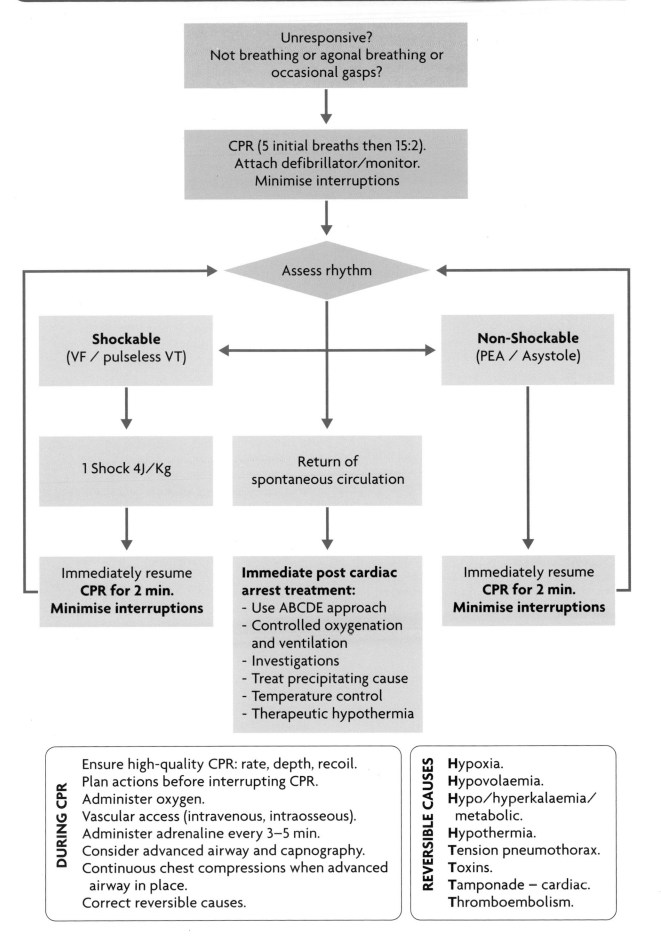

Figure 2.11 – Advanced life support algorithm – modified from the Resuscitation Council (UK) Guidelines 2010 algorithm for the JRCALC Resuscitation Supplement 2010 (www.resus.org.uk).

Foreign Body Airway Obstruction (Child) [47]

1. Introduction

The majority of choking events in infants and children occur during play or whilst eating when a carer is usually present.

Events are frequently witnessed and interventions are usually initiated when the child is conscious.

Foreign body airway obstruction (FBAO) is characterised by the sudden onset of respiratory distress associated with coughing, gagging or stridor (Table 2.13).

Table 2.13 – GENERAL SIGNS OF FOREIGN BODY AIRWAY OBSTRUCTION

- Witnessed episode.
- Coughing or choking.
- Sudden onset.
- Recent history of playing with or eating small objects.

Ineffective coughing
- Unable to vocalise.
- Quiet or silent cough.
- Unable to breathe.
- Cyanosis.
- Decreasing level of consciousness.

Effective coughing
- Crying or verbal response to questions.
- Loud cough.
- Able to breathe before coughing.
- Fully responsive.

Similar signs and symptoms may also be associated with other causes of airway obstruction such as laryngitis or epiglottitis, which require different management.

Recognition of FBAO

When a foreign body enters the airway, the child reacts immediately by coughing in an attempt to expel it.

A spontaneous cough is likely to be more effective and safer than any manoeuvre a rescuer might perform.

If coughing is absent or ineffective and the object completely obstructs the airway, the child will rapidly become asphyxiated.

Active interventions to relieve FBAO are only required when coughing becomes ineffective, but when required they should be commenced confidently and rapidly.

Suspect FBAO if:

- the onset was very sudden
- there were no other signs of illness
- there are other clues to alert the rescuer, e.g. a history of eating or playing with small items immediately prior to the onset of symptoms.

2. Assessment and Management

For the assessment and management of foreign body airway obstruction refer to Table 2.14 and Figure 2.12.

NOTES ON TECHNIQUES

BACK BLOWS – infant:

- Support the infant in a head-down, prone position, to allow gravity to assist the removal of the foreign body.
- A seated or kneeling rescuer should be able to support the infant safely across their lap.
- Support the infant's head by placing the thumb of one hand at the angle of the lower jaw, with one or two fingers from the same hand at the same point on the other side of the jaw.
- Do not compress the soft tissues under the infant's jaw, as this will exacerbate the airway obstruction.
- Deliver up to 5 sharp back blows with the heel of one hand in the middle of the back between the shoulder blades, aiming to relieve the obstruction with each blow rather than to give all five.

BACK BLOWS – child over 1 year of age:

- Back blows are more effective if the child is positioned head down.
- A small child may be placed across the rescuer's lap as with an infant. If this is not possible, support the child in a forward-leaning position and deliver the back blows from behind.

CHEST and ABDOMINAL THRUSTS

- If back blows fail to dislodge the object and the child is still conscious, use chest thrusts for infants or abdominal thrusts in older children.
- Abdominal thrusts **must not** be used in infants.

Chest thrusts for infants:

- Turn the infant into a head-down, supine position (this can be safely achieved by placing the free arm along the infant's back and encircling the occiput with the hand).
- Support the infant down your arm, which is placed down (or across) your thigh.
- Identify the landmark for chest compression (lower sternum, approximately a finger's breadth above the xiphisternum).
- Deliver 5 chest thrusts (if required).
- These are similar to external chest compressions but sharper in nature and delivered at a slower rate.

Abdominal thrusts for children over 1 year:

- Stand or kneel behind the child. Place your arms under the child's arms and encircle their torso.
- Clench your fist and place it between the umbilicus and the xiphisternum. Grasp this hand with the other hand and pull sharply inwards and upwards.
- Repeat up to 5 times (if required).
- Ensure that pressure is not applied to xiphoid process or lower rib cage (may result in abdominal trauma).

Foreign Body Airway Obstruction (Child)

RE-ASSESSMENT

Following chest or abdominal thrusts, re-assess the child:

- If object has not been expelled and victim is still conscious, continue the sequence of back blows and chest (for infant) or abdominal (for children) thrusts.
- Do not leave the child at this stage. Arrange transfer to hospital.
- If the object is expelled successfully, assess the child's clinical condition. It is possible that part of

the object may remain in the respiratory tract and cause complications.

- Abdominal thrusts may cause internal injuries and all victims so treated should be assessed further.

Methodology

For details of the methodology used in the development of this guideline refer to the guideline webpage.

[Further related reading includes 61, 64]

Table 2.14 – ASSESSMENT and MANAGEMENT of:

Foreign Body Airway Obstruction (Child)

ASSESSMENT	MANAGEMENT
Assess safety Assess for severity of obstruction refer to Table 2.13	• Do not place yourself in danger and consider the safest action to manage the choking child.
• Effective coughing	• Encourage the child to cough but do nothing else. • Monitor continuously. • Transport rapidly to hospital.
• Ineffective coughing or cough becoming ineffective	• Summon help if appropriate. • Determine the child's conscious level.
CONSCIOUS CHILD • Conscious child with ineffective coughing or cough becoming ineffective	• Give back blows. • If back blows do not relieve the FBAO, give chest thrusts (infants) or abdominal thrusts (children). These manoeuvres increase intrathoracic pressure and may dislodge the foreign body. • Alternate these until the obstruction is relieved or the child loses consciousness.
UNCONSCIOUS CHILD • If the child is or becomes unconscious:	• Place them on a firm, flat surface. **Open the airway:** • Open the mouth and look for any obvious object. If one is seen and you think you can grasp it easily, make an attempt to remove it with a single finger sweep. **DO NOT** attempt blind or repeated finger sweeps – these can cause injury and impact the object more deeply into the pharynx. **Attempt ventilation.** • Open the airway and make 5 attempts to ventilate the lungs. • Assess the effectiveness of each ventilation. • If the chest does not rise, reposition the head before making the next attempt.
• Commence CPR if there is no response to 5 attempts at ventilation (moving, coughing, spontaneous breaths). Proceed to chest compressions without further assessment of the circulation	**Commence CPR.** • Follow the sequence for single rescuer CPR for approximately 1 minute. Start with compressions. • When the airway is opened for attempted ventilation, look to see if the foreign body can be seen in the mouth. • If an object is seen, attempt to remove it with a single finger sweep. • If it appears that the obstruction has been relieved, open and check the airway as above. • Perform ventilations if the child is not breathing. • If the child regains consciousness and exhibits spontaneous effective breathing, place them in the recovery position. Monitor breathing and conscious level and transfer to hospital.

Foreign Body Airway Obstruction (Child)

KEY POINTS

Foreign Body Airway Obstruction (Child)

- FBAO is a potentially treatable cause of death that often occurs whilst playing or eating.
- It is characterised by the sudden onset of respiratory distress.
- If the child is coughing effectively, encourage them to continue to cough.
- If coughing is ineffective, back blows should initially be given.
- If coughing is ineffective and back blows have failed to relieve the FBAO, use chest thrusts in infants and abdominal thrusts in children.
- Abdominal thrusts may cause serious internal bleeding – such patients require further hospital assessment.
- Avoid blind finger sweeps.

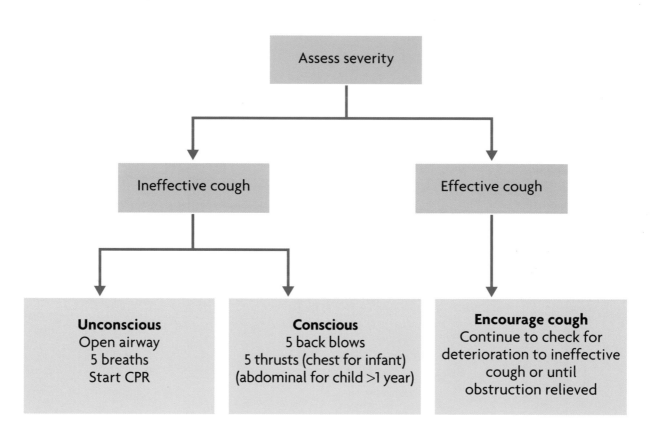

Figure 2.12 – Foreign body airway obstruction in children – modified from the Resuscitation Council (UK) Guidelines 2010 algorithm for the JRCALC Resuscitation Supplement 2010 (www.resus.org.uk).

3

Medical

3a
Undifferentiated Complaints

3b
Specific Conditions

1. Introduction

- Abdominal pain is a common presenting symptom to ambulance services. The specific cause can be difficult to identify in prehospital care and a definitive diagnosis may require in-hospital investigations.
- The nature, location and pattern of the pain together with associated symptoms, may indicate a possible cause (refer to Table 3.1). It is important to consider life-threatening causes.
- The elderly, alcoholics and immunosuppressed patients may have atypical presentations.

- Abdominal pain can arise from both acute and chronic abdominal conditions:
  - **Acute conditions:** e.g. appendicitis, cholecystitis, intestinal obstruction, ureteric colic, gastritis, perforated peptic ulcer, gastroenteritis, pancreatitis, diverticular disease, leaking or ruptured abdominal aortic aneurysms and gynaecological disorders.
  - **Chronic conditions:** e.g. irritable bowel syndrome (IBS), inflammatory bowel syndromes (Ulcerative Colitis and Crohn's disease), gastric and duodenal ulcers and intra-abdominal malignancy.

Table 3.1

Common Causes of Abdominal Pain

CONDITION	CHARACTERISTICS OF PAIN	ASSOCIATED SYMPTOMS
Leaking or Ruptured Abdominal Aortic Aneurysms (AAA) Consider AAA in patients >50 years who present with the symptoms listed. Most deaths occur in the elderly.	• Sudden severe abdominal pain or backache. • Renal colic type pain – a new diagnosis of renal colic in a patient over 50 years of age raises the concern of abdominal aortic aneurysm even in the absence of a palpable mass. NB Given that <25% of all AAA patients present with classic signs and symptoms there is a risk of misdiagnosis.	• Collapse. • Hypotension with bilateral lower limb ischaemia or mottling (a late sign). • History of smoking. • Hypertension and hypercholesterolaemia.
Appendicitis Frequently misdiagnosed. Approximately one-third of women of childbearing age with appendicitis are considered as having pelvic inflammatory disease or UTI.	• A constant pain, increasing in intensity often starting in the peri umbilical area. • The pain may settle in the right lower quadrant; but the location may vary in the early stages. • There is rebound tenderness in the right iliac fossa and coughing and walking may exacerbate the pain. • Older patients may present with generalised pain, distension, and decreased bowel sounds.	• Nausea. • Vomiting. • Loss of appetite. • Constipation. • Increased temperature >37.5°C. • Diarrhoea.
Acute cholecystitis Accounts for approximately 30% of patients attending ED for acute abdominal pain.	• A sharp pain in the right upper quadrant of the abdomen. • May experience right shoulder-tip pain. • The pain is worse when breathing deeply and on palpation of the right upper quadrant.	• Nausea and vomiting. • Increased temperature >38°C. • History of fat intolerance.
Intestinal obstruction A partial or complete obstruction of the small or large intestine.	• Abdominal pain that is cramping in nature.	• Abdominal distension. • Nausea and vomiting. • Absolute constipation (late stage).
Urinary tract pathology Infection arising from the kidneys, ureters, bladder and/or urethra. Urinary tract obstruction.	• Pain in the lower abdomen and/or back. • Cramping.	• Pain/burning sensation when urinating, • Needing to urinate frequently. • Urinary frequency and nocturia. • Nausea and vomiting. • Cloudy/bloody urine with a malodour. • If the infection involves the kidneys the patient may have increased temperature >38°C, and fatigue. • Rigors may be present.

Section 3 Medical Undifferentiated Complaints

Table 3.1

Common Causes of Abdominal Pain *continued*

CONDITION	CHARACTERISTICS OF PAIN	SIGNS AND SYMPTOMS
Gastritis An inflammation of the gastric lining can be caused by medication (aspirin, non-steroidal anti-inflammatory drugs), alcohol, *Helicobacter pylori*, or stress.	● Upper abdominal pain. ● Lower/central chest pain/epigatric pain.	● Nausea and vomiting. ● Loss of appetite. ● Haematemesis.
Peptic ulcer An erosion of the lining of the stomach or small intestine forming an ulcer.	● Central burning abdominal pain. ● Back pain. ● Perforation may lead to abrupt onset epigastric pain.	● Nausea and vomiting – haematemesis. ● Fatigue. ● Weight loss.
Gastroenteritis Common infection of the stomach or bowel caused by viruses or bacteria.	● Abdominal pain and cramps.	● Nausea and vomiting. ● Diarrhoea. ● Fatigue. ● Weight loss.
Acute pancreatitis Inflammation of the pancreas.	● Constant pain in the upper left quadrant or middle of the abdomen. ● The pain may radiate to the patient's back.	● Abdominal tenderness. ● Hypotension. ● Nausea and vomiting. ● Dehydration. ● Shock. ● History of alcohol abuse or gallstones.
Diverticular disease Inflammation of diverticula in the large intestine.	● Abdominal pain in the lower left quadrant.	● Nausea and vomiting. ● Altered bowel habit. ● Bloating. ● Increased temperature >38°C.
Ectopic pregnancy Pregnancy not implanted in the uterus. It affects 1 pregnancy in 80 and accounts for 13% of all pregnancy-related deaths.	● Pain in the lower abdomen, pelvic area or back. NB Patients may present atypically but pain is almost always present.	● Nausea. ● Missed last menstrual period (though can occur before this). ● History of pelvic inflammatory disease. ● Previous ectopic pregnancy. If the pregnancy ruptures patients may report: ● Severe lower abdominal pain. ● Shoulder tip pain. ● Feeling faint/collapse.
Pelvic Inflammatory Disease A common cause of abdominal pain in females but rarely presents as an acute collapse.	● Pain in the lower abdomen, pelvic area or back. ● Abdominal tenderness.	● Vaginal discharge. ● Nausea. ● Fever
Intussusception Most commonly found in infants; another peak in incidence occurs at 6 years of age. An inward telescoping of the intestine that may cause an obstruction.	● intermittent colicky pain associated with bouts of screaming and drawing legs up.	● Vomiting. ● 'Currant jelly stool' – blood and mucus.

Table 3.2 – ASSESSMENT and MANAGEMENT of:

Abdominal Pain

ASSESSMENT	MANAGEMENT

● Assess ABCD	● If any of the following **TIME CRITICAL** features present:
	  – major **ABCD** problems
	  – suspected leaking or ruptured aortic aneurysm
	  – ectopic pregnancy
	  – sepsis resulting from perforation
	  – traumatic disruption of abdominal organs e.g. liver, spleen, then:
	● Start correcting **A** and **B** and undertake a **TIME CRITICAL** transfer to nearest appropriate receiving hospital – for patients with suspected leaking or ruptured aortic aneurysm follow local care pathway.
	● Provide an alert/information call.
	● Continue patient management en-route.

	NB For indigestion type pain have a high index of suspicion that it may be cardiac in origin.
● History of pain	Ascertain the: ● Site of pain and whether it radiates to other areas. ● Onset of pain and whether this is a new pain. ● Character of the pain e.g. constant or intermittent; improving or worsening. ● Radiates – does pain radiate elsewhere? ● Associated symptoms e.g. nausea, vomiting dizziness. ● Timing – how long have they been in pain? ● Abnormal or absent bowel sounds may indicate the presence of a serious condition. Medical history: ● Previous abdominal surgery. ● Current drug treatment if any. ● Recent travel. ● Presence of similar symptoms in others.
● Associated symptoms/ conditions	● Altered bowel habit. ● Nausea and vomiting – haematemesis/malaena may indicate gastrointestinal pathology – **refer to gastrointestinal bleeding guideline**. ● Vaginal bleeding/pregnancy/previous ectopic pregnancy – **refer to relevant obstetric and gynaecology guidelines**. ● Burning on urination. ● Menstrual and sexual history in females of childbearing age (is there any possibility of prenancy?). NB For details of signs and symptoms of specific conditions refer to Table 3.1.
● Oxygen	If oxygen is indicated refer to oxygen therapy guideline.
● ECG	● Undertake a 12-lead ECG for elderly patients and those with cardiac risk factors presenting with upper abdominal pain.
● Fluid	● If fluid resuscitation is indicated refer to intravascular fluid therapy guideline.
● Pain management	● Measure the patient's reported pain. ● If analgesia is required refer to **pain management guideline**. NB Opiate administration does not affect later clinical management.
● Transfer to further care	● Transfer to further care (consider most appropriate centre). ● Transfer all children <1 year with bile stained (green) vomit. ● A new diagnosis of renal colic in a patient over 50 years of age raises the concern of abdominal aortic aneurysm even in the absence of a palpable mass. ● Provide an alert/information call as indicated. ● Continue patient management en-route.

Medical
Undifferentiated
Complaints

SECTION 3

2. Severity and Outcome

- The most common diagnosis of patients presenting to emergency departments (ED) with abdominal pain is non-specific abdominal pain, followed by renal colic.

- Many cases are relatively minor in nature e.g. constipation, urinary tract infection (UTI), however, 25% of patients contacting the ambulance service with abdominal pain have serious underlying conditions.

- In patients >65 years there is a 6–8 times higher mortality rate due to atypical clinical presentations and the presence of comorbidities.

3. Incidence

Abdominal pain is a common presenting complaint accounting for 10% of attendances to ED. In patients over 65 years it is the main complaint in up to 13% of admissions to ED. Of those patients who present by ambulance approximately 50% are admitted for further investigation and observation.

4. Pathophysiology

Abdominal pain can be localised and referred, due to overlapping innervations of the organs contained in the abdomen e.g. small and large intestines.

5. Assessment and Management

For the assessment and management of abdominal pain refer to Table 3.2.

Methodology

For details of the methodology used in the development of this guideline refer to the guideline webpage.

KEY POINTS

Abdominal Pain

- **The most important diagnoses to consider are those that are life threatening, either as the result of internal haemorrhage or perforation of a viscus and sepsis.**
- **For indigestion type pain have a high index of suspicion that it may be cardiac in origin. Obtain 12-lead ECG for elderly patients and patients with cardiac risks presenting with upper abdominal pain.**
- **If a patient is in pain, adequate analgesia should be given.**
- **A precise diagnosis of the cause of abdominal pain is often impossible without access to tests and investigations in hospital.**

SECTION **3** Medical Undifferentiated Complaints

Cardiac Rhythm Disturbance [58, 60, 74, 105]

1. Introduction

- Cardiac arrhythmia is a common complication of acute myocardial ischaemia or infarction and may precede cardiac arrest or complicate the early post-resuscitation period.

- Rhythm disturbance may also present in many other ways and be unrelated to coronary heart disease.

- The management of disorders of cardiac rhythm is a specialised subject, often requiring detailed investigation and management strategies that are not available outside hospital.

- Diagnosis of the precise rhythm disturbance may be complicated and the selection of optimal treatment difficult. Very often, expert advice will be required, yet this expertise is rarely immediately available in the emergency situation.

2. Principles of Treatment

- Management is determined by the condition of the patient as well as the nature of the rhythm. Manage the patient using the standard ABCDE approach.

- In all cases follow the oxygen guideline and aim for a target saturation within the range of 94–98%.

- Gain venous access.

- Always take a defibrillator to any patient with suspected cardiac rhythm disturbance.

- Establish cardiac rhythm monitoring as soon as possible.

Document the arrhythmia. This should be done with a 12-lead ECG whenever possible. If only a 3-lead ECG is available, lead II provides the best waveform for arrhythmia analysis.

- Provide a printout for the hospital, and if possible archive the record electronically so that further copies can be available at a later time if needed. Repeat the recording if the rhythm should change at any time. Record the ECG rhythm during any intervention (vagotonic procedures or the administration of drugs).

- If patients are not acutely ill there may be time to seek appropriate advice.

- The presence of adverse signs or symptoms will dictate the need for urgent treatment. The following adverse factors indicate a patient who is unstable because of the arrhythmia:
  - evidence of low cardiac output: pallor, sweating, cold clammy extremities, impaired consciousness or hypotension (SBP <90 mmHg)
  - excessive tachycardia, defined as a heart rate of >150 bpm
  - excessive bradycardia, defined as a heart rate of <40 bpm
  - heart failure implies the arrhythmia is compromising left ventricular function. This may cause breathlessness, confusion and hypotension or other features of reduced cardiac output
  - ischaemic chest pain implies that the arrhythmia (particularly tachyarrhythmia) is producing myocardial ischaemia. It is particularly important if there is underlying coronary disease or

structural heart disease in which ischaemia is likely to lead to life-threatening complications including cardiac arrest.

3. Bradycardia

Introduction

- A bradycardia is defined as a ventricular rate below 60 bpm, but it is important to recognise patients with a relative bradycardia in whom the rate is inappropriately slow for their haemodynamic state.

4. Risk of Asystole

Assessment and Management

For the assessment and management of bradycardia and risk of asystole refer to Table 3.3.

5. Tachycardia

Introduction

- These guidelines are intended for the treatment of patients who maintain a cardiac output in the presence of the tachycardia.

- Pulseless ventricular tachycardia is treated according to the cardiac arrest algorithm for the treatment of pulseless VT/VF.

- Broad complex tachycardia.

- Narrow complex tachycardia.

Assessment and Management

For the assessment and management of tachycardia, broad complex tachycardia, and narrow complex tachycardia refer to Table 3.4.

Cardiac Rhythm Disturbance

Table 3.3 – ASSESSMENT and MANAGEMENT of:

Bradycardia and Risk of Asystole

Bradycardia: A ventricular rate below 60 bpm, but it is important to recognise patients with a relative bradycardia in whom the rate is inappropriately slow for their haemodynamic state.

ASSESSMENT	MANAGEMENT
Assess to determine if one or more adverse signs are present: – Systolic blood pressure <90 mmHg. – Ventricular rate <40 bpm. – Ventricular arrhythmias compromising BP requiring treatment. – Heart failure.	**If one or more signs are present:** ● Follow oxygen guidelines – aim for target saturation within the range 94–98%. ● Gain IV access. ● Administer atropine[a] (**refer to atropine guideline**) and repeat after 3–5 minutes if necessary, or transcutaneous pacing. ● Undertake a 12 lead ECG. ● Transfer to further care.

Risk of asystole: If the patient is initially stable (i.e. no adverse signs are present) or a satisfactory response is achieved with atropine, next determine the risk of asystole.

Assess for risk of asystole – this is indicated by:	If there is a risk of asytole

Assess for risk of asystole – this is indicated by:
– Previous episode of asystole.
– Möbitz II AV block.
– Complete (third degree) AV block, especially with a broad QRS complex or an initial ventricular rate <40 bpm.
– Ventricular standstill >3 seconds.
	If there is a risk of asytole (i.e. one or more signs are present) or the patient shows adverse signs and has not responded satisfactorily to atropine, transvenous pacing is likely to be required. One or more of the following interventions may improve the patient's condition during transport:
	● Transcutaneous pacing should be undertaken if available.
	If transcutaneous pacing is not available:
	● Fist pacing may produce ventricular contraction – give serial rhythmic blows with the closed fist over the lower left sternal edge to pace the heart at a rate of 50–70 bpm.
	NOTES:
	a. **Do not** give atropine to patients with cardiac transplants; their hearts will not respond to vagal blocking by atropine and paradoxical high degree AV block or sinus arrest may result.
	b. Complete heart block with a narrow QRS complex escape rhythm may not require pacing. The ectopic pacemaker (which is situated in the atrioventricular junction) may provide a stable rhythm at an adequate rate.
	c. Initiate transcutaneous pacing (if equipment is available):
	  – if there is no response to atropine
	  – if patient is severely symptomatic, particularly when high degree block (Möbitz type II or third degree AV block) is present.
	NB Transcutaneous pacing may be painful; use analgesia. Verify mechanical capture. Monitor the patient carefully; try to identify the cause of the bradycardia.

[a] Caution – Doses of atropine lower than 500 mcg may paradoxically cause further slowing of ventricular rate. Use atropine cautiously in acute myocardial ischaemia or infarction; an increased rate may worsen ischaemia.

Methodology

For details of the methodology used in the development of this guideline refer to the guideline webpage.

[Further related reading includes 61, 63, 65, 75, 106]

KEY POINTS

Cardiac Rhythm Disturbance

● **In all cases give high concentration oxygen.**
● **Gain venous access.**
● **Always take a defibrillator to any patient with suspected cardiac rhythm disturbance.**
● **Establish cardiac rhythm monitoring as soon as possible preferably with a 12-lead ECG.**
● **Record the ECG rhythm during any intervention and archive. Ensure all ECGs are safely handed over to receiving staff and archive so further copies can be retrieved if necessary.**

Cardiac Rhythm Disturbance

Table 3.4 – ASSESSMENT and MANAGEMENT of:

Tachycardia, Broad Complex Tachycardia and Narrow Complex Tachycardia

ASSESSMENT	MANAGEMENT
Tachycardia ● These guidelines are intended for the treatment of patients who maintain a cardiac output in the presence of the tachycardia. ● **Pulseless** ventricular tachycardia is treated with immediate attempts at defibrillation following the algorithm for the treatment of pulseless VT/VF.	1. Support the ABCs. 2. Administer high levels of supplemental oxygen – aim for a target saturation 94-98%. 3. Gain IV access. 4. Establish cardiac rhythm monitoring. 5. Record and monitor BP and SpO_2. 6. Record a 12-lead ECG if possible, if not, record a rhythm strip. 7. If the rhythm changes at any time, make a further recording. 8. Make a continuous record of the rhythm during any therapeutic intervention (whether a drug or physical manoeuvre like carotid sinus massage). 9. The response to treatment can provide important additional information about the arrhythmia. 10. Identify and treat reversible causes; give analgesia if indicated. 11. Try to define the cardiac rhythm from the ECG. Determine the QRS duration and determine whether the rhythm is regular or irregular. If the QRS duration is 120 msec or more, the rhythm is a broad complex tachycardia. If less than 120 msec, the rhythm is a narrow complex tachycardia.
Broad complex tachycardia	● The rhythm is likely to be ventricular tachycardia, particularly in the context of ischaemic heart disease, patients showing adverse signs (reduced consciousness, SBP <90 mmHg, chest pain or heart failure), or in the peri-arrest situation. ● In all cases, maintain the supportive measures above and monitor the patient during transport. ● Provide an alert/information call according to local guidelines. ● Atrial fibrillation with aberrant conduction may produce an irregular broad complex tachycardia, but the diagnosis is difficult to make with certainty and often requires expert examination of the ECG. This emphasises the importance of recording the ECG when the arrhythmia is present. Ambulance personnel may greatly assist the subsequent diagnosis and management of patients by obtaining good quality ECG recordings. It is advantageous if these can also be archived electronically so that additional copies are available in the future.

Narrow complex tachycardia	If the rhythm is narrow complex (QRS <120 msec) **AND REGULAR**, it is likely to be either:
	  – sinus tachycardia. This is a physiological response, for example to pain, fever, blood loss or heart failure. Treatment is directed towards the cause. Trying to slow the rate is likely to make the situation worse
	  – supraventricular tachycardia (SVT). This is often seen in patients without other forms of heart disease. There may be a history of previous attacks
	  – atrial flutter with regular AV conduction (often 2:1 and a rate of 150 bpm).
	● In cases of SVT, start with vagal manoeuvres. In some cases the patient may be aware of techniques that have terminated previous episodes. The Valsalva manoeuvre (forced expiration against a closed glottis) may be effective and is conveniently achieved (especially in supine patients) by asking the patient to blow into a 20 ml syringe with sufficient force to push back the plunger. If this fails, perform carotid sinus massage provided no carotid bruit is heard on auscultation. A bruit may indicate the presence of atheromatous plaque, rupture of which may cause cerebral embolism and stroke.
	● Record the ECG (preferably multi-lead) during each manoeuvre. If the arrhythmia is successfully terminated by vagal procedures, it is very likely to have been SVT. If the rhythm is atrial flutter, slowing of ventricular rate may occur and allow the identification of flutter waves on the ECG.
	● Maintain the supportive measures above and monitor the patient during transport.
	● **AN IRREGULAR** narrow complex rhythm is most commonly atrial fibrillation, less commonly atrial flutter with variable block. Maintain the supportive measures above and monitor the patient during transport.
	● In all cases, ensure the patient is received into a suitable emergency department maintaining cardiac monitoring throughout. Ensure detailed hand-over to appropriate staff and that ECGs are safely handed over.

1. Introduction

- Patients presenting in prehospital care with an altered level of consciousness (ALoC) provide a major challenge.

- In patients with ALoC it is important to undertake a rapid assessment for **TIME CRITICAL** conditions.

- It is important to understand, where possible, the cause of altered consciousness which can range from diabetic collapse, to factitious illness (refer to Table 3.5 and Table 3.6).

- The patient history may provide valuable insight into the cause of the current condition. Consider the following in formulating your diagnosis; ask relatives or bystanders:

  - is there any history of recent illness or pre-existing chronic illness e.g. diabetes, epilepsy?

  - any past history of mental health problems?

  - any preceding symptoms such as headache, fits, confusion?

  - any history of trauma?

NOTE: Remember, an acute condition may be an exacerbation of a chronic condition or a 'new' illness superimposed on top of a pre-existing problem.

However, often there is little available information – in these circumstances the scene may provide clues to assist in formulating a diagnosis:

- Environmental factors, e.g. extreme cold, possible carbon monoxide sources?

- Evidence of tablets, ampoules, pill boxes, syringes, including domiciliary oxygen (O_2), or administration devices, e.g. nebuliser machines?

- Evidence of alcohol, or medication abuse?

Table 3.5 – RED FLAG CONDITIONS

Condition

Stroke/TIA (**refer to stroke/TIA guideline**).

Head injury (**refer to head trauma guideline**).

Epilepsy (**refer to convulsion guideline**).

Hypoglycaemia (**refer to glycaemic emergencies**).

Hyperglycaemia (**refer to glycaemic emergencies**).

Subarachnoid haemorrhage (**refer to headache**).

Overdose (**refer to overdose and poisoning**).

Table 3.6 – SOME CONDITIONS THAT MAY RESULT IN DLoC (Decreased level of consciousness)

Alterations in pO_2 (hypoxia) and/or pCO_2 (hyper/hypocapnoea)

Inadequate airway.

Inadequate ventilation or depressed respiratory drive.

Persistent hyperventilation.

Table 3.6 – SOME CONDITIONS THAT MAY RESULT IN DLoC *continued*

Inadequate Perfusion

Hypovolaemia.

Cardiac arrhythmias.

Distributive shock.

Neurogenic shock.

Raised intracranial pressure.

Altered metabolic states

Hypoglycaemia and hyperglycaemia.

Intoxication or poisoning

Drug overdose.

Alcohol intoxication.

Carbon monoxide poisoning.

Medical conditions

Stroke.

Subarachnoid haemorrhage.

Epilepsy.

Meningitis.

Hypo/hyperthermia.

Head injury

This guideline contains guidance for managing patients with transient loss of consciousness (section 1) and coma (section 2).

2. SECTION 1 – Transient loss of consciousness (TLoC)

- Transient loss of consciousness (TLoC) may be defined as spontaneous loss of consciousness with complete recovery i.e. full recovery of consciousness without any residual neurological deficit.

- An episode of TLoC is often described as a 'blackout' or a 'collapse'. There are various causes of TLoC, including:

  - cardiovascular disorders (which are the most common)

  - neurological conditions such as epilepsy, and psychogenic attacks.

- The diagnosis of the underlying cause of TLoC is often inaccurate and delayed.

Assessment and Management

For the assessment and management of transient loss of consciousness refer to Table 3.7.

3. SECTION 2 – Coma

Introduction

- Coma is defined as U on the AVPU scale or a Glasgow Coma Score (GCS) (see Appendix) of 8 or less; however, any patient presenting with a decreased level of consciousness (GCS<15) mandates further assessment and, possibly, treatment.

Altered Level of Consciousness

Table 3.7 – ASSESSMENT and MANAGEMENT of:

Transient Loss of Consciousness

ASSESSMENT (ADULTS)	MANAGEMENT (ADULTS)
● Assess ABCD	● If any of the following **TIME CRITICAL** features are present: – major **ABCD** problems – unexpected OR persistent loss of consciousness, then: ● Start correcting any **ABCD** problems. ● Undertake a **TIME CRITICAL** transfer to nearest appropriate receiving hospital. ● Continue patient management en-route. ● Provide an alert/information call.
● Assess for TIME CRITICAL features	
● Ascertain from the patient or witnesses what happened before, during, and after the event	**Record details about:** ● Circumstances of the event. ● The patient's posture immediately before loss of consciousness. ● Prodromal symptoms (such as sweating or feeling warm/hot). ● Appearance (for example, whether eyes were open or shut) and colour of the patient during the event. ● Presence or absence of movement during the event (for example, limb-jerking and its duration). ● Any tongue-biting (record whether the side or the tip of the tongue was bitten). ● Injury occurring during the event (record site and severity). ● Duration of the event (onset to regaining consciousness). ● Presence or absence of confusion during the recovery period. ● Weakness down one side during the recovery period.
● If TLoC is confirmed:	Assess and record: ● Details of any previous TLoC, including number and frequency. ● The patient medical history and any family history of cardiac disease (for example, personal history of heart disease or family history of sudden cardiac death). ● Current medication that may have contributed to TLoC (for example, diuretics). ● Routine observations e.g. pulse rate, respiratory rate and temperature) – repeat if clinically indicated. ● Lying and standing blood pressure if clinically appropriate. ● Other cardiovascular and neurological signs.
● Assess for concomitant injuries	Refer to relevant guideline.
● Assess heart rhythm	Undertake a 12-lead ECG using automated interpretation (refer to local guidelines).
● If an underlying cause is suspected:	● Undertake relevant examinations and investigations, for example, check blood glucose levels if hypoglycaemia is suspected – refer to relevant guideline.
● Assess for uncomplicated faint and situational syncope	Diagnose uncomplicated faint (uncomplicated vasovagal syncope) on the basis of the initial assessment when: ● There are no features that suggest an alternative diagnosis (NOTE: that brief seizure activity can occur during uncomplicated faints and is not necessarily diagnostic of epilepsy). **AND** ● There are features suggestive of uncomplicated faint (the 3 'P's) such as: – **posture** – prolonged standing, or similar episodes that have been prevented by lying down. – **provoking** factors (such as pain or a medical procedure). – **prodromal** symptoms (such as sweating or feeling warm/hot before TLoC). Diagnose situational syncope on the basis of the initial assessment when: ● There are no features from the initial assessment that suggest an alternative diagnosis **AND** ● Syncope is clearly and consistently provoked by straining during micturition (usually while standing) or by coughing or swallowing.
● Care pathway	● Only patients with a GCS 15, with normal blood sugar and responsible adult supervision present may be left at scene e.g. if a diagnosis of uncomplicated faint or situational syncope is made, and there is nothing in the initial assessment to raise clinical or social concern. ● **Advise the patient to take a copy of the patient report form and the ECG record to their GP and follow local protocols to safely hand over clinical responsibility.**

Section 3 Medical Undifferentiated Complaints

Altered Level of Consciousness

- There are a number of causes of coma; refer to Tables 3.5 and 3.6.

Assessment and Management

For the assessment and management of coma refer to Table 3.8.

Table 3.8 – ASSESSMENT and MANAGEMENT of:

Coma (GCS <8)

ASSESSMENT (ADULTS)	MANAGEMENT (ADULTS) NOTE: TAKE A DEFRIBILLATOR TO THE INCIDENT – many calls to unconscious patients are cardiac arrests.
• Assess **ABCD**	• Start correcting any **ABCD** problems. • Undertake a **TIME CRITICAL** transfer to the nearest appropriate receiving hospital. • Continue patient management en-route. • Provide an alert/information call.
• Oxygen	• Administer high levels of supplementary oxygen and aim for a target saturation within the range of 94–98% (**refer to oxygen guideline**).
• Assess for hypoxia	• Apply pulse oximetry. • Obtain IV access if appropriate.
• Assess heart rhythm for arrhythmias	• Undertake a 12-lead ECG.
• Assess level of consciousness	• Assess using the AVPU scale or Glasgow Coma Scale (GCS) (refer to Appendix): A – Alert V – Response to voice P – Responds to painful stimulus U – Unresponsive. • Assess and note pupil size, equality and response to light. • Check for purposeful movement in all four limbs and note sensory function.
• Assess blood glucose level	• If hypoglycaemic (<4.0 mmol/l) or suspected **refer to glycaemic emergencies**.
• Blood pressure	• Measure blood pressure.
• Assess for significant injury especially to the head	• If trauma detected or suspected immobilise spine and **refer to neck and back trauma**.
• Assess for other causes	• Breath for ketones, alcohol and solvents. • Evidence of needle tracks/marks. • Medic alert type jewellery (bracelets or necklets) which detail the patient's primary health risk (e.g. diabetes, anaphylaxis, Addison's disease etc.) – also list a 24-hour telephone number to obtain a more detailed patient history. • Warning stickers, often placed by the front door or the telephone, directing the health professional to a source of detailed information (one current scheme involves storing the patient details in a container in the fridge, as this is relatively easy to find in the house). • Patient-held warning cards, for example, those taking monoamine oxidase inhibitor (MAOI) medication. **For management refer to relevant guideline(s).**
• Assess for respiratory depression	• In cases of severe respiratory depressions **refer to airway and breathing management guideline**. • If the level of consciousness deteriorates or respiratory depression develops in cases where an overdose with opiate-type drugs may be a possibility, consider naloxone (**refer to naloxone guideline**). • In a patient with fixed pinpoint pupils suspect opiate use/overdose. NOTE: any patient with a decreased level of consciousness may have a compromised airway.
• Re-assess ABCD	• Document any changes/note trends in: – GCS – altered neurological function – base line observations..

Altered Level of Consciousness

Appendix

GLASGOW COMA SCALE

Category	Element	Score
Eyes Opening	Spontaneously	4
	To speech	3
	To pain	2
	None	1
Motor Response	Obeys commands	6
	Localises pain	5
	Withdraws from pain	4
	Abnormal flexion	3
	Extensor response	2
	No response to pain	1
Verbal Response	Orientated	5
	Confused	4
	Inappropriate words	3
	Incomprehensible sounds	2
	No verbal response	1

Methodology

For details of the methodology used in the development of this guideline refer to the guideline webpage.

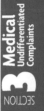

KEY POINTS

Decreased Level of Consciousness

- Maintain patent airway.
- Support ventilation if required.
- Address treatable causes.
- History – obtain as much information as possible.
- Consider an alert/information call.

Dyspnoea [112–119]

1. Introduction

- Dyspnoea is defined as *'a subjective experience of breathing discomfort that consists of qualitatively distinct sensations that vary in intensity'*.
- Dyspnoea is an important clinical symptom that may indicate underlying pathology for a large range conditions (Table 3.9), particularly those affecting the respiratory and cardiac systems.
- Acute episodes of dyspnoea often have a pulmonary or cardiac cause. Asthma, cardiogenic pulmonary oedema, Chronic Obstructive Pulmonary Disease (COPD), pneumonia, cardiac ischaemia, and interstitial lung disease are common causes and account for approximately 85% of all ED cases of dyspnoea. In 15% of cases dyspnoea is unexplained.

2. Incidence

- Dyspnoea is the most common reason for Emergency Department (ED) attendance. Approximately 25–50% of dyspnoea patients presenting to the ED are admitted to hospital.

3. Severity and Outcome

- Dyspnoea is an important clinical symptom which in some circumstances can be severe or life-threatening. Dyspnoea varies in intensity and can be a distressing symptom, especially for patients at the end of life. **For details of the severity and outcome for specific conditions refer to individual guidelines.**

4. Pathophysiology

- Dyspnoea is multi-dimensional process involving physiological and psychological systems.
- The respiratory system is designed to match alveolar ventilation with metabolic demand. Disruption of this process may lead to the conscious awareness of breathing and dyspnoea. Dyspnoea is an uncomfortable sensation and may include chest tightness, air hunger, effortful breathing, the urge to cough and a sense of suffocation.

5. Assessment and Management

- Diagnosis of the underlying cause of the patient's presenting illness can be difficult, and may require in-hospital investigations. Assessment must include a detailed history and a thorough physical examination. For the assessment and management of patients with dyspnoea refer to Table 3.11.

Table 3.9 – CAUSES OF DYSPNOEA

Pulmonary causes	Cardiac causes	Other causes
Acute exacerbation of asthma.	Cardiac arrhythmia.	Anaphylaxis.
Acute heart failure.	Cardiac tamponade.	Chemicals/Poisons.
Bronchiectasis.	Ischaemic heart disease.	Diabetic ketoacidosis.
Acute exacerbation of COPD.	Myocardial infarction.	Diaphragmatic splinting.
Flail chest.	Valvular dysfunction.	Hyperventilation.
Interstitial lung disease.	Pericarditis.	Panic attack/anxiety.
Lung/lobar collapse.		Severe hypovolaemia.
Massive haemothorax.		Metabolic causes.
Pleural effusion.		Obesity.
Pneumonia.		Pain.
Pneumothorax.		Severe anaemia.
Pulmonary embolism.		
Upper airway obstruction.		

Table 3.10 – DIFFERENTIAL DIAGNOSIS FOR COMMON CONDITIONS

Condition	Symptoms	Signs	Asculation sounds	History
Acute Asthma (refer to asthma guideline)	Dyspnoea Cough Unable to complete sentences	Wheeze Tachypnoea Tachycardia Pulsus paradoxus Hyperresonant chest Accessory muscle use	Decreased or absent breath sounds if severe	Previous asthma Recent increase in inhaler use Allergen exposure
Acute Coronary Syndrome (refer to acute coronary syndrome guideline)	Central chest pain for >15 minutes constricting or crushing that radiates to left arm/neck	Wheeze Tachycardia Arrhythmia	Crackles	Symptoms suggestive of ischaemic heart disease and previous investigations for chest pain
Acute Heart Failure (refer to heart failure guideline)	Dyspnoea especially on exertion Orthopnoea/paroxysmal nocturnal dyspnoea Cough producing frothy, white, or pink phlegm	Peripheral oedema Tachycardia	Rales Heart murmur Crepitations	IHD Hypertension History of heart failure
Anaphylaxis (refer to allergic reactions including anaphylaxis guideline)	Dyspnoea Dysphagia Chest tightness	Tachycardia Tachypnoea Wheeze Erythema Urticaria Angioedema	Decreased breath sounds	Allergen exposure
Chronic Obstructive Pulmonary Disease (COPD) (refer to COPD guideline)	Progressive dyspnoea Wheezing Chest tightness Cough – purulent sputum	Wheeze Cyanosis	Rales	Smoking >35 years of age
Foreign Body Airway Obstruction (FBAO) (refer to FBAO guideline)	Dyspnoea	Wheeze Clutching at neck Silent cough	Audible stridor	Eating – especially fish, meat, or poultry
Pneumonia (refer to medical emergencies guideline)	Dyspnoea Fever Cough	Tachycardia	Rhonchi	Smoking IHD
Pneumothorax (refer to thoracic trauma guideline)	Dyspnoea Sudden onset pleuritic chest pain	Dyspnoea Sudden onset pleuritic chest pain	Decreased breath sounds	Trauma Previous pneumothorax COPD Asthma Smoking
Pulmonary Embolism (refer to pulmonary embolism guideline)	Dyspnoea Pleuritic chest pain Cough Possible DVT Leg oedema	Tachycardia Tachypnoea Fever ECG: Non-specific ST wave changes	Focal rales	Prolonged immobilisation Recent surgery Thrombotic disease

Dyspnoea

Table 3.11 – ASSESSMENT and MANAGEMENT of:

Dyspnoea

NB Take a defibrillator at the earliest opportunity and keep with the patient until hand-over

ASSESSMENT	MANAGEMENT
● Assess **ABCD**	● If any of the following **TIME CRITICAL** features present: – major **ABCD** problems. – extreme breathing difficulty (**refer to medical emergencies guideline**) – cyanosis (**refer to medical emergencies guideline**) – hypoxia – SpO$_2$ <95% or not responding to oxygen therapy (**refer to oxygen guideline**) – features of life-threatening asthma (**refer to asthma guideline**) – features of tension pneumothorax or major chest trauma (**refer to thoracic trauma guideline**) – acute myocardial infarction (**refer to acute coronary syndrome guideline**) – anaphylaxis (**refer to allergic reactions including anaphylaxis guideline**) – loss of consciousness (**refer to altered level of consciousness guideline**), then: ● Start correcting **A** and **B** and undertake a **TIME CRITICAL** transfer to nearest receiving hospital. ● Continue patient management en-route. ● Provide an alert/information call.
● Ask the patient if they have an individualised treatment plan	● Follow the treatment plan if available. ● The patient will often be able to guide their care.
● If non-**TIME CRITICAL** – obtain a thorough history to help identify cause of dyspnoea	**Specifically assess:** ● Respiratory rate. ● Effort and effectiveness of ventilation – rate and depth. ● Degree of dyspnoea. ● Length of difficulty breathing – sudden or gradual onset? ● Pain associated with breathing – any pattern of breathing/depth of respiration? ● Do certain positions exacerbate breathing, e.g. unable to lie down, must sit upright? ● Does the patient have a cough? ● If yes, is the cough productive: – **sputum or bubbling:** consider infection or heart failure – **frothy white/pink sputum:** consider acute heart failure – **yellow/green sputum:** consider chest infection – **haemoptysis:** consider PE, chest infection, or carcinoma of the lung. ● Has the patient increased their medication recently? ● Signs of anaphylaxis: – itchy rash – facial swelling – circulatory collapse.
● Percuss the chest	● To determine if there are collections of fluid in the lungs.
● Auscultate the chest	● To determine adequacy of air entry on both sides of the chest. ● To determine chest sounds: – audible wheeze on expiration – consider asthma, ACS, anaphylaxis, COPD or heart failure (especially in older patients with no history of asthma) – audible stridor (upper airway narrowing) consider anaphylaxis, or FBAO – crepitations (fine crackling in lung bases) – ACS, heart failure – rhonchi (harsher, rattling sound) indicating collections of fluid in larger airways – pneumonia.

Consider possible causes (refer to Table 3.9 and 3.10) if there is a history of:

Consider specific respiratory problems:	● Asthma – consider acute exacerbation (**refer to asthma guideline**). ● COPD – consider acute exacerbation (**refer to COPD guideline**). ● Pulmonary embolism (**refer to PE guideline**). ● Heart failure e.g. left ventricular failure, right ventricular failure, congestive heart failure, cor pulmonale, hypertension – consider acute exacerbation (**refer to heart failure guideline**). ● Other respiratory disorder? ● Smoking.

Table 3.11 – ASSESSMENT and MANAGEMENT of:

Dyspnoea *continued*

ASSESSMENT	MANAGEMENT
Consider specific cardiovascular problems:	● Acute coronary syndrome e.g. STEMI, NSTEMI? NB Some patients with acute myocardial infarction may have breathlessness as their only symptom (**refer to ACS guideline**). ● Constricting pain (**refer to ACS guideline**). ● Angina (**refer to ACS guideline**). ● Ischaemic heart disease. ● Valvular dysfunction/congenital heart problems.
Consider other conditions:	● Recent trauma (**refer to thoracic trauma guideline**). ● Recent surgery or immobilisation (**refer to PE guideline**). ● Hyperventilation – often accompanied by numbness and tingling in the limbs and around the mouth (**refer to hyperventilation syndrome guideline**) NB Ensure other more serious conditions are excluded before considering this diagnosis.
● Known cause	● If cause of dyspnoea known follow relevant guideline.
● Unknown cause	● If cause of dyspnoea unknown **refer to medical emergencies guideline** and follow management below.
● ECG	● Undertake a 12-lead ECG.
● Oxygen	● Administer supplemental oxygen if indicated (refer to oxygen guideline).
● Ventilation	Consider assisted ventilation at a rate of 12–20 breaths per minute if (**refer to airway and breathing management guideline**): ● SpO_2 is <90% on high concentration O_2. ● Respiratory rate is <10 or >30. ● Expansion is inadequate.
● Fluid	● Administer fluid as required (refer to intravascular fluid therapy guideline).
● Pain management	● Administer pain relief if indicated (**refer to pain management guideline**).
● Position	● Position for comfort – usually sitting upright.
● Degree of dyspnoea	● Re-assess the response to using the visual analogue scale or other locally agreed scale.
● Transfer to further care	● All patients with an unexplained cause of dyspnoea. ● Where the cause is known refer to the relevant guideline for care pathway.

Methodology

For details of the methodology used in the development of this guideline refer to the guideline webpage.

KEY POINTS

Dyspnoea

● **Is breathlessness of respiratory, cardiac, both or other causes?**
● **Consider time critical causes.**
● **Assess degree of dyspnoea and response to treatment using a visual analogue score.**
● **Consider possible causes and refer to relevant guidelines for assessment and management.**

Headache [120–123]

1. Introduction
- Headache is a common condition presenting in pre-hospital care.
- Most headaches are simple and not serious, but care must be taken to ensure that **TIME CRITICAL** conditions are not missed. A **detailed history is vital** when dealing with headache, as aetiology may go back hours, days, months (or even years in relation to family history or childhood illness; for example, tumours).

2. History
- Exclude the following or refer to the specific guidelines for:
  - **stroke**
  - **head injury**
  - **glycaemic episode**.
- Assess the **SOCRATES** of the pain:
  - **S**ite – where exactly is the pain
  - **O**nset – what was the patient doing when the pain came on
  - **C**haracter – what does the pain feel like
  - **R**adiates – where does the pain spread to
  - **A**ssociated symptoms – e.g. nausea, dizziness
  - **T**iming – how long has the patient had pain
  - **E**xacerbating/relieving factors – what makes it better or worse
  - **S**everity – obtain an initial pain score.
- Key questions for patients with headache:
  - Is this the worst headache ever?
  - Is it different from your usual headache?
  - Is this a new headache?

Headaches can be broadly defined as primary or secondary.

Primary headaches are those which occur spontaneously (simple headache); in response to a lifelong condition (e.g. migraine); 'tension type' headaches (various aetiologies[a]) or cluster headache (severe short lasting headache). These should not considered as being pathophysiological; that being normal for the patient.

Secondary headaches are secondary to illness or injury and are pathological in origin, for instance; head trauma (skull fracture), infective origin (i.e. meningitis); intracranial haemorrhage (i.e. spontaneous subarachnoid bleed or sub dural bleed following trauma) or vascular (i.e. temporal arteritis).

- It is difficult to accurately differentiate between a simple headache, which requires no treatment, and a potentially more serious condition. Table 3.12 lists **'red flag'** symptoms that require the patient to undergo hospital assessment. NB This does not mean that any patient presenting without these symptoms is automatically safe to be left at home.

Consideration should be given to transferring all first presentations of severe headache to the emergency department for further investigation.

[a] Tension type or chronic daily headaches can be caused by medication overuse or withdrawal. These should be considered to be secondary headache.

Table 3.12 – RED FLAG SIGNS AND SYMPTOMS

Signs and symptoms

Headache of severe, sudden (thunderclap) onset.

Headache localised to the vertex.

Escalating headache of unusual nature.

Changed visual acuity.

Meningeal irritation.

Changed mental state and inappropriate behaviour.

Newly presenting ataxia.

NB Multiple red flags increase significantly the risk of serious pathology.

3. Incidence
Refer to Table 3.13 for details of the incidence of different types of primary headache.

Table 3.13 – INCIDENCE BY TYPE FOR PRIMARY HEADACHES

Type	Incidence
Migraine	6–8% in Men 15–18% in Women
(Episodic) Tension Type Headache	Up to 70% of whole population During life Most prevalent up to age of 30
Cluster Headache	Less than 1 in every 1000 people

- Secondary headache data is not meaningful in the emergency setting as the intention is not to exclude these potentially more serious presentations in the prehospital environment.

4. Severity and Outcome
- The severity of headaches varies from patient to patient in terms of the pain the patient experiences. Although the pain may be the primary concern of the patient, it may belie the true severity of the underlying cause.
- The outcome for patients presenting through the 999 system for headache will be varied as the cause of the headache, the clinical significance of the headache and the progression are all dependent on the presenting factors.
- Patients may deteriorate rapidly if they have a space occupying condition (e.g. haemorrhage resulting in mass effect).
- Clinicians must ensure that the patient receives the safest pathway of care and it is always better to be cautious, especially in children and those patients who are on their own.
- It is preferable to be cautious when dealing with patients with headaches, as diagnosis can be challenging.

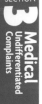

SECTION **3** Medical Undifferentiated Complaints

Headache

- Where patients are not conveyed, follow-up care MUST be arranged. Always liaise with the patient's GP (or out-of-hours doctor) to discuss onward care. Ensure that, where practicable, the patient is not left alone whilst awaiting follow-up.

5. Assessment and Management

- For the assessment and management of headache refer to Table 3.14.

Methodology

For details of the methodology used in the development of this guideline refer to the guideline webpage.

KEY POINTS

Headache

- **Crescendo headaches are significant.**
- **Headaches with different or unusual characteristic are significant.**
- **Migraineurs are at risk of serious intracranial events.**
- **In headache, blood pressure must be checked.**
- **Any persistent headache or any headache associated with altered conscious levels or unusual behaviour is significant.**
- **Sinister headaches may or may not be accompanied by neurology. Do not exclude simply based on physical examination – HISTORY IS KEY.**

Table 3.14 – ASSESSMENT and MANAGEMENT of:

Headache

ASSESSMENT	MANAGEMENT
● Assess ABCD	● Start correcting any ABCD problems – **refer to medical emergencies guideline**.
● Specifically assess:	
Levels of consciousness	● Assess AVPU: NB The only normal GCS is 15. A – Alert V – Responds to voice P – Responds to painful stimulus U – Unresponsive.
Temperature	
Pulse rate	● Do not administer supplemental oxygen unless the patient is hypoxaemic (SpO_2 <94%) (**refer to oxygen guideline**).
Respiratory rate	
Blood pressure	● Measure systolic/diastolic.
Blood glucose level	
Record pain score	● Consider symptomatic pain relief for clinically benign headaches using appropriate drug. ● **Avoid morphine** due to potential side effects which could worsen the patient's condition and/or hinder further assessment: – Respiratory depression – Nausea and vomiting – Drowsiness – Pupillary constriction.

Table 3.14 – ASSESSMENT and MANAGEMENT of:

Headache *continued*

ASSESSMENT	MANAGEMENT
Assess for: ● Any evidence of a rash. ● Neck stiffness and photophobia (light sensitivity of eyes). ● Loss of function or altered sensation. ● Flushed face but cool, pale trunk and extremities.	
● Assess for red flag symptoms (refer to Table 3.12)	● Undertake a **TIME CRITICAL** transfer to nearest suitable receiving hospital. ● Provide an alert/information call.

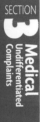

Mental Disorder [18, 19, 124–130]

1. Introduction

Definitions

- Problems and disorders that affect people's mental health are often referred to colloquially as 'mental health problems'. Such broad use of this term gives little indication of the severity of their conditions or of the likely courses of events in particular patients' circumstances. Sometimes, people who have a severe mental disorder are described as having a mental illness.

- This guideline uses the term 'mental disorder' to distinguish those conditions that are primarily related to people's mental ill health from the very common and understandable anxieties and emotional reactions of people who are casualties or who require ambulance services for any other reason. These more general and frequent psychosocial responses to accidents, injuries and illness are better referred to as 'distress' rather than calling them mental health problems or disorders. People who are distressed should be managed according to principles of psychological first aid.

- This guideline provides general advice about matters related to people who have mental disorders. There have been rapid developments in recent years of knowledge and agreement about the most effective ways to care for people who are distressed. Therefore the future intention is to develop several additional guidelines relating to distress, public mental health, and mental disorders.

The Prevalence and Nature of Mental Disorders

- Mental disorders are very common at all ages. They affect one person in four at some point during their lives. They vary from mild anxiety, phobic states and mild depression to severe disorders including, unipolar and bipolar affective disorders (otherwise termed depression, hypomania and mania), serious problems from misuse of alcohol and drugs, and schizophrenia. Some of the severe disorders may be recurrent, relapsing and remitting, and enduring. Comorbidity (having more than one disorder) is common. Many disorders, for example, are provoked by, maintained by, or associated with consumption of alcohol and other substances. Not uncommonly, people who develop mental disorders may present first to the emergency and ambulance services. Commonly, ambulance services meet people who have had a mental disorder previously, but who develop a new episode or an exacerbation of a chronic problem. Ambulance services may also be called to people who are currently in care and treatment with the mental health services.

2. Assessment

- Most patients have insight into their problems. Others may have impaired insight or lack it. Some patients may have physical diseases or substance-related (including conditions related to prescribed, and non-prescribed licit or illicit substances) causes for their altered mental states that, usually, resolve with treatment of the underlying problem.

- Some patients may agree voluntarily to accept help whether or not they have insight and/or capacity.

However, other people may need to be persuaded to receive an assessment and treatment, and, possibly compelled to do so against their will, usually using powers given by the Mental Health Act 1983 (if in England or Wales).

Approach

- Some patients may be upset, distressed, anxious, suspicious, disorientated or agitated when faced by ambulance clinicians. While considering their own safety, the approach taken by ambulance crews to patients whose behaviour appears concerning should be calm and gradual, relying on their persuasive powers to achieve a conversation and then to conduct an assessment. Non-verbal indicators such as patients' appearances or levels of agitation should be noted as part of the assessments of risk, and patients' conditions and needs. Additionally, the environments in which patients are found may give important clues (e.g. the presence of certain types of medication or chaotic living conditions).

- Do not rush. Distressed people and people who have a mental disorder may react badly to rush and hurry. Take time to explain your actions to both the patients and their relatives and always endeavour to be honest about what you are going to do and what is likely to happen.

History

- As with all assessments, a history outlining the nature of the complaint or problem is required. This should be carefully explored, with particular reference to previous mental health service involvement, medication that has been prescribed and whether or not the patient has been taking it, level of alcohol use and possible substance use or misuse. Details of the nature of the problem, the patient's mood or affect, any unusual beliefs, the presence of hallucinations or delusions (and whether visual or auditory), and the patient's thoughts about their experiences and problems are key.

Examination

- Physical illnesses can present as an apparent mental disorder and vice versa. Furthermore, research shows that people who have enduring mental disorders may also have comorbid physical disorders and that their physical healthcare may be less good than that of other people in the general population. These are all important reasons why someone who appears to have a mental disorder should have a thorough clinical examination of both their physical state and their mental state. Testing is required to exclude causes of changed behaviour such as hypoglycaemia, intoxication, head injury, meningitis, or encephalitis. As part of the assessment of mental state, note should be taken of the features given below:

ABNORMAL APPEARANCE, FEELINGS OR BEHAVIOUR

- Anxiety.
- Agitation.
- Low, very low, or apparently raised mood.
- Problems with orientation in time, place and/or person.

- Poor attention, concentration or distraction.
- Poor memory.
- Unusual form and/or content of speech.
- The thoughts that the patient expresses.
- Any strongly held beliefs that a patient expresses that are out of keeping with their culture, background and the present circumstances that might raise the possibility of delusion.
- Any apparently unusual perceptions that the patient might be experiencing that might indicate intoxication, drug effects, hallucinations, or brain injury.

- A physical examination should be undertaken and recorded. Other findings are established from the nature of the consultation, other contextual circumstances and events and by observation. They should be recorded. All of these observations, even if apparently normal, provide very important comparative information for other clinicians who examine the same patient later.

CAPACITY AND CONSENT

- Each ambulance service should have a formal process or protocol for establishing the capacity of patients to consent to assessment and to being transported for further care (for example, the requirements that apply to assessing capacity in England and Wales, are stated in the Mental Capacity Act 2005 and its code of practice).

- There is little difficulty when patients are willing to accept the assistance that they are offered. If they have capacity and decide that they do not wish to accept the assessment or treatment offered, then, usually, their decision must be respected. It is good practice to inform the patient's general practitioner, and their community psychiatric nurse and social worker, if there is one, about this decision. The process should be thoroughly documented using the relevant Ambulance Trust's processes.

Application for powers to compulsorily assess and treat mentally disordered patients in the face of their refusal

- Readers should be aware that there are different laws relating to capacity and consent, and different mental health primary and secondary legislation in England and Wales, Northern Ireland, and Scotland. This guideline cannot cover in detail any of that legislation, the associated codes of practice and governmental guidance. Furthermore, there is also the Human Rights Act 1998 to consider. Therefore, this guideline provides a very brief overview of some facets of the process in England and Wales.

- The Mental Health Act 1983 (England and Wales) was substantially amended in 2007. The secondary legislation to that amended Act is different in England and Wales. Readers are referred to the amended Act, the separate codes of practice for England and Wales, and a short guide published in 2011 for more information about the Act and its application.

- In England and Wales, application for patients' detention, and compulsory assessment and treatment does not turn directly on tests of capacity, but on certain features of the nature and degree of their mental state, any mental disorder thought to be present at initial assessment, and certain circumstances relating to their needs and risks to themselves and others. Most patients who are detained using the Mental Health Act 1983 as subsequently amended in 2007 do have impaired capacity, for their mental disorder at least, but it is possible that some may not. Also, some incapacitous patients may not satisfy the conditions for compulsion. Therefore, assessment of patients in this regard is a specialised matter. Ambulance clinicians should seek the advice of a doctor and/or an Approved Mental Health Professional (AMHP) if they think that a patient is in this situation.

- In the event of a patient refusing to consent, and, provided that certain specific conditions are satisfied, legislation allows for compulsory admission of patients to an appropriate facility for assessment under a section of the Mental Health Act 1983 (England and Wales as subsequently amended in 2007) or by using legislation for similar purposes in Northern Ireland and Scotland. However, the job titles, processes, and conditions differ across the jurisdictions that comprise the United Kingdom.

- Most applications for assessment and treatment under compulsion in England and Wales are made by AMHPs after their own assessments. Application also requires recommendations from at least one, but usually two medical practitioners. In the majority of circumstances, at least one of the medical practitioners is required to have special experience in assessing and managing mental disorders that is substantiated by their recognition under section 12 of the Mental Health Act 1983 (England and Wales).

- Conducting the process of application can take time. Due note should be taken of capacity or its impairment in particular cases as a component of assessments of patients' mental states and the potential requirement for application for compulsory powers.

- Reasonable and proportionate steps can be taken to prevent patients from immediately harming themselves or posing a risk to others while awaiting assessment, but if physical restraint is required, the police should be involved. In England and Wales, authority to move patients against their will must come from the AMHP who acquires the power to convey patients and to request the support of ambulance staff and/or the police once they have made a formal application using the Act. Moving some patients may require the assistance of the police.

3. Management

Risk Assessment

- A full risk assessment usually involves a thorough mental state examination and physical examination. Ambulance clinicians may not be able to carry out all aspects in emergency circumstances.

- One of the most common and concerning aspects of risk assessment relates to a patient's potential for self-harm and, possibly, suicide. This guideline includes a brief method for assessing these risks in the Appendix.

Violence

- Ambulance clinicians should assess their personal risk when approaching upset, distressed, disorientated, agitated, or threatening patients. If the risk is considered significant, the police should be called to assist. Safe restraint can only be provided safely with sufficient trained people. The police should be called.

Specific Mental Disorders

ANXIETY, AFFECTIVE AND OBSESSIVE COMPULSIVE DISORDERS

- Anxiety and affective (mood) disorders are the most common groups of problems. Sometimes, they may appear to represent the extremes of normal emotions and behaviours. Anxiety disorders, panic disorder, phobias, depression, and obsessional conditions fall into this category. They may all cause considerable distress.

PSYCHOSIS

- Psychosis is a general term that describes a group of disorders in which patients tend to be severely distressed and may not appear to be rational. Sometimes, they may interpret events in a manner that does not appear to be appropriately in touch with reality. They may have strongly-held beliefs that are unusual or unsubstantiated by events. In this situation, they may be described as having delusions. Patients may perceive voices that are not heard by others (called auditory hallucinations). Thus, delusions, hallucinations, and impaired insight may appear to assessors to be core symptoms. However, before ascribing these experiences to mental disorder, ambulance clinicians should be aware that a selection of them might occur in the case of serious physical disorders.

MANIA AND HYPOMANIA

- People who have hypomania and mania are often overactive. Some of them may have not slept properly for days. They tend to be persistent in their behaviour. They have rapid thought processes and tend to tire their relatives and friends. Patients with mania often suffer from delusions, including delusions of grandeur.

SCHIZOPHRENIA

- Schizophrenia is a common and often severe mental illness. It may present acutely with severe change in behaviour or insidiously as a slow, but progressive change over a period of time. Patients may be deluded. This means that they may hold strong beliefs that appear inappropriate to the assessor in the context of the patient's life, culture, and circumstances. Auditory hallucinations (false perceptions in which the patient can hear voices, not heard by others, that are talking to them or to another about them) may be a feature, and can cause great distress. Their behaviour may be reported by other people as seriously disordered or irrational, or the patient may show patterns of behaviour and speech that suggest that they might have thought disorder, delusions, and/or hallucinations, or patients may report these experiences.

- As stated earlier, ambulance clinicians should be aware that some of these features can also occur in the presence of physical disease, intoxication with licitly or illicitly obtained substances, and as a consequence of taking psychotropic drugs.

PARANOIA

- Paranoia can be a feature of depression, schizophrenia and other severe mental disorders. As usually defined, the term describes a state in which a patient suffers delusions of persecution or has delusions associated with great sensitivity and wariness of other people and their intentions. People so affected may be extremely suspicious and they can react unpredictably, aggressively or violently. Care should be taken to avoid provoking them.

PSYCHOTROPIC DRUGS THAT ARE USED TO TREAT PEOPLE WHO HAVE MENTAL DISORDERS

- Table 3.15 provides a very brief overview of three categories of drugs that are used to treat people who have mental disorders.

- Some of the more modern drugs may require close supervision of certain parameters of the physical health of people who take them.

- The brevity of this table and the possible side effects of psychotropic medications are two reasons why ambulance clinicians are strongly advised to consult the British National Formulary or another source of information that is approved by their employers when they assess people who are taking psychotropic medications.

Table 3.15 – DRUGS USED IN MENTAL HEALTH

Anxiolytics

Benzodiazepines are among the most frequently used drugs in this category. They can be used to induce sleep and also to reduce anxiety. In excess, they are principally sedative.

Antidepressants

This category of medication includes a number of different groups of drugs that are used over weeks and months rather than days, and some types may take up to three weeks to begin to show an effect. Some of the older drugs, the tricyclic antidepressants, are very dangerous in excess. Agitation followed by sedation and cardiac arrhythmias are the most significant effects in poisoning. The newer antidepressants, such as the selective serotonin reuptake inhibitors (SSRIs) are used much more often now. They too can cause significant side effects. Monoamine oxidase inhibitors (MAOIs) are now used rarely and only then by people who are resistant to more recently developed drugs. However, this group of antidepressants is raised here because it has an important range of severe drug interactions and, in the ambulance context, morphine must be avoided. When they interact with other drugs, they can cause a dangerous increase in blood pressure.

Table 3.15 – DRUGS USED IN MENTAL HEALTH *continued*

Antipsychotics

These drugs are also known as neuroleptics. They can be taken orally or given by injection and are powerful tranquillisers. They can be used in acute situations to sedate, but are most frequently used in the medium- to long-term management of people who have disorders such as schizophrenia and other psychoses.

COMPULSORY ASSESSMENT, TREATMENT AND DETENTION USING POWERS AFFORDED BY LEGISLATION RELATING TO CONSENT AND MENTAL HEALTH

- This guideline stresses the importance of ambulance service staff conducting themselves in accordance with the law that applies in the jurisdiction in which they work.

- However, this guideline does not include more than very general information and advice relating to consent or advice about legislation for caring for, assessing, treating, and transporting non-capacitous or mentally ill people under compulsion. Instead, this guideline recommends that staff of ambulance services should proceed in accordance with advice on legal matters and consent that is provided by their employers.

- The decision to restrict advice in this domain has been made because there are four legal jurisdictions and four governments in the UK that are responsible for setting policy on consent and related matters in their countries. As a result, there are a number of different legal measures and powers, policies, frameworks, and codes of practice that apply in the jurisdictions that comprise the UK. Also, the differing provisions for children and adults across the jurisdictions complicate the situation regarding providing brief advice that is applicable across the UK.

- The position taken in this guideline is that staff of the ambulance services should refer to their employers any questions or concerns that they might have as regards gaining lawful consent from their patients, application of the mental health legislation and associated codes of practice that apply in the jurisdiction in which they work for assessing, caring for and treating apparently incapacitous persons.

Methodology

For details of the methodology used in the development of this guideline refer to the guideline webpage.

KEY POINTS

Mental Disorder

In a situation in which there is a distressed patient who appears to be suffering from a mental disorder:

- **Ambulance clinicians should consider their personal safety before approaching the patient.**
- **History and examination should include an assessment of both the mental state and the physical state of the patient.**
- **Capacity to consent must be assessed.**
- **In certain circumstances in which risk of harm to the patient or to others is thought to be related to a disordered mental state, the patient should be protected from causing further harm to themselves or others (in England and Wales, for example, if a patient refuses consent to assessment, treatment or care, an AMHP and a doctor should be asked to assess the patient and consider application for the patient's assessment and care under compulsion using the powers given by a section of the Mental Health Act 1983 as amended in 2007 – there are similar provisions available, although the terms used and the laws and legal tests used may be different in Northern Ireland and Scotland).**

Appendix – Suicide and Self-Harm Risk Assessment Form

Item	Value	Patient Score
Sex: female	0	
Sex: male	1	
Age: less than 19 years old	1	
Age: greater than 45 years old	1	
Depression/hopelessness	1	
Previous attempts at self-harm	1	
Evidence of excess alcohol/illicit drug use	1	
Rational thinking absent	1	
Separated/divorced/widowed	1	
Organised or serious self-harm	1	
No close/reliable family, job or active religious affiliation	1	
Determined to repeat or ambivalent	1	

Total score of patient

< 3 = Low Risk
3–6 = Medium Risk
> 6 = High Risk

1. Introduction

Although the care of a wide range of medical conditions will be quite specific to the presenting condition, there are general principles of care that apply to most medical cases, regardless of underlying condition(s).

2. Patient Assessment

In order to gather as much relevant information as possible, without delaying care, the accepted format of history taking is as follows:

- Presenting complaint — why the patient or carer called for help at this time.

- The history of presenting complaint — details of when the problem started, exacerbating factors and previous similar episodes.

- Direct questioning about associated symptoms, by system. Ask about all appropriate systems.

- Past medical history, including current medication.

- Family history.

- Social history.

Combined with a good physical examination (primary and secondary survey), this format of history taking should ensure that you correctly identify those patients who are time critical, urgent or routine. The history taken must be fully documented. In many cases, a well-taken history will point to the diagnosis.

The presence of 'Medic Alert' type jewellery (bracelets or necklets) can provide information on the patient's pre-existing health risk that may be relevant to the current medical emergency.

I. A primary survey should be undertaken for **ALL** patients as this will rapidly identify patients with actual or potential **TIME CRITICAL** conditions.

II. A secondary survey is a more thorough 'head-to-toe' assessment of the patient. It should be undertaken following completion of the primary survey, where time permits. The secondary survey will usually be undertaken during transfer to further care; however, in some patients with time critical conditions, it may not be possible to undertake the secondary survey before arrival at further care.

I. Primary Survey

- The primary survey should take 60–90 seconds for assessment and follow **ABCD** approach (Table 3.17). Document the vital signs and the time the observations were taken.

- Assessment and Management should proceed in a 'stepwise' manner and abnormalities should be managed as they are encountered, i.e. do not move onto breathing and circulation until the airway is managed (**refer to airway and breathing management guideline**). Every time an intervention has been carried out, re-assess the patient.

- If any of the features/conditions listed in Table 3.16 are identified during the primary survey or immediately un-correctable ABCD problems, then the patient should be considered **TIME CRITICAL. CORRECT A AND B PROBLEMS ON SCENE, THEN**

UNDERTAKE A TIME CRITICAL transfer **TO NEAREST SUITABLE RECEIVING HOSPITAL**.

- If airway and breathing cannot be corrected, or haemorrhage cannot be controlled, evacuate immediately, continuing resuscitation as appropriate en-route.

- Provide an alert/information call.

- Continue patient assessment and management en-route.

Table 3.16 – TIME CRITICAL FEATURES/CONDITIONS

- **Adrenal crisis (including Addisonian crisis)** – is a life-threatening condition resulting from adrenal insufficiency – **refer to hydrocortisone guidelines**.

- **Airway impairment.**

- **Anaphylaxis** – is a life-threatening condition resulting from an immune response to an allergen – **refer to allergic reactions including anaphylaxis guideline**.

- Any patient with **GCS <15** – check the airway and blood glucose levels in all patients with a decreased GCS.

- **Cardiac chest pain.**

- **Cardiogenic shock.**

- **Sepsis** – is a life-threatening condition resulting from infection. Suspect sepsis in patients who have signs and symptoms of infection, a systolic blood pressure below 90 mmHg and tachypnoea – **refer to intravascular fluid guidelines**.

- **Failing ventilation.**

- **Severe breathlessness** – unable to complete a sentence.

- **Severe haemorrhage** – **refer to trauma emergencies in adults overview guideline** and gastrointestinal bleeding.

- **Severe hypotension** – due to bradycardia or extreme tachycardia.

- **Status epilepticus** – is a life-threatening condition defined as a convulsion lasting >30 minutes – **refer to convulsion guidelines**.

NB This list is not inclusive; patients with other signs may also be time critical; this is where the clinical judgement of the paramedic is important.

Table 3.17 – ASSESSMENT and MANAGEMENT of:

Medical Emergencies

- All stages should be considered but some may be omitted if not considered appropriate.

At each stage consider the need for:
- **TIME CRITICAL** transfer to further care.
- Early senior clinical support.

STAGE	ASSESSMENT	MANAGEMENT
A	**AIRWAY** – assess the airway (**refer to airway and breathing guideline**). **Look for** obvious obstructions e.g. teeth/dentures, foreign bodies, vomit, blood. **Listen for** noisy airflow e.g. snoring, gurgling or no airflow. **Feel for** air movement.	Correct any airway problems immediately by: ● Positioning – head tilt, chin lift, jaw thrust. ● Suction (if available and appropriate). ● Oropharyngeal airway. ● Nasopharyngeal airway. ● Laryngeal mask airway (if appropriate). ● Endotracheal intubation (if appropriate). ● Needle cricothyroidotomy.

B

BREATHING – expose the chest and assess (**refer to airway and breathing guideline**).

Look for:
- Respiratory rate (<10 or >30).
- Respiratory depth.
- Breaths per minute.
- Adequacy and depth of chest movements.
- Symmetry of chest movement.
- Equality of air entry.
- Effectiveness of ventilation.
- Canosis or pallor peripherally and centrally.
- Position of trachea in suprasternal notch.

Feel for:
- Any instability of chest wall and note any areas of tenderness and note depth and equality of chest movement.

Note any:
- Wheezing, noisy respiration on inspiration or expiration.
- Stridor (higher pitched noise on inspiration), suggestive of upper respiratory obstruction.

Listen for:
- Altered breathing patterns with a stethoscope – ask the patient to take deep breaths in and out briskly through their mouth if possible – listen on both sides of the chest:
    - above the nipples in the mid-clavicular line
    - laterally in the mid-axillary line
    - below the shoulder blade (front and back).
- Auscultate to assess air entry and compare sides.
- Wheezing on expiration.
- Percuss for dullness or hyperresonance.
- Crepitations at the rear of the chest (crackles, heard low down in the lung fields at the rear – may indicate fluid in the lung in heart failure).
- Additional crackles and wheeze on inspiration may be associated with inhalation of blood or vomit.

Percuss for:
- Dullness or hyperresonance.

MANAGEMENT (B)
- Correct any breathing problems immediately.
- If breathing is absent refer to appropriate resuscitation guidelines. If the breathing is inadequate **refer to airway and breathing guideline**.
- Treat underlying cause of unilateral chest movement if tension pneumothorax.
- Administer supplemental oxygen if the patient is hypoxaemic – aim for target saturation (SpO_2) within the range of 94–98% except for patients with COPD or other risk factors for hypercapnia (refer to oxygen guideline).
- In patients with a decreased level of consciousness (Glasgow Coma Scale (GCS) <15) administer the initial supplemental oxygen dose until the vital signs are normal, then reduce the oxygen dose and aim for a target saturation (SpO_2) within the range of 94–98%.
- In patients with sickle cell crisis administer supplemental oxygen via an appropriate mask/cannula until a reliable SpO_2 measurement is available; then adjust the oxygen flow to aim for target saturation within the range of 94–98%.

Consider assisted ventilation at a rate of 12–20 respirations per minute if any of the following are present:
- Oxygen saturation (SpO_2) <90% on levels of supplemental oxygen.
- Respiratory rate <10 or >30 bpm.
- Inadequate chest expansion.

NB **Restraint (positional) Asphyxia** – If the patient is required to be physically restrained (e.g. by police officers) in order to prevent them injuring themselves or others, or for the purpose of being detained under the Mental Health Act, then it is paramount that the method of restraint allows both for a patent airway and adequate respiratory volume. **Under these circumstances it is essential to ensure that the patient's airway and breathing are adequate at all times.**

Table 3.17 – ASSESSMENT and MANAGEMENT of:

Medical Emergencies *continued*

STAGE	ASSESSMENT	MANAGEMENT
	• Assess for evidence of external haemorrhage e.g. epistaxis, haemoptysis, haematemesis, melaena.	• Arrest external haemorrhage. • In cases of internal or uncontrolled haemorrhage undertake a **TIME CRITICAL** transfer to further care; provide an alert/information call. • Patients with sepsis will benefit from early fluid therapy and an appropriate hospital alert/information call.

C

ASSESSMENT

• Assess skin colour and temperature.
• Palpate for a radial pulse – if present this implies adequate perfusion of vital organs, but this is highly variable. If absent feel for a carotid pulse. NB The estimation of blood pressure by pulse is inaccurate and unreliable; however, the presence of a radial suggests adequate profusion of major organs. The presence of a femoral pulse suggests perfusion of the kidneys, while a carotid pulse and coherent mentation suggests adequate profusion of the brain.
• Assess pulse rate, volume and rhythm.
• Check capillary refill time centrally (forehead or sternum – normal <2 seconds).

Consider hypovolaemic shock and be aware of its early signs:
• Pallor.
• Cool peripheries.
• Anxiety, abnormal behaviour.
• Increased respiratory rate.
• Tachycardia.

Recognition of Shock
Shock is difficult to diagnose. In certain groups of patients the signs of shock appear late e.g. pregnant women, patients on medication such as beta blockers, and the physically fit.

Blood loss of 750–1000 ml will produce little evidence of shock; blood loss of 1000–1500 ml is required before more classical signs of shock appear. NB This loss is from the circulation **NOT** necessarily visable externally.

MANAGEMENT

Fluid Therapy
• If fluid replacement is indicated refer to intravascular fluid therapy guideline.
• Rapid fluid replacement into the vascular compartment can overload the cardiovascular system particularly where there is pre-existing cardiovascular disease and in the elderly. Gradual rehydration over many hours rather than minutes is indicated. NB Monitor fluid replacement closely in these cases.

D

ASSESSMENT

DISABILITY (mini neurological examination)
Note the initial level of responsiveness on AVPU scale, and time of assessment.
• **A** – Alert
• **V** – Responds to voice
• **P** – Responds to painful stimulus
• **U** – Unresponsive

Assess and note pupil size, equality and response to light.

• Check for purposeful movement in all four limbs.
• Check sensory function.

• Assess blood glucose levels in all patients with a history of diabetes, impaired consciousness, convulsions, collapse or alcohol consumption.

MANAGEMENT

Check blood glucose level to rule out hypo or hyperglycaemia as the cause – **refer to glycaemic emergencies guideline in adults**.

II. Secondary Survey

- A secondary survey should only commence after the primary survey has been completed and an assessment of the patient's critical status has been made.
- The secondary survey is a more thorough 'head-to-toe' assessment of the patient including their past medical history (Table 3.18). It is important to monitor the patient's vital signs during the survey.
- The secondary survey will usually be undertaken during transfer to hospital; however, in some patients with critical conditions, it may not be possible to undertake the secondary survey before arrival at further care.

Table 3.18 – SECONDARY SURVEY

Assessment

HEAD
- Re-assess airway, breathing, and circulation.
- Re-assess levels of consciousness (AVPU), pupil size and activity.
- Establish Glasgow Coma Scale (refer to Table 3.19).

CHEST
- Re-assess rate and depth of breathing.
- Re-listen for breath sounds in all lung fields, and record.
- Assess for pneumothorax – in small pneumothorax no clinical signs may be detected. A pneumothorax causes breathlessness, reduced air entry and chest movement on the affected side. If this is a tension pneumothorax, then the patient will have increasing respiratory distress, distended neck veins, and tracheal deviation (late sign) away from affected side may also be present.
- Assess skin colour, temperature, and record.
- Assess heart sounds and heart rate.
- Obtain a blood pressure reading using a sphygmomanometer.
- Document and record all results.
- Record pulse oximeter reading.
- Re-assess and continue management as appropriate en-route to further care.

ABDOMEN
- Feel for tenderness and guarding in all four quadrants.
- Check for bowel sounds.
- Listen and asculate.

LOWER/UPPER LIMBS
Check for MSC in **ALL** four limbs:
- **MOTOR** – Test for movement and power.
- **SENSATION** – Apply light touch to evaluate sensation.
- **CIRCULATION** – Assess pulse and skin temperature.

MANAGEMENT
Correcting:
- Airway
- Breathing
- Circulation
- Disability (mini neurological examination).

- Ensure adequate oxygen therapy and support ventilation if required.
- Apply ECG and pulse oximetry monitoring, as required.
- Consider patient positioning, e.g. sitting upright for respiratory problems.
- Check blood glucose levels in all patients with history of diabetes, impaired consciousness, seizures, collapse or alcohol/drug consumption. Provide drug therapy as required; refer to appropriate drug guidelines. In adrenal crisis **refer to hydrocortisone guideline**.
- If the level of consciousness deteriorates or respiratory depression develops in cases where an overdose with opiate type drugs may be a possibility, consider administering naloxone (**refer to naloxone guideline**).
- In patients with fixed pinpoint pupils suspect opiate use. Follow ADDITIONAL MEDICAL guidelines as indicated by the patient's condition, e.g. cardiac rhythm disturbance:
  - correct A and B problems on scene
  - undertake a **TIME CRITICAL** transfer to nearest suitable further care
  - provide an alert/information call required
  - provide a comprehensive verbal hand-over and a completed patient report form to the receiving staff.

ADDITIONAL INFORMATION

- The patient history can provide valuable insight into the cause of the current condition.

The following may assist in determining the diagnosis:

- Relatives, carers or friends with knowledge of the patient's history.
- Packets or containers of medication (including domiciliary oxygen) or evidence of administration devices, e.g. nebuliser machines.
- Medic alert type jewellery (bracelets or necklets) which detail the patient's primary health risk (e.g. diabetes, anaphylaxis, Addison's disease etc.) but also list a 24-hour telephone number to obtain a more detailed patient history.
- Warning stickers, often placed by the front door or the telephone, directing the health professional to a source of detailed information (one current scheme involves storing the patient details in a container in the fridge, as this is relatively easy to find in the house).
- Patient-held warning cards denoting previous thrombolysis, at-risk COPD patients, or those taking monoamine oxidase inhibitor (MAOI) medication.
- Patients' individualised treatment plans.
- Patients on long-term steroids or who have adrenal insufficiency may deteriorate rapidly because of steroid insufficiency. If significantly unwell, the patient should be given hydrocortisone and fluids if required.

Appendix

Table 3.19 – GLASGOW COMA SCALE

Category	Element	Score
Eyes Opening	Spontaneously	4
	To speech	3
	To pain	2
	None	1
Motor Response	Obeys commands	6
	Localises pain	5
	Withdraws from pain	4
	Abnormal flexion	3
	Extensor response	2
	No response to pain	1
Verbal Response	Orientated	5
	Confused	4
	Inappropriate words	3
	Incomprehensible sounds	2
	No verbal response	1

Methodology

For details of the methodology used in the development of this guideline refer to the guideline webpage.

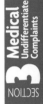

KEY POINTS

Medical Emergencies in Adults (Overview)

- Detect TIME CRITICAL problems early.
- Minimise time on scene.
- Continuously re-assess ABCD, AVPU.
- Initiate treatments en-route if deterioration.
- Provide an alert/information call for TIME CRITICAL patients.

1. Introduction

- Chest pain is one of the most common symptoms of acute coronary syndrome (ACS).
- It is also a common feature in many other conditions such as aortic dissection chest infection with pleuritic pain, pulmonary embolus, reflux oesophagitis, indigestion, and simple musculoskeletal chest pain.
- There must be a high index of suspicion that any chest pain is cardiac in origin.
- **Taking and assessing a history** – there are a number of specific factors that may help in reaching a reasoned working diagnosis, and applying appropriate management measures to the patient. ACS cannot be excluded on clinical examination (**refer to ACS guideline**).
- Do not assess symptoms differently in women and men or patients from different ethnic groups.

2. Incidence

It is estimated that over 360,000 patients attend emergency departments with acute chest pain each year.

3. Severity and Outcome

Some cases of chest pain may be life-threatening e.g. aortic dissection.

4. Assessment and Management

For the assessment and management of non-traumatic chest pain/discomfort refer to Table 3.21.

Methodology

For details of the methodology used in the development of this guideline refer to the guideline webpage.

Table 3.20 – FEATURES OF DIFFERENT TYPES OF PAIN

Features which suggest a diagnosis of myocardial ischaemia include:
- Central chest pain.
- Crushing or constricting in nature.
- Persists for >15 minutes.
- Pain may also present in:
  - the shoulders
  - upper abdomen
  - referred to the neck, jaws and arms.

Features which suggest a diagnosis of stable angina include:
- Pain is typically related to exertion and tends to last minutes but should it persist for >15 minutes, or despite usual treatment ACS is more likely.

Features of pleuritic type pain:
- Stabbing.
- Generally one-sided.
- Worse on breathing in.
- Usually have cough with sputum.
- Raised temperature (>37.5°C).

Features of indigestion type pain:
- Central.
- Related to food.
- May be associated with belching and burning.
NB Some patients with ACS may also suffer indigestion type pain and belching.

Features of muscular type pain:
- Sharp/stabbing.
- Worse on movement.
- Often associated with tenderness.

KEY POINTS

Non-Traumatic Chest Pain/Discomfort
- **Most chest pain is not Acute Coronary Syndrome – but this possibility needs to be excluded rapidly.**
- **Is there another life-threatening cause e.g. aortic dissection?**
- **Have a low threshold for recording a 12–lead ECG.**
- **A normal ECG cannot reliably exclude ACS.**

Table 3.21 – ASSESSMENT and MANAGEMENT of:

Non-Traumatic Chest Pain/Discomfort

NB A defibrillator must always be taken at the earliest opportunity to patients with symptoms suggestive of a heart attack and remain with the patient until hand-over to hospital staff.

ASSESSMENT	MANAGEMENT
● Assess **ABCD**	If any of the following **TIME CRITICAL** features are present: ● Major ABC problems. ● Suspected acute coronary syndrome especially ST-segment-elevation myocardial infarction (STEMI) (**refer to acute coronary syndrome guideline**). ● Pulmonary embolism. ● Aortic dissection. ● Pneumonia. ● Respiratory rate <10 or >30 breaths per minute. ● Oxygen saturation (SpO$_2$) <95% on air. ● Start correcting any **ABC** problems. ● Undertake a **TIME CRITICAL TRANSFER**. Provide an alert/information call. ● Continue management en-route.
● Assess whether the chest pain may be cardiac	● For the features of specific types of pain refer to Table 3.20 ● Note time of onset, duration, characteristics (type including radiation and aggravating and alleviating factors). ● Ask the patient if they have a previous history of coronary heart disease.
● Assess for accompanying features	● Nausea ● Vomiting. ● Sweating. ● Pallor. ● Cough. ● Radiation of pain to the arm(s). ● Breathlessness – NB If breathlessness is a predominant symptom/sign with tightness in the chest then causes of breathlessness must also be considered.
● Undertake a clinical assessment specifically for:	● Haemodynamic problems. ● Heart failure. ● Cardiogenic shock. ● Other non-coronary causes e.g. aortic dissection.
● Other conditions	● If clinical examination and a 12-lead ECG make a diagnosis of ACS less likely, assess for other acute conditions (pulmonary embolism, aortic dissection, pneumonia). **NB DO NOT exclude an acute coronary syndrome when patients have a normal resting 12-lead ECG – a normal ECG cannot reliably exclude ACS.**
● Measure and record	● Respiratory rate. ● Pulse. ● Blood pressure. ● Monitor with ECG for arrhythmias. ● Undertake and assess a 12-lead ECG. Where facilities exist for telemetry transmit ECG to appropriate hospital department according to local protocols.
● Assess oxygen saturation	● Closely monitor the patient's SpO$_2$ but do not administer oxygen unless the patient is hypoxaemic on air (SpO$_2$ <94%) (**refer to oxygen guidelines**).
● Assess patient's pain	● Measure and record pain score (**refer to pain management guideline**). ● Consider analgesia (**refer to pain management guideline**).
● Documentation	● Complete documentation.[49]

3 Medical Undifferentiated Complaints
SECTION

1. Introduction

- Recognising (and acting upon) the signs and symptoms of serious illness in a child is much more important than reaching the correct diagnosis.

- Good patient assessment will allow potentially life-threatening illnesses or injuries to be recognised sooner, allowing treatments and interventions to be given at the earliest opportunity. (This includes the need for rapid hospital transfer when urgent assessment and further treatments are required.)

- Assessment priorities include the detection of respiratory distress, circulatory impairment or decreased consciousness.

Cardiac Arrest

- Adults often suffer sudden cardiac arrest while well perfused and in a relatively normal metabolic state, because the heart suddenly stops with an arrhythmia.

- In contrast, cardiac arrest in children is much more likely to occur as a result of unrecognised or prolonged hypoxia. As a consequence of hypoxia and acidosis, the heart becomes bradycardic and can result in asystole. Hypoxia and acidosis decrease the likelihood of successful resuscitation and so it is essential that serious childhood illnesses are recognised long before this chain of events can occur if child deaths are to be avoided.

- Recognition of the seriously ill or injured child involves the identification of a number of key signs affecting the child's airway, breathing, circulatory and neurological systems.

- If any of these signs are present, the child must be regarded as time critical.

2. Assessment
Primary Assessment

AIRWAY – Assessment of the Airway
Check the airway for obstruction, foreign material or vomit.

Position the Head to Open the Airway
The younger the child the less neck extension will be required. A newborn's head should be placed in the neutral position whilst older children should be extended into a 'sniffing the morning air' position.

Abnormal Upper Airway Sounds Should be Sought:
- Inspiratory noises (stridor) suggest an airway obstruction near the larynx.

- A snoring noise (stertorous breathing) may be present when there is obstruction in the pharynx e.g. massive tonsils.

3. Breathing – Assessment and Recognition of Potential Respiratory Impairment

Measure the Respiratory Rate
- A rapid respiratory rate (tachypnoea) at rest in a child indicates a need for increased ventilation and suggests:
  - an airway problem
  - a lung problem

- a circulatory problem, or
- a metabolic problem.

Table 3.22 – NORMAL RESPIRATORY RATES

Age	Respiratory Rate
<1 year	30–40 breaths per minute
1–2 years	25–35 breaths per minute
2–5 years	25–30 breaths per minute
5–11 years	20–25 breaths per minute
>12 years	15–20 breaths per minute

Recession (indrawing, retraction)
- Children have pliable rib cages so when respiratory effort is high, indrawing is seen between the ribs (intercostal recession) and along the costal margins where the diaphragm attaches (subcostal recession). The sternum itself may even be drawn in (sternal recession) in tiny babies but as children get older, the rib cage becomes less pliable and other signs of accessory muscle use (other than recession) will be seen (see below). If recession is seen in older children, it suggests severe respiratory difficulty.

Accessory Muscle Use
- As in adult life, when the work of breathing is increased, the sternocleidomastoid muscle may be used as an accessory respiratory muscle. In infants this may cause the head to bob up and down with each breath.

Flaring of the Nostrils
- This is a subtle sign that is easily missed. It indicates significant respiratory distress.

Inspiratory or Expiratory Noises
- Wheezing indicates lower airway narrowing and is most commonly heard on expiration. The volume of wheeze is **NOT** an indicator of severity and may diminish with increasing distress because less air is being moved.

Inspiratory Noises (stridor)
- Suggests an imminent danger to the airway due to reduction in airway circumference to approximately 10% of normal. Again, the volume of stridor does **NOT** reflect severity and may also diminish with increasing distress as less air is moved.

Grunting
- Is produced by exhalation against a partially closed laryngeal opening (glottis). This is more likely to be seen in infants and is a sign of severe respiratory distress.

Effectiveness of Breathing – chest expansion and breath sounds
Note the degree of expansion on both sides of the chest and whether it is equal.

Auscultate the Chest with a Stethoscope
A silent chest is a pre-terminal sign, as it indicates that very little air is moving in or out of the chest.

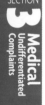

Pulse Oximetry

This can be used at all ages to measure oxygen saturation (readings are less reliable in the presence of shock, hypothermia and other conditions such as carbon monoxide poisoning and severe anaemia).

Table 3.23 – THE EFFECTS OF RESPIRATORY INADEQUACY ON OTHER SYSTEMS

Heart Rate
- Tachycardia (or eventually bradycardia) may result from hypoxia and acidosis.
- Bradycardia in a sick child is a pre-terminal sign.

Skin Colour
- Flushing of the skin (vasodilation) is seen in early respiratory distress due to elevated carbon dioxide levels.
- Hypoxia causes vasoconstriction and skin pallor.
- Cyanosis is a pre-terminal sign of hypoxia.

Mental Status
- Hypoxia makes children agitated and drowsy.
- Agitation may be difficult to recognise due to the child's distress. Use parents to help make this assessment.
- Drowsiness gradually progresses leading to unconsciousness.

---

4. Circulation – Recognition of Potential Circulatory Failure (Shock)

- Circulatory assessments in children are difficult as each physical sign may have a number of confounding variables.
- When assessing whether a child is shocked, it is important to assess and evaluate each of the signs below.

Heart Rate
- Tachycardia results from loss of circulatory volume. Heart rates, particularly in Infants, can be very high (up to 220 beats per minute) (heart rates greater than 220 bpm are seen in supraventricular tachycardia).
- Bradycardia becomes apparent before cardiac arrest (see above).

Table 3.24 – NORMAL HEART RATES

Age	Heart Rate
<1 year	110–160 beats per minute
1–2 years	100–150 beats per minute
2–5 years	95–140 beats per minute
5–11 years	80–120 beats per minute
>12 years	60–100 beats per minute

Pulse Volume
- Peripheral pulses become weak and then absent as shock advances.
- Children peripherally vasoconstrict their extremities as shock progresses, initially cooling skin distally and then more proximally as shock advances.
- There is no validated relationship between the presence of certain peripheral pulses and the systemic blood pressure in children.

Capillary Refill
- This should be measured on the forehead or the sternum.
- A capillary refill time of >2 seconds indicates poor perfusion, although this is influenced by a number of factors, including cold and poor lighting conditions.

Blood Pressure
- Varies with age.
- Is difficult to reliably measure, increasing on-scene times, and, as a result, is not routinely measured in prehospital practice.
- Hypotension is a very late (and pre-terminal) sign in shocked children and so other signs of circulatory inadequacy will manifest (and should have been recognised!) long before hypotension occurs.

Table 3.25 – THE EFFECTS OF CIRCULATORY INADEQUACY ON OTHER SYSTEMS

Respiratory Rate
- The combination of both rapid respiratory rate but no recession may indicate circulatory insufficiency.
- Tachypnoea occurs as the body tries to correct metabolic derangements.

Skin
- Mottled, cold, pale skin reflects poor perfusion.

Mental Status
- Agitation is seen in early shock, progressing to drowsiness as shock advances.
- Poor cerebral perfusion may ultimately result in loss of consciousness.

---

5. Disability – Recognition of Potential Central Neurological Failure

Level of Consciousness/Alertness/the 'AVPU' score:

A Alert

V Responds to voice

P Responds to painful stimulus

U Unresponsive

Response to a Painful Stimulus

Pinch a digit or pull frontal hair. A child who is unconscious or who only responds to pain has a significant degree of coma (refer to Glasgow Coma Scale – Appendix).

Posture: Observe the child's posture
- Children may be:

- Floppy (hypotonia) – recent floppiness in a child suggests serious illness.
- Stiffness (hypertonia) or back arching (opisthotonus)
  - new onset stiffness suggests severe cerebral disturbance
  - decerebrate or decorticate postures suggests a serious underlying cerebral abnormality.

Pupils

- Test pupil size and reaction.
- Pupils should be equal, of normal size and react briskly to light.
- Any abnormality or change in pupil size or reaction may be significant.

Table 3.26 – THE EFFECTS OF NEUROLOGICAL IMPAIRMENT ON OTHER SYSTEMS

Respiratory System
Brain insults produce abnormal breathing patterns e.g. hyperventilation, Cheyne-Stokes breathing or apnoea.

Circulatory System
Bradycardia may be a result of dangerously raised intracranial pressure.

NOTE: the whole assessment should take less than two minutes unless intervention is required.

Frequent re-assessment of ABCDs is necessary to assess the response to treatment or to detect deterioration. (Blood glucose levels should be measured in any seriously ill child.)

6. Management

Any child believed to have a serious problem involving:

- Airway.
- Breathing.
- Circulation.
- Disability.

must be considered to have a **TIME CRITICAL** condition and receive immediate management of airway, breathing and circulation, and be rapidly transferred to an appropriate receiving hospital with a suitable pre-alert message.

Remember: **A** and **B** problems should be addressed on scene and **C** problems managed en-route to further care.

7. Airway Management

- The child's airway should be managed in a stepwise manner.
- If epiglottitis is possible then extreme caution must be exercised (**refer to respiratory illness in children guideline**).

Manual Extension Manoeuvres, Head Tilt, Chin Lift or Jaw Thrust

- Do not to place pressure on the soft tissues under the chin or in front of the neck as this can obstruct the airway.

Aspiration, Foreign Body Removal

- Avoid blind finger sweeps as they may push material further down the airway or damage the soft palate.
- Use paediatric suction catheters where available.

Oropharyngeal Airway (OPA)

- Ensure the OPA is of the appropriate size (**refer to page for age**) and inserted using the correct technique. Discontinue insertion or remove if the child gags (**refer to paediatric resuscitation guidelines**).

Nasopharyngeal Airway

- Correct sizing is essential (**refer to page for age**).
- In small children, a smaller size may be required.
- Care should be taken not to damage tonsillar/adenoidal tissues.

Endotracheal Intubation

- The hazards associated with intubation in children are considerable and usually outweigh the advantages. It should **ONLY** be attempted where other more basic methods of ventilation have failed (**refer to paediatric resuscitation charts (or page for age) for ET sizes**).

Needle Cricothyroidotomy

- Surgical airways should not be performed in children under the age of 12 years.
- Needle cricothyroidotomy is a method of last resort.
- The initial oxygen (O_2) flow rate in litres per minute should be set equal to the child's age in years and gradually increased until adequate chest wall movements are seen (**refer to foreign body airway obstruction in children guideline**).

8. Breathing Management

- **Ensure adequate oxygenation** (**refer to oxygen guideline**).
- All sick children require adequate oxygenation.
- Administer high levels of supplemental oxygen (O_2) via a non-rebreathing mask.
- In children with sickle cell disease or cardiac disease, high levels of O_2 should be administered routinely, whatever their oxygen saturation.
- If the child finds the facemask distressing, ask the parent to help by holding the mask as close to the child's face as possible. If this still produces distress, wafting O_2 across the face directly from the tubing (with the facemask detached from the tubing) is better than nothing.
- Consider assisted ventilation at a rate equivalent to the normal respiratory rate for the age of the child (**refer to paediatric resuscitation charts for normal values**) if:
  - the child is hypoxic (SpO_2 <90%) and remains so after 30–60 seconds on high concentration O_2
  - respiratory rate is <50% normal or >3 times normal (see Table 3.22)
  - expansion is inadequate.
- Use an appropriately sized mask to ensure a good seal.

SECTION **3** Medical Undifferentiated Complaints

- Try to avoid hyperventilation to minimise the risks of i) gastric insufflation or ii) barotrauma. The bag-valve-mask should have a pressure release valve as an added safety measure. If this is not available extreme care must be taken not to overexpand the lungs. No bag smaller than 500 ml volume should be used for bag-valve-mask ventilation unless the child is <2.5 kg (preterm baby size).

Wheezing

The management of asthma is discussed elsewhere (**refer to asthma in children guideline**).

9. Circulation Management

Arrest External Haemorrhage

NB Do not waste time attempting to gain intravenous (IV) or intraosseous (IO) access at the scene. Obtain access en-route unless delay is unavoidable.

Cannulation

Attempt cannulation with the widest bore cannula that can be confidently placed. The vehicle can be stopped briefly to allow for venepuncture and disposal of the sharp with transport being recommenced before applying the IV dressing.

The intraosseous route may be required where venous access has failed on two occasions or no suitable vein is apparent within a reasonable timeframe. The intraosseous route is the preferred route for vascular access in all cases of cardiac arrest in young children.

Blood glucose level should be measured in i) all children in whom vascular access is being obtained and ii) any child with decreased conscious level (**refer to altered level of consciousness guideline**).

Fluid Administration

- Use sodium chloride 0.9% to treat shock.
- Fluids should be measured in millilitres and documented as volume administered – not the volume of fluid chosen.
- Fluids should be administered as boluses rather than 'run in'.

Hand-over at the receiving unit must include details of volume and type of fluid administered.

Fluid volumes

Children found to have shock (circulatory failure*) as a result of medical illness are usually resuscitated with 20 ml/kg boluses of sodium chloride 0.9%, to restore vital signs to normal.

No more than two boluses should be given except on medical advice (**refer to intravascular fluid and sodium chloride 0.9% guidelines**).

Exceptions

- In diabetic ketoacidosis, fluids are administered more cautiously to reduce the risk of cerebral oedema. (**refer to glycaemic emergencies in childhood guideline**).

* The signs of circulatory failure (cold peripheries, delayed capillary refill time, mottled skin, a weak thready pulse) are detailed above.

- In diabetic ketoacidosis, fluid should be withheld unless severe shock is present when 10 ml/kg should be administered over 10–15 minutes (**refer to glycaemic emergencies in childhood guideline**).
- If a child has heart failure or renal failure give a 10 ml/kg bolus but stop if the patient deteriorates. Transfer to hospital as a priority.
- Where exceptional circumstances are present, e.g. long transfer time, medical advice should be obtained.

10. Disability Management

The aim of management of any child with a cerebral insult is to minimise further insult by optimising their circumstances.

This usually concerns management strategies designed to:

- prevent hypoxia (see above).
- normalise circulation (without causing fluid overload).
- identifying and treating hypoglycaemia (**refer to glycaemic emergencies in childhood guideline**).

Other conditions which can be treated before hospital and are discussed elsewhere include:

- convulsions (**refer to childhood convulsions guideline**).
- opiate poisoning (refer to naloxone guideline).
- meningococcal septicaemia (**refer to meningococcal septicaemia guideline**).

Summary

The Primary Assessment of the child should establish whether the child is **TIME CRITICAL or not**.

Immediate correction of **A** and **B** problems must be undertaken without delay at the scene.

C problems can be corrected en-route to hospital.

Children who are found to be seriously ill must be considered **TIME CRITICAL** and **MUST BE** taken to the nearest suitable receiving hospital without delay.

A hospital alert/information call should be made whenever a seriously ill child is transported.

NB Paediatric drug doses are expressed in 'mg/kg' (refer to specific drug guidelines for dosages and information).

Drug doses MUST be checked prior to ANY drug administration, no matter how confident the practitioner may be.

Additional Information

Remember that the child/parent's history provides invaluable insights into the cause of the current condition.

The following may be of great help in making an assessment:

- Relatives, carers or friends with knowledge of the child's history.
- Packets or containers of medication or evidence of administration devices e.g. inhalers, spacers etc.

- Medic Alert® type jewellery e.g. bracelets, which detail the child's primary health risk (e.g. diabetes, anaphylaxis, drug allergy etc.) as well as a 24-hour telephone number to obtain a more detailed patient history.
- Child protection concerns may become apparent during the initial medical assessment and should be appropriately dealt with (**refer to safeguarding children guideline**).

KEY POINTS

Medical Emergencies

- **The child/parent's history will provide a valuable insight into the cause of the child's current condition.**
- **Emergency airway management rarely requires intubation.**
- **Hypoxia and hypovolaemia need urgent correction.**
- **Check the blood glucose in all seriously ill children and those with a decreased level of consciousness.**
- **A and B should be corrected on scene and C problems managed en-route to further care.**

Methodology

For details of the methodology used in the development of this guideline refer to the guideline webpage.

Appendix

Glasgow Coma Scale and modified Glasgow Coma Scale.

GLASGOW COMA SCALE

Item		Score
Eyes Opening:		
	Spontaneously	4
	To speech	3
	To pain	2
	None	1
Motor Response:		
	Obeys commands	6
	Localises pain	5
	Withdraws from pain	4
	Abnormal flexion	3
	Extensor response	2
	No response to pain	1
Verbal Response:		
	Orientated	5
	Confused	4
	Inappropriate words	3
	Incomprehensible sounds	2
	No verbal response	1

MODIFICATION OF GLASGOW COMA SCALE FOR CHILDREN UNDER <4 YEARS OLD

Item	Score
Eyes Opening:	As per adult scale
Motor Response:	As per adult scale
Best Verbal Response:	
Appropriate words or social smiles, fixes on and follows objects	5
Cries, but is consolable	4
Persistently irritable	3
Restless, agitated	2
Silent	1

SECTION
3
Medical
Undifferentiated
Complaints

Minor Illness in Children [For references, refer to individual medical guidelines]

1. Introduction

- Traditional ambulance priorities 'focused' on the recognition and management of both serious illness and major injury prior to hospital transfer (**refer to medical emergencies in children – overview guideline**).

- Recent changes in prehospital care mean that children with less serious illnesses are now increasingly managed either at home or in the community rather than in Emergency Departments or on 'Children's Units', as before.

- Fever is the commonest reason for parents to seek medical attention for their child and usually suggests an underlying infection.

- Thereafter, respiratory illnesses and episodes of gastroenteritis make up a large proportion of the remaining acute paediatric presentations.

Paediatric Considerations

i) The Paediatric Population

- Children should not simply be viewed as 'little adults'. They pose many pitfalls for the unwary and inexperienced and present healthcare providers with significant challenges wherever the setting.

- Children display important differences in their anatomy, their physiology, their immunity, the illnesses they encounter, as well as the ways in which these conditions present, develop and progress.

- Difficulties verbalising and communicating their condition further add to these challenges.

ii) 'Major' and 'Minor' Illnesses

- Before considering 'minor' illnesses in children, it is crucial to both appreciate and understand that 'major' childhood illnesses – including life-threatening conditions such as meningococcal disease – rarely present in extremis, but more commonly present with relatively innocent features that can easily be mistaken for minor illnesses.

- Children with advanced major illness (or significant injury) typically have deranged vital signs that are usually readily detected. Earlier in their illness, these children may well have had normal physiology and appeared relatively well – if assessed early in their illness, these children might be misdiagnosed as only having a minor illness.

- Using the febrile child as an example, children with '**RED**' traffic light features clearly require transfer to hospital. Disease progression is much harder to predict in those with '**GREEN**' or '**AMBER**' features. These children will most probably have a minor illness but (as described above) they may be within the early stages of a more significant infection, when their symptoms and signs have not progressed and fully developed, hiding the seriousness of the evolving, underlying condition.

- This scenario is not uncommon in early meningococcal disease which classically presents with non-specific signs e.g. fever, sore throat, lethargy, vomiting, diarrhoea, decreased appetite etc., mimicking either an upper respiratory tract infection or gastroenteritis.

- Identifying a child with a serious infection early in their illness significantly improves their outcome and so it is essential that the very subtle, early signs of serious illness are sought (**refer to febrile illnesses in children guideline**).

2. Assessment and Management

- Refer to the following guidelines that facilitate the assessment and management of children with minor illnesses, offering i) clinical management strategies, and ii) guidance to help identify the group of children with relatively insignificant symptoms that are masking a more serious underlying illness, requiring further medical assessment and intervention.

See following guidelines on:
i)   **febrile illness in children**
ii) **respiratory illnesses in children**
iii) gastroenteritis in children.

Methodology

For details of the methodology used in the development of this guideline please refer to the guideline webpage.

KEY POINTS

Minor Illness in Children

- **Prehospital practices are changing.**
- **Children should not be viewed simply as 'little adults'.**
- **Childhood febrile illnesses, respiratory illnesses and gastroenteritis are frequently encountered.**
- **Major illnesses (e.g. meningococcal septicaemia) will often mimic otherwise trivial conditions.**
- **See guidelines on febrile illness in children, respiratory illnesses in children, gastroenteritis in children, and meningococcal septicaemia.**

1. Introduction

- Sick children are notoriously difficult to assess except for the times when they are obviously very ill or injured, with grossly deranged vital signs. (The younger the child the more difficult the assessment.)

- In critically ill children, temperature is not routinely recorded as part of the 'ABC' assessment as it delays treatment without altering management.

- Temperature should however be measured in the less ill child, where it forms part of the picture of their illness and is essential in informing decision making.

- Staff should be familiar with NICE's published guidance on this topic (on which this guideline is based).

Fever

- Normal body temperature is 37°C. A temperature of 38°C and above is likely to be significant.

- Fever is part of the immune system's response to infection and is not thought to be harmful (although lay people often assume that it is).

- It can herald a significant underlying infection hence the importance of identifying its cause.

- Throughout most of childhood, the height of the fever bears little relationship to the gravity of the illness, although in babies aged <6 months, a high temperature is much more likely to be significant.

- When facing serious infections, small babies often have unstable body temperatures and may paradoxically present with a low body temperature.

- Febrile illnesses in children aged between 6 months and 6 years can produce a seizure – a febrile convulsion – following a rapid rise in body temperature (**refer to convulsions in children guideline**).

2. Incidence

- Febrile illness is the commonest medical problem in childhood and suggests an underlying infection. Younger children are the most vulnerable due to the immaturity of their immune systems. By the age of 18 months, an otherwise healthy child would be expected to have had around 8 acute febrile illnesses.

3. Severity and Outcome

- Infectious diseases are a major cause of childhood mortality and morbidity.

- Most febrile illnesses are due to self-limiting viral infections requiring little or no intervention. However, fever is a common presenting feature of serious bacterial infections (SBI) such as meningitis, septicaemia, urinary tract infections and pneumonia and distinguishing between a simple viral infection and a more serious bacterial infection can be a real diagnostic challenge. 1% of the UK's under-5 population will have an SBI each year.

4. Assessment

a) TEMPERATURE MEASUREMENT
Do not take temperatures orally in the under 5s. Even in older children, it may be easier to avoid using the oral method.

The best method to measure a small baby's temperature (aged <1 month) is an electronic axillary thermometer.

Between 1 month and 5 years, both chemical 'dot' thermometers and aural tympanic thermometers are reliable and are equally effective.

The thermometer must be left in place for at least the minimum recommended time, otherwise it may well under-record.

Chemically sensitive strips placed on the forehead are inaccurate and should not be used.

Mercury-containing, glass thermometers are no longer used for safety reasons.

If a parent states that their child has been feverish this should be accepted as evidence of fever and taken seriously (even if they had not measured the temperature with a thermometer at the time).

b) FEBRILE CHILD ASSESSMENT
Carry out a primary survey immediately on any ill child to exclude any evidence of life-threatening illness.

Assuming this is negative, take and record a full history of the illness, including at a minimum:

1) Length of illness.

2) Other symptoms besides fever, specifically asking about:
   - Urinary symptoms.
   - Abdominal pain.
   - Headache, photophobia, neck stiffness.
   - Abnormal skin colour, cold hands and feet, muscle pains, or
   - Other complaints such as a painful joints, sore throat, ear pain etc.

3) Is fluid intake adequate? A febrile child needs extra fluids to prevent dehydration.

   If they are vomiting, they may:

   i) become dehydrated and ii) be unable to absorb medication. Diarrhoea also increases fluid losses, increasing the risk of dehydration.

4) Underlying (chronic) medical problems, including advice that the parent may have been given by specialists regarding actions to be taken if their child develops a fever. (This should include whether the child is under current investigation or management by a doctor.)

5) Medications, antibiotics or steroids (or other drugs reducing immunity). To assess a child properly, you will need to be aware of the action of any drug that they are taking as this may be relevant. If in doubt, this must be checked.

6) Any other illness in the family, the nursery or school etc?

7) Recent foreign travel – consider malaria or other tropical illness.

Febrile Illness in Children

Examination

Following the history, perform a detailed examination including:

1) Overall assessment/general impression – lively, miserable, disinterested, playful, floppy etc.

2) Physiological parameters – measure respiratory rate[a], heart rate[a], capillary refill time (CRT) and temperature. Oxygen saturations and an AVPU score may also be useful.

Important clinical points

As a general rule, **tachycardia** accompanies fever and raises the possibility of sepsis, whilst **tachypnoea** suggests an underlying respiratory illness.

A child's resting heart rate increases 10 bpm for every 1°C rise in body temperature.

A **disproportionate tachycardia** – i.e. above the accepted normal range (refer to Table 3.27) having taken account of the fever – is seen in early sepsis and meningococcal disease. Such children must receive further medical assessment.

Other features suggesting sepsis include cold hands and feet, abnormal skin colour and muscle pains in the legs.

Infants and small children with meningococcal disease rarely exhibit 'classical' textbook signs **(neck stiffness, photophobia** and **non-blanching rash)**, but more commonly present with features that might suggest a non-specific viral illness such as an upper respiratory tract infection (URTI) or gastroenteritis.

In such circumstances, seek (and document) evidence to rule out the possibility of meningococcal disease.

1) Assessment of dehydration (**refer to gastroenteritis in children guideline**).

2) Examine all other systems (including skin) to determine the source of the fever and estimate the disease severity.

A positive sign must be 'seen' rather than assumed – e.g. otitis media cannot be diagnosed on a history of 'earache' alone. (Direct visualisation of the tympanic membrane using an auroscope is required to make the diagnosis!)

NB It is possible for a child to have a common infection as well as a more serious underlying one; a child with coryza and runny nose could still have meningitis.

3) Perform a **'Traffic Light'** assessment (refer to Table 3.28–3.30). This tool was developed by NICE to prioritise febrile children into three groups according to the presence of certain symptoms and signs:

'**Green**' is low risk,

'**Amber**' is intermediate risk and,

'**Red**' is high risk.

Note: The traffic light system does not seek to make a specific diagnosis but simply identifies which symptoms and signs should receive the highest priority, guiding subsequent management.

[a]These signs must be documented and interpreted using the age-specific, normal ranges for that child, listed in Table 3.27.

c) SPECIFIC FEBRILE ILLNESSES

The following potential diagnoses must each be specifically considered:

- **Meningococcal septicaemia** – often the child may not present as acutely as tradition would have it.
- **Meningitis (under one year olds do not always have neck stiffness).**
- **Urinary tract infection (UTI)** – particularly common in babies and young children and can cause permanent kidney damage. UTIs can also progress to life-threatening septicaemia. Symptoms can again be very non-specific and include: poor feeding, lethargy and abdominal pains. In hospital practice, clean catch urine samples are collected on every febrile child to exclude UTIs.
- **Pneumonia** – typical chest signs may be absent.
- **Herpes simplex encephalitis** – classical pointers include focal neurological signs and focal seizures.
- **Septic arthritis/osteomyelitis** – fever plus very tender swollen joint(s)/bone(s), refusal to weight-bear.
- **Kawasaki's disease** – a collection of signs including: fever for >5 days; cervical lymphadenopathy; mucosal changes in the upper respiratory tract e.g. redness and cracked lips; peripheral changes in the distal limbs – e.g. oedema, peeling skin; a non-specific, blanching 'measles-like' rash; bilateral conjunctival redness.

5. Management

Giving an **antipyretic** such as paracetamol or ibuprofen purely to treat the fever is not necessary, but parental sensitivities should be observed.

An analgesic/antipyretic may help relieve misery and other unpleasant symptoms that often accompany febrile illnesses e.g. aches, pains and other symptoms which the child is often unable to fully describe.

Antipyretics do not protect against febrile convulsions. Giving antipyretics to a child who has either just had a seizure or who is thought to be at risk of having a seizure has not been shown to be beneficial.

Note: Antipyretics are effective, even in children with serious bacterial infections. It would therefore be wrong to assume that a clinical improvement seen following an antipyretic excludes a serious underlying infection.

Combinations of **both** paracetamol and ibuprofen taken together may be more effective than taking one or the other individually but care must be taken to ensure carers understand the dosing and timing differences between these two medicines if this is done. (Follow instructions on the bottle.)

Antibiotics should not be given to a febrile child where the diagnosis is not known. This can delay the subsequent diagnosis of a serious infection such as meningitis.

6. Referral Pathway

Febrile children fulfilling the following criteria **must** be transported to hospital:

- Any child <5 years old fulfilling **RED** criteria, no matter how well they may otherwise appear.
- Any febrile baby <1 month old (irrespective of the absolute temperature).
- Any febrile child <3 months old without an obvious cause (as a minimum, an urgent urine sample will be required).
- Those aged <3 years without an obvious cause, if a urine sample cannot be arranged at the time through the GP.
- Those with any signs of serious illness (**refer to medical emergencies in children guideline**).
- Any child with a significant fever but no localising symptoms or signs, who has received antibiotics within the last 48 hours (signs of meningitis can be masked by antibiotic use; so called 'partially-treated' meningitis).
- Any child on steroids or other medication known to suppress the immune system.
- Any child, regardless of age, where there is any doubt that they could be seriously ill.
- Any child where the social or psychological environment suggests that they may not receive adequate supervision or care if left at home.
- Those with a medical protocol saying that this is necessary.

Other categories (includes **AMBER** and **GREEN** groups).

Give serious consideration to transporting any child <5 years old that meets **AMBER** criteria to hospital, no matter how well they appear (see below).

Note: if a child fulfils **AMBER** criteria and a decision is made **not** to transport the child OR a child falls into the **GREEN** category but a cause for the fever has not been found, one of the following 'safety nets' **MUST** be put in place:

Safety Netting

a) Provide written information on warning symptoms to the parent/carer with advice regarding further management and how further healthcare can be accessed. A parental information sheet detailing suitable advice is available in the NICE Feverish Child quick reference guide. (NICE suggest either 'verbal or written' advice, but an anxious parent/carer absorbs verbal information poorly so written instructions should be given.)

b) Make urgent follow-up arrangements for any child fulfilling **AMBER** criteria with a GP or other paediatric healthcare professional giving a specified time and place e.g. for the child to be seen within the next 2–6 hours (exact timing to be decided by the attending staff).

Direct verbal hand-over to the doctor is important but may not always be possible.

The arrangements must be made by the attending ambulance staff.

It is not adequate to tell the parents to make their own arrangements to see the GP.

c) Liaison with other healthcare professionals such as the GP or out-of-hours service, to ensure the parent or carer has direct access to them if they are worried.

Finally, if in any doubt about your decision, consult the doctor responsible for the child (either their GP or out-of-hours doctor).

Methodology

For details of the methodology used in the development of this guideline refer to the guideline webpage.

KEY POINTS

Febrile Illness in Children

- **Febrile illness is the commonest paediatric presentation and suggests underlying infection.**
- **Always seek the underlying cause of the fever.**
- **All febrile children must be assessed with a full history and examination.**
- **Physiological parameters must be measured, documented and compared against age-specific, 'normal' values.**
- **Significant tachycardia suggests sepsis.**
- **Use the NICE 'traffic light' system.**
- **Early non-specific features are common in serious infections e.g. meningococcal disease often mimics URTIs and gastroenteritis.**
- **Small children rarely exhibit the 'classical' meningococcal signs – neck stiffness, photophobia or non-blanching rash; these features are more likely in older children and teenagers. In all age groups important early features include fever, cold hands and feet, abnormal skin colour and muscle pains or confusion.**
- **Improvement following antipyretics does not rule out a serious underlying infection.**
- **Do not blindly give antibiotics to a febrile child where the diagnosis is not known.**
- **Where a justifiable clinical reason not to transport a child to hospital has been found and a decision made to stay at home, these decisions must be carefully documented.**
- **Provide a 'safety net,' with written information, to any febrile child not transferred to hospital.**
- **If uncertain, seek advice from either their GP or out-of-hours doctor.**
- **The GP should be routinely informed of any consultation.**

Table 3.27 – 'NORMAL' PAEDIATRIC PHYSIOLOGICAL VALUES

Age	Respiratory rate (bpm)	Heart rate (bpm)
< 1 year	30–40	110–160
1–2 yrs	25–35	100–150
2–5 yrs	25–30	95–140
5–12 yrs	20–25	80–120
Over 12 yrs	15–20	60–100

Table 3.28 – GREEN: NICE 'TRAFFIC LIGHTS' CLINICAL ASSESSMENT TOOL

Colour	Normal colour of skin, lips and tongue
Activity	Responds normally to social cues Content/smiles Stays awake or awakens quickly Strong/normal cry/not crying
Hydration	Normal skin and eyes Moist mucous membranes
Other	No amber or red symptoms or signs

Table 3.29 – AMBER: NICE 'TRAFFIC LIGHTS' CLINICAL ASSESSMENT TOOL

Colour	Pallor reported by parent/carer
Activity	Not responding normally to social cues Wakes only with prolonged stimulation Decreased activity No smile
Respiratory	Nasal flaring Tachypnoea: ● RR >50/min age 6–12 months ● RR >40/min age >12 months O_2 sat ≤ 95% in air Crackles
Hydration	Dry mucous membranes Poor feeding in infants Capillary Refill Time (CRT) ≥3 seconds ↓Urinary output
Other	Fever for ≥5 days Swelling of a limb or joint Non-weight bearing/not using an extremity A new lump >2 cm

Table 3.30 – RED: NICE 'TRAFFIC LIGHTS' CLINICAL ASSESSMENT TOOL

Colour	Pale/mottled/ashen/blue
Activity	No response to social cues Appears ill to a healthcare professional Unable to rouse, or if roused, does not stay awake Weak/high pitched/continuous cry
Respiratory	Grunting Tachypnoea: RR >60/min Moderate or severe chest indrawing
Hydration	Reduced skin turgor
Other	0-3 months, temp ≥38°C 3–6 months, temp ≥39°C Non blanching rash Bulging fontanelle Neck stiffness Status epilepticus Focal seizures Focal neurological signs Bile-stained vomiting

Section 3 Medical Undifferentiated Complaints

Introduction

Childhood respiratory illnesses include:
1. Asthma.
2. Bronchiolitis.
3. Croup.
4. URTIs (tonsillitis, otitis media).
5. Pneumonia.

1. Asthma

For the management of mild, moderate, severe and life-threatening asthma **refer to the asthma in children guideline**.

2. Bronchiolitis

2.1 Introduction
Bronchiolitis is an acute, self-limiting respiratory infection that is usually caused by Respiratory Syncytial Virus (RSV) and occurs predominantly in the autumn and winter months. It is characterised by inflammation of the bronchioles.

2.2 Assesment
- Clinical presentation: a coryzal baby (peak age 2–5 months) with their first wheezy episode.

- Irregular breathing and apnoeas are frequently reported.

- During the first 72 hours, bronchiolitic infants may deteriorate clinically, before symptomatic improvements are seen.

- The baby's parents and siblings often have concurrent respiratory illnesses and may report sore throats or dry coughs.

- Examination may reveal:
  - ↓oxygen saturations
  - ↑respiratory rate
  - recession
  - fine, bilateral inspiratory crackles
  - high-pitched expiratory wheezes
  - low grade fever
  - high fevers (temp >38.5 °C) suggest bacterial pneumonia rather than bronchiolitis.

- Premature babies, those with chronic lung disease, children with congenital heart disease, cystic fibrosis, congenital or acquired immune deficiency (HIV), and those either aged <2 months or having apnoeas are at highest risk and **must** be transferred to further care.

- Previously well babies with diminished feeding, irregular breathing, hypoxia (O_2 saturations <95% on air), tachypnoea or tachycardia should also be transferred to further care where they will receive respiratory support and help with feeding/hydration.

2.3 Management
- Treatments aim to provide respiratory support and support feeding/hydration.

- Antivirals, antibiotics, steroids, nebulisers, physiotherapy, steam treatments, nasal decongestants, homeopathy and complementary therapies have not been shown to be effective.

- Acute bronchiolitis lasts approximately two weeks from its onset, but can last up to four weeks.

- Ongoing cough and persisting wheeze are not uncommonly seen after the initial illness has passed but should prompt further medical assessment.

3. Croup

3.1 Introduction
- Croup is a common, acute, respiratory illness of gradual onset, characterised by stridor that typically is mild and self-limiting.

3.2 Incidence
- Croup mostly affects children between the ages of 6 months and 6 years.
- It can occur all year round but peaks are seen in both spring and autumn.

3.3 Pathophysiology
- Croup results from viral infections, most commonly Parainfluenza, but also RSV, Influenza A and B, as well as *Mycoplasma pneumoniae*.
- Stridor, hoarseness and a barking 'seal-like' cough result from inflammation and narrowing around the subglottic region of larynx. (This is the narrowest point of the paediatric airway.)

NB Stridor may also be caused by epiglottitis, bacterial tracheitis, retropharyngeal abscesses, foreign bodies, anaphylaxis and angio-oedema, blunt trauma, glandular fever, inhalation of hot gases and diphtheria; all children with these conditions **must** be transferred to further care.

3.4 Assessment
- The child with croup may have mild clinical features in keeping with a simple, upper respiratory tract infection although they can present with more worrying features including respiratory distress, respiratory failure and respiratory arrest.
- (The features of respiratory distress – increased respiration rate, increased work of breathing, recession, nasal flaring, grunting, use of accessory muscles and stridor – are described in the **medical emergencies in childhood guideline**).
- The Modified Taussig Score is a simple clinical assessment tool that can be used to determine the severity of croup and the need for medication by scoring i) stridor and ii) recession (Table 3.31).

Table 3.31 – MODIFIED TAUSSIG CROUP SCORE

		Score*
Stridor	None	0
	Only on crying, exertion	1
	At rest	2
	Severe (biphasic)	3
Recession	None	0
	Only on crying, exertion	1
	At rest	2
	Severe (biphasic)	3

* Mild: 1–2; Moderate: 3–4; Severe: 5–6

- Hypoxia (O_2 saturations <95% on air), cyanosis, physical exhaustion (quietening stridor, reduced recession in a child that is becoming more unwell), restlessness, irritability and altered consciousness are ominous signs.
- Croup (and the differentials listed above) can cause: respiratory distress, but may also progress exceedingly rapidly, to produce complete upper airway obstruction and respiratory arrest. Therefore

all children with stridor must be transferred to further care for further medical assessment and observation.

- Keep the child in a position of comfort, sat upright and supported on a parent's lap – children often 'know' how to maintain their own airways in an optimal position (they often adopt a so-called 'tripod' posture).
- At all times, a calm approach is to be encouraged. Any intervention likely to upset the child – examining their ears, nose or throat, blood sugar measurement, cannulation, and even nebulisation (see below) – must be avoided, as distressing the child can precipitate an acute deterioration and complete airway obstruction. This is of increased importance in prehospital settings as skills for expert airway intervention will not be immediately available.

3.5 Severity and outcome

- Using the Modified Taussig Score, croup can be described as mild (1–2), moderate (3–4) or severe (5–6) (see Table 3.30).

3.6 Management

- **Steroids** are the mainstay of treatment – usually oral dexamethasone (nebulised budesonide may alternatively be used but may distress the child adversely worsening their symptoms) – and work by relieving subglottic inflammation.
- Children with moderate or severe croup (Modified Taussig Score ≥3), may benefit from early steroid treatment but must still be transferred to further care for subsequent observation.
  - Oral dexamethasone (**refer to dexamethasone guideline**) is preferred to nebulised Budesonide, as nebulisation frequently distresses small children, producing further airway narrowing.
  - NB The intravenous preparation of **dexamethasone** is administered **ORALLY** (**refer to Dexamethasone guideline**).

3.7 Referral pathway

As above, irrespective of whether steroids are given, all children with stridor must still be transferred to further care for subsequent observation, even if clinical improvements are noted at home.

4. Upper Respiratory Tract Infections (URTIs) e.g. tonsillitis (sore throat, acute pharyngitis, acute exudative tonsillitis), otitis media, etc.

4.1 Introduction

Upper respiratory tract infections (URTIs) are one of the commonest reasons for paediatric presentation, especially during the winter months.

4.2 Incidence

25% of all under 5-year olds see their GPs each year for tonsillitis.

4.3 Assessment

- Children with URTIs may complain of:
  - sore throat
  - cough
  - fever
  - headache
  - earache
  - systemic illness
  - anorexia and lethargy.
- Physical examination may reveal:
  - cervical lymphadenopathy
  - offensive breath
  - inflamed, purulent tonsils.

Breathing may also be compromised by either stridor or respiratory distress. In these circumstances, avoid attempts to examine the throat (see Croup guidance above) and transfer urgently to further care.

Children with 'muffled' voices that sound as if they have something hot in their mouths must also be transferred to further care, to exclude quinsy (peritonsillar abscess).

Tenderness behind the ear (over their mastoid process) in a child with otitis media, whose ear may/may not be starting to 'stickout' suggests mastoiditis (a dangerous infection of the bone around the ear) and must be transferred to further care.

The child's hydration status should be estimated as fluid intake can be significantly decreased.

4.4 Management

URTIs are usually self-limiting. Parents should be offered advice about managing their child's symptoms (rest, extra fluids, analgesia, antipyretics etc.) and informed about the likely duration of their child's illness (see Table 3.32).

Antibiotics are not prescribed routinely. Most URTIs are viral and so do not respond to antibiotics. Bacteria (e.g. Streptococci) also cause URTIs but even in these cases antibiotics are rarely needed; they don't improve the child's symptoms and they can often cause diarrhoea, vomiting and rashes.

Table 3.32 – TYPICAL DURATION OF ACUTE RESPIRATORY ILLNESSES

Condition	Duration
acute otitis media	4 days
acute sore throat/ pharyngitis/ tonsillitis	1 week
common cold	1½ weeks
acute rhinosinusitis	2½ weeks
acute cough/ bronchitis	3 weeks

GPs tend to use one of three antibiotic strategies:

a. **no prescribing** – no antibiotics are needed where the URTI is thought likely to clear up on its own.
b. **delayed prescribing** – delayed antibiotics are useful when symptoms fail to improve or even worsen.
c. **immediate prescribing** – immediate antibiotic prescriptions are reserved for the most severe cases, including:

- Under-2s with acute bilateral otitis media.
- Children with acute otitis media and otorrhoea (ear discharge).

- Children with acute streptococcal URTIs (no cough but fever, pustular tonsils and tender lymph nodes).

Antibiotics are also prescribed for children who are:
- Systemically very unwell.
- At high risk of serious complications because of pre-existing illnesses (heart, lung, renal, liver or neuromuscular disease, diabetes, cystic fibrosis, prematurity, immunosuppression or previous hospitalisations).

Cough mixtures: over-the-counter cough and cold preparations often contain sedatives and antihistamines that are dangerous if taken accidentally by small children in overdose. As a result, these medicines are no longer available for children aged 2 years or under. Children in this age group with colds and fever should now only be offered paracetamol or ibuprofen to manage their temperature, if needed.

Simple cough syrups containing glycerol, and honey and lemon may still be given, as well as vapour rubs and inhalant decongestants (see individual labelling).

4.5 Referral pathway
Hospital admission may also be indicated when:
- There is diminished fluid intake e.g. young child with severe tonsillitis and teenagers with glandular fever, and
- Where concerns regarding the diagnosis persist (NB early **meningococcal disease** is frequently misdiagnosed as an URTI in small children – where this diagnosis cannot be excluded, arrangements for an urgent medical opinion should be made). (**Refer to febrile illness in children guideline.**)

4.6 Non-conveyance
As when managing the febrile child, if a decision not to transfer a child to further care has been reached, a clinically justifiable reason should be present and properly documented.

'Safety netting,' with written advice, should again be encouraged and follow-up arrangements should be provided.

Where doubts persist seek senior advice or review.

Again, remember that early **meningococcal disease** is frequently misdiagnosed in small children simply as an URTI.

5. Pneumonia (lower respiratory tract infections, 'chest infections')

Children with pneumonia are likely to have the following signs and symptoms:
- Fever.
- Cough.
- Tachypnoea.
  - RR > 60 breaths/min, age 0–5 months
  - RR > 50 breaths/min, age 6–12 months
  - RR > 40 breaths/min, age > 12 months
- Nasal flaring.
- Chest indrawing.
- Oxygen saturations ≤95%.
- Crackles in the chest.

- Cyanosis.

Such children are likely to require antibiotics and possibly additional oxygen and should be seen by either their GP or a paediatrician.

Methodology

For details of the methodology used in the development of these guidelines refer to the guideline webpage.

KEY POINTS

Respiratory Illness
- **Childhood respiratory illnesses are common and usually self-limiting.**
- **Antibiotics are rarely indicated.**
- **Children with underlying conditions e.g. prematurity, chronic lung disease, congenital heart disease, cystic fibrosis, congenital or acquired immune deficiency (HIV), cerebral palsy, are especially vulnerable and must be seen either by their GP or in hospital.**
- **Tachypnoea is seen in all respiratory illnesses.**
- **Respiratory distress causes increased respiration rate, increased work of breathing, recession, nasal flaring, grunting, use of accessory muscles and stridor.**
- **Exhaustion suggests respiratory failure and respiratory arrest may rapidly follow.**
- **Stridor can progress rapidly to complete upper airway obstruction and respiratory arrest.**
- **Approach a child with stridor calmly and gently. Sit them upright, in a position of comfort and avoid painful/distressing procedures.**
- **Transfer all children with stridor for further medical assessment and observation.**
- **Steroids (dexamethasone) are used in moderate and severe croup.**
- **Children with pneumonia require antibiotics and possibly oxygen therapy. They should be seen by either their GP or a paediatrician.**
- **Whilst URTIs are very common, early meningococcal disease can easily be misdiagnosed as an URTI. (When unable to exclude this diagnosis, make arrangements for an urgent second opinion.)**
- **Provide a 'safety net' (with written information) for all children with respiratory illness not transferred to hospital.**
- **If uncertain, seek advice from either the child's GP or the out-of-hours doctor.**

1. Introduction

- Heat related illness is a relatively uncommon presenting condition to ambulance services but it can be life-threatening.
- Heat related illness can be **exogenous**, caused by environmental factors (e.g. the sun) or **endogenous** (e.g. drugs and exercise).
- Heat related illness is a continuum of heat related conditions (Figure 3.1).

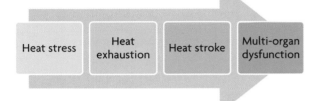

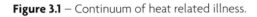

Figure 3.1 – Continuum of heat related illness.

The management of heat related illness is supportive: refer to Table 3.36.

Heat stress

- Heat stress is a mild form of heat illness, characterised by the features below (Table 3.33). This level of heat disorder is often self-managed, but if left untreated can progress to more serious conditions.

Table 3.33 – FEATURES OF HEAT STRESS (EUROPEAN RESUSCITATION COUNCIL GUIDELINES)

Heat stress
Temperature: normal or mildly elevated.
Heat oedema: swelling of feet and ankles.
Heat syncope: vasodilation and dehydration causing hypotension.
Heat cramps: sodium depletion causing cramps.

Heat exhaustion

- A less severe heat illness than heat stroke, lacking the defining neurological symptoms of this condition. Symptoms are mainly due to excess fluid loss and electrolyte imbalance.

Table 3.34 – FEATURES OF HEAT EXHAUSTION (ERC)[60]

Heat exhaustion
Systemic reaction to prolonged heat exposure (hours to days).
Temperature >37°C and <40°C.
Headache, dizziness, nausea, vomiting, tachycardia.
Hypotension, sweating, muscle pain, weakness and cramps.

Table 3.34 – FEATURES OF HEAT EXHAUSTION (ILCOR) continued

Heat exhaustion
Haemoconcentration.
Hyponatraemia or hypernatraemia.
May progress rapidly to heat stroke.

Heat stroke

- A 'systemic inflammatory response' to a core body temperature >40.6°C in addition to a change in mental status and organ dysfunction (European Resuscitation Council Guidelines)[60].

There are two types of heat stroke:

a. **Non-exertional heat stroke** due to very high external temperatures and/or high humidity; it tends to be more common in very hot climates. It tends to occur in the:
   - elderly
   - very young
   - chronically ill.

b. **Exertional heat stroke** is due to excess heat production. This tends to occur in:
   - athletes including marathon and fun-runners
   - manual workers
   - firefighters
   - military recruits.

Table 3.35 – FEATURES OF HEAT STROKE (ERC)[60]

Heat stroke
Core temperature ≥40°C.
Hot, dry skin (sweating is present in about 50% of cases of exertional heat stroke).
Early signs and symptoms, e.g., extreme fatigue, headache, fainting, facial flushing, vomiting and diarrhoea.
Cardiovascular dysfunction including arrhythmias and hypotension.
Respiratory dysfunction including ARDS.
Central nervous system dysfunction including seizures and coma.
Liver and renal failure.
Coagulopathy.
Rhabdomyolysis.

2. Incidence

The exact incidence of heat stroke is unknown with many sufferers self-managing their condition. Mortality, in the absence of a heat wave is relatively low; in the United Kingdom it is estimated to be 40 deaths per million annually.

A variety of medications may predispose to the development of heat illness. In addition, individuals who take drugs of abuse (e.g. cocaine, ecstasy, amphetamines) and then engage in vigorous dancing in crowded 'rave' settings may also develop heat illness.

3. Severity and Outcome

- Heat stroke is a life-threatening emergency that requires prompt appropriate treatment, with estimates of mortality of 10–50%. Recovery from heat stroke even after appropriate treatment and rehabilitation may be incomplete and leave patients with persistent functional impairment.

- **Systemic effects** – heat stroke can lead to a variety of life-threatening systemic conditions including: disseminated intravascular coagulation, rhabdomyolysis, renal failure, hepatic necrosis, metabolic acidosis, decreased tissue perfusion, in addition to cerebral and cerebellar damage.

4. Pathophysiology

- In heat illnesses there is an imbalance in the metabolic production and subsequent loss of heat by the body. This increase in core body temperature has multiple undesirable effects on many body systems. Systemically this increased temperature leads to swelling and degeneration at both cellular and tissue levels.

- **Cellular changes** – at increased temperatures cellular organelles swell and stop functioning properly. Cell membranes become distorted, leading to unwanted increased permeability and inappropriate movement of ions into and out of cells. Red blood cells also change shape at elevated temperatures and their capacity to carry oxygen is decreased. At higher temperatures cells will also undergo inappropriate apoptosis and die.

5. Assessment and Management

- For the assessment and management of heat related illness refer to Table 3.36.

Methodology

For details of the methodology used in the development of this guideline, refer to the guideline webpage.

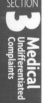

SECTION **3** **Medical** Undifferentiated Complaints

KEY POINTS

Heat Related Illness

- **Heat exhaustion/heat stroke occurs in high external temperatures, as a result of excess heat production and with certain drugs. The higher the level of activity the lower the environmental temperature required to produce heat stroke.**

- **Do not assume that collapse in an athlete is due to heat – check for other causes.**

- **In heat exhaustion the patient may present with flu-like symptoms, such as headache, nausea, dizziness, vomiting, and cramps: the temperature may not be elevated.**

- **In heat stroke the patient will have neurological symptoms such as decreased level of consciousness, ataxia, and convulsions and the temperature will usually be elevated, typically >40°C.**

- **Remove the patient from the hot environment or remove cause, if possible, remove clothing and cool.**

Table 3.36 – ASSESSMENT and MANAGEMENT of:

Heat Related Illness

ASSESSMENT	MANAGEMENT

● Assess ABCD	● If any of the following **TIME CRITICAL** features are present:
	  – major **ABC** problems
	  – haemodynamic compromise
	  – decreased level of consciousness, then:
	● Start correcting **A** and **B** problems.
	● Undertake a **TIME CRITICAL** transfer to nearest appropriate receiving hospital.
	● Provide an alert/information call.
	● Continue patient management en-route.

● Assess	Undertake physical examination and assess for the presence of features of heat related illness (Tables 3.32–3.35) ● Remove the patient from the hot environment or remove cause if possible. ● Remove to an air-conditioned vehicle where available. ● Remove all clothing. ● Commence cooling with fanning, tepid sponging, water misting or with a wet sheet loosely over the patient's body. NB Consider other potential causes e.g. diabetes or cardiac problems.
● Temperature	Measure and record: ● The patient's core temperature. ● If possible and time allows measure the environmental temperature. NB The core temperature may or may not be elevated, but patients may be tachycardic, hypotensive and/or sweating excessively.
● Heat stroke	Heat stroke is potentially fatal and the patient needs to be cooled as an emergency. ● If cold or iced water is used, massaging of the skin may be needed to overcome cold induced vasoconstriction and ensure effective heat loss. ● Apply ice packs if available wrapped in a thin cloth or towel to the patient's neck, axilla and groin. NB Ice packs applied directly to the skin can cause frostbite. ● Transfer the patient with air conditioning turned on or with windows open. NB Immersion in ice water is effective but usually not possible in the prehospital environment.
● GCS	● Check Glasgow Coma Score.
● Oxygen	● If the patient is hypoxaemic, administer high levels of supplemental oxygen and aim for a target saturation within the range of 94–98% – refer to oxygen guideline.
● Fluid therapy	● If fluid therapy is indicated refer to intravascular fluid therapy guidelines. ● **DO NOT** delay on scene for fluid replacement; administer en-route.
● Blood glucose	● Measure blood glucose – **refer to glycaemic emergencies guidelines**.
● Vital signs	● Monitor vital signs. ● Monitor ECG.
● Transfer	● Transfer patients to nearest appropriate receiving hospital. ● Continue management en-route. ● Complete documentation.[49]

3 Medical Undifferentiated Complaints
SECTION

Hyperventilation Syndrome [238–249]

1. Introduction

- Hyperventilation syndrome (HVS) is a common presentation in prehospital care.
- It is defined as 'a rate of ventilation exceeding metabolic needs and higher than that required to maintain a normal level of plasma carbon dioxide (CO_2)'.
- Hyperventilation can occur in a number of conditions, including life-threatening conditions such as:
  - pulmonary embolism
  - diabetic ketoacidosis
  - asthma
  - hypovolaemia.

The cause of hyperventilation cannot always be determined in the prehospital environment, especially in the early stages.

2. Incidence

- It is estimated that 6–11% of primary care patients may suffer from some form of HVS. The condition is more common in women.
- HVS most commonly occurs between 15 and 55 years of age, although it can occur at any age, but it is rare in children where the most likely cause is physical illness .

3. Severity and Outcome

- Although death is rare, the condition can be debilitating with physical signs and symptoms and is distressing.

4. Pathophysiology

- The cause of HVS is unknown but it is hypothesised that stress may result in an exaggerated respiratory response. Stressors may include: psychological distress, caffeine, isoproterenol, cholecystokinin and deficiencies in sodium lactate metabolism. Other causes include elevated level of CO_2, and some have argued that sufferers have a lower threshold trigger for the 'fight-flight response'.
- HVS presents in two forms, acute and chronic. Acute HVS accounts for 1% of cases.

- Over-breathing results in hypocapnia (decreased level of carbon dioxide in the blood) causing respiratory alkalosis and a decreased level of serum-ionised calcium, resulting in a number of physical and psychological signs and symptoms. Patients may present with one or more of the signs and symptoms listed in Table 3.37.

Table 3.37 – PRESENTING FEATURES

Signs and Symptoms

Breathing:
- Sudden dyspnoea.
- Hyperpnoea.
- Tachypnoea.

Electrolyte imbalance:
- Tetany due to calcium imbalance.
- Paraesthesia (numbness and tingling of the mouth and lips and extremities).
- Carpopedal spasm.

Psychological:
- Acute agitation and anxiety.

Other:
- Chest pain – may resemble angina pectoris.
- Palpitations.
- Tachycardia and electrocardiographic changes.
- Aching of the muscles of the chest.
- Feeling of light-headedness or dizziness.
- Weakness and fatigue.
- Frequent sighing.
- Non-diaphragmatic respiratory effort.

Assessment and Management

For the assessment and management of hyperventilation syndrome refer to Table 3.38 and Figure 3.2.

Methodology

For details of the methodology used in the development of this guideline refer to the guideline webpage.

KEY POINTS

Hyperventilation Syndrome
- **HVS is a diagnonsis of exclusion.**
- **Medical conditions can cause hyperventilation.**
- **In children a medical cause is more likely than stress.**
- **Administer supplemental oxygen if hypoxaemic (SpO$_2$ <94%)**
- **Tetany, paraesthesia and carpopedal spasm may occur.**

Hyperventilation Syndrome

Table 3.38 – ASSESSMENT and MANAGEMENT of:

Hyperventilation Syndrome

ASSESSMENT	MANAGEMENT

● Assess ABCD	● If any of the following **TIME CRITICAL** features present:
	  − major **ABCD** problems
	  − cyanosis
	  − reduced level of consciousness − **refer to decreased level of consciousness guideline**.
	  − hypoxia − refer to oxygen guideline.
	● Start correcting **A** and **B** problems.
	● Undertake a **TIME CRITICAL** transfer to nearest receiving hospital.
	● Continue patient management en-route.
	● Provide an alert/information call.
	NB If any of the **TIME CRITICAL** features listed above are present, it is unlikely to be due to hyperventilation syndrome but is more likely to be physiological hyperventilation, secondary to an underlying pathological process.

Ask the patient if they have an individualised treatment plan	● Follow individualised treatment plan if available. ● The patient will often be able to guide their care.
Specifically assess: History	⚠ **Always presume hyperventilation is secondary to hypoxia or other underlying respiratory or metabolic disorder until proven otherwise and such is a diagnosis of exclusion.** ● Cause of hyperventilation. ● Previous episodes of hyperventilation. ● Previous medical history. ● Features of hyperventilation syndrome refer to Table 3.37.
Differential diagnosis	Consider differential diagnosis such as: ● Heart failure − **refer to heart failure guideline**. ● Acute asthma − **refer to asthma guidelines**. ● Chest infection − **refer to medical emergencies guideline**. ● Pulmonary embolism − **refer to pulmonary embolism guideline**. ● Diabetic ketoacidosis or other causes of metabolic acidosis − **refer to glycaemic emergencies guideline**. ● Pneumothorax − **refer to thoracic trauma guideline**. ● Drug overdose − **refer to overdose and poisoning guidelines**. ● Acute myocardial infarction − **refer to acute coronary syndrome guideline**.
Oxygen saturation	● Apply pulse oximeter. ● **DO NOT** administer supplemental oxygen unless hypoxaemic (SpO_2 <94%) − refer to oxygen guideline. NB Low SpO_2 is not a presenting feature of HVS and will indicate an underlying clinical condition.
Breathing	● Consider auscultation of breath sounds during assessment of breathing. ● Aim to restore a normal level of pCO_2 over a period of time by reassuring the patient and coaching them regarding their respirations. ● Try to remove the source of the patient's anxiety − this is particularly important in the management of children. ● **Refer to dyspnoea guideline**.
● Transfer	Transfer to further care: ● Patients experiencing their first episode. ● Known HVS sufferers whose symptoms have not settled, or re-occur within 10 minutes. ● Patients who have an individualised care plan and a responsible adult present may be considered for non conveyance and managing at home according to local protocols. Provide details of local care pathways if symptoms re-occur.

Hyperventilation Syndrome

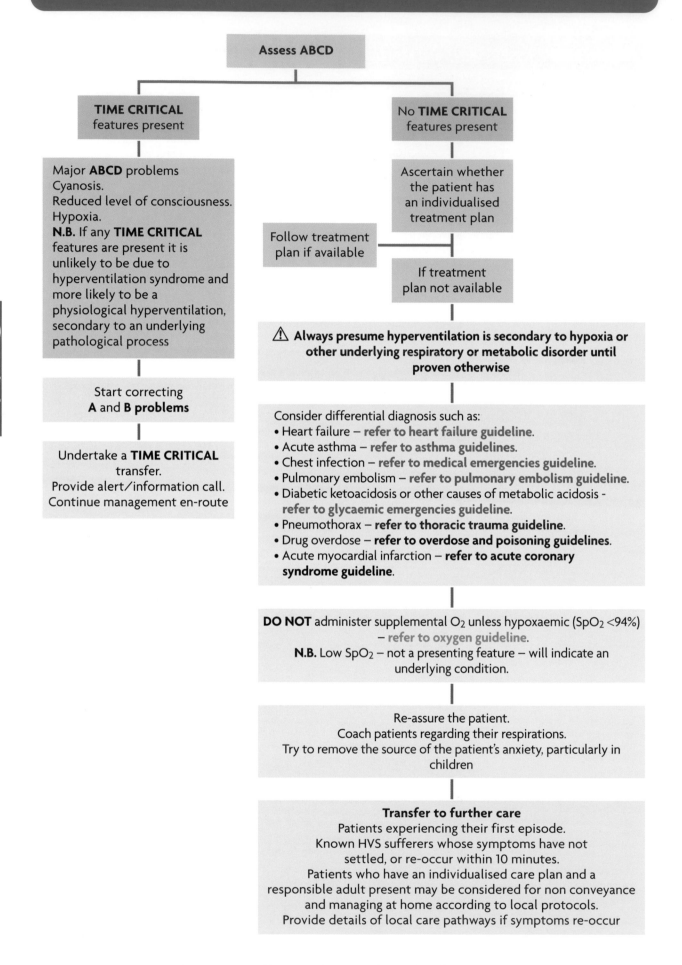

Assess ABCD

TIME CRITICAL features present

Major **ABCD** problems
Cyanosis.
Reduced level of consciousness.
Hypoxia.
N.B. If any **TIME CRITICAL** features are present it is unlikely to be due to hyperventilation syndrome and more likely to be a physiological hyperventilation, secondary to an underlying pathological process

Start correcting **A** and **B problems**

Undertake a **TIME CRITICAL** transfer.
Provide alert/information call.
Continue management en-route

No **TIME CRITICAL** features present

Ascertain whether the patient has an individualised treatment plan

Follow treatment plan if available

If treatment plan not available

⚠ **Always presume hyperventilation is secondary to hypoxia or other underlying respiratory or metabolic disorder until proven otherwise**

Consider differential diagnosis such as:
• Heart failure – **refer to heart failure guideline**.
• Acute asthma – **refer to asthma guidelines**.
• Chest infection – **refer to medical emergencies guideline**.
• Pulmonary embolism – **refer to pulmonary embolism guideline**.
• Diabetic ketoacidosis or other causes of metabolic acidosis - **refer to glycaemic emergencies guideline**.
• Pneumothorax – **refer to thoracic trauma guideline**.
• Drug overdose – **refer to overdose and poisoning guidelines**.
• Acute myocardial infarction – **refer to acute coronary syndrome guideline**.

DO NOT administer supplemental O_2 unless hypoxaemic (SpO_2 <94%) – refer to oxygen guideline.
N.B. Low SpO_2 – not a presenting feature – will indicate an underlying condition.

Re-assure the patient.
Coach patients regarding their respirations.
Try to remove the source of the patient's anxiety, particularly in children

Transfer to further care
Patients experiencing their first episode.
Known HVS sufferers whose symptoms have not settled, or re-occur within 10 minutes.
Patients who have an individualised care plan and a responsible adult present may be considered for non conveyance and managing at home according to local protocols.
Provide details of local care pathways if symptoms re-occur

Figure 3.2 – Assessment and management of hyperventilation syndrome algorithm.

1. Introduction

- Hypothermia is defined as a core body temperature below 35°C (Figure 3.3). It is a potentially life-threatening condition.

- There are three main types of hypothermia depending on the speed at which a person loses heat:

  i. **Acute hypothermia (immersion hypothermia)**

  - This occurs when a person loses heat very rapidly e.g. by falling into cold water. It is associated with near-drowning. Acute hypothermia may also occur in a snow avalanche when it may be associated with asphyxia.

  ii. **Subacute hypothermia (exhaustion hypothermia)**

  - This typically occurs in a hill walker who is exercising in moderate cold who becomes exhausted and is unable to generate any heat. Heat loss will occur more rapidly in windy conditions or if the patient is wet or inadequately clothed. It may be associated with injury or frostbite. Do not forget that if one person in a group of walkers is hypothermic, others in the party who are similarly dressed and who have been exposed to identical conditions may also be hypothermic.

  iii. **Chronic hypothermia**

  - In chronic hypothermia heat loss occurs slowly, often over days or longer. It most commonly occurs in the elderly person living in an inadequately heated house or the person who is sleeping rough. It can be associated with injury or illness e.g. the patient who falls or has a stroke and who is on the floor overnight.

- Mixed forms of hypothermia may occur; e.g. the exhausted walker who collapses and falls into a stream.

Diagnosis

- In order to measure core body temperature accurately and make a diagnosis, a low-reading thermometer is required. In the prehospital environment, measuring the patient's temperature using an oesophageal, bladder or rectal, approach may not be practical. However, tympanic thermometry in cold environments may not be reliable (as the probe is not well insulated) and if the patient is in cardiac arrest, with no blood flow in the carotid artery.

- Because of the difficulty of diagnosing hypothermia in the prehospital environment, patients should be treated as having hypothermia if there is clinical suspicion of the diagnosis based on the risk factors in Table 3.39, the clinical history, examination, and the presence of concurrent injuries or illness which may suggest hypothermia.

Table 3.39 – RISK FACTORS FOR HYPOTHERMIA

Factors
● Older patients > 80 years due to impaired thermoregulation.
● Children due to their proportionately larger body surface area.
● Some medical conditions e.g. hypothyroidism, stroke etc. due to impaired thermoregulation.
● Intoxicated patients e.g. alcohol, recreational drugs.
● In association with near-drowning and in patients exposed to cold, wet and windy environments especially if inadequately dressed.
● Patients suffering from exhaustion.
● Injury and immobility.
● Decreased level of consciousness.

2. Incidence

- The true incidence is unknown but the ONS report fewer than 400 deaths per annum in England and Wales. However, it is suggested that hypothermia may be under-diagnosed in temperate climates such as the UK.

- Death from hypothermia is more common in women than men and in people over 80 years old.

3. Pathophysiology

As the core body temperature falls there may be:

- Progressive decrease in the level of consciousness (**refer to altered level of consciousness guideline**).

- Other brain dysfunction e.g. slurring of speech, muscular incoordination.

- Slowing heart rate.

- Slowing respiratory rate.

- Development of cardiac arrhythmias (sinus bradycardia → atrial fibrillation → ventricular fibrillation → asystole).

- Cooling the body decreases oxygen demand and is protective for the brain and vital organs; therefore **DO NOT STOP CARDIAC RESUSCITATION IN THE FIELD** as good outcomes have resulted from prolonged resuscitation of hypothermic patients.

4. Severity and Outcome

The severity of hypothermia can be classified into mild, moderate and severe depending on the patient's core body temperature (Figure 3.3).

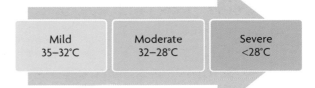

| Mild 35–32°C | Moderate 32–28°C | Severe <28°C |

Figure 3.3 – Severity of hypothermia.

Medical Undifferentiated Complaints — SECTION 3

Hypothermia

- However, in the prehospital environment, core temperature is difficult to measure, and it may be better to define the severity clinically (Table 3.40).

5. Assessment and Management

For the assessment and management of hypothermia refer to Table 3.41.

Methodology

For details of the methodology used in the development of this guideline, please refer to the guideline webpage.

Table 3.40 – CLINICAL STAGES OF HYPOTHERMIA

Stage	Clinical Signs
I	Clearly conscious and shivering.
II	Impaired consciousness without shivering.
III	Unconscious.
IV	No breathing.
V	Death due to irreversible hypothermia.

Table 3.41 – ASSESSMENT and MANAGEMENT of:

Hypothermia

ASSESSMENT	MANAGEMENT
Assess ABCD	<ul><li>If any of the following **TIME CRITICAL** features are present:</li><li>Major ABC problems.</li><li>Haemodynamic compromise.</li><li>Decreased level of consciousness.</li><li>Cardiac arrest, then:</li></ul>Start correcting **A** (with cervical spine protection if indicated) and **B** problems. Undertake a **TIME CRITICAL** transfer to nearest appropriate receiving hospital. Provide an alert/information call. Continue patient management en-route.
Assess	Undertake physical examination and assess for the presence of features of hypothermia (Table 3.40): early symptoms are non-specific and include: ataxia, slurred speech, apathy, irrational behaviour, and decrease in the level of consciousness (**refer to decreased level of consciousness guideline**), heart rate and rhythm, and respiratory rate.
Temperature	Measure and record the patient's core temperature – temperature measurement in the field is difficult, therefore it is important to suspect and treat hypothermia from the history and circumstances of the situation. NB Shivering occurs early but will cease when the temperature falls further (Table 3.40); the patient will feel cold to the touch.
Warming	**PREVENT FURTHER HEAT LOSS** as in the mildly hypothermic patient, preventing further heat loss will enable the patient to warm up by their own metabolism.<ul><li>Place in vehicles.</li><li>When sheltered e.g. in the ambulance, gently cut off wet clothes and dry the patient before covering them with blankets. **DO NOT** wrap cold patients in foil blankets – you will insulate them and keep them cold.</li><li>If the patient is conscious provide a hot drink/food if available and appropriate.</li><li>**DO NOT** rub the patient's skin as this causes vasodilatation and may increase heat loss.</li><li>**DO NOT** give the patient alcohol as this causes vasodilatation and may increase heat loss.</li><li>Manage co-existing trauma or medical condition as they arise (refer to appropriate **trauma/medical** guidelines).</li></ul>
Resuscitation	**BEWARE:** Hypothermia may mimic death with very slow and weak or undetectable pulse, very slow and shallow respiration, fixed dilated pupils, and increased muscle tone.<ul><li>Airway – clear the airway.</li><li>Ventilation – if there are no signs of respiration, ventilate with high concentrations of oxygen (**refer to appropriate resuscitation guidelines**).</li><li>Signs of life – look for signs of life (palpate central artery, ECG monitoring etc.) for up to 1 minute.</li><li>Cardiac arrest – **refer to appropriate resuscitation guidelines** and additional information below.</li><li>Rough handling can invoke cardiac arrhythmias (including VF and pulseless VT) so handle patients carefully.</li><li>Cardiac arrythmias (except VF) will usually revert spontaneously with re-warming and do not need treatment unless they persist after re-warming.</li></ul>

Table 3.41 – ASSESSMENT and MANAGEMENT of:

Hypothermia *continued*

ASSESSMENT	MANAGEMENT
Oxygen	• If the patient is hypoxaemic, administer high levels of supplemental oxygen and aim for a target saturation within the range 94–98% – **refer to oxygen guideline**.
Fluid therapy	• If fluid therapy is indicated, refer to **intravascular fluid therapy guidelines**. NB The use of cold fluids should be avoided if possible. • **DO NOT** delay on scene for fluid replacement; administer en-route.
Blood glucose	• Measure blood glucose level if <4.0 mmol/L treat for hypoglycaemia (**refer to glycaemic emergencies guidelines**).
Vital signs	• Monitor ECG. • Respiratory rate may be very slow – measure for 10 seconds.
Transfer	• Transfer patients to nearest appropriate receiving hospital. • In severe hypothermia, the fastest way to re-warm patients is by extracorporeal warming: – this may not be available in every hospital so follow any local care pathways. • Continue management en-route. • Complete documentation.[49]
	Additional information for cardiac arrest in hypothermia: Follow the usual procedure (**refer to appropriate resuscitation guidelines**) with the following minor changes: • **Signs of life** – because the heart rate and respiratory rate may be slow and difficult to detect, look for signs of life (palpate central artery, ECG monitoring etc.) for up to 1 minute. • Hypothermia may cause chest wall stiffness and ventilations and compressions may be more difficult. • Drugs are less likely to be effective at low body temperatures: do not give drugs if the core temperature is below 30°C. • Defibrillation is less likely to be effective at low body temperatures: if VF persists after three shocks, delay further defibrillation until the core temperature is above 30°C. • **DO NOT STOP CARDIAC RESUSCITATION IN THE FIELD**, hypothermia is protective and good outcomes have resulted from prolonged resuscitation of hypothermic patients. **Trauma (refer to appropriate trauma guidelines)** – hypothermia worsens the prognosis of trauma patients, so it is important that patients who are initially normothermic, are not allowed to become hypothermic. This may occur e.g. during a prolonged extrication from a road traffic collision or from the cooling of burns.

KEY POINTS

Hypothermia

• **Hypothermia is defined as a core body temperature below 35°C.**
• **There are three main classifications depending on the speed at which a person loses heat: acute, subacute, and chronic hypothermia.**
• **Prevent further heat loss; wrap the patient appropriately, do not rub the skin or give alcohol.**
• **Patients with decreased level of consciousness may develop VF or pulseless VT and should be immobilised and managed horizontally.**
• **Cardiac arrest is treated in the usual way, bearing in mind that drugs/defibrillation are less likely to be effective at low body temperatures.**

3 **Medical** Undifferentiated Complaints SECTION

1. Introduction

- Sickle cell disease is a hereditary condition affecting the haemoglobin contained within red blood cells.

- A previous history of sickle cell disease and sickle cell crisis will be present in most cases, with the patient almost always being aware of their condition.

- The signs and symptoms include (**any of those listed below may apply**):
  - severe pain, most commonly in the long bones and/or joints of the arms and legs, but also in the back and abdomen
  - stroke
  - high temperature
  - difficulty in breathing, reduced oxygen (O_2) saturation, cough and chest pain may indicate Acute Chest Syndrome
  - pallor
  - tiredness/weakness
  - dehydration
  - headache
  - priapism.

2. Incidence

- There are different types of sickle cell disease found mainly in people of African or Afro-Caribbean origin, but can also affect people of Mediterranean, Middle Eastern and Asian origin. In the United Kingdom it is estimated that 15,000 adults and children suffer from sickle cell disease with 1 in every 2,000 babies born with the condition.

3. Severity and Outcome

- These painful crises can result in damage to the patient's lungs, kidneys, liver, bones and other organs and tissues. The recurrent nature of these acute episodes is the most disabling feature of sickle cell disease, and many chronic problems can result, including leg ulcers, blindness and stroke. Acute Chest Syndrome[a] is the leading cause of death amongst sickle cell patients.

4. Pathophysiology

- The red cells of patients with sickle cell disease are prone to assuming a permanently sickled shape when exposed to a variety of factors including hypoxia, cold or dehydration. These cells are prone to mechanical damage, hence the haemolytic anaemia in this group of patients, and to occluding the microvasculature leading to tissue hypoxia and pain and end organ damage.

- A crisis may follow as a result of an infection, during pregnancy, following surgery or a variety of other causes including mental stress.

5. Assessment and Management

For the assessment and management of patients with sickle cell crisis refer to Table 3.42 or Figure 3.4.

Methodology

For details of the methodology used in the development of this guideline refer to the guideline webpage.

KEY POINTS

Sickle Cell Crisis

- **Sickle cell disease is a hereditary condition affecting the haemoglobin contained within red blood cells; the cells are irregular in shape and occlude the microvasculature leading to tissue ischaemia.**

- **Sickle cell crises can result in damage to the lungs, kidneys, liver, bones and other organs and tissues.**

- **Sickle cell crises can be very painful and patients should be offered pain relief.**

- **Administer supplemental oxygen to all patients including those with chronic sickle lung disease.**

- **Patients with sickle cell disease can be dangerously ill but in no pain (e.g. aplastic crisis, stroke, hepatic sequestration, PE, etc.).**

- **Acute Chest Syndrome is a leading cause of death amongst sickle cell patients and is characterised by hypoxia and tachypnoea.**

---

[a]**Acute Chest Syndrome (also known as chest crisis)**. This is a common and potentially life-threatening complication of painful crises, and is often precipitated by a chest infection. The patient becomes breathless, hypoxic and tachypnoeic/tachycardic over a short period of time. Chest pain is often present, and the hypoxia responds poorly to inhaled oxygen. Crackles are often present in the lung bases and will ascend rapidly to involve the whole lung fields in severe cases. Radiological changes follow late and patients may be critically ill with near normal radiology. If a chest crisis is suspected, treatment should be initiated with inhaled oxygen and intravenous fluids. In hospital, intravenous antibiotics and urgent exchange transfusion are likely to be instituted after discussion with the haematology team. Intensive care and mechanical ventilation may be required in some cases. Pulmonary embolus is an important differential diagnosis.

Sickle Cell Crisis

Table 3.42 – ASSESSMENT and MANAGEMENT of:

Sickle Cell Crisis

ASSESSMENT	MANAGEMENT

● Assess ABCD	● If any of the following **TIME CRITICAL** features present:
	  – major **ABCD** problems
	  – ᵃacute chest syndrome, then:
	● Start correcting **A** and **B** and undertake a **TIME CRITICAL** transfer to nearest receiving hospital.
	● Continue patient management en-route.
	● Provide an alert/information call.

● Ask the patient if they have an individualised treatment plan	● Follow the treatment plan if available. ● The patient will often be able to guide their care. ● Follow **medical emergencies guideline** in addition to the specific management detailed below.
● Oxygen	Administer supplemental oxygen to **ALL** patients including those with chronic sickle lung disease; oxygen helps to counter tissue hypoxia and reduce cell clumping. ● **Adults** – administer supplemental oxygen via an appropriate mask/cannula until a reliable SpO₂ measurement is available; then adjust the oxygen flow to aim for target saturation within the range of 94–98%. ● **Children** – administer high levels of supplemental oxygen. ● Apply pulse oximeter. NB It is safer to over-oxygenate until a reliable SpO₂ measurement is available.
● ECG	● Undertake a 12-lead ECG in patients with chest pain to exclude obvious cardiac causes (**refer to acute coronary syndrome guideline**).
● Fluid	Patients with a sickle cell crisis will not have acute fluid loss, but may present with dehydration if they have been ill for an extended period of time. ● If fluid resuscitation is indicated (refer to intravascular fluid therapy guideline).
● Pain management	● Offer **ALL** patients pain relief. ● **Entonox** – administer initially but do not administer for extended periods (refer to Entonox guideline). ● **Opiate analgesia** – administer orally or subcutaneously rather than intravenously if possible (refer to morphine guidelines). The dose should be guided by the patient's hand-held record if available, otherwise **refer to pain management guidelines**.
● Transfer to further care	● Transfer to specialist unit where the patient is usually treated. ● Patients should not walk to the ambulance as this will exacerbate the effects of hypoxia in the tissues.

ᵃ**Acute Chest Syndrome (also known as chest crisis)**. This is a common and potentially life-threatening complication of painful crises, and is often precipitated by a chest infection. The patient becomes breathless, hypoxic and tachypnoeic/tachycardic over a short period of time. Chest pain is often present, and the hypoxia responds poorly to inhaled oxygen. Crackles are often present in the lung bases and will ascend rapidly to involve the whole lung fields in severe cases. Radiological changes follow late and patients may be critically ill with near normal radiology. If a chest crisis is suspected, treatment should be initiated with inhaled oxygen and intravenous fluids. In hospital, intravenous antibiotics and urgent exchange transfusion are likely to be instituted after discussion with the haematology team. Intensive care and mechanical ventilation may be required in some cases. Pulmonary embolus is an important differential diagnosis.

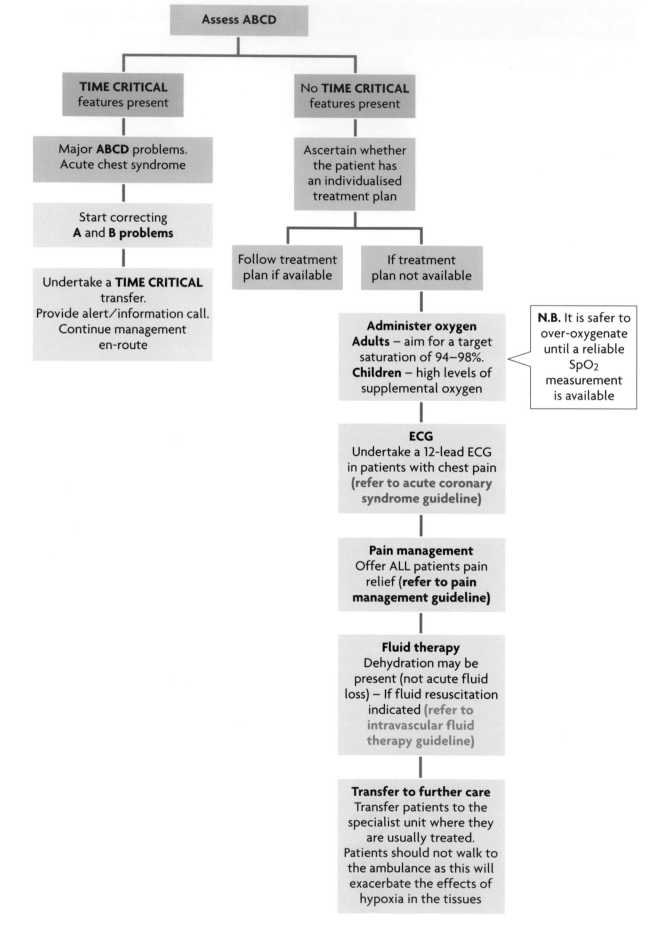

Figure 3.4 – Assessment and management algorithm for sickle cell crisis.

1. Introduction

- Meningococcal disease is the leading cause of death by infection in children and young adults and can kill a healthy person of any age within hours of their first symptoms.

2. Incidence

- There are 1,200 confirmed cases of meningococcal disease in England and Wales each year, although the true figure is probably twice this number.

3. Pathophysiology

- Two clinical categories are described although they often overlap:
  - i.   meningitis.
  - ii. septicaemia.
- In meningitis, the meninges covering the brain and spinal cord are infected by bacteria causing inflammation.
- In septicaemia, bacteria invade the bloodstream, releasing toxins and producing a clinical picture of shock and circulatory collapse. Deterioration can be rapid and may be irreversible, with treatment becoming less effective by the minute. Early recognition and prompt treatment improves clinical outcomes.

4. Severity and Outcome

- The mortality from septicaemia can be up to 40% but if recognised early, resuscitated aggressively and managed on ITU, mortalities of less than 5% can be achieved.

5. Assessment

- **Refer to medical emergencies in adults or children**.
- The 'classical features' – **neck stiffness, photophobia** and **haemorrhagic rash** – should be sought and are useful clinical discriminators when present, but less helpful and potentially falsely reassuring when absent.
- These features are more common in adults, older children and teenagers but quite rare in pre-school children. Small children often present with non-specific signs such as nausea, vomiting, loss of appetite, sore throat and coryzal symptoms – features that might otherwise suggest a diagnosis of viral illness.

Airway:

- Added sounds e.g. grunting.
- Upper airway obstruction e.g. coma, fitting.

Breathing:[a]

- Respiratory rate.
- Breathing effort.
- Oxygen saturations (SaO_2).

Circulation:[a]

- Pulse.
- Capillary refill time.

[a]For the 'normal' paediatric age-related respiratory and cardiovascular parameters **refer to medical emergencies in children – overview guideline**.

Disability:

A   Alert
V   Responds to voice
P   Responds to painful stimulus
U   Unresponsive

Expose:

- Examine for rashes (see below).
- Measure temperature if appropriate.

The patient may have been previously unwell with non-specific symptoms e.g.

- Irritability.
- Pyrexia.
- 'Flu-like' symptoms.

THE RASH

Presentation – the classical, haemorrhagic, non-blanching rash (may be petechial or purpuric) is seen in approximately 40% of infected children.

In pigmented skin it can be helpful to look at the conjunctiva under the lower eyelid.

In an unwell patient, a non-blanching rash suggests meningococcal septicaemia.

The 'Glass' or 'Tumbler' test

A petechial or purpuric rash does **NOT** blanch/fade when pressed with a glass tumbler, **remaining visible through the glass**.

If the 'glass' test is negative, do not assume that meningococcal disease has been excluded; often there will be **NO** rash.

If meningococcal disease is suspected in any patient (irrespective of the presence or absence of a rash) undertake a TIME CRITICAL transfer (refer to Figure 3.5).

CLINICAL FINDINGS

The patient may be 'unwell' and deteriorate rapidly. Clinical features include:

- Fever (may be masked by peripheral shutdown or antipyretics).
- Cold, mottled skin (especially extremities) (the skin may rarely be warm and flushed; features of 'warm shock').
- Vomiting, abdominal pain and diarrhoea.
- Pain in joints, muscles and limbs.
- Rash – progressive petechial rash becoming purpuric – like a bruise or blood-blister. (NB These rashes are often **absent** at presentation.)
- Raised respiratory rate and effort.
- O_2 saturations – reduced or unrecordable (poor perfusion).
- Raised heart rate.
- Capillary refill time >2 seconds.
- Rigors.
- Seizures.

Level of consciousness:

- Alert/able to speak during early stages of shock.
- As shock advances:
  - **babies:** limp, floppy, drowsy, fitting
  - **older children and adults:** difficulty walking / standing, drowsiness, confusion, convulsions.

6. Management

- Open airway.

Oxygen:

- **Children:** administer high levels of supplemental oxygen (O$_2$).
- **Adults:** administer high levels of oxygen via a non re-breathing mask, ensuring oxygen saturations (SpO$_2$) of >95%.
- Consider assisted ventilation (rate: 12–20 breaths/min.) if:
  - SpO$_2$ is <90% on high concentration O$_2$
  - respiratory rate is <10 or >30
  - expansion is inadequate.
- Correct **A** and **B** problems at scene then **DO NOT DELAY TRANSFER** to nearest receiving hospital.
- When meningococcal septicaemia is suspected (e.g. a non-blanching rash is seen), administer **benzylpenicillin EN-ROUTE** to further care (**refer to Figure 3.5 and to benzylpenicillin guideline**). NB Meningococcal septicaemia can progress rapidly – the sooner antibiotics are administered the better.

Fluid therapy:

Hypovolaemia occurs in meningococcal septicaemia and requires fluid resuscitation (**refer to intravascular fluid therapy guidelines**).

- **DO NOT** delay at scene for fluid replacement; cannulate and give fluid **EN-ROUTE TO HOSPITAL** wherever possible.
- Measure blood glucose level and treat if necessary.
- Provide hospital alert message (include child's age if paediatric) en-route, repeat ABC assessments and manage as necessary.

7. Risk of Infection to Ambulance Personnel

- Meningococcal bacteria are very fragile and do not survive outside the nose and throat.
- Ambulance personnel directly exposed to large respiratory particles, droplets or secretions from patients with meningococcal disease should be offered preventative antibiotics. Such exposure is unlikely to occur unless working in very close proximity to the patient e.g. inhaling droplets coughed or sneezed by the patient, or when undertaking airway management.
- If a case of meningococcal disease is confirmed, Public Health will provide antibiotics for exposed contacts who may otherwise be at increased risk of infection.

Methodology

For details of the methodology used in the development of this guideline refer to the guideline webpage.

KEY POINTS

Meningococcal Meningitis and Septicaemia

- Meningococcal disease is the leading cause of death from infection in children and young adults. It can kill a healthy person of any age within hours of their first symptoms.
- Two clinical categories are described – meningitis and septicaemia - although they often overlap.
- Non-specific symptoms, such as pyrexia or a 'flu-like' illness may be the only clinical features at first presentation.
- Look for a rash; a non-blanching rash suggests meningococcal septicaemia (but is not universally present).
- Whenever meningococcal disease is suspected (irrespective of the presence or absence of a rash) undertake a TIME CRITICAL transfer.
- Administer benzylpenicillin if septicaemia is suspected. The illness progresses rapidly and early antibiotics improve outcomes.

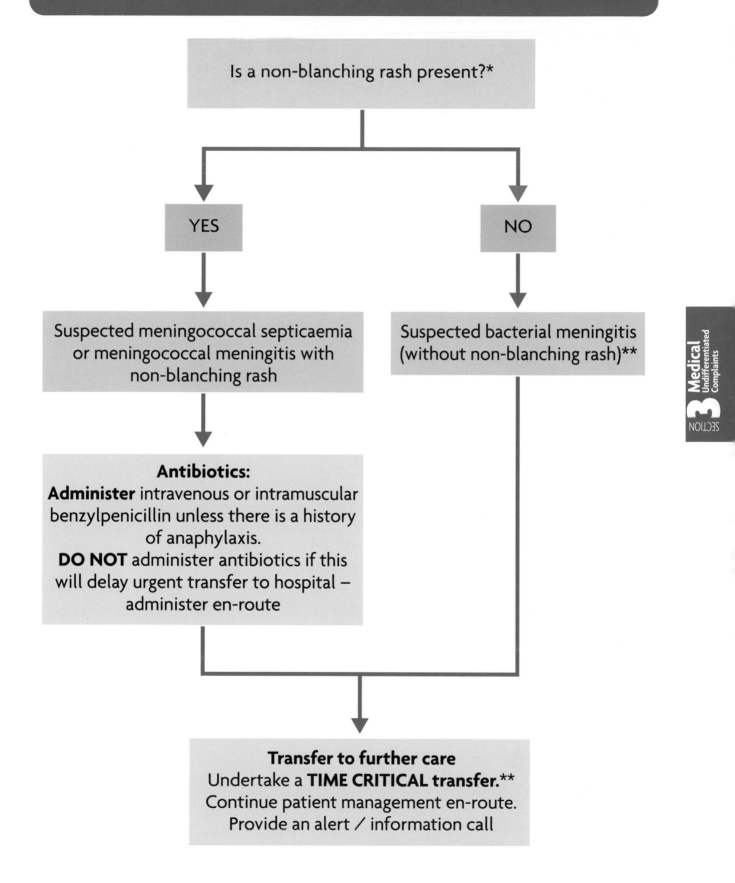

Figure 3.5 – Management algorithm for patients with suspected meningococcal disease.

*The term non-blanching rash is interchangeable with 'haemorrhagic rash', 'petechial rash' and 'purpuric rash'.
**If bacterial meningitis is suspected and urgent transfer is not possible, administer antibiotics even in the absence of a non-blanching rash.

Acute Coronary Syndrome [106, 108, 294–300]

1. Introduction

- Acute Coronary Syndrome (ACS) covers a range of conditions including:
  i. unstable angina
  ii. non-ST-segment-elevation myocardial infarction (NSTEMI)
  iii. ST-segment-elevation myocardial infarction (STEMI).

Chest pain is a cardinal, but not the only, symptom of ACS or 'heart attack' (Table 3.43).

Table 3.43 – FEATURES OF DIFFERENT TYPES OF PAIN

Features which suggest a diagnosis of Myocardial Ischaemia include:
- Central chest pain.
- Crushing or constricting in nature.
- Persists for >15 minutes.
- Pain may also present in:
  - the shoulders
  - upper abdomen
  - referred to the neck, jaws and arm.

Features which suggest a diagnosis of stable angina include:
- Pain is typically related to exertion and tends to last minutes but should it persist for >15 minutes, or despite usual treatment, ACS is more likely.

- Coronary heart disease (CHD) is a major single cause of death in the UK.
- **Time is of the essence in restoring coronary blood flow in patients with ST segment elevation myocardial infarction (STEMI).**
- **The benefits of reperfusion with primary percutaneous coronary intervention (PPCI) or thrombolytic treatment are time-dependent.**
- **PPCI is now the most common form of reperfusion treatment.**
- Patients with STEMI who are ineligible for thrombolysis have a high mortality rate and should be referred for PPCI where facilities exist.

2. Incidence

- In 2010/11 the MINAP database recorded 79,863 heart attacks of which 40% were STEMI, but this is possibly an underestimation.

3. Severity and Outcome

- Approximately two-thirds of STEMI patients will die before they reach hospital.
- The risk of cardiac arrest from ventricular fibrillation (VF) or other arrhythmia is highest in the first few hours from symptom onset. VF can occur without warning.
- Survival from VF occurring in the presence of ambulance personnel with a defibrillator immediately available is as high as 40%. This falls rapidly to 2% or less if the defibrillator is not immediately available.
- Patients with NSTEMI and unstable angina manifestations of ACS are at significant risk of death and should be treated as medical emergencies.

4. Pathophysiology

- ACS occurs when there is an abrupt reduction in blood supply to the muscle of the heart; leading to myocardial ischaemia.
- Myocardial ischaemia is usually caused by a disruption of the internal artery wall, at the site of an atheroma plaque, causing a blood clot to form, occluding the coronary artery.

5. Assessment and Management

For assessment and management of ACS refer to Table 3.44 and Figure 3.6.

Methodology

For details of the methodology used in the development of this guideline refer to the guideline webpage.

KEY POINTS

Acute Coronary Syndrome
- Acute Coronary Syndrome refers to a spectrum of conditions.
- Always take defibrillator to the patient.
- Patients with ECG evidence of STEMI should be assessed for suitability for reperfusion with PPCI or thrombolysis according to local care pathways.
- Patients with NSTEMI remain at high risk and should be treated as a MEDICAL EMERGENCY.

Acute Coronary Syndrome

Table 3.44 – ASSESSMENT and MANAGEMENT of:

Acute Coronary Syndrome

NB A defibrillator must always be taken at the earliest opportunity to patients with symptoms suggestive of a heart attack and remain with the patient until hand-over to hospital staff.

ASSESSMENT	MANAGEMENT

• Assess ABCD	• If any of the following **TIME CRITICAL** features are present:
	  – major ABC problems
	  – 12-lead ECG shows STEMI or LBBB with other clinical features suggestive of ACS
	  – suspected acute coronary syndrome with haemodynamic instability, then:
	• Start correcting any **ABC** problems.
	• Undertake a time **CRITICAL TRANSFER. NB For patients with STEMI undertake a direct admission to a 'cardiac facility'** (access to cardiological advice).
	• Provide an alert/information call.
	• Continue management en-route:
	  – send a 12-lead ECG for expert review where possible
	  – patients with ECG evidence of STEMI should be assessed for suitability for reperfusion treatment (Figure 3.6)
	  – administer aspirin as soon as possible (refer to the aspirin guideline)
	  – administer **clopidogrel** (refer to the clopidogrel guideline) – follow local guidelines
	  – administer **glyceryl trinitrate (GTN)** for patients with ongoing ischaemic discomfort (refer to the GTN guideline).

• Assess whether the chest pain may be cardiac	• Pain typically comes on over seconds and minutes rather than starting abruptly – 'classical presentation' is detailed in Table 3.43. NB Many patients do not have 'classical presentation' as described above and some people, especially the elderly, and those with diabetes, may not experience pain as their chief complaint. This group have a high mortality rate.
• Assess for accompanying features	• Nausea and vomiting. • Marked sweating. • Breathlessness. • Pallor. • Combination of chest pain associated with haemodynamic instability. • Feelings of impending doom. • Skin that is clammy and cold to the touch. **NB These may not always be present.**
• ECG	• **DO NOT exclude an ACS where patients have a normal resting 12-lead ECG.** • Use clinical judgement as to whether a repeat 12-lead ECG is required after normal or equivocal ECG but history suggestive of ACS (continuing or worsening pain or heamodynamic instability).
• Assess oxygen saturation	• Closely monitor the patient's SpO$_2$ but do not administer oxygen unless the patient is hypoxaemic on air (SpO$_2$ <94%) (refer to oxygen guidelines).
• Undertake further assessment and management in the order appropriate to the circumstances	• Monitor ECG for arrhythmias. • Obtain intravenous access if clinically indicated. • Monitor vital signs. • Repeat dose of GTN if chest discomfort persists. • 12-lead ECG (as above).
• Assess patient's pain	• Measure and record pain score (**refer to pain management guideline**). • Consider analgesia (**refer to pain management guideline**).
• Documentation	• Complete documentation.[49]
	Additional Information: • The treatment of patients with ACS is a rapidly developing area of practice. • National and international standards and guidelines for ACS care consistently emphasise the importance of rapid access to defibrillation and reperfusion and specialist cardiological care. • Pre-alerting the hospital can speed up appropriate treatment of STEMI patients. • Prehospital thrombolysis may be an option where PPCI is not available, but patients can subsequently be transferred to a PPCI capable hospital.

Acute Coronary Syndrome

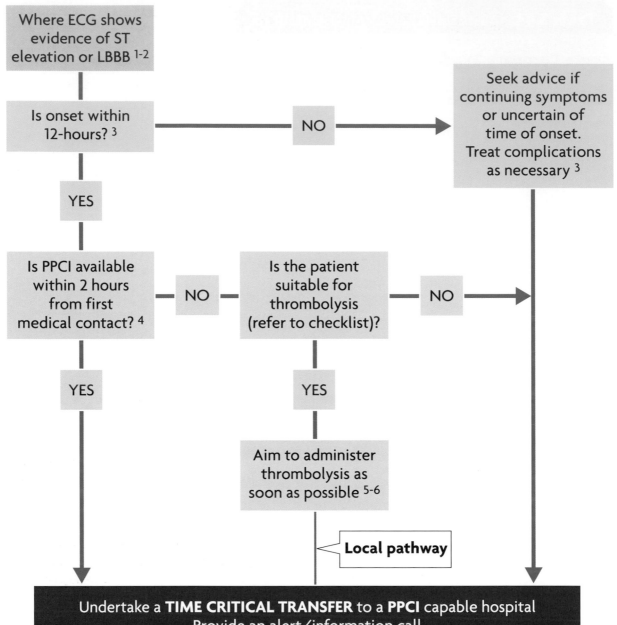

Where ECG shows evidence of ST elevation or LBBB [1-2]

Is onset within 12-hours? [3]

NO → Seek advice if continuing symptoms or uncertain of time of onset. Treat complications as necessary [3]

YES

Is PPCI available within 2 hours from first medical contact? [4]

NO → Is the patient suitable for thrombolysis (refer to checklist)?

NO →

YES

YES

Aim to administer thrombolysis as soon as possible [5-6]

Local pathway

Undertake a TIME CRITICAL TRANSFER to a PPCI capable hospital
Provide an alert/information call
Administer aspirin and clopidogel unless contra-indicated as per local policy

---

1. Up to a third of patients with MI will have atypical presentations such as shortness of breath or collapse, without chest pain. This is particularly so in patients with diabetes or the elderly. **Have a low threshold for performing a 12-lead ECG in any patient presenting as 'unwell'.** Seek advice in 'atypical' patients who have ST elevation or LBBB (see below) as urgent reperfusion may still be indicated.

2. ECG criteria for reperfusion include ST segment elevation (≥ 2mm in 2-standard or 2 adjacent precordial leads, not including V1) or **LBBB** in patients with other clinical features suggestive of ACS. Patients who have ST depression rather than elevation are a high risk group who need urgent specialist assessment. **Seek advice.**

3. If there is uncertainty about the time of symptom onset, or any ongoing chest pain/discomfort or haemodynamic upset beyond 12 hours, seek advice as urgent reperfusion may still be indicated.

4. Refer to local policies for target 'call to balloon' time.

5. Thrombolytic treatment should not be regarded as the end of the emergency care of a STEMI patient. Rapid transfer to an appropriate hospital for timely therapy to prevent re-infarction, and assessment of the need for rescue PPCI, is essential.

6. Refer to reteplase or tenecteplase guidelines for the checklist to identify eligibility for prehospital thrombolysis.

Figure 3.6 – The management of patients presenting with STEMI or LBBB.

Allergic Reactions including Anaphylaxis (Adults) [53, 60, 63, 301–313]

1. Introduction
- The incidence of allergic reactions continues to rise.
- The symptoms range from mild to life-threatening and include:
  - urticaria (hives)
  - itching
  - angio-oedema (swelling of the face, eyelids, lips and tongue)
  - a petechial or purpuric rash
  - dyspnoea
  - wheeze
  - stridor
  - hypoxia
  - hypotension
  - abdominal pain
  - diarrhoea/vomiting.
- The most common triggers are food, drugs and venom (Table 3.45) but in 30% of cases the trigger is unknown.
- Injected allergens commonly result in cardiovascular compromise, with hypotension and shock predominating.
- Slow release drugs prolong absorption and exposure to the allergen.

Table 3.45 – COMMON TRIGGERS OF ALLERGIC REACTIONS

1 – Foods
Nuts (e.g. peanuts, walnut, almond, brazil, and hazel), pulses, sesame seeds, milk, eggs, fish/shellfish.

2 – Venom – insect sting/bites
Insect stings and bites (e.g. wasp and bees).
NB Bees may leave a venom sac which should be scraped off (not squeezed).

3 – Drugs
Antibiotics (e.g. penicillin, cephalosporin, amphotericin, ciprofloxacin, and vancomycin), non-steroidal anti-inflammatory drugs, angiotensin converting enzyme inhibitor, gelatins, protamine, vitamin K, etoposide, acetazolamide, pethidine, local anaesthetic, diamorphine, streptokinase.

4 – Other causes
Latex[a], hair dye, semen and hydatid.

2. Incidence
- It is estimated that allergic reactions affect 30% of adults with anaphylaxis estimated to affect up to 2% of the population.

3. Severity and Outcome
- The severity of symptoms varies from a localised urticaria to life-threatening pulmonary and/or cardiovascular compromise – anaphylaxis.
- Generally, the longer it takes for anaphylactic symptoms to develop, the less severe the overall reaction.

[a] Latex allergy has implications for equipment use.

- Some patients relapse after an apparent recovery (biphasic response), therefore, patients who have experienced an anaphylatic reaction should be transferred to hospital for further evaluation.
- The mortality associated with anaphylaxis is estimated to be <1%. Death occurs quickly (venom: 10–15 minutes; food: 30–35 minutes) after contact with the trigger usually as a result of respiratory arrest from airway obstruction.

4. Assessment and Management
For the assessment and management of anaphylaxis and allergic reactions refer to Figure 3.7.

Patients with previous episodes:
- May wear 'Medic Alert' bracelets/necklets.
- Carry an adrenaline pen.
- May experience panic attacks.

Methodology
For details of the methodology used in the development of this guideline refer to the guideline webpage.

KEY POINTS

Allergic Reactions Including Anaphylaxis
- **Remove from trigger if possible.**
- **Anaphylaxis can occur despite a long history of previously safe exposure to a potential trigger.**
- **Consider anaphylaxis in the presence of acute cutaneous symptoms and airway or cardiovascular compromise.**
- **Anaphylaxis may be rapid, slow or biphasic.**
- **Adrenaline is key in managing anaphylaxis.**
- **The benefit of using appropriate doses of adrenaline far exceeds any risk.**

Allergic Reactions including Anaphylaxis (Adults)

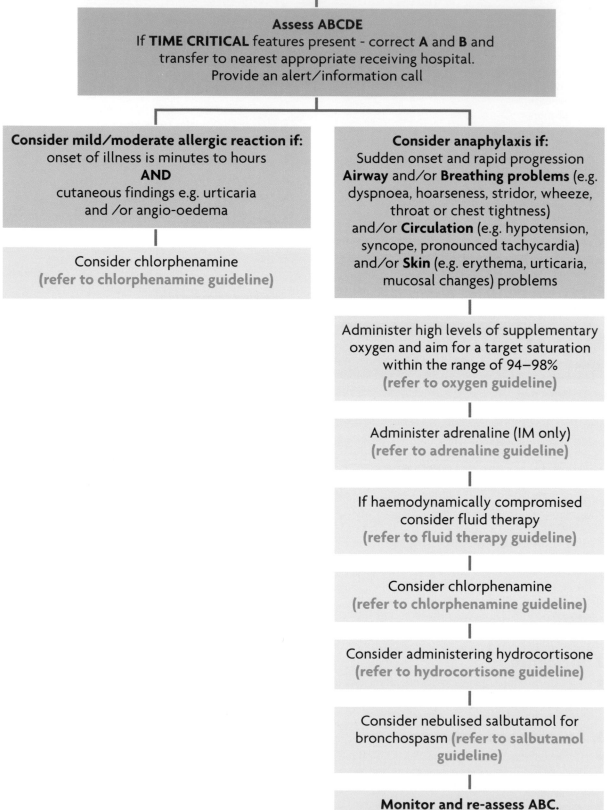

Quickly remove from trigger if possible e.g. environmental, infusion etc.
DO NOT delay definitive treatment if removing trigger not feasible

Assess ABCDE
If **TIME CRITICAL** features present - correct **A** and **B** and transfer to nearest appropriate receiving hospital.
Provide an alert/information call

Consider mild/moderate allergic reaction if:
onset of illness is minutes to hours
AND
cutaneous findings e.g. urticaria and /or angio-oedema

Consider chlorphenamine
(refer to chlorphenamine guideline)

Consider anaphylaxis if:
Sudden onset and rapid progression
Airway and/or **Breathing problems** (e.g. dyspnoea, hoarseness, stridor, wheeze, throat or chest tightness)
and/or **Circulation** (e.g. hypotension, syncope, pronounced tachycardia)
and/or **Skin** (e.g. erythema, urticaria, mucosal changes) problems

Administer high levels of supplementary oxygen and aim for a target saturation within the range of 94–98%
(refer to oxygen guideline)

Administer adrenaline (IM only)
(refer to adrenaline guideline)

If haemodynamically compromised consider fluid therapy
(refer to fluid therapy guideline)

Consider chlorphenamine
(refer to chlorphenamine guideline)

Consider administering hydrocortisone
(refer to hydrocortisone guideline)

Consider nebulised salbutamol for bronchospasm **(refer to salbutamol guideline)**

Monitor and re-assess ABC.
Monitor ECG, PEFR (if possible), BP and pulse oximetry en-route

Figure 3.7 – Allergic reactions including anaphylaxis algorithm.

1. Introduction

- Asthma is one of the commonest of all medical conditions. Asthma has varying levels of severity and patients usually present to prehospital care with one of four presentations: mild/moderate, severe, life-threatening, and near fatal (Table 3.46).
- Typically in patients requiring hospital admission the symptoms will have developed gradually over a number of hours (>6 hours). Usually patients are known asthmatics and may be on regular inhaler therapy for this. Patients may have used their own treatment inhalers and in some cases will have used a home-based nebuliser.
- Patients may report a history of increased wheezy breathlessness, often worse at night or in the early morning, associated either with infection, allergy or exertion as a trigger.

2. Incidence

- Asthma is rare in the elderly population and practitioners should be aware that many people will describe a range of other respiratory conditions as 'asthma', and therefore other causes of breathlessness need to be considered.
- In adults, asthma may often be complicated and mixed in with a degree of bronchitis, especially in smokers. This can make the condition much more difficult to treat, both routinely and in emergencies. The majority of asthmatic patients take regular 'preventer' and 'reliever' inhalers.

3. Severity and Outcome

- The obstruction in its most severe form can be **TIME CRITICAL** and some 2,000 people a year die as a result of asthma. Patients with severe asthma and one or more risk factor(s) (Table 3.47) are at risk of death.
- In patients ≤40 years, deaths from asthma peak in July/August in contrast to patients aged >40 years where deaths peak in December/January.

4. Pathophysiology

- Asthma is caused by a chronic inflammation of the bronchi, making them narrower. The muscles around the bronchi become irritated and contract, causing sudden worsening of the symptoms. The inflammation can also cause the mucus glands to produce excessive sputum which further blocks the air passages.
- The obstruction and subsequent wheezing are caused by three factors within the bronchial tree:
  i.   increased production of bronchial mucus
  ii. swelling of the bronchial tube mucosal lining cells
  iii. spasm and constriction of bronchial muscles.

  These three factors combine to cause blockage and narrowing of the small airways in the lung. Because inspiration is an active process involving the muscles of respiration, the obstruction of the airways is overcome on breathing in. Expiration occurs with muscle relaxation, and is severely delayed by the narrowing of the airways in asthma. This generates the wheezing on expiration that is characteristic of this condition.

- Asthma is managed with a variety of inhaled and tablet medications. Inhalers are divided into two broad categories: preventer and reliever.

Table 3.46 – FEATURES OF SEVERITY

Near-fatal asthma
- Raised $PaCO_2$ and/or requiring mechanical ventilation with raised inflation pressures.

Life-threatening asthma
Any one of the following in a patient with severe asthma:
- Altered conscious level.
- Exhaustion.
- Arrhythmia.
- Hypotension.
- Cyanosis.
- Silent chest.
- Poor respiratory effort.
- PEF <33% best or predicted.
- SpO_2 <92%.
- PaO_2 <8 kPa.
- 'Normal' $PaCO_2$ (4.6–6.0 kPa).

Acute severe asthma
Any one of:
- PEF 33–50% best or predicted.
- Respiratory rate ≥25/minute.
- Heart rate ≥110/minute.
- Inability to complete sentences in one breath.

Moderate asthma exacerbation
- Increasing symptoms.
- PEF >50–75% best or predicted.
- No features of acute severe asthma.

Table 3.47 – RISK FACTORS FOR DEVELOPING NEAR-FATAL ASTHMA

Medical
- Previous near-fatal asthma, e.g. previous ventilation or respiratory acidosis.
- Previous hospital admission for asthma especially if in the last year requiring three or more classes of asthma medication.
- Heavy use of β2 agonist.
- Repeated emergency department attendance for asthma care especially if in the last year.
- Brittle asthma.

Psychological/Behavioural
- Non-compliance with treatment or monitoring.
- Failure to attend appointments.
- Fewer GP contacts.
- Frequent home visits.
- Self discharge from hospital.
- Psychosis, depression, other psychiatric illness or deliberate self harm.
- Current or recent major tranquilliser use.
- Denial.
- Alcohol or drug abuse.
- Obesity.
- Learning difficulties.
- Employment problems.
- Income problems.
- Social isolation.
- Childhood abuse.
- Severe domestic, marital or legal stress.

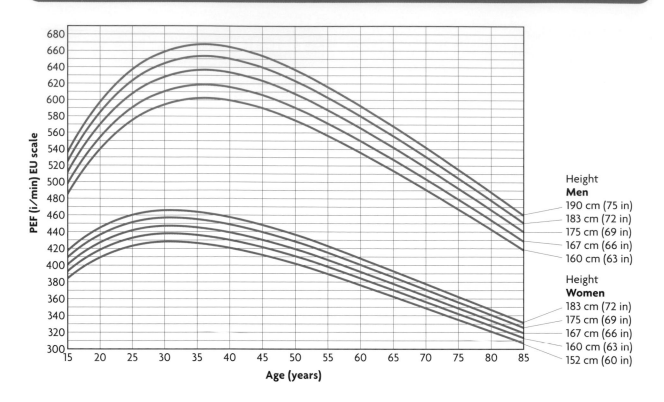

Figure 3.8 – Peak flow charts – Peak expiratory flow rate – normal values. For use with EU/EN13826 scale PEF meters only.[a]

[a] Adapted by Clement Clarke for use with EN13826 / EU scale peak flow meters from Nunn AJ Gregg I, Br Med J 1989:298;1068-70.

1. The preventer inhalers are normally anti-inflammatory drugs and these include steroids and other milder anti-inflammatories such as Tilade. The common steroid inhalers are beclomethasone (Becotide), budesonide (Pulmicort) and luticasone (Flixotide). These drugs act on the lung over a period of time to reduce the inflammatory reaction that causes the asthma. Regular use of these inhalers often eradicates all symptoms of asthma and allows for a normal lifestyle.

2. The reliever inhalers include salbutamol (Ventolin), terbutaline (Bricanyl), tiotropium (Spiriva) and ipratropium bromide (Atrovent). These inhalers work rapidly on the lung to relax the smooth muscle spasm when the patient feels wheezy or tight chested. They are used in conjunction with preventer inhalers. Inhalers are often used through large plastic spacer devices, such as the Volumatic. This allows the drug to spread into a larger volume and allows the patient to inhale it more effectively. In mild and moderate asthma attacks some patients may be treated with high doses of 'relievers' through a spacer device. This has been shown to be as effective as giving a salbutamol nebuliser.

5. Assessment

*   Assess **ABCD** as per medical emergencies in adults overview, but specifically assess for the severity of the asthma attack (refer to asthma algorithm – Figure 3.9 and Table 3.46).

6. Management

*   Refer to the asthma algorithm (Figure 3.9 and Table 3.48) for the management of mild/moderate, severe, life-threatening, and near-fatal.

For less severe attacks:

*   Where possible the patient's own β2 agonist should be given (ideally using a spacer) as first line treatment. Increase the dose by two puffs every two minutes according to response up to ten puffs.

*   If symptoms are not controlled by ten puffs then start nebulised salbutamol whilst transferring to the emergency department.

*   Patients (or friends/bystanders) who have previously experienced a severe asthma attack may be more likely to call for help early in the development of an attack, and the symptoms may appear mild on arrival of the ambulance.

*   Some patients may be appropriate for alternative care pathways, for example, early referral to a general practitioner. However, apparently minor symptoms should not preclude onward referral especially where an alternative pathway is not readily accessible. Local care pathways should be followed where patients are considered for non conveyance. However, caution should be exercised in known severe asthmatics and robust safety netting of patients must be in place.

Peak Expiratory Flow Rate (PEFR)

*   Peak flow is a rapid measurement of the degree of obstruction in the patient's lungs. It measures the maximum flow on breathing out, or expiring and therefore can reflect the amount of airway obstruction. Whenever possible, peak flow should be performed before and after nebulised treatment. Many patients now have their own meter at home and know what their normal peak flow is. Clearly, when control is good, their peak flow will be

SECTION **3** Medical Undifferentiated Complaints

Asthma (Adults)

Table 3.48 – ASSESSMENT and MANAGEMENT

Asthma

ASSESSMENT	MANAGEMENT
• Assess **ABCD** Specifically assess for the severity of the asthma attack (refer to Figure 3.9)	• If any of the following **TIME CRITICAL** features present: – major ABCD problems – extreme difficulty in breathing or requirement for assisted ventilations – exhaustion – cyanosis – Silent chest – SpO$_2$ <92% – PEF <33% best or predicted. • Start correcting A and B problems. • Undertake a **TIME CRITICAL** transfer to nearest receiving hospital. • Continue patient management en-route. • Provide an alert/information call.
• Mild/moderate asthma Increasing symptoms, PEF >50–75% best or predicted, no features of acute severe asthma	• Move to a calm quiet environment. • Encourage use of own inhaler, using a spacer if available. Ensure correct technique is used (refer to Figure 3.9). • If unresponsive: – administer high levels of supplementary oxygen – administer nebulised salbutamol (refer to salbutamol guideline).
• Severe asthma Any one of: – PEF 33–50% of best or predicted – Respiratory rate >25/minute – Heart rate >110/minute – Inability to complete sentences in one breath	• Administer high levels of supplementary oxygen. • Administer nebulised salbutamol (refer to salbutamol guideline). • If no improvement administer ipratropium bromide (refer to ipratropium bromide guideline). • Administer steroids (refer to relevant steroids guideline). • Continuous salbutamol nebulisation may be administered unless clinically significant side effects occur (refer to salbutamol guideline).
• Life threatening asthma Any one of – Altered conscious level – Exhaustion – Arrhythmia – Hypotension – Cyanosis – Silent chest – Poor respiratory effort – PEF<33% best or predicted – SpO$_2$ <92%	• Continuous salbutamol nebulisation may be administered unless clinically significant side effects occur (refer to salbutamol guideline). • Administer adrenaline 1 in 1000 IM only (refer to adrenaline guideline).
• Near fatal asthma – Requiring bag-valve-mask ventilation with raised inflation pressures – Transfer	• Positive pressure ventilation using a nebulising T piece. Assess for bilateral tension pneumothorax. • Transfer rapidly to nearest receiving hospital. • Provide an alert/information call. • Continue patient management en-route. • For cases of mild asthma that respond to treatment consider alternative care pathway where appropriate. Note: exercise caution in known severe asthmatics.

equivalent to a normal patient's measurement, but during an attack it may drop markedly (Figure 3.8).

Methodology

For details of methodology used in the development of this guideline refer to the guideline webpage.

KEY POINTS

Asthma in Adults

● **Asthma is a common life-threatening condition.**

● **Its severity is often not recognised.**

● **Accurate documentation is essential.**

● **A silent chest is a pre-terminal sign.**

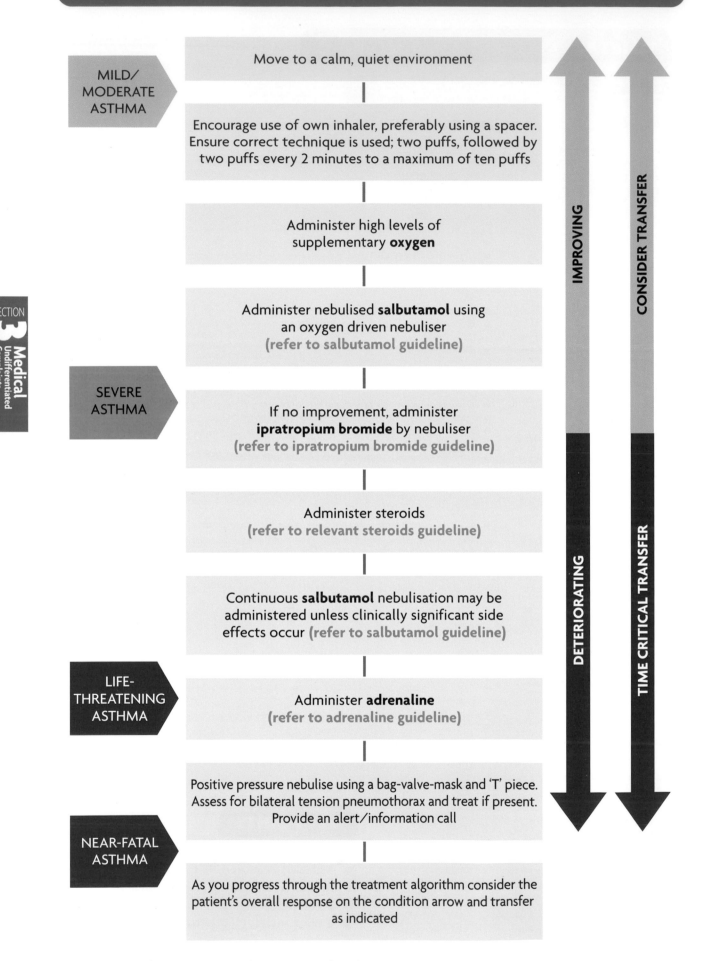

MILD/ MODERATE ASTHMA

Move to a calm, quiet environment

Encourage use of own inhaler, preferably using a spacer. Ensure correct technique is used; two puffs, followed by two puffs every 2 minutes to a maximum of ten puffs

Administer high levels of supplementary **oxygen**

Administer nebulised **salbutamol** using an oxygen driven nebuliser **(refer to salbutamol guideline)**

SEVERE ASTHMA

If no improvement, administer **ipratropium bromide** by nebuliser **(refer to ipratropium bromide guideline)**

Administer steroids **(refer to relevant steroids guideline)**

Continuous **salbutamol** nebulisation may be administered unless clinically significant side effects occur **(refer to salbutamol guideline)**

LIFE-THREATENING ASTHMA

Administer **adrenaline** **(refer to adrenaline guideline)**

Positive pressure nebulise using a bag-valve-mask and 'T' piece. Assess for bilateral tension pneumothorax and treat if present. Provide an alert/information call

NEAR-FATAL ASTHMA

As you progress through the treatment algorithm consider the patient's overall response on the condition arrow and transfer as indicated

IMPROVING

CONSIDER TRANSFER

DETERIORATING

TIME CRITICAL TRANSFER

SECTION 3 Medical Undifferentiated Complaints

Figure 3.9 – Asthma assessment and management algorithm.

Chronic Obstructive Pulmonary Disease [314, 316–325]

1. Introduction

- Chronic Obstructive Pulmonary Disease (COPD) is a chronic progressive disorder characterised by airflow obstruction ('*reduced post-bronchodilator FEV 1 /FVC ratio (where FEV 1 is forced expiratory volume in 1 second and FVC is forced vital capacity), such that FEV 1 /FVC is less than 0.7*').

- A diagnosis of COPD is usually made in the presence of airflow obstruction in people >35 years of age, who are or were previously smokers and may have one or more risk factors (Table 3.49).

Table 3.49 – SIGNS/SYMPTOMS OF COPD

Signs/symptoms

- Exertional breathlessness.
- Chronic cough.
- Regular sputum production.
- Frequent winter 'bronchitis'.
- Wheeze.
- No clinical features of asthma.

- Patients with COPD usually present to the ambulance service with an acute exacerbation of the underlying illness. COPD is a concomitant/secondary illness in many incidents with other chief complaints.

- Some patients with severe COPD may have an individualised treatment plan to assist in their care. This can be used to guide therapy.

2. Incidence

- It is estimated that approximately 3 million people have COPD affecting 2–4% of the population over 45 years of age. However, only 1.5% of the population are diagnosed with the condition.

- In the UK, COPD is the fifth leading cause of death and it is estimated that by 2020 it will be the third leading cause of death worldwide.

3. Severity and Outcome

- COPD results in disability and impaired quality of life leading to 30,000 deaths per annum in the UK.

- COPD is the second leading cause of emergency admission, with 130,000 cases per annum, in the UK and direct costs estimated at £800 million and indirect costs of £24 million.

4. Pathophysiology

- Airflow obstruction is the result of airway and parenchymal damage due to chronic inflammation.

- COPD increases the risk of co-morbidities such as lung cancer and cardiovascular disease.

- An acute exacerbation refers to a worsening of the patient's symptoms (Table 3.50). There is no one feature that defines an exacerbation, although there are a number of known causes (Table 3.52), however, in 30% of cases the cause is unknown.

- COPD patients generally have lower than normal SpO_2 levels and British Thoracic Society oxygen guidelines should be followed to maintain an SpO_2 of 88–92%

- Some exacerbations are mild and self-limiting whilst others are more severe, potentially life-threatening, and require intervention – not all features will be present (Table 3.50).

- Some conditions may present with symptoms similar to an exacerbation of COPD – consider these when diagnosing an exacerbation of COPD (Table 3.51).

5. Assessment and Management

Assessment and management of Chronic Obstructive Pulmonary Disease refer to Table 3.53 and Figure 3.10.

Methodology

For details of the methodology used in the development of this guideline refer to the guideline webpage.

Table 3.50 – FEATURES OF AN ACUTE EXACERBATION OF COPD

Features

- Increased dyspnoea   particularly on exertion.
- Increased sputum volume/purulence.
- Increased cough.
- Upper airway symptoms (e.g. colds and sore throats).
- Increased wheeze.
- Chest tightness.
- Reduced exercise tolerance.
- Fluid retention.
- Increased fatigue.
- Acute confusion.
- Worsening of a previously stable condition.

Severe features

- Marked dyspnoea.
- Tachypnoea.
- Purse lip breathing.
- Use of accessory respiratory muscles (sternomastoid and abdominal) at rest.
- Acute confusion.
- New-onset cyanosis.
- New-onset peripheral oedema.
- Marked reduction in activities of daily living.

Table 3.51 – CONDITIONS WITH SIMILAR FEATURES TO AN ACUTE EXACERBATION OF COPD

Features

- Asthma.
- Pneumonia.
- Pneumothorax.
- Left ventricular failure/pulmonary oedema.
- Pulmonary embolus.
- Lung cancer.
- Upper airway obstruction.
- Pleural effusion.
- Recurrent aspiration.

Table 3.52 – CAUSES OF EXACERBATION OF COPD

Infections
- Rhinoviruses (common cold).
- Influenza.
- Parainfluenza.
- Coronavirus.
- Adenovirus.
- Respiratory Syncytial Virus.
- *C. pneumoniae.*
- *H. influenzae.*
- *S. pneumoniae.*
- *M. catarrhalis.*
- *S. aureus.*
- *P. aeruginosa.*

Pollutants
- Nitrogen dioxide.
- Particulates.
- Sulphur dioxide.
- Ozone.

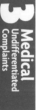

SECTION
3
Medical
Undifferentiated
Complaints

KEY POINTS

Chronic Obstructive Pulmonary Disease
- Early respiratory assessment (including oxygen saturation) is vital.
- If in doubt, provide oxygen therapy, titrating en-route, aiming for oxygen saturation of 88–92%.
- Provide nebulisation with salbutamol and assess response.

Table 3.53 – ASSESSMENT and MANAGEMENT of:

Chronic Obstructive Pulmonary Disease

ASSESSMENT	MANAGEMENT
● Assess ABCD	● If any of the following **TIME CRITICAL** features present: – major **ABCD** problems – extreme breathing difficulty (by reference to patient's usual condition) – cyanosis (although peripheral cyanosis may be 'normal' in some patients) – exhaustion – hypoxia (oxygen saturation <88%) unresponsive to oxygen (O_2) – COPD patients normally have a lower than normal oxygen saturation (SpO_2). ● Start correcting **A** and **B** problems. ● Undertake a **TIME CRITICAL** transfer to nearest receiving hospital. ● Continue patient management en-route. ● Provide an alert/information call.
● Ask the patient if they have an individualised treatment plan	● Follow the individualised treatment plan if available. ● The patient will often be able to guide their care.
Specifically assess: **Diagnosis**	● Assess whether this is an acute exacerbation of COPD – refer to Table 3.50 for the features of COPD. ● Or another condition – refer to Table 3.51 for conditions with similar features to an acute exacerbation of COPD. NB Chest pain and fever are uncommon symptoms of COPD – therefore consider other possible causes.
Airway	● Maintain airway patency. NB Noises (e.g. 'bubbling' or wheeze) associated with breathing indicating respiratory distress.
Breathing	● Note and monitor respiratory rate and effort.
● Bronchodilators	● Administer nebulised salbutamol (refer to salbutamol guideline). ● If inadequate response after five minutes, a further dose of nebulised salbutamol may be administered concurrently with ipratropium bromide (refer to ipratropium bromide guideline). Ipratropium can only be administered **ONCE**; salbutamol may be repeated at regular intervals unless the side effects of the drug become significant. ● NB Limit nebulisation to **six** minutes.
● Position	● Position patient for comfort and ease of respiration – often sitting forwards – but be aware of potential hypotension.
● Oxygen[a]	● Measure oxygen saturation.[b] ● Administer supplemental oxygen; aim, for a target saturation within the range of 88–92% or the prespecified range – refer to the patients individualised treatment plan if available. NB The aim of oxygen therapy is to prevent life-threatening hypoxia – administer cautiously, as a proportion of COPD sufferers are chronically hypoxic and when given oxygen may develop increasing drowsiness and loss of respiratory drive. If this occurs, reduce oxygen concentration and support ventilation if required.
● ECG	● Undertake a 12-lead ECG.
● Ventilation	● Consider non-invasive ventilation if not responding to treatment.
● Cardiorespiratory arrest	● Be prepared for cardio-respiratory arrest – **refer to appropriate resuscitation guideline**.
● Transfer	● Transfer rapidly to nearest receiving hospital. ● Provide an alert/information call. ● Continue patient management en-route. ● Consider alternative care pathway where appropriate.

Medical
Undifferentiated Complaints
SECTION 3

[a] If the primary illness in a patient with COPD requires high concentration oxygen (refer to oxygen guideline) then this should **NOT BE WITHHELD**. The patient should be continually monitored closely for changes in respiratory rate and depth and the inspired concentration adjusted accordingly. In the short time that a patient is in ambulance care, hypoxia presents a much greater risk than hypercapnia in most cases.

[b] Pulse oximetry, whilst important in COPD patients, will not indicate carbon dioxide (CO_2) levels which are assessed by capnometry or more commonly, blood gas analysis in hospital.

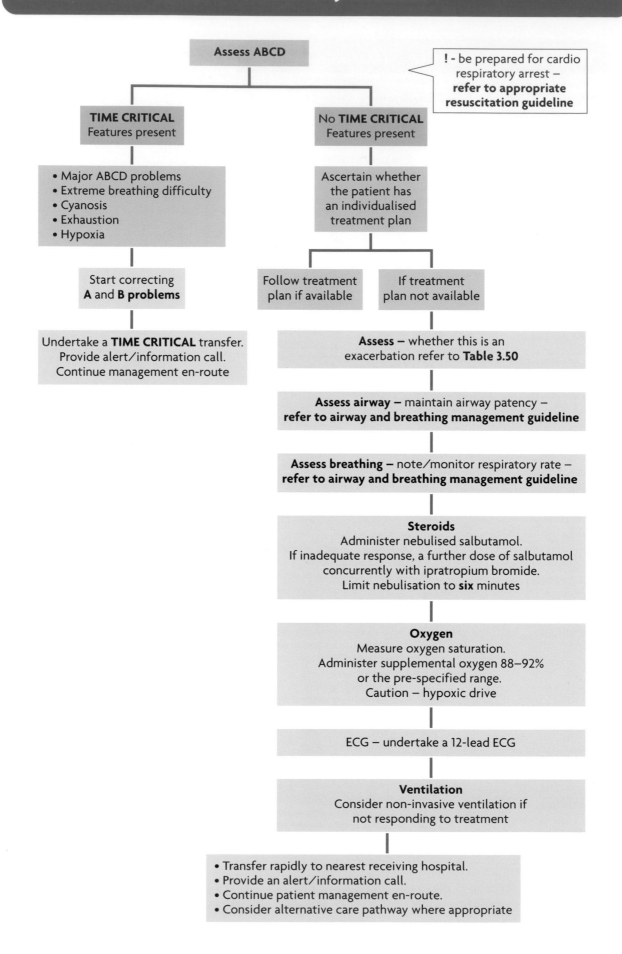

Assess ABCD

! - be prepared for cardio respiratory arrest – **refer to appropriate resuscitation guideline**

TIME CRITICAL Features present

No **TIME CRITICAL** Features present

- Major ABCD problems
- Extreme breathing difficulty
- Cyanosis
- Exhaustion
- Hypoxia

Ascertain whether the patient has an individualised treatment plan

Start correcting **A** and **B problems**

Follow treatment plan if available

If treatment plan not available

Undertake a **TIME CRITICAL** transfer. Provide alert/information call. Continue management en-route

Assess – whether this is an exacerbation refer to **Table 3.50**

Assess airway – maintain airway patency – **refer to airway and breathing management guideline**

Assess breathing – note/monitor respiratory rate – **refer to airway and breathing management guideline**

Steroids
Administer nebulised salbutamol.
If inadequate response, a further dose of salbutamol concurrently with ipratropium bromide.
Limit nebulisation to **six** minutes

Oxygen
Measure oxygen saturation.
Administer supplemental oxygen 88–92% or the pre-specified range.
Caution – hypoxic drive

ECG – undertake a 12-lead ECG

Ventilation
Consider non-invasive ventilation if not responding to treatment

- Transfer rapidly to nearest receiving hospital.
- Provide an alert/information call.
- Continue patient management en-route.
- Consider alternative care pathway where appropriate

Figure 3.10 – Assessment and management of chronic obstructive pulmonary disease algorithm.

1. Introduction

- Convulsion, seizure, and fit are all terms used to describe an 'an abnormal and excessive depolarisation of a set of neurons in the brain'.

- Clinical presentation depends on the area of the brain affected by the depolarisation, the cause and age. Often patients experience a period of involuntary muscular contraction, followed by a **post-ictal** recovery period, often characterised by lethargy and confusion and, in some cases, profound sleep. It is not uncommon for patients to act out of character when in the post-ictal state. This may include verbal or physical aggression. Oxygen therapy, in line with BTS guidelines, and a calm approach are important.

- There are a number of types of convulsion:
  - **epileptic** – neurological condition resulting in recurrent convulsions. Persistent and continual convulsions lasting >30 minutes are termed **status epilepticus and are potentially life-threatening**
  - **eclamptic** – occurs peri-natally and is often associated with pregnancy induced hypertension.

2. Incidence

2.1 Epilepsy

- Epilepsy affects 50 per 100,000 per annum in the UK. Convulsions affect 60% of patients with two-thirds experiencing focal and one-third generalised tonic-clonic convulsions.

- Approximately 30% of sufferers develop chronic epilepsy; the remainder will experience a period of remission, being convulsion-free for five years.

  The number of convulsions experienced varies:
  - 33% – <1 per year
  - 33% – 1–12 per year
  - 33% – 1 per month.

- Patients with chronic epilepsy may present regularly to the Ambulance Service.

2.2 Eclamptic convulsion

- For information regarding the incidence of eclamptic convulsion **refer to pregnancy induced hypertension (including eclampsia)**.

3. Severity and Outcome

- In 80% of cases convulsions will have stopped after ten minutes. However, seizures lasting five minutes or more and serial seizures of three or more in an hour are medical emergencies.

3.1 Epilepsy

- In a few cases, sudden death, termed 'sudden unexpected death in epilepsy (SUDEP)', can occur during a convulsion and results in 500 deaths per year in the UK. This is often due to non-compliance with medication.

- In patients recently diagnosed with epilepsy, death is generally a result of an underlying disease, e.g. vascular disease, tumour.

3.2 Fever

- A fever can reduce the threshold for a convulsion when there is underlying pathology. Investigation and treatment are indicated to prevent recurrence.

3.3 Eclamptic convulsion

- For information regarding the severity and outcome of eclamptic convulsion **refer to pregnancy induced hypertension (including eclampsia)**.

4. Pathophysiology

- The classification of convulsion is based on clinical presentation and underlying neurological disorder.

4.1 Epilepsy

- There are a number of causes of epilepsy (see above). However, in some cases the cause remains unknown. In newly diagnosed, or suspected epilepsy, 60% of cases the cause is unknown.

- The commonest presentation to ambulance services is the tonic/clonic seizure, previously known as 'grand mal'.

4.2 Eclamptic convulsion

- See above.

5. Assessment and Management

- For the assessment and management of convulsion in adults refer to Table 3.54 and Figure 3.11.

KEY POINTS

Convulsions in Adults

- **Most tonic/clonic convulsions are self-limiting and do not require drug treatment.**

- **Convulsions may be caused by other medical conditions e.g. hypoxia, hypoglycaemia, which may be easily treated.**

- **Administer drugs if convulsion lasts longer than five minutes.**

- **Assume eclampsia as a cause of the convulsion in the peri-natal patient.**

- **Only consider leaving a patient at home who makes a full recovery following a convulsion if they are known to suffer from epilepsy, and can be supervised adequately.**

- **Consider referral to local epilepsy service for review/follow-up.**

Methodology

For details of the methodology used in the development of this guideline refer to the guideline webpage.

Convulsions (Adults)

Table 3.54 – ASSESSMENT and MANAGEMENT of:

Convulsions in Adults

NB Always take a defibrillator to a convulsing patient – this may be the presenting sign of circulatory arrest at the onset of sudden cardiac arrest.

ASSESSMENT	MANAGEMENT

● Assess **ABCD**	● If any of the following **TIME CRITICAL** features present:
	  – major **ABCD** problems – **hypoxia may cause convulsions**
	  – serious head injury
	  – status epilepticus – following failed treatment
	  – underlying infection, e.g. meningococcal septicaemia (refer to benzylpenicillin guideline), then:
	  – eclampsia – **refer to pregnancy induced hypertension (including eclampsia)**, then:
	● Start correcting **A** and **B** problems.
	● Check blood glucose to ensure hypoglycaemia is identified and treated.
	● Undertake a **TIME CRITICAL** transfer to nearest receiving hospital if the patient can be moved despite convulsing – it is important to reach hospital for definitive care as rapidly as possible.
	● Continue patient management en-route.
	● Provide an alert/information call.

If not **TIME CRITICAL**	● Take a history from patient/eyewitness – if possible, to ascertain if a convulsion has occurred.
If the patient is known to suffer from epilepsy, check if they have an individualised treatment plan	● Follow the individualised treatment plan if available. ● Patients are usually on anti-epileptic medication such as phenytoin, sodium valproate (Epilim), carbamazepine (Tegretol), and lamotrigine (Lamictal).
Specifically assess:	
Type of convulsion	Ascertain type of convulsion if still convulsing: ● Epileptic. ● Eclamptic convulsion (**refer to pregnancy induced hypertension (including eclampsia) guideline**).
Blood glucose level	● Convulsion may be a presenting sign of **HYPOGLYCAEMIA** – consider in **ALL** cases. ● Check blood glucose level if <4.0 mmol/l or clinically suspected, administer glucose (**refer to glycaemic emergencies guideline**; glucose 10% guideline and glucagon guideline).
Heart rate and rhythm	● Monitor heart rate and rhythm for **ARRHYTHMIA** (**refer to cardiac rhythm disturbance guideline**) e.g. a burst of rapid ventricular tachycardia may drop the blood pressure, and cause transient cerebral **HYPOXIA**, giving rise to a convulsion.
Temperature	● A raised temperature and any sign of a rash may indicate meningococcal septicaemia (**refer to meningococcal septicaemia guideline**). NB Patients often feel warm to touch following generalised convulsions due to the heat generated by excessive muscular activity.
Blood pressure	● Severe hypotension can trigger a convulsion e.g. with syncope or a vasovagal attack where the patient remains propped up. ● In these instances there will usually be a clear precipitating event and no prior history of epilepsy. Once the patient lies flat and the blood pressure is restored the convulsion may stop.
Alcohol/drug usage	● Convulsions are more common in alcoholics, are associated with hypoglycaemia and can be triggered by a number of prescription or illegal drugs (e.g. tricyclic antidepressants) – **refer to glycaemic emergencies guideline**.
Injury	● Assess for mouth/tongue injury – often accompanies an epileptic convulsion. ● Is there any history of head injury? ● Dislocated shoulder. ● Road Traffic Collision may have resulted from a convulsion – **refer to appropriate trauma guideline**. NB Wherever possible, obtain contact details of any witnesses and pass this to the receiving hospital.
Incontinence	● Often accompanies a convulsion.
● Airway	**DO NOT** attempt to force an oropharyngeal airway into a convulsing patient. A nasopharyngeal airway is a useful adjunct in such patients – **NB Caution in patients with suspected basal skull fracture or facial injury.**

Table 3.54 – ASSESSMENT and MANAGEMENT of:

Convulsions in Adults *continued*

ASSESSMENT	MANAGEMENT
● Position	● Position patient for comfort and protect from dangers, especially the head.
● Oxygen	**ACTIVE CONVULSION** ● Administer 15 litres per minute until a reliable SpO_2 measurement can be obtain and then adjust oxygen flow to aim for a target saturation within the range of 94–98% – as a convulsion occurs the brain is acutely starved of oxygen. **POST-ICTAL** ● Apply pulse oximeter. ● Measure oxygen saturation. ● Administer supplemental oxygen if hypoxaemic (SpO_2 of <94%) (refer to oxygen guideline).

● Medication	Most tonic/clonic convulsions are self-limiting and do not require drug treatment. Establish if any treatment has already been administered.
	
	Midazolam – refer to patient's own midazolam instructions.
	● If a grand-mal convulsion is still continuing ten minutes **after the first dose of midazolam**:
	  – the ambulance clinician can advise the carer to administer a second dose of midazolam
	  – ambulance paramedics and technicians can administer the patient's own prescribed midazolam – if they are competent to administer medication via the buccal or intranasal route and are familiar with the indications, actions and side effects of midazolam
	  – a paramedic can administer a single dose of diazepam intravenously (IV) or rectally (PR).
	NB Due to the time taken to cannulate and administer intravenous diazepam and the time it takes for rectal diazepam to act, a second dose of midazolam is preferable.
	
	If the patient does not have their own midazolam:
	
	Diazepam
	● Administer diazemuls. Rectal diazepam (stesolid) may be given when IV access cannot be obtained (refer to diazepam guideline) for:
	  – fits lasting >5 minutes and **STILL FITTING**
	  – repeated fits in close succession – not secondary to an uncorrected hypoxia or hypoglycaemic episode
	  – status epilepticus
	  – eclamptic fits lasting >2-3 minutes or recurrent.
	If a grand-mal convulsion continues ten minutes after the second dose, medical advice should be sought. **Refer to eclampsia guideline**.

● Transfer	Transfer to further care: ● Patients suffering from serial convulsions (three or more in an hour). ● Patients suffering from an eclamptic convulsion (**refer to pregnancy induced hypertension (including eclampsia) guideline**). ● Patients suffering their first convulsion. ● Difficulties monitoring the patient's condition. NB Known epileptics who make a full recovery, are not at risk and can be supervised adequately, can be managed at home following local guidelines. For these patients: ● Measure and record vital signs with the explanation given to the patient. ● Advise the patients and carer to contact the general practitioner (GP) if the patient feels generally unwell or 999 if there are repeated convulsions. ● Document the reasons for the decision not to transfer to further care and this must be signed by the patient and/or carer. ● Ensure contact is made with the patient's GP particularly where the patient has made repeated calls. ● Provide an information sheet. NB It is important not to label a patient as epileptic unless there is a known diagnosis.

3 Medical Undifferentiated Complaints — SECTION

Convulsions (Adults)

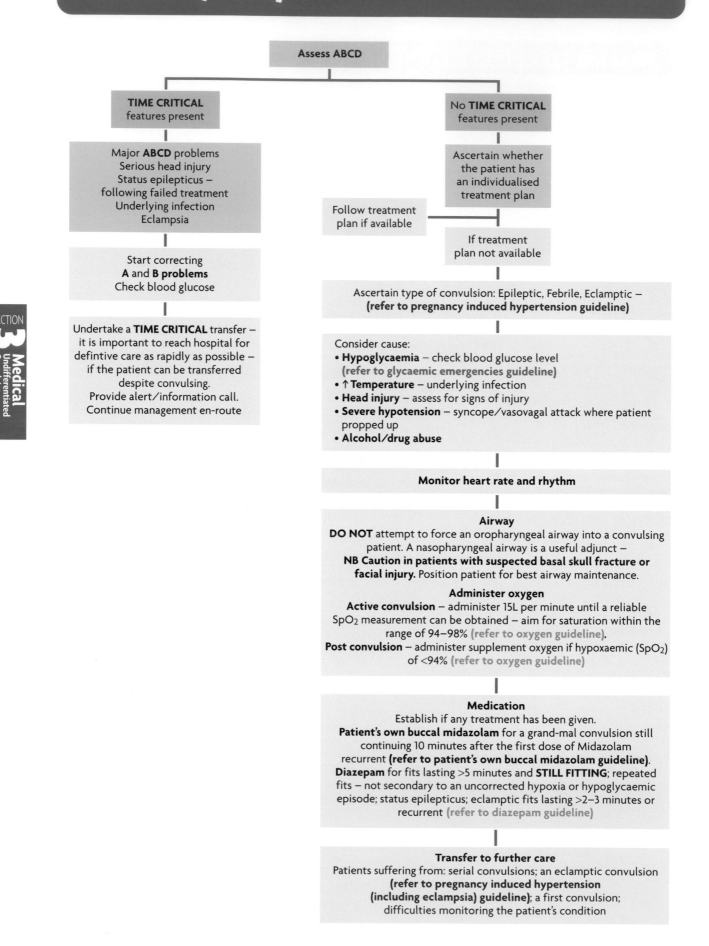

Assess ABCD

TIME CRITICAL features present

Major **ABCD** problems
Serious head injury
Status epilepticus –
following failed treatment
Underlying infection
Eclampsia

Start correcting
A and **B problems**
Check blood glucose

Undertake a **TIME CRITICAL** transfer –
it is important to reach hospital for
defintive care as rapidly as possible –
if the patient can be transferred
despite convulsing.
Provide alert/information call.
Continue management en-route

No **TIME CRITICAL** features present

Ascertain whether
the patient has
an individualised
treatment plan

Follow treatment
plan if available

If treatment
plan not available

Ascertain type of convulsion: Epileptic, Febrile, Eclamptic –
(refer to pregnancy induced hypertension guideline)

Consider cause:
• **Hypoglycaemia** – check blood glucose level
(refer to glycaemic emergencies guideline)
• **↑ Temperature** – underlying infection
• **Head injury** – assess for signs of injury
• **Severe hypotension** – syncope/vasovagal attack where patient
propped up
• **Alcohol/drug abuse**

Monitor heart rate and rhythm

Airway
DO NOT attempt to force an oropharyngeal airway into a convulsing
patient. A nasopharyngeal airway is a useful adjunct –
**NB Caution in patients with suspected basal skull fracture or
facial injury.** Position patient for best airway maintenance.

Administer oxygen
Active convulsion – administer 15L per minute until a reliable
SpO$_2$ measurement can be obtained – aim for saturation within the
range of 94–98% **(refer to oxygen guideline)**.
Post convulsion – administer supplement oxygen if hypoxaemic (SpO$_2$)
of <94% **(refer to oxygen guideline)**

Medication
Establish if any treatment has been given.
Patient's own buccal midazolam for a grand-mal convulsion still
continuing 10 minutes after the first dose of Midazolam
recurrent **(refer to patient's own buccal midazolam guideline)**.
Diazepam for fits lasting >5 minutes and **STILL FITTING**; repeated
fits – not secondary to an uncorrected hypoxia or hypoglycaemic
episode; status epilepticus; eclamptic fits lasting >2–3 minutes or
recurrent **(refer to diazepam guideline)**

Transfer to further care
Patients suffering from: serial convulsions; an eclamptic convulsion
**(refer to pregnancy induced hypertension
(including eclampsia) guideline)**; a first convulsion;
difficulties monitoring the patient's condition

Figure 3.11 – Assessment and management of convulsions in adults algorithm.

1. Introduction

Gastrointestinal (GI) bleeding is a common medical emergency accounting for 7,000 admissions per year in Scotland alone.

Gastrointestinal haemorrhage is commonly divided into:

- **Upper gastrointestinal bleeding.**
- **Lower gastrointestinal bleeding.**

2. Incidence

- Upper gastrointestinal bleeding is more common than lower gastrointestinal bleeding and is more prevalent in socioeconomically deprived areas.
- UPPER GI BLEEDING accounts for up to 85% of gastrointestinal bleeding events.

3. Severity and Outcome

- The severity of gastrointestinal bleeding can range from clinically insignificant blood loss to significant life-threatening haemorrhage.
- Death is uncommon in patients less than 40 years of age, it is estimated that the overall mortality rate in the UK for patients admitted with acute GI bleeding is approximately 7%. The majority of deaths occur in the elderly, particularly those with comorbidities. There are many factors that are associated with a poor outcome including liver disease, acute haemodynamic disturbance, clotting abnormalities, continued bleeding, haematemesis, haematochezia, and elevated blood urea.
- Upper gastrointestinal bleeding tends to be more severe and in extreme circumstances can rapidly lead to hypovolaemic shock.

4. Pathophysiology

- The upper gastrointestinal tract comprises the oesophagus, stomach and duodenum. For common causes of bleeding refer to Table 3.55.
- The lower gastrointestinal tract comprises of the lower part of the small intestine, the colon, rectum and anus. Common causes of bleeding include diverticular disease, inflammatory bowel disease, haemorrhoids, and tumour.

ACUTE UPPER GI BLEEDING

- More than 50% of cases are due to peptic ulcers which, together with oesophagitis and gastritis, account for up to 90% of all upper GI bleeding in the elderly. 85% of deaths associated with upper GI bleeding occur in persons older than 65 years.
- Patients presenting with upper GI bleeding may have a history of aspirin or non-steroidal anti-inflammatory drug (NSAID) use.
  - Only 50% of patients present with haematemesis alone, 30% with melaena and 20% with haematemesis and melaena
  - Patients with haematemesis tend to have greater blood loss than those with melaena alone. Patients older than 60 years account for up to 45% of all cases (60% of these women).

Table 3.55 – COMMON CAUSES OF UPPER GASTROINTESTINAL BLEEDING

Common causes
Peptic ulcers: – Duodenal ulcers – Gastric ulcers
Oesophageal varices
Gastritis
Oesophagitis
Mallory-Weiss tears
Caustic poison
Tumour

Peptic ulcers

- Peptic ulcers are commonly associated with the use of aspirin, non-steroidal anti-inflammatory drugs, corticosteroids, anticoagulants, alcohol and cigarettes.

Oesophageal varices

- It is estimated that variceal bleeding is the cause of 10% of cases. These patients can bleed severely with up to 8% dying within 48 hours from uncontrolled haemorrhage. It is commonly associated with alcoholic cirrhosis and increased portal pressure (causing progressive dilation of the veins and protrusion of the formed varices into the lumen of the oesophagus). Spontaneous rupture of the varices will cause the patient to become haemodynamically unstable within a very short period of time due to large volumes of blood loss.

Mallory-Weiss tears

- Approximately 10% are caused by oesophageal tears, which are more common in the young. Predisposing factors include hiatal hernia and alcoholism. Initiating factors are persistent coughing or severe retching and vomiting, often after an alcoholic binge; haematemesis presents after several episodes of non-bloody emesis. Bleeding can be mild to moderate.

- **Gastritis** – drugs, infections, illnesses, and injuries can cause inflammation of the lining of the stomach and lead to bleeding.

- **Oesophagitis** – Gastroesophageal reflux disease or alcohol can lead to inflammation and ulcers in the lining of the oesophagus which may lead to bleeding.

- **Tumour** – in the oesophagus, stomach or duodenum can cause bleeding.

ACUTE LOWER GI BLEEDING

Patients with a lower GI bleed commonly present with bright red blood/ dark blood with clots per rectum (PR); bright red blood PR in isolation excludes upper GI bleeding in over 98% of cases (unless the patient appears hypovolaemic). Lower GI bleeding are less likely to present with signs of haemodynamic compromise, are more prevalent in men and also have a common history of aspirin or NSAID use. The mean age for lower GI bleeding is 63 to 77 years with mortality around 4% (even serious cases have rarely resulted in death). Common causes include:

Diverticular disease

● Diverticular bleeding accounts for up to 55% of cases. Patients commonly present with an abrupt but painless PR bleed. The incidence of diverticular bleeding increases with age.

Inflammatory bowel disease

● Major bleeding from ulcerative colitis and Crohn's disease is rare. Inflammatory bowel disease accounts for less than 10% of cases.

Haemorrhoids

● Haemorrhoids account for less than 10% of cases. Bleeding is bright red and usually noticed on wiping or in the toilet bowl. The incidence is high in pregnancy, a result of straining associated with constipation and hormonal changes. Further evaluation may be needed if the patient complains of an alteration of bowel habit and blood mixed with the stool.

Tumour

● Tumour in the large bowel can cause bleeding.

Differential Diagnosis

● Post rectal bleeding can cause significant embarrassment for the patient and care must be taken when assessing female patients that PV bleeding is excluded.

5. Assessment and Management

For the assessment and management of gastrointestinal bleeding refer to Table 3.56.

Methodology

For details of the methodology used in the development of this guideline refer to the guideline webpage.

KEY POINTS

Gastrointestinal Bleeding

● Haematemesis or melaena indicates an upper GI source.
● Bright red or dark blood with clots per rectum indicates a lower GI source.
● Almost all deaths from GI bleeds occur in the elderly.
● Approximately 80% of all GI bleeds stop spontaneously or respond to conservative management.

Table 3.56 – ASSESSMENT and MANAGEMENT of:

Gastrointestinal Bleeding

ASSESSMENT	MANAGEMENT

● Assess ABCD	● If any of the following **TIME CRITICAL** features are present:
	  – major **ABCD** problems
	  – haematemesis – large volume of bright red blood
	  – haemodynamic compromise
	  – decreased level of consciousness.
	● Start correcting **A** and **B** problems
	● Undertake a **TIME CRITICAL** transfer to nearest receiving hospital.
	● Provide an alert/information call.
	● Continue patient management en-route.

● Assess blood loss	Where does the bleeding originate – upper or lower GI tract? ● **Haematemesis** – vomited fresh/dark red/brown/black or 'coffee ground' blood (depending on how long it has been in the stomach). Did this occur after an increase in intra-abdominal pressure e.g. retching or coughing. ● Ascertain how many episodes of non-bloody emesis. ● **Melaena** – malodorous, liquid, black stool or bright red/dark blood with clots per rectum (PR). It can be difficult to estimate blood loss when mixed with faeces. ● Estimate blood loss – if not visible ask the patient or relatives/carers to estimate colour/volume – PR blood loss is difficult to estimate. (NB The blood acts as a laxative, but repeated blood-liquid stool, or just blood, is associated with more severe blood loss than maroon/black solid stool.) ● Has the patient suffered unexplained syncope – this may indicate concealed GI bleeding. Ensure PV bleeding is excluded in females.

● History	● **When did the bleeding begin?**
	● Is/has the patient:
	  – currently taking or recently taken aspirin or NSAID?
	  – currently taking iron tablets?
	  – consumed food or drink containing red dye(s)?
	  – currently taking beta blockers or calcium-channel blockers – may mask tachycardia in the shocked patient?
	  – currently taking or recently taken anticoagulatory or antiplatelet therapy?
	
	● **Is there a history of:**
	  – bleeding disorders?
	  – liver disease?
	  – abdominal surgery in particular abdominal aortic surgery?
	  – alcohol abuse?
	  – syncope?

● Oxygen	● Administer supplemental oxygen if the patient is hypoxaemic (SpO_2 <94%).
● Vital signs	● Monitor vital signs. ● Monitor ECG.
● IV access	● Obtain if analgesia or fluid therapy are indicated.
● Pain management	● GI bleeding is not generally associated with pain. ● If pain relief is indicated **refer to pain management guidelines**.
● Fluid	● If fluid resuscitation indicated (refer to intravascular fluid therapy guideline).
● Transfer to further care	● Continue patient management en-route. ● Provide an alert/information call.

3 Medical Undifferentiated Complaints SECTION

Glycaemic Emergencies (Adults)

1. Introduction
- A non-diabetic individual maintains their blood glucose level within a narrow range from 3.0 to 5.6 mmol per litre.
- This is achieved by a balance between glucose entering the blood stream (from the gastrointestinal tract or from the breakdown of stored energy sources) and glucose leaving the circulation through the action of insulin.

SECTION 1 – Hypoglycaemia
- A low blood glucose level is defined as <4.0 mmol/L, but the clinical features of hypoglycaemia may be present at higher levels and clinical judgement is as important as a blood glucose reading.
- Correction of hypoglycaemia is a medical emergency.
- If left untreated hypoglycaemia may lead to the patient suffering permanent brain damage and may even prove fatal.
- Hypoglycaemia occurs when glucose metabolism is disturbed – see Table 3.57 for risk factors.
- Any person whose level of consciousness is decreased, who is having a convulsion, is seriously ill or traumatised should have hypoglycaemia excluded.
- Signs and symptoms can vary from patient to patient (Table 3.58) and the classical symptoms may not be present.
- Some patients are able to detect the early symptoms for themselves, but others may deteriorate rapidly and without apparent warning.
- Abnormal neurological features may occur, for example, one-sided weakness, identical to a stroke.
- Symptoms may be masked due to medication or other injuries, for example, with beta-blocking agents.

2. Assessment and Management
For the assessment and management of hypoglycaemia refer to Table 3.59 and or Figure 3.12.

SECTION 2 – Hyperglycaemia
- Hyperglycaemia is the term used to describe high blood glucose levels.
- Symptoms include unusual thirst (polydipsia), urinary frequency, and tiredness (Table 3.60). They are usually of slow onset in comparison to those of hypoglycaemia.

Diabetic ketoacidosis (DKA)
- A relative lack of circulating insulin means that cells cannot take up glucose from the blood and use it to provide energy. This forces the cells to provide energy for metabolism from other sources such as fatty acids.
- This produces acidosis and ketones. The body tries to combat this metabolic acidosis by hyperventilation to blow off carbon dioxide. High blood glucose level means glucose spills over into the urine dragging water and electrolytes with it causing dehydration and glycosuria.
- New onset diabetes type 1 may present with DKA.

Table 3.57 – RISK FACTORS FOR HYPOGLYCAEMIA

Medical
- Insulin or other hypoglycaemic drug treatments.
- Tight glycaemic control.
- Previous history of severe hypoglycaemia.
- Undetected nocturnal hypoglycaemia.
- Long duration of diabetes.
- Poor injection technique.
- Impaired awareness of hypoglycaemia.
- Preceding hypoglycaemia (< 3.5 mmol/L).
- Severe hepatic dysfunction.
- Renal dialysis therapy.
- Impaired renal function.
- Inadequate treatment of previous hypoglycaemia.
- Terminal illness.
- Metabolic illness.
- Endocrine illness (including Addisonian crisis).
- Drug ingestion e.g. oral hypoglycaemic drugs, beta-blockers, alcohol.
- Sudden cessation of peritoneal dialysis.
- Hypothermia.
- Sudden cessation of tube or IV feeding.

Lifestyle
- Inadequate carbohydrate intake.
- Increased exercise (relative to usual)/excessive physical activity.
- Irregular lifestyle.
- Increasing age.
- Excessive or chronic alcohol intake.
- Early pregnancy.
- Breast feeding.
- Injection into areas of lipohypertrophy.
- Inadequate blood glucose monitoring.

Table 3.58 – SIGNS AND SYMPTOMS OF HYPOGLYCAEMIA

Autonomic	Neurological
Sweating	Confusion
Palpitations	Drowsiness
Shaking	Odd behaviour
Hunger	Speech difficulty
	In-coordination
	Aggression
General malaise	Fitting
Headache	Unconsciousness
Nausea	

- More frequently it complicates intercurrent illness in a known diabetic. Infections, myocardial infarction (which may be silent) or a CVA may precipitate the condition.
- Omissions or inadequate dosage of insulin or other hypoglycaemic therapy may also contribute or be responsible. Some medications, particularly steroids may greatly exacerbate the situation.
- Patients may present with one or more signs and symptoms (Table 3.60) and this should alert the pre-hospital provider to the possibility of hyperglycaemia and DKA.

Medical – specific conditions

Table 3.59 – ASSESSMENT and MANAGEMENT of:

Hypoglycaemia in Adults

ASSESSMENT	MANAGEMENT
● Undertake ABCD assessment	● Start correcting ABC problems (**refer to medical overview guideline**).
● Consider and look for medical alert/information signs (alert bracelets, chains and cards)	
● Assess blood glucose level	● Measure and record blood glucose level (pre-treatment measure).
● Treatment	● When treating hypoglycaemia, use all available clinical information to help decide between glucagon IM, oral glucose gel (40%), or glucose 10% IV.
SEVERE: patient unconscious (GCS ≤8)/convulsing, very aggressive	● Keep nil by mouth as there is an increased risk of aspiration/choking. ● Administer IV glucose 10% by slow IV infusion (**refer to glucose 10% guideline**). ● Titrate to effect – an improvement should be observed rapidly. ● Re-assess blood glucose level after 10 minutes. ● If <5.0 mmol/L administer a further dose of IV glucose – if IV route not possible administer IM glucagon (onset of action 5–10 minutes). ● Re-assess blood glucose level after a further 10 minutes. ● Transfer immediately to the nearest suitable receiving hospital. ● Continue patient management en-route. ● Provide an alert/information call.
MODERATE: Patient with impaired consciousness: uncooperative, an increased risk of aspiration or choking	● If capable and cooperative, administer 15–20 grams of quick acting carbohydrate (sugary drink, chocolate bar/biscuit or glucose gel). ● If NOT capable and cooperative, but able to swallow, administer 1–2 tubes of Dextrose Gel 40% or intra-muscular glucagon. ● Re-assess blood glucose level after a further 10 minutes. ● Ensure blood glucose level has improved to at least 5.0 mmol/L in addition to an improvement in level of consciousness. ● If no improvement, repeat treatment up to three times. ● If no improvement after three treatments, consider intravenous glucose 10%. ● Refer to care pathway below.
MILD: Patient consciousness, orientated, able to swallow	● Administer 15–20 grams of quick acting carbohydrate (sugary drink, chocolate bar/biscuit or glucose gel). ● Ensure blood glucose level has improved to at least 5.0 mmol/L. ● If no improvement, repeat treatment up to three times. ● If no improvement after three treatments, consider intravenous glucose 10%. ● Refer to care pathway below.
	Care Pathway: **The following patients may be appropriate to leave at home:** ● Patients whose episode was mild or moderate and who are now fully recovered after treatment, with a blood glucose level of > 5.0 mmol/L, who have been able to eat/drink a glucose and carbohydrate containing food, and are in the care of a responsible adult. ● Advise patients to call for help if any symptoms of hypoglycaemia recur. ● Ambulance services must arrange locally for a message to be forwarded to the local diabetic nurse/primary healthcare team. ● Leave an advice sheet. **Transfer the following patients to further care – continue patient management en-route:** ● Those who have had recurrent treatment within previous 48 hours. ● Those patients taking **glibenclamide**. ● Those patients with no previous history of diabetes and have suffered their first hypoglycaemic episode. ● Those patients with a blood glucose level <5.0 mmol/L after treatment. ● Those patients who have not returned to normal mental status within 10 minutes of IV glucose. ● Those patients with any additional disorders or other complicating factors, e.g. renal dialysis, chest pain, cardiac arrhythmias, alcohol consumption, dyspnoea, seizures or focal neurological signs/symptoms. ● Those patients with signs of infection (urinary tract infection, upper respiratory tract infections) and/or unwell (flu-like symptoms).

Glycaemic Emergencies (Adults)

- Diabetic patients may present with significant dehydration resulting in reduced fluid in both the vascular and tissue compartments. Often this has taken time to develop and will take time to correct. Rapid fluid replacement into the vascular compartment can compromise the cardiovascular system particularly where there is pre-existing cardiovascular disease and in the elderly. Gradual rehydration over hours rather than minutes is indicated.
- Ketone measurement (blood or urine) is useful in the diagnosis of DKA.

3. Assessment and Management

For the assessment and management of hyperglycaemia refer to Table 3.61.

Methodology

For details of the methodology used in the development of this guideline refer to the guideline webpage.

Table 3.60 – SIGNS AND SYMPTOMS OF HYPERGLYCAEMIA

Symptoms
- Polyuria
- Polydipsia
- Increased appetite

Signs
- Fruity odour of ketones on the breath (resembling nail varnish remover)

NB Not everyone can detect this odour
- Lethargy, confusion and ultimately unconsciousness
- Dehydration, dry mouth and possible circulatory failure due to hypovolaemia
- Hyperventilation
- Kussmaul breathing
- Weight loss

Table 3.61 – ASSESSMENT and MANAGEMENT of:

Hyperglycaemia in Adults

ASSESSMENT	MANAGEMENT
Undertake ABCD assessment	Start correcting ABC problems (**refer to medical overview guideline**).
If the patient is **TIME CRITICAL**	Correct life-threatening conditions, airway and breathing on scene. Then commence transfer to nearest suitable receiving hospital. NB These patients have a potentially life-threatening condition – they require urgent hospital treatment including insulin and fluid/electrolyte therapy.
Consider and look for medical alert/information signs (alert bracelets, chains and cards)	
Assess for blood glucose level	Measure and record blood glucose level.
Assess for signs of dehydration	**Signs may include:** The skin of the forearm remains tented following a gentle pinch, only returning to its normal position slowly. Dry mouth. In severe cases this may lead to hypovolaemic shock – If the patient is shocked, with poor capillary refill, tachycardia, reduced Glasgow Coma Score (GCS) and hypotension, then refer to the intravascular fluid therapy guideline. **DO NOT** delay at scene for fluid replacement.
Assess heart rhythm	Undertake ECG.
Measure oxygen saturation (SpO$_2$)	Administer supplemental oxygen if the patient is hypoxaemic SpO$_2$ <94%. Refer to oxygen guideline.
	Provide a pre-alert/information message. If the patient has records of their blood or urine glucose levels, ensure these accompany the patient.

KEY POINTS

Glycaemic Emergencies in Adults

- **Clean skin prior to obtaining blood glucose reading (using either soapy solution or an alcohol wipe, allowing the finger to dry).**
- **If blood glucose reading of <4.0 mmol/L treat with oral solids (glucose drinks, chocolate or hypostop solutions) if GCS >13.**
- **If GCS ≤13 consider IM glucagon or 10% IV glucose 100 ml bolus and review patient's condition titrate to effect.**
- **Consider fluid therapy to counteract the effects of dehydration.**

MILD

Patient conscious, orientated and able to swallow.

Administer 15–20 grams of quick acting carbohydrate (sugary drink, chocolate bar/biscuit or glucose gel).

Test blood glucose level if <4 mmol/L, repeat up to 3 times.

Consider intravenous glucose 10% or 1 mg glucagon.

MODERATE

Patient conscious, but confused/ disorientated or aggressive and able to swallow.

If capable and cooperative, administer 15–20 grams of quick acting carbohydrate (sugary drink, chocolate bar/biscuit or glucose gel). Test blood glucose level.

Continue to test after 15 minutes and repeat up to 3 times consider intravenous glucose 10%. (Repeat up to 3 times until BGL above 4 mmol/L.)

Test blood glucose level, if <4 mmol/L administer 15–20 grams of quick acting carbohydrate.

Continue to test after 15 minutes and repeat up to 3 times, consider intravenous glucose 10% (Repeat up to 3 times until BGL above 4 mmol/L.)

SEVERE

Patient unconscious/ convulsing or very aggressive or nil by mouth or where there is an increased risk of aspiration/choking.

Assess ABCD Measure and record blood glucose level.

Administer IV glucose 10% by slow IV infusion (refer to glucose 10% guideline) – titrate to effect.

Re-assess blood glucose level after 10 minutes.

If <5 mmol/L administer a further dose of IV glucose – if IV not possible administer IM glucagon (onset of action 5–10 minutes).

Re-assess blood glucose level after a further 10 minutes.

If no improvement transfer immediately to nearest suitable receiving hospital. Provide alert/ information call.

Medical
Undifferentiated Complaints
3 SECTION

Figure 3.12 – Hypoglycaemic emergencies algorithm.

1. Introduction

- Heart failure is not a specific disease entity, rather it is a clinical syndrome characterised by a number of clinical signs, symptoms and diagnostic findings. It occurs as a consequence of diastolic or systolic dysfunction resulting in the inability of the heart to provide adequate cardiac output for the body's metabolic needs.

- Acute Heart Failure (AHF) represents new or worsening signs or symptoms consistent with an underlying deterioration in ventricular function. It is characterised by dyspnoea resulting from acutely elevated cardiac filling pressures often, though not always, leading to rapid accumulation of fluid within the lung's interstitial and alveolar spaces (cardiogenic pulmonary oedema).

2. Incidence

- The overall prevalence of heart failure varies between 1 and 2%; it is the leading reason for hospital admission in patients over 65 years of age in westernised countries. Of heart failure cases, 80% are diagnosed following admission to hospital as an acute emergency.

3. Severity and Outcome

- The 60-day mortality following hospital admission because of an exacerbation of heart failure varies with estimates between 8–20%. Approximately 30% of heart failure patients will be re-admitted to hospital each year as a result of an acute exacerbation.

- The overall prehospital mortality rate for cases of acute cardiogenic pulmonary oedema has been reported at 8%.

4. Pathophysiology

- The pathophysiology underlying the worsening ventricular function is often coronary artery disease. Diseased coronary arteries become inelastic and intravascular pressures rise as a consequence – coronary artery perfusion will reduce unless mean arterial pressures are raised to ensure adequate coronary artery blood flow.

- As mean arterial pressures rise so too does cardiac afterload that will lead to an increased end diastolic volume unless the force of ventricular contraction is raised. These combined processes initiate a spiral of increasing mean arterial pressures, increasing afterload and increasing preload.

> **Risk Factors**
> - Advancing age
> - History of CHF
> - Hypertension

- Acute Heart Failure patients will often present with clinical signs of vascular congestion and the formation of oedema. The pathophysiology underlying the formation of oedema can vary depending on cause; however in Acute Heart Failure acute oedema occurs as a result of fluid shifts from the vascular compartment into the interstitial space.

- Left Ventricular Failure (LVF) may precipitate formation of pulmonary oedema as a result of reduced cardiac output and increasing pulmonary hypertension. As pulmonary vascular pressures rise, so increasing amounts of fluid will shift from the pulmonary vascular compartment into the lung interstitial spaces and alveoli. Pulmonary oedema occurs as a result of the accumulation of this fluid in the alveoli which decreases gas exchange across the alveoli, resulting in decreased oxygenation of the blood and, in some cases, accumulation of carbon dioxide (CO_2).

- The pathophysiology of pulmonary oedema can be thought of in terms of three factors (Table 3.62):
  i. flow
  ii. fluid
  iii. filter.

Table 3.62 – PULMONARY OEDEMA

i. Flow
The ability of the heart to eject the blood delivered to it depends on three factors:
1. the amount of blood returning to the heart (preload)
2. the co-ordinated contraction of the myocardium
3. the resistance against which it pumps (afterload).
Preload may also be increased by over-infusion of IV fluid or fluid retention. Coordinated contraction fails following heart muscle damage (Myocardial Infarction (MI), heart failure) or due to arrhythmias. Afterload increases with hypertension, atherosclerosis, aortic valve stenosis or peripheral vasoconstriction.

ii. Fluid
The blood passing through the lungs must have enough 'oncotic' pressure to 'hold on' to the fluid portion as it passes through the pulmonary capillaries. As albumin is a key determinant of oncotic pressure, low albumin states can also lead to the formation of pulmonary oedema, e.g. burns, liver failure, nephrotic syndrome.

iii. Filter
The capillaries through which the fluid passes may increase in permeability, e.g. acute lung injury (as in smoke inhalation), pneumonia or drowning.

- Right Ventricular Failure (RVF) may precipitate formation of peripheral oedema as a result of increasing right ventricular filling pressures, reduced right venticular output and increasing systemic congestion. Peripheral oedema occurs as a result of the accumulation of fluid in the interstitial spaces and is most commonly noted in the lower legs and sacrum.

- The signs and symptoms of heart failure vary depending upon the extent of failure and underlying physiologic cause. However, three symptoms are common to nearly all forms; fatigue (including exercise intolerance), dyspnoea and congestion. It can be difficult to differentiate heart failure from other causes of breathlessness, such as exacerbation of Chronic Obstructive Pulmonary Disease (COPD), pulmonary embolism or pneumonia. Therefore, a thorough history and physical examination are required.

5. Assessment and Management

For the assessment and management of heart failure refer to Table 3.63.

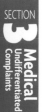

SECTION **3** Medical Undifferentiated Complaints

Heart Failure

Table 3.63 – ASSESSMENT and MANAGEMENT

Heart Failure

ASSESSMENT	MANAGEMENT
Undertake ABCD assessment If the patient is **TIME CRITICAL** 1. Assess PERFUSION status Signs of ADEQUATE perfusion: ● Normal mentation ● Peripheral pulses present ● Systolic blood pressure >90 mmHg ● **NOT** pale ● Capillary Bed Refill Time <2 sec	● Start correcting ABC problems (**refer to medical emergencies overview**). ● Correct life-threatening conditions, airway and breathing on scene. ● Then commence transfer to nearest suitable receiving hospital. Refer to Figure 3.13.
Signs of **INADEQUATE** perfusion: ● Reduced consciousness ● Systolic blood pressure <90 mmHg ● Pallor ● Capillary Bed Refill Time >2 sec	Refer to Figure 3.13.
2. Assess CONGESTION status Signs of congestion: ● Pulmonary oedema ● Peripheral oedema ● Elevated jugular venous pulse	Refer to Figure 3.13. ● If pulmonary oedema is evident position the patient sitting upright if possible.
Record a 12-lead ECG	● It is uncommon for patients with heart failure to have a normal ECG. Where no ECG abnormalities are identified clinicians should consider the possibility of an alternative diagnosis. ● Where the ECG indicates that heart failure may be due to Acute Coronary Syndrome manage as per the **ACS guideline**.

Table 3.64

Clinical Indicators of Potential Heart Failure

Pulmonary oedema
● Fine crackling sounds are suggestive of pulmonary oedema, commonly heard in the lung bases, but may be heard over other lung fields as well.
● Often accompanied by the coughing up of frothy sputum, white or pink (blood stained) in colour.

Peripheral oedema
● Although peripheral oedema is a common sign of chronic heart failure, it is not specific to heart failure and may be seen as a consequence of numerous pathologies. It usually only becomes apparent when the extracellular volume exceeds 5 litres.

Third heart sound
● An auscultated third heart sound (S3), or gallop rhythm, in an adult patient is usually a pathological indicator of reduced ventricular compliance.
● It is strongly associated with elevated atrial pressure; consequently it can be an important indicator of left ventricular failure and dilation.
Although a third heart sound is not sensitive (24%) for heart failure, it is highly specific (99%).

Jugular venous pressure
● Jugular venous pressure (JVP) provides an estimation of right atrial filling pressure as there are no valves between the right atrium and the internal jugular vein.
● Jugular venous pressure is assessed while the patient is supine with the upper body at a 30–45° angle from the horizontal plane.
● The vertical height of the crest of the internal jugular venous pulsation above the sternal angle determines the height of the venous pressure and provides the estimate of right atrial filling pressure.
● Any measurement greater than 3 cm suggests elevated right atrial filling pressure.
Elevated jugular venous pressure is a specific (90%) but not sensitive (30%) indicator of elevated left ventricular filling.

Medical Undifferentiated Complaints — SECTION 3

Heart Failure

Table 3.65

Therapies in Heart Failure

GTN
- The use of nitrates in pulmonary oedema is associated with improved survival to hospital discharge.
- Buccal nitrates produce an immediate reduction in preload, comparable with IV GTN.
- Nitrates have some benefit as the first-line treatment in acute pulmonary oedema.

Furosemide
- There is little high-level evidence for or against the use of furosemide (refer to furosemide protocol for dosage and information) in the treatment of acute pulmonary oedema, but it has been standard treatment for many years.
- There is some evidence that furosemide can have a transient adverse vasoconstrictor effect; it is unclear whether this is beneficial or harmful.
- The acute vasodilator effect of furosemide is inhibited by aspirin.
- Prehospital trials comparing repeated furosemide vs. repeated nitrates favour the use of nitrates.

Furosemide should only be given after nitrates (which act on both preload and after-load).

Salbutamol
- The effectiveness of salbutamol in the treatment of pulmonary oedema presenting in the acute setting is unclear.
- Studies addressing the use of bronchodilators in chronic heart failure suggest worse outcomes following their use, however a number of prehospital trials of combination drug therapies (including salbutamol) indicate improved outcomes.

Owing to the diagnostic uncertainty and possibility for misdiagnosis, salbutamol may still be considered in the management of heart failure where wheeze is present; this may avoid depriving COPD/asthma patients of vital bronchodilators.

Morphine
- Morphine and diamorphine are commonly used in the in-hospital emergency management of pulmonary oedema.

The drugs act by reducing preload (venodilation) and also serve to decrease anxiety.
- Despite their widespread use, there is no conclusive trial evidence showing symptomatic improvement or mortality benefit.

Analysis of large heart failure registries suggest that the use of opiates in heart failure increases mortality; therefore they should not routinely be used unless they are being used to manage ACS and the patient is complaining of chest pain.

CPAP
- Non-invasive positive pressure ventilation (NiPPV) comprises two main treatment modalities – continuous positive airway pressure (CPAP) and bilevel positive airways pressure (BiPAP). The fundamental difference between these two modalities is the level of pressure maintained throughout the patient's respiratory cycle. In CPAP therapy pressure remains constant through the inspiratory and expiratory phases; in BiPAP therapy pressure is reduced during the expiratory phase and increases during the inspiratory phase.
- The objective of non-invasive positive pressure ventilation (NiPPV) is two-fold. First is to 'splint' open collapsing alveoli and increase intra-alveolar pressure. The increase in pressure helps shift fluid present in the alveoli back into the pulmonary capillaries thereby reducing pulmonary oedema. Second is to raise intrathoracic pressure throughout the respiratory cycle. This increase in intrathoracic pressure increases pressure in the vena cavae, and consequently serves to reduce filling pressures. Combined, these two actions serve to reduce congestion.
- Prospective randomised controlled trials have demonstrated that CPAP improves survival to hospital discharge, decreased intubation rates and fewer complications.
- Prehospital studies exist suggesting CPAP is feasible in this setting, and may reduce severity of acute LVF, increase SpO_2 levels and improve survival to hospital discharge.

Expert opinion has recommended CPAP for use in the prehospital environment.

Methodology

For details of the methodology used in the development of this guideline refer to guideline webpage.

KEY POINTS

Heart Failure

- **Pulmonary oedema can be difficult to differentiate from other causes of breathlessness, such as exacerbation of COPD, pulmonary embolism or pneumonia; therefore, a thorough history and physical examination are needed.**
- **Symptoms include dyspnoea, worsening cough, pink frothy sputum, waking at night gasping for breath, breathlessness on lying down (sleeping on more pillows recently?), and anxiousness/restlessness.**
- **Sit the patient upright where possible.**
- **Early nitrate administration is the cornerstone of early treatment.**
- **Furosemide administration MUST be secondary to nitrate administration and should only be considered in cases with adequate perfusion and evidence of oedema.**
- **Morphine should be avoided unless there are signs of ACS.**
- **CPAP should be utilised where equipment and suitably trained personnel are available.**

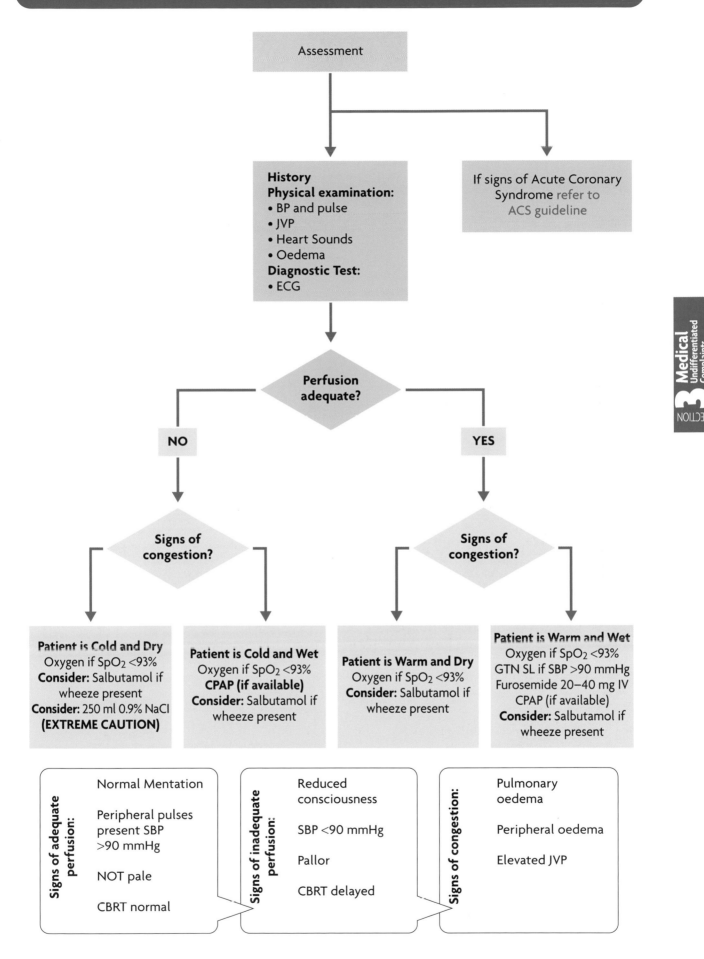

Figure 3.13 – Assessment and management algorithm of Acute Heart Failure.

1. Introduction

The Implantable Cardioverter Defibrillator (ICD) has revolutionised the management of patients at risk of developing a life-threatening ventricular arrhythmia. Several clinical trials have testified to their effectiveness in reducing deaths from sudden cardiac arrest in selected patients, and the devices are implanted with increasing frequency.

ICDs are used in both children and adults.

ICD systems consist of a generator connected to electrodes placed transvenously into cardiac chambers (the ventricle, and sometimes the right atrium and/or the coronary sinus) (Figure 3.14). The electrodes serve a dual function allowing the monitoring of cardiac rhythm and the administration of electrical pacing, defibrillation and cardioversion therapy. Modern ICDs are slightly larger than a pacemaker and are usually implanted in the left subclavicular area (Figure 3.14). The ICD generator contains the battery and sophisticated electronic circuitry that monitors the cardiac rhythm, determines the need for electrical therapy, delivers treatment, monitors the response and determines the need for further therapy.

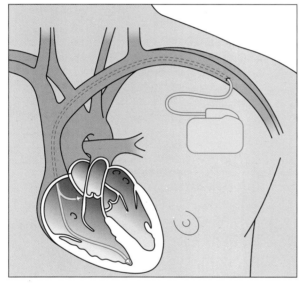

Figure 3.14 – Usual location of an ICD.

The available therapies include:

- Conventional programmable pacing for the treatment of bradycardia.
- Anti-tachycardia pacing (ATP) for ventricular tachycardia (VT).
- Delivery of biphasic shocks for the treatment of ventricular tachycardia and ventricular fibrillation (VF).
- Cardiac resynchronisation therapy (CRT) (biventricular pacing) for the treatment of heart failure.

These treatment modalities and specifications are programmable and capable of considerable sophistication to suit the requirements of individual patients. The implantation and programming of devices is carried out in specialised centres. The patient should carry a card or documentation which identifies their ICD centre and may also have been given emergency instructions.

The personnel caring for such patients in emergency situations are not usually experts in arrhythmia management or familiar with the details of the sophisticated treatment regimes offered by modern ICDs. Moreover, the technology is complex and evolving rapidly. In an emergency patients will often present to the ambulance service or Emergency Department (ED) and the purpose of this guidance is to help those responsible for the initial management of these patients.

2. General Principles

Some important points should be made at the outset.

On detecting VF/VT the ICD will usually discharge a maximum of eight times before shutting down. However, a new episode of VF/VT will result in the recommencing its discharge sequence. A patient with a fractured ICD lead may suffer repeated internal defibrillation as the electrical noise is misinterpreted as a shockable rhythm.

These patients are likely to be conscious with a relatively normal ECG rate.

When confronted with a patient fitted with an ICD who has a persistent or recurring arrhythmia, or where the ICD is firing, expert help should be summoned at the outset. Outside hospital this will normally be from the ambulance service, who should be summoned immediately by dialling 999.

When confronted with a patient in cardiac arrest the usual management guidelines are still appropriate (**refer to cardiac arrest and arrhythmia guidelines**). If the ICD is not responding to VF or VT, or if shocks are ineffective, external defibrillation/cardioversion should be carried out. Avoid placing the defibrillator electrodes/pads/paddles close to or on top of the ICD; ensure a minimum distance of 8 cm between the edge of the defibrillator paddle pad/electrode and the ICD site. Most ICDs are implanted in the left sub-clavicular position (see Figure 3.14) and are usually readily apparent on examination; the conventional (apical/right subclavicular) electrode position will then be appropriate. The anterior/posterior position may also be used, particularly if the ICD is right sided.

Whenever possible, record a 12-lead electrocardiogram (ECG) and record the patient's rhythm (with any shocks). Make sure this is printed out and stored electronically (where available) for future reference. Where an external defibrillator with an electronic memory is used (whether for monitoring or for therapy) ensure that the ECG report is printed and handed to appropriate staff. Again, whenever possible, ensure that the record is archived for future reference. Record the rhythm during any therapeutic measure (whether by drugs or electricity). All these records may provide vital information for the ICD centre that may greatly influence the patient's subsequent management.

The energy levels of the shocks administered by ICDs (up to 40 Joules) are much lower than those delivered with

The Implantable Cardioverter Defibrillator

external defibrillators (120–360J). **Personnel in contact with the patient when an ICD discharges are unlikely to be harmed, but it is prudent to minimise contact with the patient while the ICD is firing.** Chest compression and ventilation can be carried out as normal and protective examination gloves should be worn as usual.

Placing a ring magnet over the ICD generator can temporarily disable the shock capability of an ICD. The magnet does not disable the pacing capability for treating bradycardia. The magnet may be kept in position with adhesive tape if required. Removing the magnet returns the ICD to the status present before application. The ECG rhythm should be monitored at all times when the device is disabled. An ICD should only be disabled when the rhythm for which shocks are being delivered has been recorded. If that rhythm is VT or VF, external cardioversion/defibrillation must be available. With some models it is possible to programme the ICD so that a magnet does not disable the shock capabilities of the device. This is usually done only in exceptional circumstances, and consequently, such patients are rare.

The manufacturers of the ICDs also supply the ring magnets. Many implantation centres provide each patient with a ring magnet and stress that it should be readily available in case of emergency. With the increasing prevalence of ICDs in the community it becomes increasingly important that emergency workers have this magnet available to them when attending these patients.

Decisions to apply a Do Not Attempt Resuscitation (DNAR) order will not be made in the emergency situation by the personnel to whom this guidance is directed. Where such an order does exist it should not be necessary to disable an ICD to enable the implementation of such an order.

Many problems with ICDs can only be dealt with permanently by using the programmer available at the ICD centre.

The guidelines should be read from the perspective of your position and role in the management of such patients. For example, the recommendation to 'arrange further assessment' will mean that the ambulance clinician should transport the patient to hospital. For ED staff however, this might mean referral to the medical admitting team or local ICD centre.

Coincident conditions that may contribute to the development of arrhythmia (for example, acute ischaemia worsening heart failure) should be managed as appropriate according to usual practice.

Maintain oxygen saturations at 94–98%.

Receiving ICD therapy may be unpleasant 'like a firm kick in the chest', and psychological consequences may also arise. It is important to be aware of these, and help should be available from implantation centres. An emergency telephone helpline may be available.

3. Management

The following should be read in conjunction with the treatment table (Table 3.66) and algorithm (Figure 3.15).

Approach and assess the patient and perform basic life support according to current BLS guidelines.

Monitor the ECG

3.1. If the patient is in cardiac arrest.

3.1.1 Perform basic life support in accordance with current BLS guidelines. Standard airway management techniques and methods for gaining IV/IO access (as appropriate) should be established.

3.1.2 If a shockable rhythm is present (VF or pulseless VT) but the ICD is not detecting it, perform external defibrillation and other resuscitation procedures according to current resuscitation guidelines.

3.1.3 If the ICD is delivering therapy (whether by anti-tachycardia pacing or shocks) but is failing to convert the arrhythmia, then external defibrillation should be provided, as per current guidelines.

3.1.4 If a non-shockable rhythm is present manage the patient according to current guidelines. If the rhythm is converted to a shockable one, assess the response of the ICD, as in 3.1.2 above, performing external defibrillation as required.

3.1.5 If a shockable rhythm is converted to one associated with effective cardiac output (whether by the ICD or by external defibrillation), manage the patient as usual and arrange further treatment and assessment.

3.2. If the patient is not in cardiac arrest.

3.2.1 Determine whether an arrhythmia is present.

3.2.2 If no arrhythmia is present.
If therapy from the ICD has been effective and the patient is in sinus rhythm or is paced, monitor the patient, give O$_2$ and arrange further assessment to investigate possibility of new myocardial infarction (MI), heart failure, other acute illness or drug toxicity/electrolyte imbalance etc.
An ICD may deliver inappropriate shocks (i.e. in the absence of arrhythmia) if there are problems with sensing the cardiac rhythm or there are problems with the leads. Record the rhythm (while shocks are delivered, if possible), disable the ICD with a magnet, monitor the patient and arrange further assessment with help from the ICD centre. Provide supportive treatment as required.

3.2.3 If an arrhythmia is present.
If an arrhythmia is present and shocks are being delivered, record the arrhythmia (while ICD shocks are delivered if possible) on the ECG. Determine the nature of the arrhythmia. Transport rapidly to hospital in all cases.

TACHYCARDIA

3.2.3.1 If the rhythm is a **supraventricular tachycardia** i.e. sinus tachycardia, atrial flutter, atrial fibrillation, junctional tachycardia, etc. and the patient is haemodynamically stable, and the patient is continuing to receive shocks, disable the ICD with a magnet. Consider possible causes, treat appropriately and arrange further assessment in hospital.

3.2.3.2 If the rhythm is **ventricular tachycardia**:

- Pulseless VT should be treated as cardiac arrest (3.1.2 above).
- If the patient is haemodynamically stable, monitor the patient and convey to the emergency department.
- If the patient is haemodynamically unstable, and ICD shocks are ineffective treat as per VT guideline.
- An ICD will not deliver anti-tachycardia pacing (ATP) or shocks if the rate of the VT is below the programmed detection rate of the device (generally 150 beats/min). Conventional management may be undertaken according to the patient's haemodynamic status.
- Recurring VT with appropriate shocks. Manage any underlying cause (acute ischaemia, heart failure etc.). Sedation may be of benefit.

INAPPROPRIATE /INEFFECTIVE ICD FIRING

3.2.3.3 A ring magnet placed over the ICD box will stop the ICD from firing and may be considered in conscious patients where the ICD shocks are ineffective and the patient is distressed. In ICDs that have a dual pacing function, the magnet will also usually change the pacing function to deliver a paced output of 50 beats/min.

Methodology

For details of the methodology used in the development of this guideline refer to guideline webpage.

[Further related reading includes references 63, 75]

SECTION

3 Medical
Undifferentiated
Complaints

KEY POINTS

Implantable Cardioverter Defibrillators (ICDs)

- **ICDs deliver therapy with bradycardia pacing, ATP and shocks for VT not responding to ATP or VF.**
- **ECG records, especially at the time that shocks are given, can be vital in subsequent patient management. A recording should always be made if circumstances allow.**
- **Cardiac arrest should be managed according to normal guidelines.**
- **Avoid placing the defibrillator electrode over or within 8 cm of the ICD box.**
- **A discharging ICD is unlikely to harm a rescuer touching the patient or performing CPR.**
- **An inappropriately discharging ICD can be temporarily disabled by placing a ring magnet directly over the ICD box.**

The Implantable Cardioverter Defibrillator

Table 3.66 – ASSESSMENT and MANAGEMENT of:

Patients Fitted with an ICD

ASSESSMENT	MANAGEMENT
If the patient is in cardiac arrest: ● Assess the patient ● Monitor the ECG	● Perform basic life support in accordance with current BLS guidelines. ● Standard airway management techniques. ● IV access (if required) should be used.
Assess rhythm: Shockable rhythm is present (VF or pulseless VT)	● **BUT** the ICD is not detecting it, perform external defibrillation and other resuscitation procedures according to current resuscitation guidelines. ● If the ICD is delivering therapy (whether by anti-tachycardia pacing or shocks) but is failing to convert the arrhythmia, then external defibrillation should be provided, as per current guidelines.
Non-shockable rhythm	● Manage the patient according to current guidelines. If the rhythm is converted to a shockable one, assess the response of the ICD, as in 3.1.2 above, performing external defibrillation as required.
If a shockable rhythm is converted to one associated with effective cardiac output (whether by the ICD or by external defibrillation):	● Manage the patient as usual and arrange further treatment and assessment.
If the patient is not in cardiac arrest:	● Determine whether an arrhythmia is present.
If no arrhythmia is present:	If therapy from the ICD has been effective, the patient is in sinus rhythm or is paced: ● Monitor the patient. ● Administer oxygen and aim for a saturation of 94–98% (**refer to oxygen guideline**). ● Arrange further assessment to investigate possibility of new myocardial infarction (MI), heart failure, other acute illness or drug toxicity/electrolyte imbalance etc. An ICD may deliver inappropriate shocks (i.e. in the absence of arrhythmia) if there are problems with sensing the cardiac rhythm or problems with the leads: ● Record the rhythm (while ICD shocks are delivered, if possible). ● Disable the ICD with a magnet. ● Monitor the patient. ● Arrange further assessment with help from the ICD centre. Provide supportive treatment as required.
If an arrhythmia is present:	If an arrhythmia is present and shocks are being delivered: ● Record the arrhythmia (while ICD shocks are delivered, if possible) on the ECG. ● Determine the nature of the arrhythmia. ● Transport rapidly to hospital in all cases.
If the rhythm is **supraventricular** i.e. sinus tachycardia, atrial flutter, atrial fibrillation, junctional tachycardia, etc:	If the patient is haemodynamically stable, and the patient is continuing to receive shocks, disable the ICD with a magnet: ● Consider possible causes, treat appropriately. Arrange further assessment in hospital.
If the rhythm is **ventricular tachycardia**:	● Pulseless VT should be treated as cardiac arrest (3.1.2 above).
	If the patient is haemodynamically stable: ● Monitor the patient. ● Convey to the emergency department. **If the patient is haemodynamically unstable, and ICD shocks are ineffective, treat as per VT guideline.** ● An ICD will not deliver anti-tachycardia pacing (ATP) or shocks if the rate of the VT is below the programmed detection rate of the device. Conventional management may be undertaken according to the patient's haemodynamic status. ● For recurring VT with appropriate shocks, manage any underlying cause (acute ischaemia, heart failure etc.). Sedation may be of benefit.

The Implantable Cardioverter Defibrillator

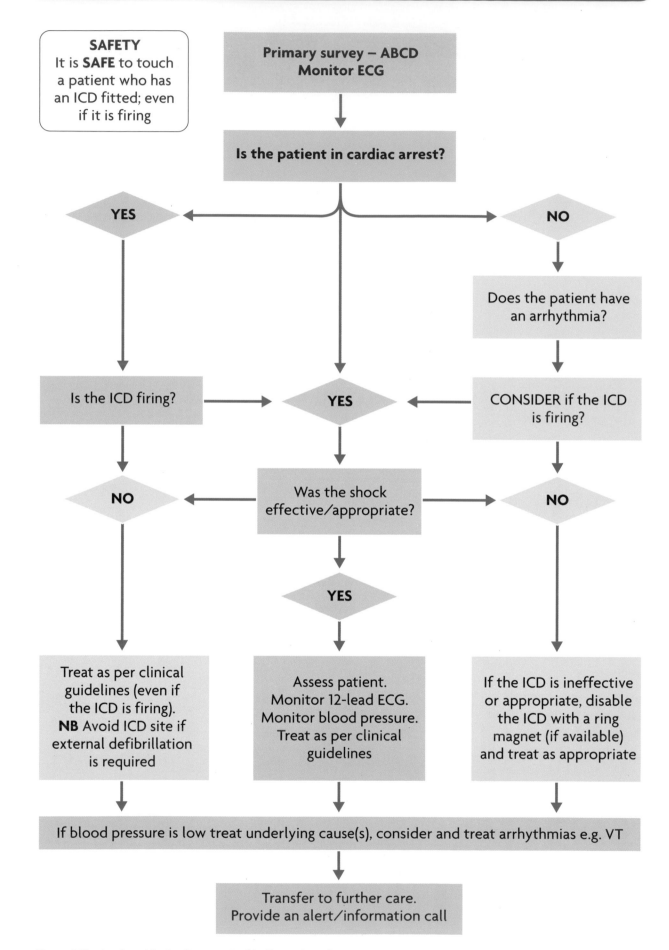

Primary survey – ABCD
Monitor ECG

Is the patient in cardiac arrest?

YES

NO

Does the patient have an arrhythmia?

Is the ICD firing?

YES

CONSIDER if the ICD is firing?

NO

Was the shock effective/appropriate?

NO

YES

Treat as per clinical guidelines (even if the ICD is firing).
NB Avoid ICD site if external defibrillation is required

Assess patient.
Monitor 12-lead ECG.
Monitor blood pressure.
Treat as per clinical guidelines

If the ICD is ineffective or appropriate, disable the ICD with a ring magnet (if available) and treat as appropriate

If blood pressure is low treat underlying cause(s), consider and treat arrhythmias e.g. VT

Transfer to further care.
Provide an alert/information call

Figure 3.15 – Implantable Cardioverter Defibrillator algorithm.

Overdose and Poisoning (Adults) [60, 128, 457–468]

1. Introduction

Overdose and poisoning is a common cause of calls to the ambulance service accounting for 140,000 hospital admissions per year.

Poisoning

Exposure by ingestion, inhalation, absorption, or injection of a quantity of a substance(s) that may result in mortality or morbidity.

Common agents include:

- **Household products** e.g. washing powders, washing-up liquids and fabric cleaning liquid/tablets, bleaches, hand gels and screen-washes, anti-freeze and de-icers, silica gel, batteries, petroleum distillates, white spirit (e.g. paints and varnishes), descalers and glues.

- **Pharmaceutical/recreational substances** e.g. paracetamol, ibuprofen, co-codamol, aspirin, tricyclic antidepressants, selective serotonin uptake inhibitors (SSRIs), beta-blockers (Atenolol, Sotalol, Propranolol), calcium channel blockers, benzodiazepines, opioids, iron tablets, cocaine and amphetamines.

- **Plants/fungi** e.g. foxglove, laburnum, laurel, iris, castor oil plant, amanita palloides, etc. For further details of poisonous plants refer to: http://www.toxbase.org.

- **Alcohol**

- **Chemicals** – for details **refer to the Chemical, Biological, Radiological and Nuclear and Explosive Incidents guideline**.

- **Cosmetics**.

Poisoning may be:
i.   accidental.
ii. intentional (self-harm), mal-intent.
iii. non-accidental.

Overdose

Exposure by ingestion, inhalation, absorption, or injection of a quantity of a substance(s) above the prescribed/known safe dose; this is a common form of poisoning, involving prescribed or illicit drugs and may be accidental or intentional.

2. Incidence

- It is difficult to estimate the exact number of overdose and poisoning incidents, as not all cases are reported. In 2009/2010 there were 49,690 poison-related queries involving patients to the National Poisons Information Service.

3. Severity and Outcome

- There are a number of factors which will affect severity and outcome following exposure, including, age, toxicity of the agent, quantity and route of exposure.

- In 2009 there were 2,878 deaths related to drug overdose and poisoning in England and Wales. In patients that self-harm death commonly results from airway obstruction and respiratory arrest, secondary to a decreased level of consciousness.

4. Pathophysiology

- The mode of action following exposure will depend primarily on the nature of the toxin. For details of the actions of specific toxins refer to: http://www.toxbase.org.

5. Assessment and Management

For the assessment and management of overdose and poisoning in adults refer to Tables 3.67–3.68.

Duty of Care

It is not uncommon to find patients who have or claim to have taken an overdose and subsequently refuse treatment or admission to hospital. An assessment of their mental health state, capacity and suicide risk should be made; **refer to mental disorder guideline**. If, despite reasonable persuasion, the patient refuses treatment, it is not acceptable to leave them in a potentially dangerous situation without any access to care.

Assistance may be obtained from the medical/clinical director or a member of the clinical team and a judgement must be made to seek appropriate advice. Attendance of the police or local mental health team may be required, particularly if the patient is at risk.

KEY POINTS

Overdose and Poisoning

- **Establish: the event, drug or substance involved, the quantity, mode of poisoning, any alcohol consumed.**
- **NEVER induce vomiting.**
- **If caustics and petroleum products have been swallowed, dilute by giving milk at the scene wherever possible.**
- **If the patient vomits, retain a sample, if possible, for inspection at hospital.**
- **Bring the substance or substances and any containers for inspection at hospital.**

Table 3.67 – ASSESSMENT and MANAGEMENT

Overdose and Poisoning

⚠ **Safety First – DO NOT put yourself in danger – carry out a dynamic risk assessment and undertake measures to preserve your own safety.**

⚠ **Avoid mouth-to-mouth ventilation in cases of poisoning or suspected poisoning by cyanide, hydrogen sulphide, corrosives and organophosphates.**

ASSESSMENT	MANAGEMENT

● Assess ABCD	● If any of the following **TIME CRITICAL** features present:
	  – major **ABCD** problems
	  – cardiac and respiratory arrest – **refer to resuscitation guidelines**
	  – decreased level of consciousness – NB Most poisons that impair conscious also depress respiration – **refer to decreased level of consciousness guideline**
	  – respiratory depression – **refer to airway management guideline**
	  – arrhythmias – **refer to cardiac rhythm disturbance guideline**
	  – hypotension <70 mmHg
	  – cardiac arrhythmias – **refer cardiac rhythm disturbance guideline**
	  – convulsions – **refer convulsion guideline**
	  – hypothermia – **refer hypothermia guideline**
	  – swallowed crack cocaine, then:
	● Start correcting **A** and **B** problems.
	● Undertake a **TIME CRITICAL** transfer to nearest appropriate receiving hospital.
	● Continue patient management en-route.
	● Provide an alert message/information call.

● Substance	● Ascertain what has been ingested/inhaled/absorbed/injected – ask relatives, friends, work colleagues etc.
	● Examine the patient for odours, needle marks, pupil abnormalities, signs of corrosion in the mouth.
	● Estimate the quantity.
	● Ascertain what if any treatment has been given.
	● Document the time the incident occurred.
	● **NEVER** induce vomiting.
	● In the case of caustic, irritant e.g. petroleum ingestion encourage the patient to drink a glass of milk, if possible.
	Refer to Table 3.68 for specific management of certain toxins.
	
	● If possible take and hand over to staff at the hospital:
	  – a sample of the ingested substance
	  – all substances found at the scene whether thought to be involved or not
	  – medicine containers
	  – a sample of vomit – if present. Important information can be gained by contacting toxbase and local protocols should be followed to enable this

● Chemical exposure	● If exposure to chemical substance is suspected – **refer to CBRNE guideline chemical section for management**.
● Oxygen	● If indicated, administer high levels of supplemental oxygen, particularly in cases of carbon monoxide poisoning or inhalation of irritant gases – refer to oxygen guideline. ● Apply pulse oximeter. NB Supplemental oxygen maybe harmful in cases of paraquat poisoning.
● ECG	● Undertake a 12-lead ECG.

● Respirations	● Monitor respirations.
	● Consider assisted ventilation if:
	  – SpO$_2$ is <90% after administering high levels of oxygen for 30–60 seconds
	  – respiratory rate is **<half normal rate OR >three times normal rate**
	  – expansion is inadequate.

● Naloxone	● Opiates such as morphine, heroin etc., can cause respiratory depression; in cases of respiratory depression consider naloxone; monitor vital signs closely. NB Repeated doses of naloxone may be required – refer to naloxone guideline.
● Blood pressure	● Hypotension is common in severe cases of poisoning. ● Monitor blood pressure.
● Intravascular fluid	● In cases of drug induced symptomatic hypotension consider intravascular fluid – refer to intravascular fluid guideline.

Table 3.67 – ASSESSMENT and MANAGEMENT of:

Overdose and Poisoning *continued*

ASSESSMENT	MANAGEMENT
● Blood glucose level	● Measure blood glucose level – especially in cases of alcohol intoxication which is a common cause of hypoglycaemia (<4.0 mmol/l). ● Correct blood glucose level – **refer to glycaemic emergencies**; other relevant guidance: **glucose 10% guideline** and **glucagon guideline** – NB Glucagon is often not effective in overdoses.
● Thermoregulation	● Hypo- or hyperthermia can occur.
● Mental health assessment	● In cases of self-harm assess the patient's emotional and mental state – undertake a rapid mental health assessment – **refer mental disorder guideline**. Do not delay treatment, but if possible, document the following information: ● The patient's home environment. ● The patient's social and family support network. ● The patient's emotional state and level of distress. ● The events leading to the incident.

● Transfer to further care	● All patients suffering an opioid overdose whether or not they have responded to naloxone – the effects of respiratory depression opioid overdose can last 4–5 hours.
	● All patients who have suffered an intentional overdose even if the substance is found to be harmless. If the patient does not require emergency treatment, but a mental health assessment may be required, consider alternative pathways e.g. specialist mental health service – as per local protocol. NB This decision should take into account the patient's preferences, and the views of the receiving service.
	
	Patients may be considered to be left at home if:
	  – The substance is verified by **TOXBASE/NPIS** as harmless.
	  – The incident is/was accidental.
	  – There is a responsible adult present.
	  – Advice given to seek medical advice if the patient becomes unwell.
	  – Arrangements have been made to inform the health visitor or GP.
	In patients that refuse transfer:
	● Assess mental capacity.
	● Explain the potential consequences of not receiving treatment.
	● If necessary seek medical advice – follow local protocol.

Table 3.68 – SPECIFIC SUBSTANCES MANAGEMENT

SUBSTANCE	MANAGEMENT ⚠ Safety First – DO NOT put yourself in danger – carry out a dynamic risk assessment and undertake measures to preserve your own safety.
Alcohol (ethanol) Nausea, vomiting, slurred speech, confusion, convulsions, unconsciousness.	• Alcohol intoxication is a common emergency, especially in young adults, and is usually a transient problem. • Alcohol intoxication may cause alcohol-induced hypoglycaemia – Correct blood glucose level – **refer to glycaemic emergencies**; other relevant guidance: **glucose 10% guideline** and **glucagon guideline** – NB Glucagon is often not effective in overdoses. • When alcohol is combined with drugs in overdose, it may pose a major problem. For example, when combined with opiate drugs or sedatives, it will further decrease the level of consciousness with increased risk of respiratory depression and aspiration of vomit. In combination with paracetamol increases the risk of liver damage.
Carbon monoxide poisoning Disorientation, decreased consciousness. Unconscious. NB The supposed cherry red skin colouration in carbon monoxide poisoning is rarely seen in practice.	• Any patient found unconscious or disorientated in an enclosed space, for example, a patient involved in a fire in a confined space, where ventilation is impaired, or where a heating boiler may be defective, **MUST** be considered at risk of carbon monoxide poisoning. • The immediate requirement is to remove the patient from the source (and administer continuous supplemental oxygen in as high a concentration as possible) as carbon monoxide is displaced from haemoglobin more rapidly the higher the concentration of oxygen. SpO_2 monitoring is of no value in carbon monoxide poisoning at it measures bound haemoglobin and makes no distinction as to whether it is bound to O_2 or CO.
Orthochlorobenzalmalononitrile (CS gas) Lacrimation, burning sensation of the eyes, excessive mucus production, nausea and vomiting.	• Carried by police forces for defensive purposes. CS spray irritates the eyes (tear gas) and respiratory tract. **AVOID** contact with the gas, which is given off from patient's clothing. Where possible keep two metres from the patient and give them self-care instructions. Symptoms normally resolve in 15 minutes but may however potentiate or exacerbate existing respiratory conditions. If symptoms are present: • Remove patient to a well ventilated area. • Remove contaminated clothes and place in a sealed bag. • If possible remove contact lenses. • **DO NOT** irrigate the eyes as CS gas particles may dissolve and exacerbate irritation. If irrigation is required use copious amounts of saline. • Patients with severe respiratory problems should be immediately transported to hospital – **refer to airway management guideline**. • Ensure good ventilation of the vehicle during transfer to further care.
Calcium-channel blockers Diltiazem, Verapamil, Dihydrocodeine	• Overdose may lead to cardiac arrest. • Overdose of sustained release preparations can lead to delayed on-set symptoms including: arrhythmias, shock, sudden cardiac collapse. • Refer to Table 3.67 for management. NB Immediate release preparations: problems are unlikely to develop in patients that are asymptomatic, and where the time interval is greater than 6 hours from time of ingestion.
Iron Nausea, vomiting blood, diarrhoea, black stools, metallic taste, convulsions, dizziness, flushed appearance, decreased level of consciousness, non-cardiac pulmonary oedema.	• Iron pills are regularly used by large numbers of the population including pregnant mothers. • They may cause extensive damage to the liver and gut and these patients will require hospital assessment and treatment. NB Charcoal is contra-indicated as it may interfere with subsequent treatment.
Cyanide Confusion, drowsiness, decreased level consciousness, dizziness, headache, convulsions.	• Cyanide poisoning requires specific treatment – seek medical advice. Provide full supportive therapy and transfer immediately to hospital. Provide an alert/information call. • Cyanide poisoning can occur in patients exposed to smoke in a confined space e.g. house fire. Remove the patient from the source and administer continuous supplemental oxygen in as high a concentration as possible. If there are signs of decreased levels of consciousness transfer immediately to hospital. Provide an alert/information call. • In cases of CBRNE the HART/SORT team will provide guidance. • Poisoning may occur in certain industrial settings. Cyanide 'kits' should be available and the kit should be taken to hospital with the patient. The patient requires injection with Dicobalt edetate **refer to dicobalt edetate guideline** or administration of the currently unlicensed drug hydroxycobalamin.

Table 3.68 – SPECIFIC SUBSTANCES MANAGEMENT *continued*

SUBSTANCE	MANAGEMENT
Paracetamol and Paracetamol containing compound drugs Nausea, vomiting, malaise, right upper quadrant abdominal pain, jaundice, confusion, drowsiness – unconsciousness may develop later. NB Presentation may be unreliable.	● There are a number of analgesic drugs that contain paracetamol and a combination of codeine or dextropropoxyphene. This, in overdose, creates two serious dangers: 1. Codeine and dextropropoxyphene are both derived from opioid drugs. This in overdose, especially if alcohol is involved, may well produce profound respiratory depression. This can be reversed with naloxone (refer to naloxone guideline). 2. Even modest doses of paracetamol may induce severe liver and kidney damage. It frequently takes 24–48 hours for the effects of paracetamol damage to become apparent and urgent blood paracetamol levels are required to assess the patient's level of risk.
Tricyclic Antidepressants Central nervous system, excitability, confusion, blurred vision, dry mouth, fever, pupil dilation, convulsions, decreased level of consciousness, arrhythmias, hypotension, tachycardia, respiratory depression.	● Poisoning with tricyclic antidepressants may cause impaired consciousness, profound hypotension and cardiac arrhythmias. They are a common treatment for patients who are already depressed. Newer antidepressants such as fluoxetine (Prozac) and paroxetine (Seroxat) have different effects. ● Establish ECG monitoring. ● Arrhythmias – **refer to cardiac rhythm disturbance guideline**. ● The likelihood of convulsions is high – **refer to convulsion guidelines**. ● Monitor closely as the patient's physical condition can rapidly change.
Beta-blockers Bradycardia, hypotension, dizziness, confusion.	● Bradycardia – **refer to cardiac rhythm disturbance guideline**.
Opioids Drowsiness, nausea, vomiting, small pupils, respiratory depression, cyanosis, decreased level of consciousness, convulsions, non-cardiac pulmonary oedema.	● Ensure the airway is open – administer supplemental oxygen – refer to oxygen guideline. ● Profound respiratory depression can be reversed with naloxone – refer to naloxone guideline.
Benzodiazepines – Diazepam, lorazepam, temazepam, flurazepam, loprazolam, etc. Decreased level of consciousness, respiratory depression, hypotension.	Refer to Table 3.67 for management.

Table 3.69

Illegal Drugs

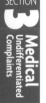

DRUG	

Cocaine
(powder cocaine, crack cocaine).
	DESCRIPTION
	Cocaine is a powerfully reinforcing psycho stimulant. Crack is made from cocaine in a process called freebasing.
	
	OUTWARD SIGNS
	Hyperexcitability, agitated, irritable and sometimes violent behaviour. Sweating. Dilated pupils.
	
	EFFECTS
	Induces a sense of exhilaration, euphoria, excitement, and reduced hunger in the user primarily by blocking the re-uptake of the neurotransmitter dopamine in the midbrain, blocks noradrenaline uptake causing vasoconstriction and hypertension.
	NB: Crack cocaine is pure and therefore more potent than street cocaine; it enters the bloodstream quicker and in higher concentrations. Because it is smoked, crack cocaine's effects are felt more quickly and they are more intense than those of powder cocaine. However, the effects of smoked crack are shorter lived than the effects of snorted powder cocaine. It is highly addictive even after only one use.
	
	ADMINISTRATION
	Cocaine comes in the form of a powder that is almost always 'cut' or mixed with other substances. It can be: snorted through the nose, rubbed into the gums, smoked or injected. Crack comes in the form of solid rocks, chips, or chunks that are smoked.
	
	SIDE EFFECTS
	The symptoms of a cocaine overdose are intense and generally short lived. Although uncommon, people do die from cocaine or crack overdose, particularly following ingestion (often associated with swallowing 'evidence').
	All forms of cocaine/crack use can cause coronary artery spasm, myocardial infarction and accelerated ischaemic heart disease, even in young people.
	Various doses of cocaine can also produce other neurological and behavioural effects such as:
	● dizziness.
	● headache.
	● movement problems.
	● anxiety.
	● insomnia.
	● depression.
	● hallucinations.
	The unwanted effects of cocaine or crack overdose may include some or all of the following:
	● tremors.
	● dangerous or fatal rise in body temperature.
	● delirium.
	● myocardial infarction.
	● cardiac arrest.
	● seizures including status epilepticus.
	● stroke.
	● kidney failure.
	
	TREATMENT
	● Transfer patient rapidly to hospital.
	● Administer supplemental oxygen – **refer to oxygen guideline**.
	● Consider assisted ventilation at a rate of 12–20 breaths per minute if:
	  – SpO$_2$ is <90% on high concentration O$_2$
	  – respiratory rate is <10 or >30
	  – expansion is inadequate.
	● Undertake a 12-lead ECG – if the patient has a 12-lead ECG suggestive of myocardial infarction and a history of recent cocaine use then administer nitrates but do not administer thrombolysis.
	● Administer aspirin and GTN if the patient complains of chest pain – **refer to aspirin and GTN guidelines**.
	● **Chest pain** – administer diazepam if the patient has severe chest pain – **refer to diazepam guideline**.
	● **Convulsions** – **refer to convulsions guideline**.
	● **Hypertension** – if systolic BP> 220 and diastolic BP > 140 mmHg in the absence of longstanding hypertension – seek medical advice.
	● **Hyperthermia** – administer paracetamol and cooling if the body temperature is elevated – **refer to paracetamol guideline**.
	NB Swallowed crack cocaine represents a severe medical emergency and needs **URGENT** transportation to hospital **EVEN IF ASYMPTOMATIC**.

Table 3.69

Illegal Drugs *continued*

DRUG
Amphetamines

(Amphetamines,
Methamphetamine)
Commonly known as:
Bennies, Billy Whizz,
Black Beauties,
Bumblebees,
Clear Rocks, Co-pilots,
Crank, Croke, Glass,
LA Turnarounds,
Mollies, Oranges,
Pep Pills, Pink
Champagne, Pink Speed,
Bombs, Rippers, Rocks,
Speed, Splash, Sulph,
Sulphate, Wake Ups,
Whizz.

DESCRIPTION
Amphetamines developed in the 1930s and have been medically prescribed in the past for diet control and as a stimulant.

OUTWARD SIGNS
Mood swings, extreme hunger, sleeplessness, and hyperactivity.

EFFECTS
Increases energy levels, confidence and sociability.

ADMINISTRATION
They can be: swallowed, sniffed or rarely injected.
Onset approximately 30 minutes. Lasts for several hours.
Used with other drugs or alcohol, the effects are magnified.

SIDE EFFECTS
Cardiovascular
- Tachycardia can lead to heart failure even in healthy individuals (**refer to cardiac rhythm disturbance guideline**).
- Hypertension can produce pinpoint haemorrhages in skin, especially on the face and even lead to stroke.

Central nervous system:
- 'High' feelings, panic, paranoia can produce mental illness picture in long-term use, poor sleep, hyperpyrexia.

Gastrointestinal
- Liver failure.

TREATMENT
- **Vital signs** – monitor pulse, blood pressure, cardiac rhythm.
- **Agitation** – seek medical advice for consideration of diazepam use for severe agitation.
- **Convulsions** – **refer to convulsions guideline**.
- **Cardiac rhythm disturbance** – narrow-complex tachycardia with cardiac output is best left untreated.
- **Hypertension** – if systolic BP >220 and diastolic BP >140 mmHg in the absence of longstanding hypertension – seek medical advice.
- **Hypotension** – correct hypotension by raising the foot of the trolley and/or the administration of intravascular fluid – **refer to intravascular fluid guideline**.
- **Hyperthermia** – rapid transfer to hospital; cooling measures may be undertaken en-route – **refer to heat related illness guideline**.

DRUG
Opiates

(Heroin, Diamorphine,
Methadone-
Amidone, Dolophine,
Methadose).

DESCRIPTION
Methadone is a synthetic opiate commonly used in the treatment of heroin addiction.

OUTWARD SIGNS
Withdrawal symptoms:
Sweating, shivering, muscle cramps, lacrimation.

EFFECTS
Reduce physical and psychological pain – relieving anxiety. The effects of Methadone are less intense.

ADMINISTRATION
Injected, snorted or smoked.

SIDE EFFECTS
Cardiovascular system
Damage to veins and lungs. Infection. It is likely that babies are born underweight.

TREATMENT
Refer to Table 3.68 for management.

Table 3.69

Illegal Drugs *continued*

DRUG

3-4 methylene dioxymethamphetamine (MDMA) – Ecstacy 'E'

Commonly known as: doves, apples, strawberries, and diamonds.

DESCRIPTION

MDMA is a psychoactive drug with hallucinogenic effects.

OUTWARD SIGNS

Sweating, dilated pupils and elevated mood.

EFFECTS

Feeling warm, energetic, and friendly, rising to a state of euphoria.

ADMINISTRATION

'E' tablets may be white embossed 'headache' sized pills, or coloured capsules.
They take 40 minutes to work, lasting for 2–6 hours.
'E' may not be addictive but is illegal.

SIDE EFFECTS

Cardiovascular system
- Tachycardia (**refer to cardiac rhythm disturbance guideline**).
- Capillary rupture, causing red marking on the face in particular.

Central nervous system
- Some patients develop hyperpyrexia which can be life-threatening. These patients need urgent transfer to hospital for specialist care. Cooling measures (**refer to heat relatred illness guideline**) may be helpful but should not delay transfer to further care.
- Depression, panic and anxiety may also occur.

Liver and kidney damage
- Liver failure and severe kidney damage may occur.

Other:
- Cystitis and heavy periods may occur in females who use 'E'.

TREATMENT
- Administer diazepam to control anxiety and agitation – refer to diazepam guideline.
- Treat convulsions with diazepam – refer to diazepam guideline.
- If the systolic BP > 220 and diastolic > 140 mmHg in the absence of longstanding hypertension give diazepam – refer to diazepam guideline.
- Correct hypotension by raising the foot of the bed and/or by giving fluids as per medical emergencies – refer to intravascular fluid guideline.
- Cooling measures (**refer to heat related illness guideline**) may be helpful but should not delay transfer to further care.
- Depression, panic and anxiety may also occur.

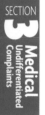

SECTION
3 Medical
Undifferentiated
Complaints

Table 3.69

Illegal Drugs *continued*

DRUG
Lysergic Acid

diethylamide (LSD)
or 'acid'.

DESCRIPTION
It is a 'mind altering drug' that alters the brain's perception of things.
It was discovered in 1943, and was used in the 1960s as a 'recreational drug'.

OUTWARD SIGNS
Agitated, unusual behaviour, clear mental disturbance.
The patient may appear distant and display anxious behaviour.
DO NOT interfere unduly as the 'trip' will self-limit, and communication is easier then. Keep the patient safe, and remember other drugs and alcohol will aggravate the effects of LSD.

EFFECTS
The alterations in perception may be pleasant or 'nightmarish', or a mix of both, and last for some 12 hours.

ADMINISTRATION
Produced on patches of blotting paper, called tabs or trips, often with printed motifs including cartoon characters.

Once swallowed they take 30–60 minutes to work. The trip will last up to 12 hours and cannot be stopped.

LSD is not addictive but is illegal.

SIDE EFFECTS
Central nervous system
- Visual hallucinations (distortion and delusions), which can cause dangerous behaviour.
- Nightmarish perceptions 'bad trips' may last for 12 hours.
- Nausea and vomiting.
- Personality changes and psychiatric illness.
- Nightmarish flashbacks that can last for years after drug use stops.
- Delusions – false sensations or visions – may affect taste, hearing and vision.
- Can trigger hidden mental illness in individuals.
- Permanent eye damage can occur.

TREATMENT
- Usually self-limiting but sedate if necessary with intravenous diazepam – refer to diazepam guideline.

Medical
Undifferentiated Complaints
SECTION 3

Pulmonary Embolism [60, 469-477]

1. Introduction

- Pulmonary embolism (PE) is an obstruction of the pulmonary vessels which usually presents as one of four types:

  1. **Multiple small pulmonary emboli** – characterised by progressive breathlessness more commonly identified at outpatients appointments than through emergency presentation due to the long-standing nature of the problem.

  2. **Segmental emboli with pulmonary infarction** – may present with pleuritic pain and/or haemoptysis but with little or no cardiovascular compromise.

  3. **Major pulmonary emboli obstruction of the larger branches of the pulmonary tree** – may present with sudden onset of shortness of breath with transient rise in pulse and/or fall in blood pressure. Often a precursor to a massive PE.

  4. **Massive pulmonary emboli** – often presenting with loss of consciousness, tachypnoea and intense jugular vein distension, and may prove immediately or rapidly (within 1 hour) fatal or unresponsive to cardiopulmonary resuscitation.

- Pulmonary embolism can present with a wide range of symptoms (Table 3.70). The presence of predisposing factors (Table 3.71) increases the index of suspicion of PE; which increases with the number of predisposing factors present. However, in approximately 30% of cases, the presentation is idiopathic.

- Symptoms such as dyspnoea, tachypnoea or chest pain have been found in >90% of cases of patients with PE; with pleuritic chest pain is one of the most frequent symptoms of presentation.

- There may be sudden collapse with no obvious physical signs, other than cardiorespiratory arrest.

- Lesser risk factors include air, coach or other travel leading to periods of immobility, especially whilst sitting, oral oestrogen (some contraceptive pills) and central venous catheterisation.

- Over 70% of patients who suffer PE have peripheral vein thrombosis and vigilance is therefore of great importance – it may not initially appear logical to check the legs of a patient with chest pain but can be of great diagnostic value in such cases.

Table 3.70 – SIGNS AND SYMPTOMS OF PE

Symptoms
- Dyspnoea.
- Pleuritic chest pain.
- Substernal chest pain.
- Apprehension.
- Cough.
- Haemoptysis.
- Syncope.

Signs
- Respiratory rate >20 breaths per minute.
- Pulse rate >100 beats per minute.
- SpO_2 <92%.
- Signs of Deep Vein Thrombosis (DVT).

Table 3.71 – PREDISPOSING FACTORS

Factor

Surgery especially recent
- Abdominal.
- Pelvic.
- Hip or knee surgery.
- Post operative intensive care.

Obstetrics
- Pregnancy.

Cardiac
- Recent acute myocardial infarction.

Limb problems
- Recent lower limb fractures.
- Varicose veins.
- Lower limb problems secondary to stroke or spinal cord injury.

Malignancy
- Abdominal and/or pelvic in particular advanced metastatic disease.
- Concurrent chemotherapy.

Other
- Risk increases with age.
- 65% ≥60 years of age.
- Previous proven PE/DVT.
- Immobility.
- Thrombotic disorder.
- Neurological disease with extremity paresis.
- Thrombophilia.
- Hormone replacement therapy and oral contraception.
- Prolonged bed rest >3 days.
- Other recent trauma.

2. Incidence

- Pulmonary embolism is a relatively common cardiovascular condition affecting approximately 21 per 10,000 per annum.

3. Severity and Outcome

- Pulmonary embolism can be life-threatening leading to death in approximately 7–11% of cases, however, treatment is effective if given early.

- Patients with a previous episode/s of PE are three times more likely to experience a recurrence.

4. Pathophysiology

- The development of a pulmonary embolism occurs when a blood clot (thrombus), comprising red cells, platelets, and fibrin, forms in a vein, subsequently dislodges (embolism) and travels in the circulation. This is known as venous thromboembolism (VTE). If the embolism is small it may be filtered in the pulmonary capillary bed, but if the embolism is large it may occlude pulmonary blood vessels. The development of a VTE can also lead to deep vein thrombosis.

- The haemodynamic problems occur when >30–50% of the pulmonary arterial bed is occluded.

Pulmonary Embolism

- The probability of a PE can be assessed using a clinical predication tool such as the Wells Criteria (Table 3.72). However a low probability cannot rule out PE.

5. Assessment and Management

For the assessment and management of pulmonary embolism refer to Table 3.73 and Figure 3.16.

Methodology

For details of the methodology used in the update of this guideline refer to the guideline webpage.

Table 3.72 – WELLS CRITERIA FOR PE

Item	Score
Clinical signs and symptoms of DVT (leg swelling and pain with palpation of the deep veins).	3
An alternative diagnosis is less likely than pulmonary embolism.	3
Pulse rate >100 beats per minute.	1.5
Immobilisation or surgery in the previous 4 weeks.	1.5
Previous DVT/pulmonary embolism.	1.5
Haemoptysis.	1
Malignancy (treatment ongoing or within previous 6 months or palliative).	1

Clinical Probability of PE		Total
high	>6 points	
moderate	2–6 points	
low	<2 points	

KEY POINTS

Pulmonary Embolism

- **Common symptoms of PE are dyspnoea, tachypnoea, pleuritic pain, apprehension, tachycardia, cough, haemoptysis, leg pain/clinical DVT.**
- **Risk factors may be identifiable from the history.**
- **Ensure ABCD assessment and apply a pulse oximetry monitor early.**
- **Patients may present with unilateral swelling of the lower limbs; they may also be warm and red.**
- **Apply oxygen and if in respiratory distress, transfer to further care as a medical emergency.**

Table 3.73 – ASSESSMENT and MANAGEMENT of:

Pulmonary Embolism

ASSESSMENT	MANAGEMENT

● Assess ABCD	● If any of the following **TIME CRITICAL** features are present:
	  – major **ABCD** problems
	  – extreme breathing difficulty
	  – cyanosis
	  – severe hypoxia (SpO$_2$) <90% – unresponsive to oxygen.
	● Start correcting **A** and **B** problems.
	● Undertake a **TIME CRITICAL** transfer to nearest appropriate hospital.
	● Provide an alert/information call.
	● Continue patient management en-route.

● Specifically assess	● Respiratory rate and effort. ● Signs and symptoms combined with predisposing factors. ● Lower limbs for unilateral swelling; may also be warm and red. ● Calf tenderness/pain may be present – extensive leg clots may also lead to femoral tenderness. ● Differential diagnoses include pleurisy, pneumothorax or cardiac chest pain. ● High index of suspicion.
● Position	● Position patient for comfort and ease of respiration – often sitting forwards – but be aware of potential hypotension.
● Cardiorespiratory arrest	● Be prepared for cardiorespiratory arrest – **refer to appropriate resuscitation guideline**.
● Oxygen	● Administer supplemental oxygen aim for a target saturation within the range of 94–98%.
● ECG	● Undertake a 12-lead ECG – be aware that the classic S1 Q3 T3 12-lead ECG presentation is often **NOT** present, even during massive PE. The commonest finding is a sinus tachycardia.
● Ventilation	● Consider assisted ventilation if indicated – **refer to airway and breathing management guideline**.
● Fluid	● If fluid therapy indicated – refer to intravascular fluid therapy guideline.
● Transfer to further care	● Transfer rapidly to nearest appropriate hospital. ● Provide an alert/information call. ● Continue patient management en-route.
	ADDITIONAL INFORMATION Whilst there is no specific prehospital treatment available, there may be a window of opportunity to manage massive PE before the patient progresses to cardiac arrest. Other in-hospital treatments may be effective including: haemodynamic and respiratory support, thrombolysis, surgical pulmonary embolectomy, percutaneous catheter embolectomy and fragmentation, and anticoagulation.

SECTION

3

Medical
Undifferentiated
Complaints

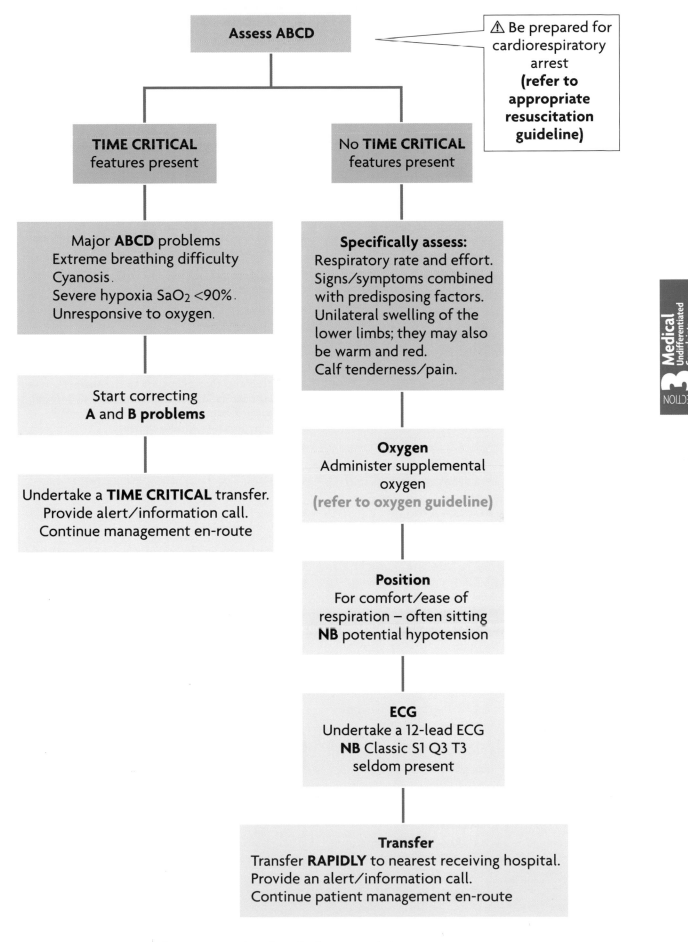

Assess ABCD

⚠ Be prepared for cardiorespiratory arrest **(refer to appropriate resuscitation guideline)**

TIME CRITICAL features present

No **TIME CRITICAL** features present

Major **ABCD** problems
Extreme breathing difficulty
Cyanosis.
Severe hypoxia SaO₂ <90%.
Unresponsive to oxygen.

Specifically assess:
Respiratory rate and effort.
Signs/symptoms combined with predisposing factors.
Unilateral swelling of the lower limbs; they may also be warm and red.
Calf tenderness/pain.

Start correcting
A and B problems

Oxygen
Administer supplemental oxygen
(refer to oxygen guideline)

Undertake a **TIME CRITICAL** transfer.
Provide alert/information call.
Continue management en-route

Position
For comfort/ease of respiration – often sitting
NB potential hypotension

ECG
Undertake a 12-lead ECG
NB Classic S1 Q3 T3 seldom present

Transfer
Transfer **RAPIDLY** to nearest receiving hospital.
Provide an alert/information call.
Continue patient management en-route

Figure 3.16 – Assessment and management algorithm of pulmonary embolism.

Medical
Undifferentiated Complaints
SECTION 3

1. Introduction

Stroke is a major health problem in the UK. Improving care for patients with stroke and transient ischaemic attack (TIA) is a key national priority, with a National Stroke Strategy published by the Department of Health in 2007, and guidelines published by the National Institute for Health and Clinical Excellence (NICE) in 2008.

1.1 Acute Stroke

Acute stroke is a medical emergency. For patients with thrombotic stroke, treatment with thrombolytic therapy (alteplase) is highly time-dependent. In order to determine suitability for treatment, patients must undergo a brain scan; therefore, patients need to be transferred to an appropriate hospital as rapidly as possible once the diagnosis is suspected.

It is important to remember that thrombolysis is not the only management proven to benefit stroke patients. Admission to a stroke unit for early specialist care is known to be life saving and to reduce disability, even if thrombolysis is not indicated.

Symptoms of stroke include:

- Numbness.
- Weakness or paralysis.
- Slurred speech.
- Blurred vision.
- Confusion.
- Severe headache.

The most sensitive features associated with diagnosing stroke in the prehospital setting are facial weakness, arm and leg weakness, and speech disturbance.

1.2 Transient ischaemic attack (TIA)

Transient ischaemic attack (TIA) is defined as stroke symptoms and signs that resolve within 24 hours. However, there are limitations to these definitions. For example, they do not include retinal symptoms (sudden onset of monocular visual loss), which should be considered as part of the definition of stroke and TIA. The symptoms of a TIA usually resolve within minutes or a few hours at most, and **anyone with continuing neurological signs when first assessed should be assumed to have had a stroke**.

The risk of a patient with TIA developing a stroke is high and symptoms should always be taken seriously.

2. Incidence

Each year in England, approximately 110,000 people have a first or recurrent stroke and a further 20,000 people have a TIA.

3. Severity and Outcome

Stroke accounted for over 56,000 deaths in England and Wales in 1999, which represents 11% of all deaths. Most people survive a first stroke, but often have significant morbidity.

More than 900,000 people in England are living with the effects of stroke, with half of these being dependent on other people for help with everyday activities.

4. Pathophysiology

The majority (70%) of strokes are ischaemic. Distinguishing between ischaemic and haemorrhagic strokes is not currently feasible in the prehospital setting.

A TIA occurs when blood supply to part of the brain is temporarily interrupted.

5. Assessment

Assess ABCDs

- Record time of onset if known.
- May have airway and breathing problems (**refer to dyspnoea guideline**).
- Level of consciousness may vary (**refer to decreased level of consciousness guideline**).

Evaluate if the patient has any TIME CRITICAL features – these may include:

- Any major ABC problem.
- Positive FAST test.
- Altered level of consciousness.

If any of these features are present, start **correcting A and B problems then transport to the nearest suitable receiving hospital. Local arrangements will determine pathways (e.g. bypassing a local hospital for the nearest 'hyperacute' stroke centre).**

- Provide an alert/information call stating clearly that the patient is FAST positive/suspected acute stroke.
- En-route – continue patient **management** (see below).
- Assess blood glucose level, as **hypoglycaemia** may mimic a stroke.

Suspected acute stroke – a positive FAST test should be considered a TIME CRITICAL condition. Perform a brief secondary survey but do not allow this to delay transport to hospital:

- Assess blood pressure to provide a baseline for hospital assessment.
- Assess Glasgow Coma Scale (GCS) on **unaffected side** – eye and motor assessments may be more readily assessed if speech is badly affected.

Table 3.74 – FAST TEST

Facial Weakness	Ask the patient to smile or show teeth. Look for NEW lack of symmetry.
Arm Weakness	Ask the patient to lift their arms together and hold for 5 seconds. Does one arm drift or fall down? The arm with motor weakness will drift downwards compared to the unaffected limb.
Speech	Ask the patient to repeat a phrase. Assess for slurring or difficulty with the words or sentence.

These components make up the **FAST** (face, arms, speech test) assessment that should be carried out on **ALL** patients with suspected stroke/TIA. A deficit in any one of the three domains is sufficient for the patient to be identified as 'FAST positive'.

6. Management

Follow **medical emergencies guideline**, remembering to: Start correcting:

- **A**irway
- **B**reathing
- **C**irculation
- **D**isability (mini neurological examination)
- oxygen therapy is not recommended unless the patient is hypoxic (**refer to oxygen guideline**).

Consider recording 12-lead ECG en-route to hospital, but **do not delay transport** for this test.

Intravenous access is not essential unless the patient requires specific interventions, and may delay transport to hospital.

Specifically:

- Check blood glucose level (**refer to glycaemic emergencies guideline**).
- Conscious patients should be conveyed in the semi recumbent position.
- Patients should be nil by mouth.

NOTE: Local policies will determine whether paramedics should use a risk score for suspected TIA patients and/or administer aspirin. In the absence of clear evidence relating to prehospital use of these interventions, JRCALC are unable to make a firm recommendation.

7. Referral Pathway

This will depend on locally commissioning arrangements. For example, bypassing local hospitals for a 'hyperacute' centre may require patients in some networks to meet specific criteria based on a positive FAST test and onset within the preceding 2 hours, so that the patient is within the 'time window' for thrombolysis.

Where possible, a witness should be asked to accompany the patient to hospital.

It is important to remember that thrombolysis is not the only management proven to benefit stroke patients. Admission to a stroke unit for early specialist care is known to be life saving and to reduce disability, even if thrombolysis is not indicated.

8. Audit Information

Ambulance services are required to monitor the use of the FAST test in patients with suspected stroke, and agree local pathways for patients with suspected stroke. Careful documentation of your assessment and management, including accurate timings are essential to improving care for this group of patients.

KEY POINTS

Stroke/Transient Ischaemic Attack (TIA)

- **Time is of the essence in suspected acute stroke.**
- **Record time of onset if known.**
- **Stroke is common and may be due to either cerebral infarction or haemorrhage.**
- **The most sensitive features associated with diagnosing stroke in the prehospital setting are facial weakness, arm and leg weakness, and speech disturbance – the FAST test.**
- **FAST test should be carried out on ALL patients with suspected stroke/TIA.**
- **Patients with TIA may be at high risk of stroke and should be taken to hospital for further assessment.**

Further Reading

Comprehensive, high-quality information on stroke is available at:

- NHS Evidence – stroke
  http://www.evidence.nhs.uk/topic/stroke
- NHS Stroke Improvement
  http://www.improvement.nhs.uk/stroke
- The Stroke Association
  http://www.stroke.org.uk

SECTION 3 Medical Undifferentiated Complaints

1. Introduction

- The incidence of allergic reactions continues to rise.
- The symptoms range from mild to life-threatening and include:
  - urticaria (hives)
  - angio-oedema (swelling of the face, eyelids, lips and tongue)
  - itching
  - dyspnoea
  - wheeze
  - stridor
  - hypoxia
  - abdominal pain
  - diarrhoea/vomiting
  - hypotension
  - pulmonary and/or cardiovascular compromise.
- The most common triggers are food, drugs and venom (Table 3.75) but in 30% of cases the trigger is unknown.
- Injected allergens commonly result in cardiovascular compromise, with hypotension and shock predominating.
- Inhaled and ingested allergens typically cause rashes, vomiting, facial swelling, upper airway swelling and wheeze.
- Slow release drugs prolong absorption and exposure to the allergen.

Table 3.75 – COMMON TRIGGERS OF ALLERGIC REACTIONS

1 – Foods
Nuts (e.g. peanuts, walnut, almond, brazil, and hazel), pulses, sesame seeds, milk, eggs, fish/shellfish.

2 – Venom – insect sting/bites
Insect stings and bites (e.g. wasp and bees).
NB Bees may leave a venom sac which should be scraped off (not squeezed).

3 – Drugs
Antibiotics (e.g. penicillin, cephalosporin, amphotericin, ciprofloxacin, and vancomycin), non-steroidal anti-inflammatory drugs, angiotensin converting enzyme inhibitor, gelatins, protamine, vitamin K, etoposide, acetazolamide, pethidine, local anaesthetic, diamorphine, streptokinase and other drugs.

4 – Other causes
e.g. Latex[a], hair dye.

[a] Latex allergy has implications for equipment use.

2. Incidence

- It is estimated that allergic reactions affect 40% of children, with anaphylaxis estimated to affect up to 2% of the population.

3. Severity and Outcome

- The severity of symptoms varies from a localised urticaria to life-threatening pulmonary and/or cardiovascular compromise, i.e. anaphylaxis.

- Generally, the longer it takes for anaphylactic symptoms to develop, the less severe the overall reaction.
- The mortality associated with anaphylaxis is estimated to be <1%. Death occurs quickly (venom: 10–15 minutes; food: 30–35 minutes) after contact with the trigger usually as a result of respiratory arrest from airway obstruction.

4. Assessment and Management

- For the assessment and management of anaphylaxis and allergic reactions refer to Figure 3.17.

Children with previous episodes:

- may wear 'Medic Alert' bracelets/necklets
- they or their carers may carry an adrenaline pen e.g. Anapen®, EpiPen®.

Methodology

For details of the methodology used in the development of this guideline refer to the guideline webpage.

KEY POINTS

Anaphylaxis/Allergic Reactions in Children

- **Remove from trigger if possible.**
- **Anaphylaxis can occur despite a long history of previously safe exposure to a potential trigger.**
- **Consider anaphylaxis in the presence of acute cutaneous symptoms and/or airway or cardiovascular compromise.**
- **Anaphylaxis may be rapid, slow or biphasic.**
- **Adrenaline is key in managing anaphylaxis.**
- **In anaphylactic reactions, the benefits of adminstering adrenaline, even at an inappropriate dose, far exceeds the risk of giving no medication at all.**

Quickly remove from trigger
if possible e.g. environmental,
infusion etc.
DO NOT delay definitive treatment
if removing trigger not feasible

Assess ABCDE
If TIME CRITICAL features present –
correct A and B and transfer to nearest
suitable receiving hospital.
Provide an alert/information call

Consider mild/moderate allergic reaction if:
Onset of illness is minutes to hours
AND
Cutaneous findings e.g. urticaria
and/or angio-oedema

Consider chlorphenamine
(refer to chlorphenamine guideline)

Consider anaphylaxis if:
Sudden onset and rapid progression
Airway and/or **Breathing** problems (e.g.
dyspnoea, hoarseness, stridor, wheeze,
throat or chest tightness) and/or
Circulation (e.g. hypotension, syncope,
pronounced tachycardia) and/or **Skin** (e.g.
erythema, urticaria, mucosal changes) problems

Administer high levels of
supplementary oxygen
(refer to oxygen guideline)

Administer adrenaline 1 in 1000 IM only
(refer to adrenaline guideline)

If haemodynamically compromised
(refer to fluid therapy guideline)

Consider chlorphenamine
(refer to chlorphenamine guideline)

Consider administering hydrocortisone
(refer to hydrocortisone guideline)

Consider nebulised salbutamol
for bronchospasm
(refer to salbutomol guideline)

Monitor and re-assess ABC
Monitor ECG, PEFR (If possible),
BP and pulse oximetry en-route

3 Medical
Undifferentiated
Complaints

SECTION

Figure 3.17 – Allergic reactions including anaphylaxis algorithm.

Asthma (Children) [60, 249, 314, 324, 485]

1. Introduction

- Asthma is one of the commonest medical conditions requiring hospitalisation.
- The severity of asthma may be subdivided into mild/moderate, severe, or life-threatening (Table 3.77).
- There may be a history of increasing wheeze or breathlessness (often worse at night or early in the morning). Respiratory infections, allergy and physical exertion are common triggers.

  Known asthmatics will be on regular medication, taking inhalers ('preventers' and/or 'relievers') and sometimes oral medications such as Montelukast (Singulair®) and theophyllines.

- Some children with asthma will have an individualised treatment plan with detailed information regarding their daily symptom control as well as what to do in an acute exacerbation.
- **Inhaled foreign body:** Consider an inhaled foreign body in a child experiencing their first wheezy episode, especially if there is a history of playing with small toys and the wheeze was of sudden onset and is unilateral. These children must be transferred for medical assessment. If they are unwell during transport, bronchodilators may provide some clinical benefit.

2. Severity and Outcome

- Children with previous hospital admissions (particularly intensive care admissions), are at risk of future severe or life-threatening episodes (and even death) — so this information should be sought.

Table 3.76 – RISK FACTORS FOR SEVERE ASTHMA

Risk Factors
- Previous severe or life-threatening episodes.
- Previous hospital admission for asthma especially if in the last year.
- Previous admission requiring intensive care.
- Back to back nebulisers with poor or no response.

3. Pathophysiology

- Asthma causes chronic bronchial inflammation which results in narrowing of the airways. In acute attacks, airway irritation causes smooth muscle contraction producing respiratory compromise. Inflammatory processes also cause i) excessive sputum production and ii) swelling of the bronchial mucosal which blocks the small airways.
- Inspiration (an active process) generates sufficient pressures to overcome airway narrowing but during expiration (a passive process) relaxation of the respiratory muscles causes airway narrowing, producing the characteristic wheeze.
- Various medications are used to treat asthma. In children, these are typically delivered using a spacer device e.g. a Volumatic® or Aerochamber®. Some children may also have a home nebuliser.

4. Assessment

Following an ABC assessment, the severity of the asthma attack should be established (refer to Table 3.77 and Asthma Algorithm – Figure 3.18).

Table 3.77 – FEATURES OF SEVERITY

Life-threatening asthma
- Silent chest.
- SpO$_2$ <92%.
- Cyanosis PEFR <33% best or predicted.
- Poor respiratory effort.
- Hypotension.
- Exhaustion.
- Confusion.

Acute severe asthma
- Can't complete sentences in one breath or too breathless to talk or feed.
- SpO$_2$ <92%.
- PEFR 33-50% best or predicted.
- Pulse:
  - >140 in children aged 2–5 years
  - >125 in children aged >5 years.
- Respiration:
  - >40 breaths/min aged 2–5 years
  - >30 breaths/min aged >5 years.

Moderate asthma exacerbation
- Able to talk in sentences.
- SpO$_2$ ≥92%.
- PEFR ≥50% best or predicted.
- Heart rate:
  - ≤140/min in children aged 2–5 years
  - ≤125/min in children >5 years.
- Respiratory rate:
  - ≤40/min in children aged 2–5 years
  - ≤30/min in children >5 years.

5. Management

The Asthma Algorithm (Figure 3.18) describes the management of mild/moderate, severe and life-threatening asthma.

Always ask if the child has an individualised asthma treatment plan and follow it, unless clinical circumstances dictate otherwise.

For some children alternative care pathways will already have been created e.g. early referral to their GP. It is well recognised however that children with apparently minor symptoms can subsequently deteriorate and practitioners should therefore have a low threshold for onward referral (especially where an alternative pathway has not already been established).

Peak Expiratory Flow Rate Measurements (PEFR): PEFR should be attempted where possible in children before and after nebulised therapy in mild to moderate asthma. However, care should be taken in severe life-threatening attacks as it could exacerbate the attack and the patient may deteriorate. Predicted PEFR are listed in Table 3.78.

Table 3.78 – PEAK EXPIRATORY FLOW CHART

Height (m)	Height (ft)	Predicted EU PEFR (L/min)
0.85	2'9"	87
0.90	2'11"	95
0.95	3'1"	104
1.00	3'3"	115
1.05	3'5"	127
1.10	3'7"	141
1.15	3'9"	157
1.20	3'11"	174
1.25	4'1"	192
1.30	4'3"	212
1.35	4'5"	233
1.40	4'7"	254
1.45	4'9"	276
1.50	4'11"	299
1.55	5'1"	323
1.60	5'3"	346
1.65	5'5"	370
1.70	5'7"	393

KEY POINTS

Asthma (Children)

- Clinical assessment should determine the severity of the attack.
- Bronchodilators (e.g. Salbutamol) are the mainstay of treatment.
- High levels of oxygen may be required during an asthma attack.
- Mild/moderate attacks should be managed with inhaled bronchodilators via a spacer device.
- Nebulised treatments should be reserved for moderate/severe attacks where oxygen is required.
- In addition to β2 agonists, ipratropium is used in severe cases.

Methodology

For details of the methodology used in the development of this guideline refer to the guideline webpage.

Section 3 — Medical Undifferentiated Complaints

Asthma (Children)

Table 3.79 – ASSESSMENT and MANAGEMENT

Asthma

ASSESSMENT	MANAGEMENT

• Assess **ABCD**
 Specifically assess for the severity of the asthma attack (refer to Figure 3.18)
	• If any of the following **TIME CRITICAL** features present:
	   – major ABCD problems
	   – extreme difficulty in breathing or requirement for assisted ventilations
	   – exhaustion
	   – cyanosis
	   – Silent chest
	   – SPO_2 <92%
	   – PEF <33% best or predicted.
	 • Start correcting A and B problems.
	 • Undertake a **TIME CRITICAL** transfer to nearest receiving hospital.
	 • Continue patient management en-route.
	 • Provide an alert/information call.

• Mild/moderate asthma
   – Able to talk in sentences
   – SpO_2 >92%
   – PEFR >50% best or predicted
   – Pulse <140 in child ages 2–5
     <125 in child >5
   – Respiration <40 in child ages 2–5
   – <30 in child ages >5
	• Move to a calm quiet environment.
	 • Encourage use of own inhaler, using a spacer if available. Ensure correct technique is used (refer to Figure 3.18).
	 • If unresponsive:
	 administer high levels of supplementary oxygen
	 administer nebulised salbutamol (**refer to salbutamol guideline**).

• Severe asthma
   – Can't complete sentences in one breath or too breathless to talk or feed
   – SpO_2 <92%
   – PEFR 33–50% best or predicted
   – Pulse >140 in child aged 2–5 years
   – >125 in child >5 years
   – Respiration >40 in child ages 2–5 years
   >30 in child aged >5 years.
	• Administer high levels of supplementary oxygen.
	 • Administer nebulised salbutamol (**refer to salbutamol guideline**).
	 • If no improvement administer ipratropium bromide (**refer to ipratropium bromide guideline**).
	 • Administer steroids (**refer to relevant steroids guideline**).
	 • Continuous salbutamol nebulisation may be administered unless clinically significant side effects occur (**refer to salbutamol guideline**).

• Life-threatening asthma
   – Silent chest
   – SpO_2 <92%
   – Cyanosis
   – PEFR<33% best or predicted (exercise caution with PEFR in this patient group)
   – Poor respiratory effort
   – Hypotension
   – Exhaustion
   – Confusion
	• Continuous salbutamol nebulisation may be administered unless clinically significant side effects occur (**refer to salbutamol guideline**).
	 • Administer adrenaline 1 in 1000 IM only (**refer to adrenaline guideline**).
	 • Positive pressure ventilation using a nebulising T piece. Assess for bilateral tension pneumothorax.

• Transfer	• Transfer rapidly to nearest receiving hospital. • Provide an alert/information call. • Continue patient management en-route.
	• For cases of mild asthma that respond to treatment consider alternative care pathway where appropriate. • **Note:** exercise caution in known severe asthmatics.

Asthma (Children)

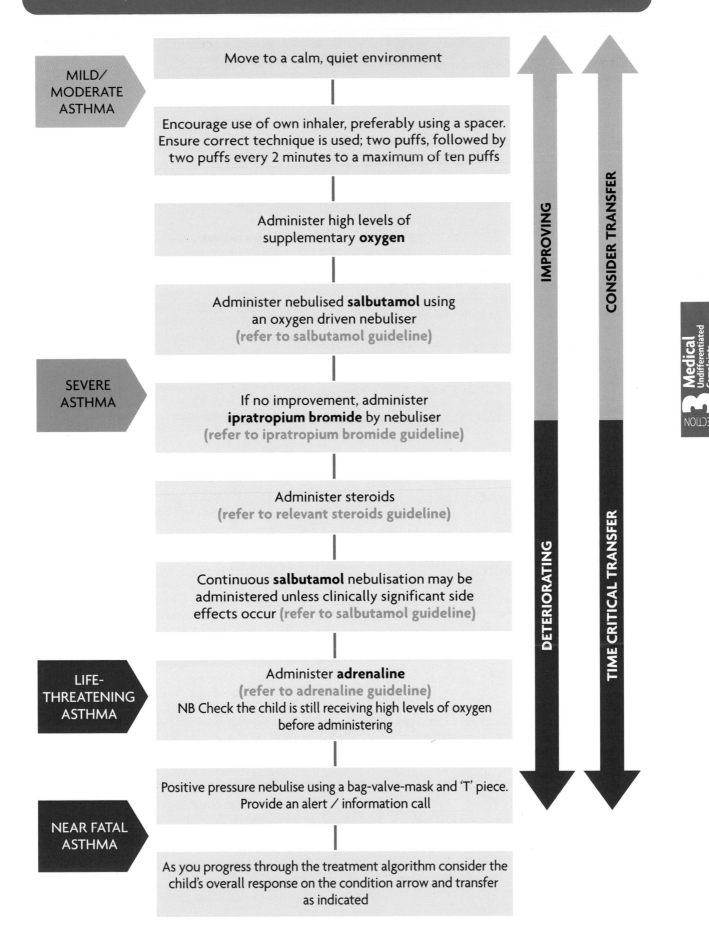

MILD/ MODERATE ASTHMA

Move to a calm, quiet environment

Encourage use of own inhaler, preferably using a spacer. Ensure correct technique is used; two puffs, followed by two puffs every 2 minutes to a maximum of ten puffs

Administer high levels of supplementary **oxygen**

Administer nebulised **salbutamol** using an oxygen driven nebuliser (refer to salbutamol guideline)

SEVERE ASTHMA

If no improvement, administer **ipratropium bromide** by nebuliser (refer to ipratropium bromide guideline)

Administer steroids (refer to relevant steroids guideline)

Continuous **salbutamol** nebulisation may be administered unless clinically significant side effects occur (refer to salbutamol guideline)

LIFE- THREATENING ASTHMA

Administer **adrenaline** (refer to adrenaline guideline) NB Check the child is still receiving high levels of oxygen before administering

Positive pressure nebulise using a bag-valve-mask and 'T' piece. Provide an alert / information call

NEAR FATAL ASTHMA

As you progress through the treatment algorithm consider the child's overall response on the condition arrow and transfer as indicated

IMPROVING

CONSIDER TRANSFER

DETERIORATING

TIME CRITICAL TRANSFER

Figure 3.18 – Asthma assessment and management algorithm.

1. Introduction

- A convulsion (seizure, fit) results from abnormal electrical activity in the brain and can occur for many reasons (including meningitis).

- A convulsion can be triggered by fever, but a febrile convulsion is not epilepsy. A child having convulsions that are not triggered by fever requires further investigation.

- Convulsions may also be triggered by other brain insults e.g. infection, head injury, hypoxia, hypoglycaemia or electrolyte imbalance. Occasionally, hypertension can cause convulsions (even in children).

- Cardiac arrest can occasionally present with a convulsion.

- Generalised convulsive (tonic–clonic) status epilepticus (CSE) is defined as a generalised convulsion lasting at least 30 minutes or a series of convulsions that occur so frequently over 30 minutes that the patient does not recover consciousness between them.

2. Incidence

- 1 in 200 people have active epilepsy. It is twice as common in children as in adults. It may be related to another underlying condition.

- Febrile convulsions are seen in children aged from 6 months to 6 years. They occur in 1 in 20 children and most occur in the first 3 years of life; 1 in 20 febrile convulsions presents with CSE.

- Convulsive status epilepticus is the commonest medical neurological emergency in children. It is seen in 1 in 20 epileptic children.

3. Severity and Outcome

Febrile convulsions

- Simple febrile convulsions have an excellent prognosis – two-thirds of children will only have one isolated febrile convulsion. The remaining third have further febrile convulsions during subsequent febrile illnesses.

Convulsive Status Epilepticus

- CSE carries a significant morbidity and mortality, which may be related to seizure duration. Neurological consequences include epilepsy, motor deficits, learning difficulties, and behavioural problems. Adverse neurological outcomes are more common in younger children.

- CSE can be fatal, but mortality in children (about 4%) is lower than that in adults.

4. Assessment (refer to Table 3.80)

- Correct hypoxia and seek the underlying cause for the seizure.

- Record the events that immediately preceded the convulsion including a history of head injury and any serious past medical history.

- If the child is febrile, this should be documented and if the child was unwell prior to the event, this should also be noted.

- When managing a child with a febrile convulsion, it is crucially important to identify the underlying infection to explain the cause for the child's fever (although this must not delay immediate treatment priorities or hospital transport).

- In any child with a convulsion (especially if they have fever), it is important to look for the typical rash of meningococcal septicaemia (and treat appropriately if present). Also remember that meningitis can present with seizures so signs of this should be sought if the child is well enough (i.e. stopped fitting).

5. Management
(refer to Table 3.80 and Figures 3.19–3.20)

- This follows ABCD priorities, treating the convulsion once ABC issues have been addressed. Often it is safest to treat the convulsion before moving the child, although if the seizure has not rapidly stopped after one dose of anticonvulsant the child will have to be moved while still convulsing.

- Manage airway, breathing and circulation as usual (also remember to measure the blood glucose as hypoglycaemia can cause seizures). An oropharyngeal airway may be helpful to maintain airway patency (alternatively, if the jaw is clenched a nasopharyngeal tube may prove useful). Administer oxygen and treat shock in the usual way. Oxygen saturation monitoring should be applied.

- Most convulsions stop spontaneously.

- Anticonvulsant treatment should be given if the convulsion lasts more than 5 minutes as it may not stop spontaneously. Prehospital treatments include **buccal midazolam** and **diazepam** (both rectal and intravenous preparations). Buccal midazolam is twice as effective as rectal diazepam but often diazepam is the only drug available. Both drugs can cause respiratory depression. (Do not delay the first dose of anticonvulsant medication whilst attempting venous access i.e. use either the buccal or rectal routes.)

- If the convulsion is continuing 10 minutes after the first dose of medication has been given, a second dose of anticonvulsant can be given. This must, however, be given intravenously or intra-osseously – not buccally or rectally e.g. **diazepam** IV/IO (**refer to diazepam guideline**). (This also applies if a carer has given the first dose of medication before the clinician arrives on scene.)

Hospital transfer

- Pre-alert the hospital if the child continues to fit during the journey or appears to be otherwise very unwell.

- All children having their first convulsion should be transported to hospital for investigation.

- If the child has fully recovered and is a known epileptic it may not be necessary to take them to hospital.

Methodology

For details of the methodology used in the development of this guideline refer to the guideline webpage.

SECTION **3** Medical Undifferentiated Complaints

Convulsions (Children)

Table 3.80 – ASSESSMENT and MANAGEMENT

Convulsions

ASSESSMENT	MANAGEMENT
Assess ABCD	Treat problems as they are found. ● The airway must be cleared. – Oropharyngeal or nasopharyngeal airways may be helpful. ● Administer high levels of supplemental oxygen – refer to oxygen guideline. ● Check blood glucose level and manage if low – **refer to hypoglycaemia emergencies in children guideline**. ● Monitor vital signs. ● Manage the convulsion (see below).

Medication	Administer anticonvulsants – first choice anticonvulsants are usually given buccally or rectally:
	   i. the fit lasts ≥5 minutes or
	   ii. the child fails to fully regain consciousness between fits.
	 Ask whether the child:
	 ● Has their own supply of medication:
	   – if the child has their own buccal midazolam this should be used
	   – ask whether they have already received a dose.
	 ● Has already received an anticonvulsant (either rectal **diazepam** or **carer administered buccal midazolam**). If the convulsion is continuing 10 minutes after this first anticonvulsant, one dose of an intravenous or intra-osseous anticonvulsant may be given e.g. **diazepam** IV/IO (refer to diazepam guideline)*.
	 ● Has their own supply of anticonvulsant medication – if not, and they have not yet received an anticonvulsant, give rectal diazepam (refer to diazepam guideline)*.
	 ● Has a convulsion that persists 10 minutes after the administration of the first anticonvulsant (buccal midazolan or rectal **diazepam**). If so, a second anticonvulsant can be given but this must be given intravenously or intra-osseously e.g. **diazepam** IV/IO (refer to diazepam guideline)*.
	 ● If it is not possible to gain vascular access for the second dose of medication, **no** further drug treatment should be used, **even if this means that the child continues to fit** i.e. do not give a second dose of buccal or rectal medication.
	 *Be ready to support ventilation as respiratory depression may occur.

Other care	● Record the child's temperature. ● If transporting to hospital, ongoing assessments of ABCDs and continuous ECG and oxygen saturation monitoring should be undertaken, continuing **oxygen** therapy as needed. ● If meningococcal septicaemia is diagnosed, treat with **benzylpenicillin** en-route to hospital (refer to benzylpenicillin guideline). ● Paracetamol may be given for fever (refer to paracetamol guideline). ● A febrile child should wear light clothing only.

Transfer to further care	The following should all be transported to hospital:
	 ● Any child who is still convulsing or in status epilepticus must be transferred to further care as soon as possible – undertake a **TIME CRITICAL** transfer, provide an alert/information call.
	 ● Any child with suspected meningococcal septicaemia or meningitis – undertake a **TIME CRITICAL** transfer, provide an alert/information call.
	 ● All first febrile convulsions even if the child has recovered.
	 ● All children with seizures who have required more than one dose of anticonvulsant.
	 ● Any child younger than 1 year old who has had a seizure (even if totally recovered).
	 ● Any child who has not fully recovered from their seizure.
	 The following children may not require transport to hospital:
	 ● Children who have a febrile convulsion:
	   – which is **not their first** and
	   – **where the carer is happy for the child not to be transported** and
	   – **who have completely recovered**
	   may be left at home, providing that urgent review by the general practitioner (GP) or out of hours (OOH) GP is arranged to establish the cause of the fever. If this cannot be arranged by the attending crew, the child must be transported to hospital.
	 ● Children who have recovered from a convulsion and **who are known to have epilepsy and have not required more than one dose of medication need not be transported** if they are otherwise well.

Follow-up	The GP or OOH service (depending on time of day) must be informed of any child left at home following a convulsion.

3 Medical Undifferentiated Complaints   SECTION

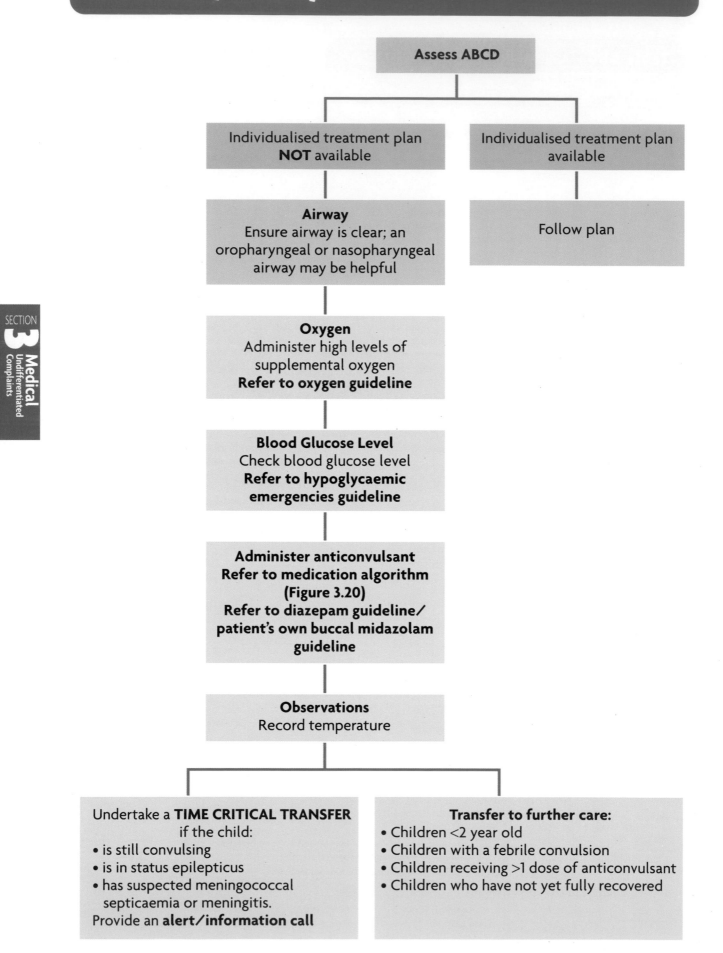

Assess ABCD

Individualised treatment plan NOT available

Individualised treatment plan available

Airway
Ensure airway is clear; an oropharyngeal or nasopharyngeal airway may be helpful

Follow plan

Oxygen
Administer high levels of supplemental oxygen
Refer to oxygen guideline

Blood Glucose Level
Check blood glucose level
Refer to hypoglycaemic emergencies guideline

Administer anticonvulsant
Refer to medication algorithm (Figure 3.20)
Refer to diazepam guideline/ patient's own buccal midazolam guideline

Observations
Record temperature

Undertake a **TIME CRITICAL TRANSFER** if the child:
• is still convulsing
• is in status epilepticus
• has suspected meningococcal septicaemia or meningitis.
Provide an **alert/information call**

Transfer to further care:
• Children <2 year old
• Children with a febrile convulsion
• Children receiving >1 dose of anticonvulsant
• Children who have not yet fully recovered

Figure 3.19 – Assessment and management algorithm of convulsions in children.

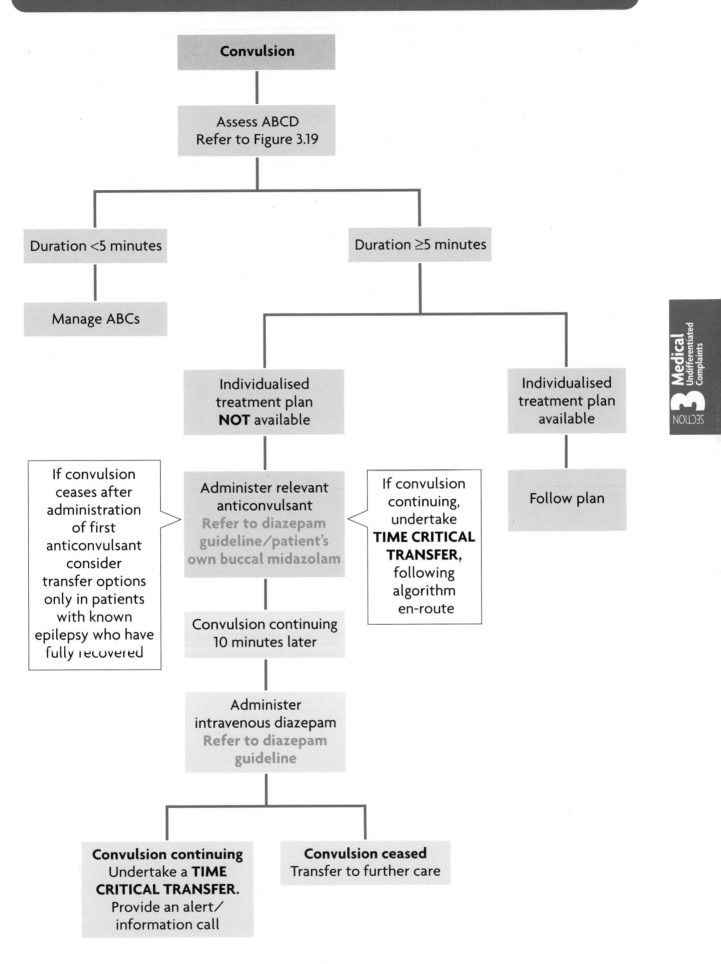

Figure 3.20 – Medication algorithm for convulsions in children.

Section 3 **Medical** Undifferentiated Complaints

KEY POINTS

Convulsions (Children)

- Most convulsions usually stop spontaneously.
- Febrile convulsions are the commonest cause for a childhood seizure and occur between the ages of 6 months and 6 years.
- A convulsion lasting more than 5 minutes should be treated with anticonvulsants.
- First choice anticonvulsants are usually given buccally or rectally.
- The second anticonvulsant should always be given intravenously e.g. diazepam.
- A child should not receive more than two doses of prehospital anticonvulsant.
- Always seek an underlying cause for the convulsion.
- All first convulsions must be transported to hospital.
- If a cause for a febrile convulsion cannot be found, the child must be taken to hospital.

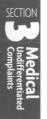

SECTION **3** Medical Undifferentiated Complaints

Childhood Gastroenteritis [77, 103, 149, 491–493]

1. Introduction

- Every year 10% of the UK's under-5s will have an episode of infective gastroenteritis.
- Characteristically they present with sudden onset of diarrhoea (with or without vomiting), which usually resolves without any specific treatment.
- When severe, dehydration can occur, which can be life-threatening. Younger children are most at risk of dehydration.

2. Severity and Outcome

In children with gastroenteritis:

i.   vomiting usually lasts 1–2 days, and stops within 3 days.

ii. diarrhoea usually lasts 5–7 days, and stops within 2 weeks.

3. Pathophysiology

Escherichia coli 0157:H7 infection

- *E. coli* 0157:H7 is a bacterium found in the intestines of healthy cattle that can cause serious human infections especially in the young and the elderly.
- It often leads to bloody diarrhoea and occasionally kidney failure (referred to as haemolytic uraemic syndrome or HUS). Outbreaks have occurred following school farm visits or following consumption of undercooked, contaminated beef. (Beef burgers are notorious as the meat comes from many animals.)
- When *Escherichia coli* 0157:H7 infection is suspected (e.g. contact with a confirmed case), urgent specialist advice must be sought.

4. Assessment

- Gastroenteritis is diagnosed on clinical findings and should be suspected where there is a sudden change in stool consistency to loose or watery stools and/or a sudden onset of vomiting.

History: consider the diagnosis when the child has had:

- recent contact with someone with acute diarrhoea and/or vomiting
- exposure to a known source of enteric infection (farm visits, contaminated water or food – see *Escherichia coli* 0157 infection above)
- recent overseas travel.

Differential Diagnosis

Apart from gastroenteritis, alternative diagnoses must be considered when the following features are found and a more experienced paediatric assessment should be sought:

- Fever:
  – temp ≥38°C in child <3 months old
  – temp ≥39°C in child ≥3 months old.
- Shortness of breath or tachypnoea.
- Altered consciousness.
- Neck stiffness.
- Bulging fontanelle in infants.
- Non-blanching rash.
- Blood and/or mucus in stool.

- Bilious (green) vomit.
- Severe or localised abdominal pain.
- Abdominal distension or rebound tenderness.

Examination: Clinical assessment for dehydration and shock

- Establish whether the child:
  – appears unwell
  – has altered responsiveness, e.g. irritability, lethargy
  – has decreased urine output
  – has pale or mottled skin
  – has cold extremities.

  Use Table 3.81 to establish whether the child is clinically dehydrated or shocked.

Children most at risk of dehydration include:

- Infants of low birth weight (i.e. <2.5 kg).
- Children <1 year, especially those aged <6 months.
- >5 diarrhoeal stools in the previous 24 hours.
- >2 vomits in the previous 24 hours.
- Those who have not been offered/not been able to tolerate oral fluids.
- Breastfed infants who have stopped feeding.
- Malnourished children.

At the end of the clinical assessment three groups of children should have been identified:

1. Those that are **not dehydrated**.
2. Those that are **clinically dehydrated**.
3. Those that are **clinically shocked**, and their management is detailed below.

Stool samples are not normally required but should be obtained in certain situations:

- Diarrhoea ≥7 days.
- Recent overseas travel.
- Possible septicaemia.
- Blood/mucus in stool.
- Immunocompromise.
- Persisting diagnostic uncertainty.

Contact the GP or out-of-hours service where this is thought to be necessary.

5. Management

Most children with gastroenteritis can be managed at home with oral fluids although dehydrated children require NG or IV fluid replacement and those in shock may require urgent intravenous fluid resuscitation. Fluid losses can be replaced either via the oral route, via a nasogastric tube or intravenously:

a) Oral (and nasogastric) fluids:
    – oral rehydration salt solutions (ORS) are given orally or via a nasogastric (NG) tube.
    – they should be given as small, frequent volumes.
    – response to oral rehydration must be monitored by regular clinical assessment.
    – commercially available ORS solutions include Dioralyte, Dioralyte Relief, Electrolade and Rapolyte.

b) Intravenous interventions (IV):
- IV fluids are required when shock is suspected or confirmed and requires urgent hospital transfer.
- when intravenous access cannot be established, intra-osseous fluids may be required.

c) Other treatments:
- antibiotics, antidiarrhoeals and anti-emetics are not routinely used in the management of gastroenteritis.

Considering the three distinct groups of children identified by clinical assessment:

1. In those children **not clinically dehydrated:**
   - fluid intake should be actively encouraged (e.g. milk, water, squash) – under-5s need approximately 10 ml of fluid every 10 minutes.
   - in infants, breastfeeding and other milk feeds should be continued.
   - in older children, fruit juices and fizzy drinks must be stopped.
   - oral rehydration salt (ORS) solutions should be offered to those at increased risk of dehydration as supplemental fluids, although toddlers and small children frequently refuse ORS because of the taste!
   - if oral intake is insufficient or if the child is persistently vomiting, they should be transferred to secondary care for NG or IV fluid replacement. (Inpatient management often includes a trial of ORS or NG fluids prior to IV fluid replacement.)

2. Any child found to be **clinically dehydrated** must be taken to hospital (refer to red flag system, ⚑ see Table 3.81). They will need additional fluids to not just **maintain** their normal body water but also to replace their fluid losses.

3. **Clinically shocked** children require intravenous fluid resuscitation and urgent hospital transfer:
   - a rapid 20 ml/kg IV of infusion **sodium chloride 0.9%** may be given but should not delay hospital transfer.
   - clinical response to fluid boluses must be monitored.
   - if shock persists, this infusion should be repeated and other causes of shock considered – **refer to 0.9% sodium chloride guideline**.

Information and advice for parents and carers

Advise parents, carers and children that:
- good handwashing is essential to prevent the spread of gastroenteritis to themselves and other family members; use soap (liquid if possible) in warm, running water followed by careful drying.
- wash hands after going to the toilet (children) or changing nappies (parents/carers) and before preparing, serving or eating food.
- infected children should not share towels.
- children should not go to school or other childcare facility while they have diarrhoea or vomiting caused by gastroenteritis and must stay away for at least 48 hours after the last episode of diarrhoea or vomiting.
- children should not swim in swimming pools for 2 weeks after the last episode of diarrhoea.

6. Referral Pathway

Children with gastroenteritis that are not dehydrated or shocked can initially be managed at home; if their condition progresses seek an additional medical opinion (GP, OOH, Emergency Department, Paediatrician) (see 'Safety Netting' below).

Hospital transfer is required if:
- Oral intake is insufficient.
- The child is persistently vomiting.
- A child is found to be clinically dehydrated.
- A child is found to be clinically shocked (Emergency Transfer).
- A child requires intravenous therapy.
- Suspecting an alternative cause for the child's symptoms e.g. UTI, meningococcal disease.
- Additionally some children's social circumstances will dictate additional/continued involvement of healthcare professionals.

Give the following advice for non dehydrated children managed at home.

Nutritional considerations

During rehydration:
- Continue breastfeeding.
- Give full-strength milk straight away.
- Continue the child's usual solid food.
- Avoid fruit juices and fizzy drinks until the diarrhoea has stopped.
- Consider giving an extra 5 ml/kg of ORS solution after each large watery stool in children at increased risk of dehydration.
- If dehydration recurs after rehydration, restart oral rehydration therapy.

'Safety netting' should be provided for children who do not require referral, giving written information to parents and carers on how to:
- Recognise developing red flag symptoms (⚑ see Table 3.81), and get immediate help from an appropriate healthcare professional if red flag symptoms develop and
- (if necessary) make arrangements for follow-up at a specified time and place i.e. face-to-face assessment.

Consider dehydration risk factors when interpreting symptoms and signs (see Table 3.81).

Within the category of 'clinical dehydration' there is a spectrum of severity indicated by increasingly numerous and more pronounced symptoms and signs.

Within the category of 'clinical shock' one or more of the symptoms and/or signs listed would be expected to be present.

Dashes (–) indicate that these clinical features do not specifically indicate shock but may still be present. Symptoms and signs with red flags (⚑) may help to identify children at increased risk of progression to shock.

If uncertain, manage as if the child has those red flag symptoms and/or signs.

Childhood Gastroenteritis

Table 3.81

Symptoms and signs of clinical dehydration and shock

Increasing severity of dehydration →

Symptoms

No clinically detectable dehydration	Clinically dehydrated	Clinically shocked
Appears well	⚑ Appears to be unwell or deteriorating	–
Alert and responsive	⚑ Altered responsiveness (for example, irritable, lethargic)	Decreased level of consciousness
Normal urine output	Decreased urine output. Output often decreased in those with normal hydration as a compensatory mechanism. Unreliable in those in nappies with diarrhoea	–
Skin colour unchanged	Skin colour unchanged	Pale or mottled skin
Warm extremities	Warm extremities	Cold extremities

Signs

No clinically detectable dehydration	Clinically dehydrated	Clinically shocked
Alert and responsive	⚑ Altered responsiveness (for example, irritable, lethargic)	Decreased level of consciousness
Skin colour unchanged	Skin colour unchanged	Pale or mottled skin
Warm extremities	Warm extremities	Cold extremities
Eyes not sunken	⚑ Sunken eyes	–
Moist mucous membranes (except after a drink)	Dry mucous membranes (except for 'mouth breather')	–
Normal heart rate	⚑ Tachycardia	Tachycardia
Normal breathing pattern	⚑ Tachypnoea	Tachypnoea
Normal peripheral pulses	Normal peripheral pulses	Weak peripheral pulses
Normal capillary refill time	Normal capillary refill time	Prolonged capillary refill time
Normal skin turgor	⚑ Reduced skin turgor	–
Normal blood pressure	Normal blood pressure	Hypotension (decompensated shock)

NB Rectal examinations should never be performed in the prehospital assessment of the paediatric acute abdomen.

Methodology

For details of the methodology used in the development of these guidelines refer to the guideline webpage.

KEY POINTS

Gastroenteritis

- Gastroenteritis is common, frequently viral and usually self-limiting.
- When severe, shock and life-threatening dehydration can occur.
- Clinical assessment determines whether dehydration or shock is present (seek Red Flag (🚩) symptoms and signs).
- Non-dehydrated children can frequently be managed at home with oral fluids or ORS.
- Failed oral rehydration requires either NG or IV fluid replacement in secondary care.
- Shocked children need urgent hospital treatment.
- Early meningococcal disease is known to mimic gastroenteritis in small children. An urgent second opinion should be sought if meningococcal disease cannot be excluded.
- Provide a 'safety net,' with written information, for all children with gastroenteritis not transferred to hospital.
- If uncertain, seek advice from either the child's GP or an out-of-hours doctor.

1. Introduction

- A non-diabetic individual maintains their blood glucose level within a narrow range from 3.0 to 5.6 mmol per litre.

- This is achieved by a balance between glucose entering the blood stream (from the gastrointestinal tract or from the breakdown of stored energy sources) and glucose leaving the circulation through the action of insulin.

- This guideline is for the assessment and management of children with glycaemic emergencies <18 years.

Section 1 – Hypoglycaemia

- Hypoglycaemia is the term used to describe low blood glucose levels.

- A low blood glucose level is defined as <4.0 mmol/l in children with diabetes and <3.0 mmol/l in non-diabetic children, but the clinical features of hypoglycaemia may be present at higher levels.

- Clinical judgement is as important as a blood glucose reading.

- Correction of hypoglycaemia is a medical emergency.

- If left untreated, hypoglycaemia may lead to the patient suffering permanent brain damage and may even prove fatal.

- Hypoglycaemia occurs when glucose metabolism is disturbed – see Table 3.82 for risk factors.

- Any child whose level of consciousness is reduced, who is having a convulsion or who is seriously ill or traumatised should have hypoglycaemia excluded.

- Signs and symptoms can vary from child to child (Table 3.83).

Table 3.82 – RISK FACTORS FOR HYPOGLYCAEMIA

Medical – diabetic
- Insulin or other hypoglycaemic drug treatments.
- Tight glycaemic control.
- Previous history of severe hypoglycaemia.
- Undetected nocturnal hypoglycaemia.
- Preceding hypoglycaemia (< 3.5 mmol/L).
- Impaired awareness of hypoglycaemia.
- Increased exercise (relative to usual).
- Irregular lifestyle /supervision.
- Inadequate carbohydrate intake.
- Inadequate blood glucose monitoring.

Medical – non-diabetic
- Very sick or traumatised children.
- Metabolic illness.
- Endocrine illness (including Addisonian crisis).
- Ketotic hypoglycaemia of infancy.
- Sudden cessation of tube or IV feeding.
- Sudden cessation of peritoneal dialysis.
- Very young babies (especially preterm).
- Hypothermia (especially in very young babies).
- Drug ingestion e.g. oral hypoglycaemic drugs, beta-blockers, alcohol.

- Some children are able to detect early symptoms for themselves, but others may be too young, or deteriorate rapidly and without apparent warning.

- Abnormal neurological features may occur, for example, one-sided weakness, identical to a stroke.

- Symptoms may be masked due to medication or other injuries.

- The classical symptoms of hypoglycaemia may **NOT** be present and children may have a variety of unusual symptoms with low blood glucose.

- In **DIABETES MELLITUS** (DM) hypoglycaemia is due to a relative excess of exogenously administered insulin over available glucose.

Table 3.83 – SIGN AND SYMPTOMS

Autonomic
- Sweating.
- Palpitations.
- Shaking.
- Hunger.

General malaise
- Headache.
- Nausea.

Neurological
- Confusion.
- Drowsiness.
- Unusual behaviour.
- Speech difficulty.
- In-coordination.
- Aggression.
- Fitting.
- Unconsciousness.

2. Assessment and Management

For the assessment and management of hypoglycaemia refer to Table 3.84. The principles of assessment and management are essentially the same in diabetic and non-diabetic children and babies.

Section 2 – Hyperglycaemia

- Hyperglycaemia is the term used to describe high blood glucose levels.

- Symptoms include unusual thirst (polydipsia), passing large volumes of urine (polyuria) and tiredness and are usually of slow onset in comparison to those of hypoglycaemia.

- Children with diabetes mellitus are very likely to develop a raised blood glucose in response to infection and will have instructions as to how to deal with this – so called 'sick day rules'.

- Hyperglycaemia may also occur transiently in children who are severely physically stressed e.g. during a convulsion.

- It is important to distinguish a simple raised blood sugar from the condition of diabetic ketoacidosis which is much more serious (see below). A raised blood glucose is not a prehospital emergency unless diabetic ketoacidosis is present. (However, the underlying reason for the raised blood sugar may, of course, be an emergency in its own right.)

Glycaemic Emergencies (Children)

Table 3 .84 – ASSESSMENT and MANAGEMENT

Hypoglycaemia in Children

SECTION **3** Medical Undifferentiated Complaints

ASSESSMENT	MANAGEMENT
● Undertake ABCD assessment. ● Measure blood glucose level.[b]	● Start correcting ABC problems (**refer to medical emergencies in children**). ● Measure and record blood glucose level (pre-treatment).
SEVERE: patient unconscious (GCS ≤8), convulsing, very aggressive	● Keep nil by mouth, increased risk of choking/aspiration. ● Administer IV glucose 10% by slow IV infusion (**refer to glucose 10% guideline**). ● Titrate to effect – an improvement in clinical state and glucose level should be observed rapidly. Do not exceed 2 ml/kg. If IV route not possible administer IM glucagon[a] (onset of action 5–10 minutes) (**refer to glucagon guideline**). ● Re-assess blood glucose level after 10 minutes. ● If <5.0 mmol/l administer a further dose of IV glucose. ● Re-assess blood glucose level after a further 10 minutes. ● Transfer immediately to the nearest suitable receiving hospital. ● Monitor vital signs and conscious level en-route. Check glucose if deteriorates, or half hourly. ● Provide an alert/information call if necessary. NB DO **NOT** administer glucose 50% as there is a risk of brain damage.
MODERATE: Patient with impaired consciousness, uncooperative	● If capable and cooperative, administer quick acting carbohydrate (sugary drink, glucose tablets (2–3), or glucose gel). Do not give chocolate as it is slower acting. ● If **NOT** capable and cooperative, but able to swallow, administer 1–2 tubes of dextrose gel 40% to the buccal mucosa, or give intra-muscular glucagon[a] (**refer to glucagon guideline**). ● Re-assess blood glucose level after a further 10 minutes. ● Ensure blood glucose level has improved to at least 5.0 mmol/l in addition to an improvement in level of consciousness. ● If blood glucose not improved to 5 mmol/l, repeat treatment up to three times. ● If no improvement after three treatments, consider intravenous glucose 10%. ● Transfer to the nearest suitable receiving hospital if requiring further treatment, otherwise can usually be safely left at home if with a responsible adult. ● Notify GP or out-of-hours provider if left at home. NB DO **NOT** administer glucose 50% as there is a risk of brain damage.
MILD: Patient conscious, orientated, able to swallow	● Administer quick acting carbohydrate (sugary drink, glucose tablets or glucose gel). Do not use chocolate (see above). ● Re-assess blood glucose level after a further 10 minutes. ● Ensure blood glucose level has improved to at least 5.0 mmol/l. ● If no improvement, repeat treatment up to three times. ● If no improvement after three treatments consider intravenous glucose 10% (**refer to glucose 10% guideline**). ● Transfer to the nearest suitable receiving hospital only if not responding to treatment. ● Notify GP or out-of-hours if left at home.

[a]Glucagon may take 5–10 minutes to take effect and requires the child to have adequate glycogen stores – thus, it may be ineffective if glycogen stores have been exhausted. This is likely in any children who have any NON diabetic causes of hypoglycaemia, although it is worth trying.
[b]Clean fingers prior to testing blood glucose levels as the child may have been in contact with sugary substances e.g. sweets.

DIABETES MELLITUS

● Diabetes mellitus can even occur in infants. These children may have blood glucose levels that are particularly difficult to control and may be very difficult to manage.

● Known diabetic children will have protocols to follow if they become unwell – if available and appropriate, always follow them.

● Type 1 (insulin dependent) DM is nearly universal in children though occasionally Type 2 (non-insulin dependent) DM is now seen, usually in association with severe obesity.

Diabetic ketoacidosis (DKA)

For the pathophysiology of this illness refer to glycaemic emergencies in adults.

● Patients may present with one or more signs as in Table 3.85.

Diabetic ketoacidosis (DKA) may occur relatively rapidly in children, sometimes without a long history of the classical symptoms. The absolute blood glucose level is not a good indicator of the presence of DKA – some children with blood glucose levels in the >20 range may appear quite well and not have DKA.

Glycaemic Emergencies (Children)

Table 3.85 – SIGN AND SYMPTOMS OF DKA

Symptoms
- Polyuria.
- Polydipsia.
- Abdominal pain.
- Vomiting.

Signs
- Weight loss.
- Lethargy, drowsiness confusion and ultimately coma and death.
- Dehydration, and occasionally circulatory failure due to hypovolaemia.
- Hyperventilation (Kussmaul breathing).
- Presence of ketones (measured) in the urine and/or blood.

- Children with DKA may present with significant dehydration – however, if IV fluid is given too fast this can lead to cerebral oedema and death. **Refer to intravascular fluid therapy guideline.** Do not give children with DKA IV fluids unless they have good evidence of hypovolaemic shock.

- True shock (circulatory failure), as opposed to dehydration, is relatively uncommon in children with DKA, but does not require IV fluid resuscitation. Volumes must not exceed 10 ml/kg.
- Do not try to give oral fluids to children with DKA – they have a very high risk of aspiration.
- Ketone measurement (blood or urine) is useful in the diagnosis of DKA.

3. Assessment and Management

If a known diabetic child is well, not vomiting, fully conscious, has a blood glucose level >16 mmol/l but a blood ketone level <3 mmol/l, the family should contact their diabetes team or GP. Do not attempt to manage the patient yourself.

Once a blood ketone level is above 3 mmol/l (or urine ketones are high) and the child is unwell with vomiting then they should be managed as having DKA.

For the assessment and management of diabetic ketoacidosis refer to Table 3.86.

Methodology

For details of the methodology used in the development of this guideline refer to the guideline webpage.

Table 3.86 – ASSESSMENT and MANAGEMENT of:

Diabetic Ketoacidosis in Children

ASSESSMENT	MANAGEMENT
• Undertake ABCD assessment	• Start correcting ABC problems (**refer to medical emergencies in children**). • Do not give IV fluids unless there is clear evidence of circulatory failure and no more than 10 ml/kg sodium chloride (**refer to intravascular fluids/0.9% saline guideline**).
• If the child is **TIME CRITICAL**	• Correct life-threatening conditions (airway and breathing on scene). • Then commence transfer to nearest suitable receiving hospital. NB DKA is a life-threatening condition requiring urgent hospital treatment.
• Measure blood glucose level	• Measure and record blood glucose level.
• Assess for signs of dehydration	• Do not give IV fluids to treat dehydration unless shocked (see above).
• Measure oxygen saturation (SpO₂)	• Administer high-flow oxygen as part of shock management. • Provide an alert/information call if necessary. • If the child has records of their blood or urine glucose levels, bring them with the patient.

KEY POINTS

Glycaemic Emergencies in Children
- **Hypoglycaemia is a medical emergency.**
- **Treat hypoglycaemia with a suitable form of glucose (this will depend on the patient's condition).**
- **Glucagon may be used intramuscularly to treat hypoglycaemia if treatment with glucose is not possible.**
- **Children, whose hypoglycaemia is not due to diabetes, may not respond well to glucagon.**
- **DKA usually requires no emergency prehospital treatment except rapid transport to hospital.**
- **IV fluids can cause cerebral oedema in children with DKA.**
- **Do not give IV fluids to children with DKA unless significant shock is present and then only limited amounts.**

Overdose and Poisoning (Children) [60, 467, 468, 502]

1. Introduction

Overdose and poisoning is a common cause of calls to the ambulance service accounting for 140,000 hospital admissions per year.

Poisoning

Exposure by ingestion, inhalation, absorption, or injection of a quality of a substance(s) that results in mortality or morbidity.

Common agents include:

- **Household products** e.g. washing powders, washing-up liquids and fabric cleaning liquid/tablets; bleaches, hand gels and screen-washes; anti-freeze and de-icers, silica gel, batteries, petroleum distillates, white spirit (e.g. paints and varnishes), descalers and glues. Exposure generally occurs as a result of ingestion but can arise from eye and skin contact; exposure can arise from multiple routes of exposure.
- **Pharmaceutical agents** e.g. paracetamol, ibuprofen, co-codamol, aspirin, tricyclic antidepressants, selective serotonin uptake inhibitors (SSRIs), beta-blockers, calcium-channel blockers, cocaine, benzodiazepines, opioids, iron tablets.
- **Plants/fungi** e.g. foxglove, laburnum, laurel, iris, castor oil plant, amanita palloides, etc. For further details of poisonous plants refer to: http://www.toxbase.org.
- **Alcohol**.
- **Chemicals**.
- **Cosmetics**.

Poisoning in children

1. **Accidental** exposure to a poisonous substance or medicine by an inquisitive child. This usually occurs in young children and ingestion of tablets is common, although, almost anything, however unpalatable to the adult palate, may be ingested. The event may not be obvious and may only be found on detailed questioning, if old enough to give a history.
2. **Intentional** poisoning (usually a medicine), as an act of deliberate self-harm. Over-the-counter medicine e.g. paracetamol, or prescribed drugs are commonly used.
3. **Non-accidental** poisoning of children is extremely unlikely to be detected by the Ambulance Service, but if it is suspected it must be reported. **Refer to the safeguarding children guideline**.

Overdose

Exposure by ingestion, inhalation, absorption, or injection of a quality of a substance(s) above the prescribed dose; this is a common form of poisoning, involving prescribed or illicit drugs and may be accidental or intentional.

2. Incidence

- It is difficult to estimate the exact number of overdose and poisoning incidents, as not all cases are reported. In 2009/2010 there were 49,690 poison-related queries involving patients to the National Poisons Information Service. Over one-third concerned children under the age of five. The majority of incidents were accidental and occurred in the home.

3. Severity and Outcome

- There are a number of factors which will affect severity and outcome following exposure, for example, age, toxicity of the agent, quantity and route of exposure.
- In 2009 there were 2,878 deaths related to drug overdose and poisoning in England and Wales.

4. Pathophysiology

- The mode of action following exposure will depend primarily on the nature of the toxin. For details of the actions of specific toxins refer to: http://www.toxbase.org

5. Assessment and Management

For the assessment and management of overdose and poisoning in children refer to Table 3.88.

Methodology

For details of the methodology used in the development of this guideline refer to the guideline webpage. Important information can be gained from toxbase and local protocols should be followed to obtain this information

KEY POINTS

Overdose and Poisoning

- **Children and adolescents with serious poisoning and deliberate overdoses must be transferred to hospital.**
- **After an accidental poisoning that was found to be non-toxic, some children (see Table 3.88) may be considered for home management.**
- **Alcohol often causes hypoglycaemia even in adolescents.**
- **NEVER induce vomiting.**
- **If the child vomits, retain a sample, if possible, for inspection at hospital.**
- **Bring the substance or substances and any containers found to the hospital for inspection.**
- **Estimate the quantity of substance ingested.**

Overdose and Poisoning (Children)

Table 3.87

Specific Substance Management

SUBSTANCE/SIGNS AND SYMPTOMS	MANAGEMENT
Alcohol (ethanol) ● Nausea, vomiting, slurred speech, confusion, convulsions, unconsciousness.	● Alcohol poisoning follows the consumption of excessive amounts of alcohol. ● It can be fatal so should be taken seriously. ● It is not uncommon in teenagers. ● Can cause severe hypoglycaemia even in teenagers. ● **ALWAYS** check the blood glucose levels in any child or young person with a decreased conscious level, especially in children and young adults who are 'drunk', as hypoglycaemia (blood glucose <4.0 mmol/l) is common and requires treatment with oral glucose or glucose 10% IV (**refer to glycaemic emergencies in children**). NOTE: Glucagon is not effective in alcohol-induced hypoglycaemia.
Tricyclic Antidepressants ● Central nervous system excitability, confusion, blurred vision, dry mouth, fever, pupil dilation, convulsions, coma, arrhythmias, hypotension, tachycardia, respiratory depression; physical condition can rapidly change.	● ECG monitoring and IV access should be established early in the treatment of tricyclic overdose. ● The likelihood of fitting is high; this should be treated following the **convulsions in children guidelines**.
Iron ● Nausea, vomiting blood, diarrhoea (black stools), metallic taste, convulsions, dizziness, flushed appearance, unconsciousness, non-cardiac pulmonary oedema.	● Iron pills are regularly used by large numbers of the population including pregnant mothers. In overdose, especially in children, they are exceedingly dangerous. They may cause extensive damage to the liver and gut and these children will require hospital assessment and treatment. NB Charcoal is contra-indicated as it may interfere with subsequent treatment.
Paracetamol ● Nausea, vomiting, malaise, right upper quadrant abdominal pain, jaundice, confusion, drowsiness – coma may develop later. NB Frequently asymptomatic, symptoms are unreliable.	● There are a number of analgesic preparations that contain paracetamol and a combination of codeine or dextropropoxyphene. This, in overdose, creates two serious dangers for the child: 1. The codeine and dextropropoxyphene are both derived from opioid drugs. This in overdose, especially if alcohol is involved, may well produce profound respiratory depression. This can be reversed with naloxone (**refer to naloxone guideline**). 2. Paracetamol, even in modest doses, is **dangerous** and can induce severe liver and kidney damage in susceptible children. Initially there are no clinical features to suggest this, which may lull the child's carers, the child, and ambulance clinicians into a false sense of security. It frequently takes 24–48 hours for the effects of paracetamol damage to become apparent and urgent blood paracetamol levels are required to assess the child's level of risk.
Opioids ● Drowsiness, nausea, vomiting, small pupils, respiratory depression, cyanosis, coma, convulsions, non-cardiac pulmonary oedema.	● May produce profound respiratory depression. This can be reversed with naloxone (**refer to naloxone guideline**).

3 Medical Undifferentiated Complaints SECTION

Table 3.88 – ASSESSMENT and MANAGEMENT of:

Overdose and Poisoning

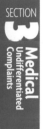

ASSESSMENT	MANAGEMENT
● Assess ABCD	● If any of the following **TIME CRITICAL** features present: – major **ABCD** problems – decreased level of consciousness – NB Most poisons that impair conscious also depress respiration – **refer to altered level of consciousness guideline** – respiratory depression – hypotension <70 mmHg – cardiac arrhythmias – **refer to cardiac rhythm disturbance guideline** – convulsions – **refer to convulsion guideline** – hypothermia – **refer to hypothermia guideline**, then: ● Start correcting **A** and **B** problems. ● Undertake a **TIME CRITICAL** transfer to nearest receiving hospital. ● Continue patient management en-route. ● Provide an alert/information call.
● Substance	● Ascertain what has been ingested. ● The time the incident occurred. ● Estimate the quantity of substance ingested/inhaled/absorbed/injected. ● What if any treatment has been administered. ● Refer to Table 3.87 for specific management. ● **NEVER** induce vomiting. ● In the case of caustic/petroleum ingestion encourage the child to drink a glass of milk, if possible. ● If possible take to hospital: – a sample of the ingested substance – medicine containers – a sample of vomit – if present. ● Consider non-accidental injury – **refer to safeguarding children guideline**.
● Chemical exposure	● If exposure to chemical substance is suspected – **refer to CBRNE guideline chemical section** for management.
● Oxygen	● Administer high levels of supplemental oxygen, particularly in cases of carbon monoxide poisoning or inhalation of irritant gases – refer to oxygen guideline. ● Apply pulse oximeter. NB Supplemental oxygen maybe harmful in cases of paraquat poisoning.
● ECG	● Undertake a 12-lead ECG.
● Respirations	● Monitor respirations. ● Consider assisted ventilation if: – SpO$_2$ is <90% after administering high levels of oxygen for 30–60 seconds – respiratory rate is <$\frac{1}{2}$ **normal rate** OR **>3 times normal rate** – expansion is inadequate. ● Opiates such as morphine, heroin can cause respiratory depression; consider naloxone – refer to naloxone guideline.
● Blood pressure	● Hypotension is common in cases of severe poisoning. ● Monitor blood pressure.
● Intravascular fluid	● If fluid is indicated refer to intravascular fluid guideline.
● Blood glucose level	● Measure blood glucose level. ● Blood glucose levels <4.0 mmol/l need correcting – refer to glucose 10% guideline. NB Glucagon is often not effective in overdoses.
● Mental health assessment	● In cases of attempted suicide undertake a rapid mental health assessment – **refer to mental disorder guideline**.
● Transfer to further care	● All children who have encountered a serious poisoning. ● All children who have taken a deliberate overdose. (Even if the substance was harmless, they need to be transferred for a hospital-based assessment of their mental health). Following an accidental poisoning, it is possible for some children to be managed at home. This option may be considered when: – the substance is/verified on **TOXBASE** as harmless – the incident is/was accidental – the carers know to seek medical advice if the child becomes unwell – arrangements have been made to inform the health visitor or GP.

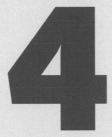

4

Trauma

Trauma

1. Introduction

- Trauma is a leading cause of death in the UK. The wide range of traumatic injuries encountered in prehospital care can present a complex challenge. Research suggests that assessing and managing patients in a systematic way can lead to improved outcomes.

- This overview will outline the process of assessment and management of trauma patients. This guideline supports the following related guidelines:
    - abdominal trauma
    - head trauma
    - limb trauma
    - neck and back trauma
    - pelvic trauma
    - thoracic trauma
    - trauma in pregnancy
    - traumatic cardiac arrest
    - airway management
    - burns and scalds
    - electrical injuries
    - fluid therapy
    - oxygen therapy
    - pain management.

This guideline uses mechanism of injury and primary survey as the basis of care for all trauma patients.

2. Incidence

- In England it is estimated that there are approximately 20,000 cases of major trauma annually. Road traffic collisions (RTC) are the most common cause.

3. Severity and Outcome

- In England major trauma accounts for approximately 5,400 deaths, with many more cases leading to significant short- and long-term morbidity. In Scotland (1992–2002) there were 5,847 deaths resulting from trauma. Major trauma is the leading cause of death in patients under 45 years of age.

4. Incident management

Overall control of the incident allows paramedics to concentrate on patient assessment and management and it is recommended that a model, such as SCENE, is used to assess the initial trauma scene so that it can be managed effectively (see Table 4.1).

5. Patient Assessment

A primary survey should be undertaken for **ALL** patients as this will rapidly identify patients with actual or potential **TIME CRITICAL** injuries (Table 4.3).

A secondary survey is a more thorough 'head-to-toe' assessment of the patient. It should be undertaken following completion of the primary survey, where time permits. The secondary survey will usually be undertaken during transfer to further care; however, in some patients with time critical trauma, it may not be possible to undertake the secondary survey before arrival at further care (Table 4.4).

5.1 Primary Survey

- The primary survey should take no more than 60–90 seconds and follow the **<C>ABCDE** approach. Document the vital signs and the time they were taken.

- Consider mechanism of injury and the possible injury patterns that may result; but be aware that mechanism alone cannot predict or exclude injury and physiological signs should be utilised as well.

- Assessment and management should proceed in a '**stepwise**' manner and life-threatening injuries should be managed as they are encountered, i.e. do not move onto breathing and circulation until the airway is secured. Every time an intervention has been carried out, re-assess the patient.

- As soon as a life-threatening injury is identified and managed, it is recommended that transport should be immediately instigated to the appropriate trauma facility according to local procedures.

- If immediate transfer is not possible, consider mobilising senior clinical support if not already done during the SCENE assessment.

Table 4.1 – SCENE

S Safety

Perform a dynamic risk assessment, are there any dangers now or will there be any that become apparent during the incident. This needs to be continually re-assessed throughout the incident. Appropriate personal protective equipment should be utilised according to local guidelines.

C Cause including MOI

Establish the events leading up to the incident. Is this consistent with your findings?

E Environment

Are there any environmental factors that need to be taken into consideration? These can include problems with access or egress, weather conditions or time of day.

N Number of patients

Establish exactly how many patients there are during the initial assessment of the scene.

E Extra resources needed

Additional resources should be mobilised now. These can include additional ambulances, helicopter or senior medical support. Liaise with the major trauma advisor according to local protocols.

MANAGEMENT OVERVIEW

If the patient has a life-threatening condition start immediate transfer to an appropriate trauma facility according to local procedures with treatment undertaken en-route to hospital.

- Provide an alert/information call.

- Continue patient re-assessment and management.

- If a patient requires IV fluids and fulfils the criteria in steps 1 or 2 of the Prehospital Major Trauma Triage tool (Appendix) then they should receive a bolus of tranexamic acid if available (**refer to tranexamic acid guideline**).

- **Pain management** – if analgesia is indicated **refer to pain management guideline**.
- Hand over – it is recommended that the patient is handed over to receiving clinicians using the ATMIST format (see Table 4.2).

If the patient is **NON-TIME CRITICAL** undertake a secondary survy (Table 4.3).

5.2 Secondary Survey

- A secondary survey should only commence after the primary survey has been completed and in critical patients only during transport.

Table 4.2 – ATMIST

A	Age
T	Time of incident
M	Mechanism
I	Injuries
S	Signs and symptoms
T	Treatment given/immediate needs

Table 4.3 – ASSESSMENT and MANAGEMENT of:

Trauma Emergencies

- **All stages should be considered but some may be omitted if not considered appropriate.**
- **To reduce clot disruption avoid unnecessary movements.**
- **When available administer tranexamic acid to all patients who require TIME CRITICAL transfer, except isolated head injuries.**

At each stage consider the need for:
- **TIME CRITICAL – transfer to nearest appropriate hospital as per local trauma care pathway.**
- **Early senior clinical support.**

STAGE	ASSESSMENT	MANAGEMENT
\<C\>	**CATASTROPHIC HAEMORRHAGE** – assess for the presence of **LIFE-THREATENING EXTERNAL BLEEDING**	Follow the management in Figure 4.1.
A	**AIRWAY** – assess the airway and **AT ALL TIMES** consider C-spine injury and the need to immobilise (**refer to neck and back trauma guideline**). **Look for** obvious obstructions e.g. teeth/dentures, foreign bodies, vomit, blood, trauma, soot/burns/oedema in burn patients. **Listen for** noisy airflow e.g. snoring, gurgling or no airflow. **Feel for** air movement.	Correct any airway problems immediately by: - Jaw thrust, chin lift (no neck extension). - Suction (if appropriate). - Nasopharyngeal airway. - Oropharyngeal airway. - Laryngeal mask airway (if appropriate). - Endotracheal intubation. - Needle cricothyroidotomy.
B	Assess rate, depth and quality of respiration Grade breathing 1–5 1. patient not breathing 2. Slow <12 per min 3. normal 12–20 but check depth 4. fast 20–30 observe very closely 5. very fast >30 Feel for depth and equality of chest movement, any instability of chest wall. Look for obvious chest injuries, wounds, bruising or flail segment. Auscultate lung fields assessing air entry on each side. Percuss the chest wall checking the pitch of the percussion note. In addition assess the chest and neck for the following using the mnemonic **TWELVE** - **T**racheal deviation - **W**ounds, bruising or swelling - **E**mphysema (surgical) - **L**aryngeal crepitus - **V**enous engorgement - **E**xcluding open/tension pneumothorax, flail segment, massive haemothorax.	Administer 100% O_2, in all patients with critical trauma to target O_2 sats of 94–98% even if there are risk factors such as COPD. - Breathing graded at 1,2 should receive O_2 via BVM as should grade 5 if clinically appropriate. - Breathing graded at 3,4 should receive supplemental 100% O_2 but be monitored very closely. - Apply non-occlusive dressing to sucking chest wounds (**refer to thoracic trauma guideline**). - Decompress a tension pneumothorax (**refer to thoracic trauma guideline**). - Flail segments should not be splinted (**refer to thoracic trauma guideline**). NB **Restraint (POSITIONAL) Asphyxia** – If the patient is required to be physically restrained (e.g. by police officers) in order to prevent them injuring themselves or others, or for the purpose of being detained under the Mental Health Act, then it is paramount that the method of restraint allows both for a patent airway and adequate respiratory volume. **Under these circumstances it is essential to ensure that the patient's airway and breathing are adequate at all times.**

SECTION **4** Trauma

Table 4.3 – ASSESSMENT and MANAGEMENT of:

Trauma Emergencies *continued*

STAGE	ASSESSMENT	MANAGEMENT
C	If massive external haemorrhage was controlled at start of assessment reassess this now. Assess for radial and carotid pulses noting rate, rhythm and volume, assess central and peripheral capillary refill time, note skin colour, texture and temperature. Remain alert to the possibility of internal bleeding and assess for signs of blood loss in five places (blood on the floor and four more). 1. External 2. Chest (already done during breathing assessment) 3. Abdomen by palpation and observation of bruising or external marks 4. Pelvis – do not manipulate the pelvis – MOI may suggest a fracture 5. Long bones – assess for but do not be distracted by limb trauma. Consider hypovolaemic shock but be aware that blood loss of 1000–1500 ml is required before classical signs start to appear. Signs of hypovolaemic shock include pallor, cool peripheries, anxiety and abnormal behaviour, increased respiratory rate and tachycardia. Signs of shock also appear much later in certain patient groups e.g. pregnant women, patients on beta blockers and the physically fit. There may well be little evidence of shock; blood loss of 1000–1500 ml is required before more classic signs of shock appear.	**MANAGEMENT** Follow the management for haemorrhage control in Figures 4.1 and 4.2. Consider splinting: ● In the critical patient, **long bone fractures** should be splinted en route to the trauma facility. ● **Pelvic fractures** should be stabilised at the earliest possible opportunity, preferably before the patient is moved – **refer to pelvic trauma guideline**. **Fluid Therapy** If fluid replacement is indicated refer to intravascular fluid therapy guideline. **TRANEXAMIC ACID** If a patient requires IV fluids and fulfils the criteria in steps 1 or 2 of the Prehospital Major Trauma Triage tool (Appendix A) then they should receive a bolus of tranexamic acid (refer to tranexamic acid guideline). In cases of internal or uncontrolled haemorrhage undertake a **TIME CRITICAL** transfer to appropriate hospital according to local procedures. To minimise clot disruption avoid unnecessary movement in victims of blunt trauma: ● Log roll should be avoided wherever possible. ● Patients should be lifted from the ground using a scoop (bivalve) stretcher. ● Once on a scoop (bivalve) stretcher patients should be transported on it. ● A long spinal board is an extrication device and should not be used unless required. Once on a long spinal board the patient should be transported on it – **refer to neck and back trauma guideline**. ● A patient with penetrating trauma who has no neurology and no possibility of direct trauma to the spinal column should NOT be imobilised.
D	**Disability** Obtain a full GCS (see Table 4.5) for the patient as this is required for the PreHospital Major Trauma Triage tool (Appendix A)	
	Assess and note pupil size, equality and response to light.	
	Altered mental status.	Check blood glucose level to rule out hypo- or hyperglycaemia as the cause – **refer to glycaemic emergencies guideline in adults**.
E	**EXPOSURE and ENVIRONMENT** At this stage further monitoring may be applied.	
	Exposure.	Ensure patient does not suffer from exposure to cold/wet conditions.
	Trapped patient.	Consider mobilising early senior clinical support.

● A secondary survey should only commence after the primary survey has been completed, and in critical patients only during transport.

● The secondary survey is a more thorough "head-to-toe" survey of the patient; however, it is important to monitor the patient's vital signs during the survey.

● In some patients with critical trauma it may not be possible to undertake a secondary survey before arriving at a trauma facility. However, in patients with altered mental status it is recommended that a BM reading should be taken during transport.

Table 4.4 – SECONDARY SURVEY

ASSESSMENT

Head
- Re-assess airway.
- Check skin colour and temperature.
- Palpate for bruising/fractures.
- Check pupil size and reactivity.
- Examine for loss of cerebrospinal fluid.
- Establish Glasgow Coma Scale (refer to Table 4.5).
- Assess for other signs of basal skull fracture.

NB For further information **refer to the head trauma guideline**.

Neck
- The collar will need to be loosened for proper examination of the neck.
- Re-assess for signs of life-threatening injury using the mnemonic 'TWELVE':
  - tracheal deviation
  - wounds, bruising, swelling
  - emphysema (surgical)
  - laryngeal crepitus
  - venous engorgement (jugular).
- Assess and palpate for spinal tenderness, particularly note any bony tenderness.

NB For further information **refer to the neck and back trauma guideline**.

Chest
- Assess rate, depth and quality of respiration and grade breathing 1–5
1. patient not breathing
2. Slow <12 per min
3. normal 12–20 but check depth
4. fast 20–30 observe very closely
5. very fast >30
- Breathing graded at 1,2 should receive O_2 via BVM as should grade 5 if clinically appropriate
- Breathing graded at 3,4 should receive supplemental 100% O_2 but should be monitored very closely
- Feel for rib fractures, instability and surgical emphysema.
- Look for contusions, seat belt marks and flail segments.
- Auscultate lung fields for signs of:
  - Pneumothorax
  - Tension pneumothorax
  - Haemothorax
  - Cardiac tamponade
  - Assess for signs of pulmonary contusion
  - Assess the front and as much of the back as is possible

N.B. for further information **refer to the thoracic trauma guideline**.

Abdomen
- Examine for open wounds, contusions and seatbelt marks
- Palpate the entire abdomen for tenderness and guarding
- Examine the front and as much of the back as is possible

N.B. for further information **refer to the abdominal trauma guideline**.

Table 4.4 – SECONDARY SURVEY *continued*

ASSESSMENT

Pelvis
- Blood loss may be visible either from the urethra or PV
- The patient may have the urge to urinate

N.B. for further information **refer to the pelvic trauma guideline**.

Lower/Upper Limbs
- Examine lower limbs then upper limbs.
- Look for wounds and evidence of fractures.
- Check for MSC in **ALL** four limbs:
  - **MOTOR** – Test for movement
  - **SENSATION** – Apply light touch to evaluate sensation
  - **CIRCULATION** – Assess pulse and skin temperature.

NB For further information **refer to the limb trauma guideline**.

6. Special Circumstances in Trauma

6.1 The Trapped Patient
Entrapment can be:

- **Relative:** trapped by difficulty in access/egress from the wreckage, including the physical injury stopping normal exit.

- **Absolute:** firmly trapped by the vehicle and its deformity necessitating specialised cutting techniques to free the patient.

All patients that have an **absolute** entrapment are at high risk of having suffered significant transfer of energy and therefore are at increased risk of severe injury.

6.2 Management
- Conduct a thorough assessment of the incident using SCENE or similar model.
- Consider mobilising senior clinical support at the earliest opportunity.
- Mobilise and liaise with other emergency services.
- Perform primary survey and manage as per trauma guideline.
- Form a rescue plan.
- Provide analgesia (**refer to pain management guidelines**).

Table 4.5 – GLASGOW COMA SCALE

Item		Score
Eyes Opening:		
	Spontaneously	4
	To speech	3
	To pain	2
	None	1
Motor Response:		
	Obeys commands	6
	Localises pain	5
	Withdraws from pain	4
	Abnormal flexion	3
	Extensor response	2
	No response to pain	1

Table 4.5 – GLASGOW COMA SCALE
continued

Item	Score
Verbal Response:	
Orientated	5
Confused	4
Inappropriate words	3
Incomprehensible sounds	2
No verbal response	1

Methodology

For details of the methodology used in the development of this guideline refer to the development website.

KEY POINTS

Trauma Emergencies Overview (Adults)

- **Overall assessment of safety: self, scene, casualties is of prime importance.**
- **The primary survey forms the basis of patient assessment, with due consideration for C-spine immobilisation.**
- **Arrest of external haemorrhage can be life saving.**
- **Consider mobilising senior clinical support at the earliest opportunity.**

Appendix – The NHS Clinical Advisory Group on Trauma Prehospital Major Trauma Triage Tool >12 years

Prehospital Major Trauma Triage Tool

The Major Trauma Triage Tool presented below is based on the American College of Surgeons Guidelines for Field Triage 2006 with minor modifications. In Step 2 'Flail chest' has been changed to 'Chest injury with altered physiology' and 'Paralysis' has been changed to 'Sensory or motor deficit (new onset following trauma)'. In Step 3 'feet' have been changed to 'metres' for distance fallen. 'Entrapment' has been added. Step 4 Burns are considered special if they are facial, circumferential or 20% Body Surface Area (BSA).

Entry criteria for use of triage is a judgement that the patient may have suffered significant trauma.

Step 1

Physiological:

- GCS < 14 (Table 4.5)
- SBP < 90 mmHg.

If any of the above factors are present, activate Major Trauma Alert and definitive care to be from Major Trauma Centre; otherwise proceed to Step 2.

Step 2

Anatomical:

- Penetrating to head/neck/torso/limbs proximal to elbow/knee.
- Chest injury with altered physiology.
- Two proximal long bone fractures.
- Crushed/degloved/mangled extremity.
- Amputation proximal to wrist/ankle.
- Pelvic fractures.
- Open or depressed skull fracture.
- Sensory or motor deficit (new onset following trauma).

If any of the above factors are present activate a Major Trauma Alert and definitive care to be from Major Trauma Centre; otherwise proceed to Step 3.

Step 3

Mechanism

- Falls
  - Fall > 6 m/2 storeys in adult
  - Fall > 3 m/2 times height in child.
- Motor vehicles
  - Intrusion > 30 cm occupant site
  - Ejection partial/complete
  - Death in same passenger compartment
  - Vehicle telemetry data consistent with high risk of injury.
- Pedestrian/cyclist versus motor vehicle thrown/run over/with significant (> 20 mph) impact.
- Motorcycle crash > 20 mph.
- Entrapment.

If any of the above factors present consider a Major Trauma Alert with further assessment by either Trauma Unit or Major Trauma Centre; otherwise proceed to Step 4.

Step 4

- Special considerations that should lower the threshold for a Trauma Alert
  - Older adults (age > 55)
  - Children (to Paediatric Trauma Centre)
  - Anticoagulation/bleeding disorders
  - Burns: full thickness facial, circumferential or 20% body surface area (BSA)
  - Time-sensitive extremity injury
  - Dialysis-dependent renal disease
  - Pregnancy > 20 weeks
  - EMS provider judgement.

If any of the above factors present consider Major Trauma Alert with further assessment by either Trauma Unit or Major Trauma Centre.

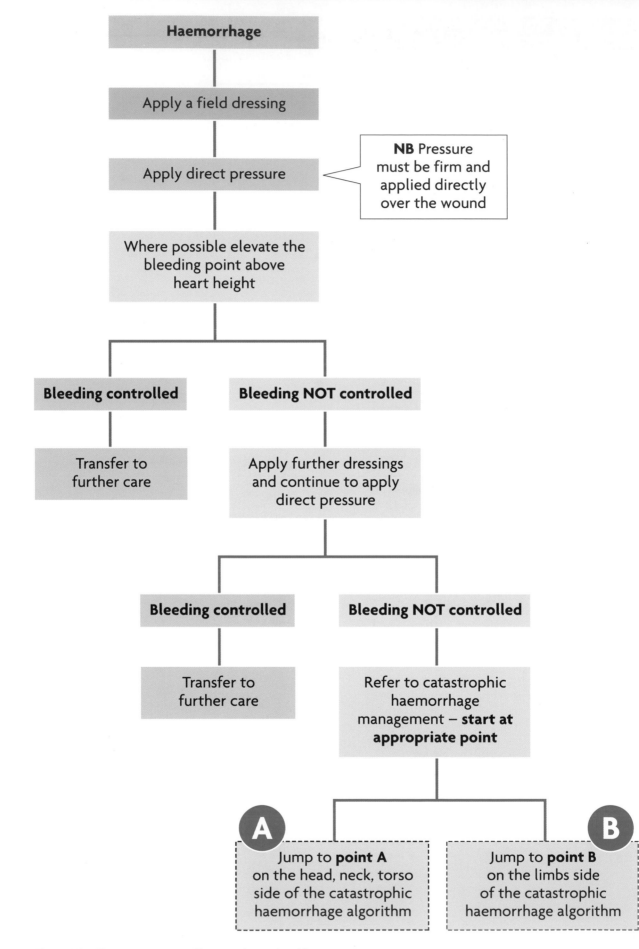

Haemorrhage

Apply a field dressing

Apply direct pressure

NB Pressure must be firm and applied directly over the wound

Where possible elevate the bleeding point above heart height

Bleeding controlled

Transfer to further care

Bleeding NOT controlled

Apply further dressings and continue to apply direct pressure

Bleeding controlled

Transfer to further care

Bleeding NOT controlled

Refer to catastrophic haemorrhage management – **start at appropriate point**

A

Jump to **point A** on the head, neck, torso side of the catastrophic haemorrhage algorithm

B

Jump to **point B** on the limbs side of the catastrophic haemorrhage algorithm

Figure 4.1 – The management of haemorrhage algorithm.

SECTION
4
Trauma

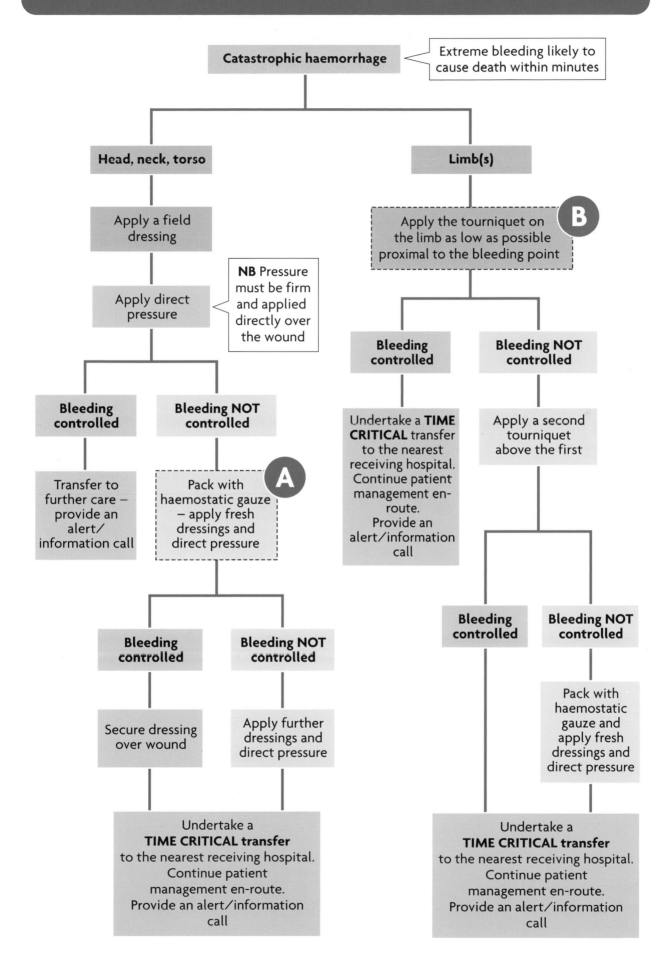

Catastrophic haemorrhage ← Extreme bleeding likely to cause death within minutes

Head, neck, torso

Apply a field dressing

Apply direct pressure

NB Pressure must be firm and applied directly over the wound

Bleeding controlled → Transfer to further care – provide an alert/information call

Bleeding NOT controlled → Pack with haemostatic gauze – apply fresh dressings and direct pressure **A**

Bleeding controlled → Secure dressing over wound

Bleeding NOT controlled → Apply further dressings and direct pressure

Undertake a **TIME CRITICAL transfer** to the nearest receiving hospital. Continue patient management en-route. Provide an alert/information call

Limb(s)

Apply the tourniquet on the limb as low as possible proximal to the bleeding point **B**

Bleeding controlled → Undertake a **TIME CRITICAL** transfer to the nearest receiving hospital. Continue patient management en-route. Provide an alert/information call

Bleeding NOT controlled → Apply a second tourniquet above the first

Bleeding controlled

Bleeding NOT controlled → Pack with haemostatic gauze and apply fresh dressings and direct pressure

Undertake a **TIME CRITICAL transfer** to the nearest receiving hospital. Continue patient management en-route. Provide an alert/information call

Figure 4.2 – The management of catastrophic haemorrhage algorithm.

Trauma

Trauma Emergencies Overview (Children)

1. Introduction

- Paediatric trauma is managed following the standard **<C>ABCDE** approach to trauma, taking into account differences in the child's anatomy, relative size and physiological response to injury. These differences are addressed below.

2. Incidence

- 700 children die as a result of accidents in England and Wales each year.

- 50% of child trauma deaths occur in motor vehicle incidents. Children travelling by car should legally be restrained but this law is not always followed and many deaths and serious injuries occur following vehicular ejection. Additionally, child deaths from cycle and pedestrian incidents are also very common.

- 30% of child trauma deaths occur at home with burns and falls being the leading causes.

- Child death reviews often identify circumstances that could potentially have been avoided had injury prevention methods been rigorously applied.

3. Assessment: The Basic Trauma Approach

3.1 SCENE

Overall control of the incident allows paramedics to concentrate on patient assessment and management and it is recommended that a model, such as SCENE, is used to assess the initial trauma scene so that it can be managed effectively (see below).

S Safety

Risk assessment. Perform a dynamic risk assessment. Are there any dangers now or will there be any that become apparent during the incident? This needs to be continually re-assessed throughout the incident. Appropriate personal protective equipment should be utilised according to local protocols.

C Cause including MOI

Establish the events leading up to the incident. Is this consistent with your findings? Read the scene/wreckage looking for evidence that children were involved e.g. toys or child seats. These may provide a clue that a child has been ejected from the vehicle or wandered off from the scene but may still require medical attention or other care. Ask if children were involved.

E Environment

Are there any environmental factors that need to be taken into consideration? These can include problems with access or egress, weather conditions or time of day.

N Number of patients

Establish exactly how many patients there are during the initial assessment of the scene

E Extra resources needed

Additional resources should be mobilised now. These can include additional ambulances, helicopter or senior medical support. Liaise with the major trauma advisor according to local protocols.

3.2 Primary Survey

- Catastrophic haemorrhage (refer to Figure 4.4).
- Airway with cervical spine control (**refer to neck and back trauma guideline**)
- Breathing.
- Circulation.
- Disability.
- Exposure.

The management of a child suffering a traumatic injury requires a careful approach, with an emphasis on explanation, reassurance and honesty. Trust of the carer by the child makes management much easier.

If possible, it is helpful to keep the child's parents/carers close by for reassurance, although their distress can exacerbate that of the child.

3.4 Stepwise Primary Survey Assessment

As for all trauma care, a systematic approach, managing problems as they are encountered before moving on is required.

4. Catastrophic Haemorrhage

Catastrophic blood loss must be arrested immediately (refer to catastrophic haemorrhage control Figure 4.4).

5. Airway

In small children, the relatively large occiput tends to flex the head forward. In order to return the head to the neutral position it may be necessary to insert a small amount of padding under the shoulders.

Vomit, blood or foreign material may obstruct the airway. Apply gentle suctioning under direct vision. Blind finger sweeps are contra-indicated.

Head tilt should be avoided in trauma and a chin lift alone or a jaw thrust used to open the airway.

If an airway adjunct is needed, then an oropharyngeal airway should be inserted under direct vision. If it is necessary to insert a nasopharyngeal airway (e.g. because of trismus) care must be taken in all head injured children in case there is an underlying skull fracture, causing a risk of misplacement through the cribriform plate into the brain. It is also important to avoid damage to the adenoidal tissue. This can cause considerable bleeding making the airway even more difficult to manage.

High concentration oxygen (O_2) (**refer to oxygen guideline**) should be administered routinely, whatever the oxygen saturation, in children sustaining major trauma or long bone fractures.

Administer high concentration O_2 via a non-rebreathing mask, to maintain an oxygen saturation of at least 95%. If a high flow mask is not tolerated, the mask (or just the oxygen tubing) may be held near the child's nose or mouth.

Airway burns are considered as a 'special case' (**refer to burns and scalds in children guideline**). Examine for soot in the nostrils and mouth, erythema and blistering of the lips and hoarseness of the voice. These suggest potential airway injury. These children require early endotracheal intubation and may deteriorate faster than adults due to the smaller diameter of their airway. Unless there is somebody at the scene who is trained in pre-hospital paediatric anaesthesia and difficult paediatric airway management who can electively intubate the child, it is best to transport the child rapidly (time critical transfer) and to pre-alert the hospital so they can have suitable experts standing by. If the airway swelling becomes life-threatening, and the airway cannot be controlled any other way, needle cricothyroidotomy may be required. Surgical airways should be avoided under the age of 12 years.

6. Cervical Spine

Cervical spinal immobilisation is essential when an injury to the neck has possibly occurred. Manual immobilisation is initially used although the subsequent use of a correctly sized cervical collar, head blocks and forehead/chin tapes and a scoop stretcher or a long board where the child has to be extricated is recommended. If the child is combative, this may not be possible and manual immobilisation may be the only possible method (**refer to neck and back trauma guideline**).

7. Breathing

A child's chest wall is readily deformable and may withstand significant force. As a result, significant intra-thoracic injuries can occur without any apparent external chest wall signs.

Auscultate the chest if practical.

Look at the chest for bruising and record the rate and adequacy of breathing. Chest wall movement and the presence of any wounds should be sought. Poor excursion may suggest an underlying pneumothorax.

Feel for rib fractures, or surgical emphysema.

This should reveal good, bilateral air entry and the absence of any added sounds. Listen specifically to the 3 areas:
i.   above the nipples in the mid-clavicular line
ii. in the mid-axilla under the armpits
iii. at the rear of the chest, below the shoulder blades when it is possible to access this area.

Table 4.6 – NORMAL RESPIRATORY RATES

Age	Respiratory Rate
<1 year	30–40 breaths per minute
1–2 years	25–35 breaths per minute
2–5 years	25–30 breaths per minute
5–11 years	20–25 breaths per minute
>12 years	15–20 breaths per minute

Assess for:
● Percuss the chest if possible assessing for hyporesonance or hyperresonance.

● Tension pneumothorax.
● Massive haemothorax.
● Sucking chest wounds (open pneumothorax).
● Flail chest.

NB **Refer to thoracic trauma guideline** for the management of these conditions.

NB Distended neck veins are very difficult to see in children and in shock may be absent.

Management

If ventilation is inadequate (see below) the child's respiratory effort may require support from bag-valve-mask ventilation and high flow oxygen. Assist ventilation at a rate equivalent to the normal respiratory rate for the age of the child (refer to Table 4.6) if:

● The child is hypoxic (SpO$_2$ <90%) and remains so after 30–60 seconds on high concentration O$_2$.
● Respiratory rate is <50% normal or >3 times normal.

Treat life-threatening chest injuries as per appropriate guideline (see above).

8. Circulation

Refer to Medical Emergencies – recognition of Circulatory Failure

Look firstly for evidence of significant external haemorrhage and treat as per haemorrhage guideline (Figures 4.3 and 4.4).
Assess the:

● Brachial or carotid pulses; record rate and volume (refer to Table 4.7):
  – tachycardia (with a poor pulse volume) suggests shock
  – bradycardia also occurs in the shocked child but is a **PRE-TERMINAL SIGN**.
● Respiratory rate: elevated due to compensatory mechanisms in shock.
● Capillary refill time: measure on the forehead or sternum.
● Colour.
● Conscious level.
● Examine the abdomen for signs of intra-abdominal bleeding (if present assume a pelvic fracture).
● Remember cardiac tamponade in a rapidly deteriorating child where chest injury has occurred and where the cause of the deterioration is not clear (**refer to thoracic trauma guideline**).

Table 4.7 – NORMAL HEART RATES

Age	Heart Rate
<1 year	110–160 beats per minute
1–2 years	100–150 beats per minute
2–5 years	95–140 beats per minute
5–11 years	80–120 beats per minute
>12 years	60–100 beats per minute

Significant blood losses are seen in long bone fractures with even greater losses (double the volume) seen when the fracture is open, when compared to a corresponding closed fracture: e.g. in a closed femoral fracture 20% of the circulating blood volume may bleed into the surrounding tissues compared to losses of 40% from an open femoral shaft fracture.

Management

Splintage, traction and full immobilisation can reduce blood loss and pain.

Where possible, vascular access can be gained en-route to hospital, reducing the time spent on scene. Use the widest possible cannula for the veins available.

In paediatric trauma **5 ml/kg fluid boluses** are used and repeated as needed to improve clinical signs (e.g. RR, HR, capillary refill, conscious level) **towards normal**.

NB Hypotensive resuscitation practices (as used in adult trauma) should not be used in children.

(Due to their physiological reserves, children maintain their systolic blood pressures in the face of major blood loss, with hypotension only occurring at a very late stage. Significant cardiovascular compromise and even cardiac arrest may occur if volume resuscitation were to be delayed until a child had reached such an advanced state of hypovolaemia).

Following IV fluid resuscitation, in paediatric major trauma with catastrophic haemorrhage, a bolus of tranexamic acid should be given, if available (**refer to tranexamic acid guideline**).

9. Disability – Assessment

Record the initial level of consciousness using the AVPU Scale (below):

A Alert

V Responds to voice

P Responds to painful stimulus

U Unresponsive

as well as:

● The time of the AVPU assessment.

● Pupil size, shape, symmetry and response to light.

● Whether the child was moving some or all limbs. If there is no movement, then ask the child to 'wiggle' their fingers and toes, paying particular note to movements peripheral to any injury site.

● Any abnormalities of posture.

If the child is not **alert** they should be considered time critical. A formal GCS (see Appendix) en-route may be valuable to the receiving hospital but should only be recorded if it can be accurately done and does not delay transfer.

9.1 Stepwise Disability Management

Confusion or agitation in an injured child may result directly from a significant head injury, but equally may be secondary to hypoxia from an impaired airway or compromised breathing or else hypoperfusion due to blood loss and shock.

The management of any child with impaired consciousness is based on ensuring an adequate airway, oxygenation, ventilation and circulation.

Always measure the blood glucose level in any child with altered consciousness. If hypoglycaemia is detected **refer to the glycaemic emergencies in children guideline for treatment**.

10. Exposure

Children will lose heat rapidly when exposed for examination and immobilised during trauma care. Do protect the child from a cold environment during your assessment.

Expose children 'piecemeal' if possible replacing a piece of clothing before removing the next as stripping a child may cause insecurity or embarrassment as well as exposing them to cold .

If the child is **TIME CRITICAL** they must be packaged appropriately (with full spinal immobilisation – or improvisation as tolerated – and pelvic splint if pelvic injury suspected) and transported rapidly to hospital.

An **alert/information call should be given for all TIME CRITICAL children** en-route.

If there is no apparent problem with the primary survey, a secondary survey may be commenced en-route. This should not delay the transfer to definitive care.

10.1   Secondary Survey

This is a systematic and careful review of each part of the injured child looking for non-critical and/or occult injuries. It is rarely possible to complete this before hospital in a seriously injured child.

Any deterioration in the child's condition mandates an immediate return to the primary survey and the problem sought and treated.

Dress and immobilise any injuries found as required. Perform a simple **MSC** check of **ALL** 4 limbs (see below):

M	MOTOR	Test for movement
S	SENSATION	Apply light touch to evaluate sensation
C	CIRCULATION	Assess pulse and skin temperature

11. Analgesia in Trauma

As would happen for an adult, a child's pain must be addressed once their life-threatening problems have been attended to (**refer to pain management in children guideline**).

Note:

Paediatric drug doses are expressed as mg/kg (**refer to specific drug protocols/Page-for-Age** for dosages and information). Drug doses **MUST** be checked prior to **ANY** drug administration, no matter how confident the practitioner may be.

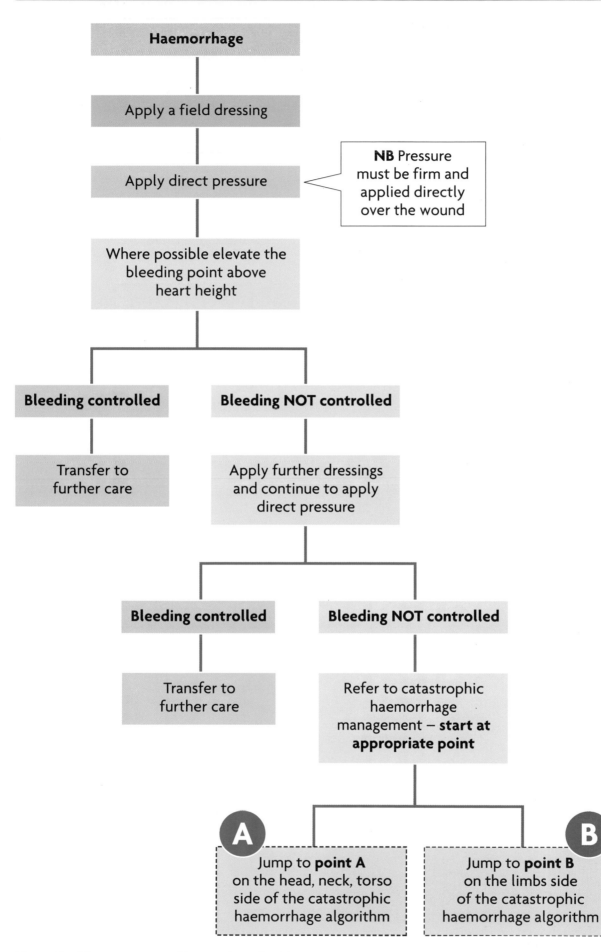

Haemorrhage

Apply a field dressing

Apply direct pressure

NB Pressure must be firm and applied directly over the wound

Where possible elevate the bleeding point above heart height

Bleeding controlled

Transfer to further care

Bleeding NOT controlled

Apply further dressings and continue to apply direct pressure

Bleeding controlled

Transfer to further care

Bleeding NOT controlled

Refer to catastrophic haemorrhage management – **start at appropriate point**

A

Jump to **point A** on the head, neck, torso side of the catastrophic haemorrhage algorithm

B

Jump to **point B** on the limbs side of the catastrophic haemorrhage algorithm

Figure 4.3 – The management of haemorrhage algorithm.

SECTION **4** Trauma

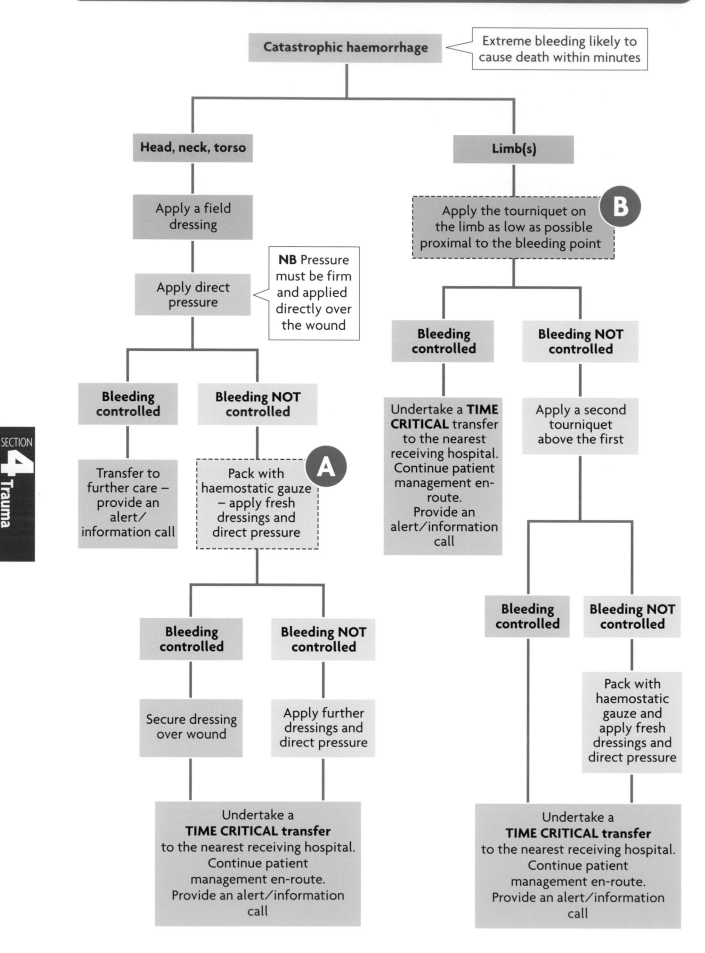

Figure 4.4 – The management of catastrophic haemorrhage algorithm.

SECTION
4
Trauma

12. Summary

Read the scene for mechanism of injury and the presence of children.

Trauma emergencies in childhood are managed using similar priorities and techniques to those used in adult practice. Remember the important anatomical and physiological differences encountered in children whilst performing Primary (and/or Secondary) Surveys.

Children may **conceal** serious underlying injuries using compensatory mechanisms so a high index of clinical suspicion is required. Agitation and/or confusion may indicate primary brain injury, but also be due to inadequate ventilation and/or cerebral perfusion.

Methodology

For details of the methodology used in the development of this guideline please refer to the guideline webpage.

KEY POINTS

Trauma Emergencies in Childhood

- Important anatomical and physiological differences exist between children and adults — a different approach will often be needed.
- Read the wreckage — toys or child seats may indicate that children have been involved in the incident.
- Assess and continuously re-assess <C>ABCDE.
- Detect time critical problems as part of the primary survey and transport urgently with a hospital pre-alert.

APPENDIX – Glasgow Coma Scale and modified Glasgow Coma Scale

Table 4.8 – GLASGOW COMA SCALE

Item	Score
Eyes Opening:	
Spontaneously	4
To speech	3
To pain	2
None	1
Motor Response:	
Obeys commands	6
Localises pain	5
Withdraws from pain	4
Abnormal Flexion	3
Extensor response	2
No response to pain	1
Verbal Response:	
Orientated	5
Confused	4
Inappropriate words	3
Incomprehensible sounds	2
No verbal response	1

Table 4.9 – MODIFICATION OF GLASGOW COMA SCALE FOR CHILDREN AGED UNDER 4 YEARS OLD

Item	Score
Eyes Opening:	As per adult scale
Motor Response:	As per adult scale
Best Verbal Response:	
Appropriate words or social smiles, fixes on and follows objects	5
Cries, but is consolable	4
Persistently irritable	3
Restless, agitated	2
Silent	1

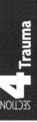

Abdominal Trauma [49, 503–517]

1. Introduction

- Trauma to the abdomen can be extremely difficult to assess even in a hospital setting. In the field, identifying which abdominal structure/s has been injured is less important than identifying that abdominal trauma itself has occurred.

- It is therefore, of major importance to note abnormal signs associated with blood loss, and establish that abdominal injury is the probable cause, rather than being concerned with, for example, whether the source of that abdominal bleeding originates from the spleen or liver.

- There may be significant intra-abdominal injury with very few, if any, initial indications of this at the time the abdomen is examined by the paramedic at the scene.

2. Severity and Outcome

The leading cause of morbidity and mortality is as a result of blunt trauma. Mortality from isolated abdominal stab wounds is approximately 1–2%.

3. Pathophysiology

The abdomen may be described as three anatomical areas:

i. **Abdominal cavity**
ii. **Pelvis**
iii. **Retro-peritoneal area.**

i. **Abdominal cavity** – extends from the diaphragm to the pelvis. It contains the stomach, small intestine, large intestine, liver, gall bladder and spleen.

   The upper abdominal organs are partly in the lower thorax and lie under the lower ribs; therefore fractures of lower ribs may damage abdominal structures such as the liver and spleen.

ii. **Pelvis** – contains the bladder, the lower part of the large intestine and, in the female, the uterus and ovaries. The iliac artery and vein overlie the posterior part of the pelvic ring and may be torn in pelvic fractures, adding to already major bleeding.

iii. **Retro-peritoneal area** – lies against the posterior abdominal wall, and contains the kidneys and ureters, pancreas, abdominal aorta, vena cava, and part of the duodenum. These structures are attached to the posterior abdominal wall, and are often injured by shearing due to rapid deceleration forces.

4. Abdominal Injuries

Blunt trauma – is the most common pattern of injury seen and results from direct blows to the abdomen or rapid deceleration. Blunt trauma may also result from all phases of a blast.

- The spleen, liver (hepatic tear), and 'tethered' structures such as duodenum are the most commonly injured. The small bowel, mesentery and aorta may also sustain injury.

Penetrating trauma – stab wounds, gunshot wounds, blast injuries and other penetrating injuries.

- **Stab wounds** – stab injures should be assumed to have caused serious damage until proved otherwise. Damage to liver, spleen or major blood vessels may cause massive haemorrhage. NB Upper abdominal stab wounds may have caused major intra-thoracic damage if the weapon was directed upwards (**refer to thoracic trauma guideline**). Similarly, chest stabbing injuries may also cause intra-abdominal injury.

- **Gunshot wounds** – tend to cause both direct and indirect injury, due to the forces involved and the chaotic paths that bullets may take. The same rules apply to associated intra-thoracic injuries.

- **Blast injuries** – can lead to both blunt and penetrating injuries. In an explosion in a confined space the blast wave can cause injuries to the bowel (perforation and haemorrhage) and penetrating ballistics can lead to organ damage.

5. Assesssment and Management

For the assessment and management of abdominal trauma refer to Table 4.10.

Methodology

For details of the methodology used in the development of this guideline refer to the guideline webpage.

KEY POINTS

Abdominal Trauma

- Abdominal trauma can be difficult to assess.
- Identifying that abdominal trauma has occurred is more important than identifying which structure/s has been injured, therefore note signs associated with blood loss.
- Observe mechanism of injury.
- Ensure ‹C›ABCs are assessed and managed; consider C-spine immobilisation.
- Transport to the nearest appropriate facility, providing an alert/information call en-route.

Abdominal Trauma

Table 4.10 – ASSESSMENT and MANAGEMENT of:

Abdominal Trauma

ASSESSMENT	MANAGEMENT

● **Assess <C>ABC**	● Control any external catastrophic haemorrhage – **refer to trauma emergencies overview**.
	 ● If any of the following **TIME CRITICAL** features are present:
	   – major **ABC** problems
	   – haemodynamic compromise
	   – decreased level of consciousness
	   – neck and back injuries – **refer to neck and back trauma guideline**, then:
	 ● Start correcting **A** and **B** problems.
	 ● Undertake a **TIME CRITICAL** transfer to nearest appropriate receiving hospital.
	 ● Provide an alert/information call.
	 ● Continue patient management en-route.

● Assess	● Ascertain the mechanism of injury: ● **Road traffic collision:** look for impact speed and severity of deceleration; seat belt and lap belt use are particularly associated with torn or perforated abdominal structures. ● **Stabbing and gunshot wound(s):** consider the length of the weapon used or the type of gun and the range. ● **Blast injuries:** blast wave injuries and penetrating ballistics. Assess the chest and abdomen – NB Some abdominal organs e.g. liver and spleen are covered by lower ribs/chest margins. **ABDOMEN:** ● Examine for signs of tenderness. ● Examine for external signs of injury e.g. contusions, seat/lap belt abrasions. ● Evisceration (protruding abdominal organs). **GENTLY** palpate the four quadrants of the abdomen for signs of tenderness, guarding and rigidity. Shoulder-tip pain should increase suspicion of injury or internal bleeding. NB Significant **INTRA-ABDOMINAL TRAUMA** may show little or no evidence in the early stages, therefore **DO NOT** rule out injury if initial examination is normal. **CHEST:** ● Fractures of the lower ribs – if confirmed or suspected **refer to thoracic trauma guideline**.
● Evisceration	● **DO NOT** push protruding abdominal organs back into the abdominal cavity. ● Cover protruding abdominal organs with warm moist dressings.
● Impaling objects	● Leave impaling objects e.g. a knife **IN-SITU**. ● Secure the object prior to transfer to further care. If the object(s) is pulsating, **DO NOT** completely immobilise it, but allow it to pulsate.
● Haemorrhage	● In the case of external haemorrhage apply a field dressing and direct pressure – **refer to trauma emergencies overview guideline**.
● Oxygen	● Administer high levels of supplemental oxygen (aim for SpO$_2$ <94–98%) – refer to oxygen guideline. ● Apply pulse oximeter.
● Ventilation	Consider assisted ventilation at a rate of 12–20 respirations per minute if: ● Oxygen saturation (SpO$_2$) is <90% on high levels of supplemental oxygen. ● Respiratory rate is <12 or >30bpm. ● Inadequate chest expansion. **Refer to airway and breathing management guideline**.
● Vital signs	● Monitor vital signs. ● Monitor ECG.
● Pelvic injuries	● Consider pelvic injuries – if suspected **refer to pelvic trauma guideline**.
● Thoracic injuries	● If the injury affects the chest **refer to thoracic trauma guideline**.
● Pain management	● If pain relief is indicated **refer to pain management guidelines**.
● Fluid	● If fluid resuscitation is indicated – refer to intravascular fluid therapy guideline. ● **DO NOT** delay on scene for fluid replacement.
● Transfer to further care	● Continue patient management en-route. ● Provide an alert/information call. ● Complete documentation.

1. Introduction

- Head trauma may occur in isolation or as part of multi-system injury. There is a significant association with cervical spinal injury and a depressed level of consciousness.

    '**NEVER** presume decreased conscious level is solely due to the effects of alcohol or drugs. Intoxicated patients commonly sustain head injuries.'

The aim of prehospital treatment is to ensure adequate perfusion of the brain by:

- Optimising oxygenation.
- Maintaining normal $EtCO_2$ by ensuring adequate ventilation and avoiding hyperventilation.
- Maintenance of mean arterial pressure to ensure adequate cerebral perfusion pressure.

2. Incidence

- Head injury is the cause of an estimated 1,000,000 hospital presentations each year in the UK, with an incidence of severe brain injury of between 10 and 15 per 100,000 population.

3. Incidence

- A history of a period of loss of consciousness may indicate an increased risk of a significant head injury.
- Retrograde amnesia (amnesia of events before the injury) of greater than 30 minutes indicates a major injury. Post-traumatic amnesia is less prognostic, but also suggests significant injury.
- There is a significant association between head and cervical spine injuries.

Mechanism of injury for Intracranial head injury:

- 'Bulls-eye' of the windscreen.
- Blood staining of the dashboard or steering wheel.
- Significant scratch or fracture damage to a protective helmet.
- Identification of a weapon that might have been used in an assault.
- A history or clues suggestive of fall from height.
- Patients with a decreased level of consciousness are at risk of airway compromise.
- Early evacuation of an intracranial haematoma is associated with a significantly improved outcome.

4. Pathophysiology

- Primary brain injury occurs at the time of injury. Prevention strategies include the wearing of motorcycle and cycle helmets, the use of vehicle restraint systems (e.g. seatbelts and airbags) and public education.
- Secondary brain injury occurs following the primary event as a result of hypoxia, hypercarbia or hypoperfusion.
- A reduced level of consciousness may lead to airway obstruction or inadequate ventilation resulting in poor oxygenation, carbon dioxide retention and acidosis.
- Blood loss from other injuries in a patient with multi-system trauma may lead to hypovolaemia, hence a fall in mean arterial pressure and consequently cerebral perfusion pressure.
- Cerebral perfusion pressure (CPP) needs to be maintained to ensure normal brain physiology and prevent oedema. It is determined by the relationship between the mean arterial pressure (MAP). This is the mean pressure during the cardiac pumping cycle pushing blood into the brain against the resistance of the intracranial pressure (ICP).

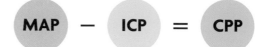

Figure 4.5 – Cerebral perfusion pressure.

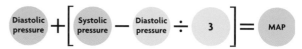

Figure 4.6 – Mean arterial pressure.

- The ICP is increased by the presence of anything that occupies the intra-cerebral space (haematoma, a neoplasm) or causes vasodilatation (hypoxia, hypercarbia) and consequent oedema.

5. Assessment

- For the assessment and management of head trauma refer to Table 4.11.

Table 4.11 – ASSESSMENT and MANAGEMENT of:

Head Injury

ASSESSMENT	MANAGEMENT
● Assess <C>ABC	● Control any external catastrophic haemorrhage – **refer to trauma emergencies overview**. ● If any of the following **TIME CRITICAL** features are present: – major **ABC** problems – haemodynamic compromise – altered level of consciousness – **refer to altered level of consciousness guideline** – neck and back injuries – **refer to neck and back trauma guideline**, then: ● Start correcting **A** and **B** problems. ● Undertake a **TIME CRITICAL** transfer to nearest appropriate receiving hospital. ● Provide an alert/information call. ● Continue patient management en-route.
Assess mechanism of injury	Gather any information from the scene about the mechanism of injury; suspect a significant head injury if: ● There are signs such as a 'bulls-eye' of the windscreen. ● Blood staining of the dashboard or steering wheel in a motor vehicle collision. ● Significant scratch or fracture damage to a protective helmet. ● A weapon that might have been used in an assault. ● A history or clues suggestive of fall from height. ● A pedestrian or cyclist struck by a motor vehicle. ● An occupant ejected from a motor vehicle.
Assess for other indicators of injury	● Boggy swelling(s). ● Trauma to the scalp or skull (never insert a finger into a head wound to feel for a fracture). ● Leakage of cerebrospinal fluid from the ears and/or nose. ● Blood from the ears. ● Bruising behind ears (late sign of basal skull fracture). ● Bilateral black eyes (late sign of basal skull fracture). ● Amnesia for events before/after injury. ● Persistent headache following injury. ● Convulsions following injury. ● Vomiting following injury. ● Consider non-accidental injury. NB Determine whether the patient is on anticoagulant therapy or has a bleeding/clotting disorder.
Assess level of consciousness	Undertake a rapid mini-neurological assessment to give a baseline against which improvement or deterioration can be measured – re-asssess every 15 minutes as the patient's condition may change over time. ● Measure Glasgow Coma Scale (Table 4.12) and record score. ● Changes over time: e.g. a period of lucidity (with or without a preceding episode of loss of consciousness) followed by decreasing conscious level might suggest the development of an extra-dural haematoma. ● Pupil size and reactivity. ● Presence of spontaneous limb movements. NB Any painful stimulus should be applied **ABOVE** the clavicles in case a cervical cord injury is present. Supra-orbital pressure, pinching the ear lobe, or pressure behind the angle of the jaw, are all acceptable; sternal rubbing should never be performed. **When recording a GCS:** ● Ensure each element is recorded separately. ● Be accurate, scoring the highest possible score for each element: e.g. if a patient does not respond to a painful stimulus on the right hand side, but localises to pain if the stimulus is applied to the left hand side then the score for localising must be recorded.
Decreased level of consciousness	Consider other causes for a decreased level of consciousness: ● **Convulsions** – a history of epilepsy might suggest the patient is post-ictal. ● **Hypo- or hyper-glycaemia** – a history of diabetes. ● **Alcohol or drugs** – intake of alcohol, recreational/prescription drug overdose. NB The presence of any of these findings does not necessarily rule out a concomitant head injury.
Wounds	● If brain matter can be seen, cover with a light dressing.

Head Trauma

Table 4.11 – ASSESSMENT and MANAGEMENT of:

Head Injury *continued*

ASSESSMENT	ADDITIONAL INFORMATION
Airway	• Patients with a decreased level of consciousness are at risk of airway obstruction because they are not be able to protect their own airway due to loss of muscle tone in the oropharyngeal structures and the loss of the gag reflex increases the risk of aspiration; this is potentially life-threatening and needs rapid intervention – **refer to airway management guideline**. NB Spinal immobilisation must be started at the same time as airway control – but does not take priority over airway control. Indications for spinal immobilisation include: GCS<15 on initial assessment, neck and back tenderness, focal neurological deficit, paraesthesia in the extremities or other clinical suspicions of cervical spine injury.
Ventilation	Consider assisted ventilation at a rate of 12–20 respirations per minute if: • Oxygen saturation (SpO$_2$) is <90% on high levels of supplemental oxygen. • Respiratory rate is <12 or >30bpm. • Inadequate chest expansion. **Refer to airway management guideline.**
Oxygen	• Administer high levels of supplemental oxygen; aim for SpO$_2$ <94–98% – refer to oxygen guideline.
Vital signs	• Monitor vital signs. • Monitor ECG.
Pain management	If pain relief is indicated **refer to pain management guidelines**. NB Pain can lead to arise in intracranial pressure.
Fluid	• Fluid therapy is not normally indicated in an isolated head injury. However if it becomes necessary – refer to intravascular fluid therapy guideline. Hypovolaemia will greatly exacerbate a serious head injury. Patients with a head injury and other injuries causing blood pressure to drop below 90 mmHg require fluid therapy. • **DO NOT** delay on scene for fluid replacement.
Combative patients	• A combative head-injured patient may be suffering from hypoxia or hypoventilation. NB Consider senior clinical input where combativeness compromises management.
Transfer to further care	• Transfer to the nearest appropriate facility according to local trauma care pathway. • Continue patient management en-route. • Provide an alert/information call. • Inform receiving staff of any relevant information from the scene about the mechanism of injury, images from the scene and changes in the patient's condition, e.g. periods of (un)consciousness, visual/speech disturbances, decreased sensation, general weakness, loss of balance, and or movement of limbs since the injury. Report any suspicions of non-accidental injury (**refer to safeguarding children guideline**). • Complete documentation.

Methodology

For full details of the methodology used in the development of this guideline refer to the guideline webpage.

Appendix – Glasgow Coma Scale

There are a number of issues in the assessment that should be considered:

- In the absence of eyelid muscle tone in a deeply unconscious person, the eyes may be open. If there is no response to stimulation, then this is recorded as 'none'.

- If there is severe facial swelling that would prevent eye opening, then this is documented as such.

- Deaf patients or those who cannot give a verbal response, such as those with a tracheostomy, are recorded as assessed, but a caveat should also be documented.

- During motor assessment, if there is a difference between the two sides of the body, the better response is recorded.

- Verbal response in small children does not fit with the scale and so a modification is utilised (Table 4.13).

Pupil response

- The pupils should be round and equal in size and respond promptly by constricting when a light is shone into them. When light is shone in one eye the other pupil should respond appropriately too. Any abnormalities should be documented.

- Abnormal findings might be due to trauma to the eye itself or pre-existing eye disease. Elderly patients may be taking medication to dilate or constrict the pupil and these can have a long duration of action. Prior administration of opiate analgesia may also be the cause. However, no unsupported assumptions should be made in the presence of head injury as abnormal pupillary response may be an indicator of significant brain injury and swelling.

Table 4.12 – GLASGOW COMA SCALE

Item		Score
Eyes Opening:		
	Spontaneously	4
	To speech	3
	To pain	2
	None	1
Motor Response:		
	Obeys commands	6
	Localises pain	5
	Withdraws from pain	4
	Abnormal flexion	3
	Extensor response	2
	No response to pain	1
Verbal Response:		
	Orientated	5
	Confused	4
	Inappropriate words	3
	Incomprehensible sounds	2
	No verbal response	1

Table 4.13 – MODIFIED GCS

Item	Score
Appropriate words, social smile, fixes and follows with eyes	5
Cries but consolable	4
Persistently irritable	3
Restless and agitated	2
None	1

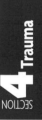

KEY POINTS

Head Trauma

- **NEVER presume a decreased conscious level is solely due to the effects of alcohol: intoxicated patients commonly sustain head injuries.**

- **Ascertain duration and depth of unconsciousness, as such findings signify the possibility of a significant injury.**

- **Unconscious patients are not capable of protecting their airway: obstruction may occur through loss of muscle tone with the tongue falling backwards, or by the accumulation of secretions or blood in the pharynx.**

- **A modified jaw thrust should be used for initial airway management due to the risk of cervical spine injury.**

- **The aim of prehospital treatment is to deliver adequate oxygen to the brain and maintain normal EtC02.**

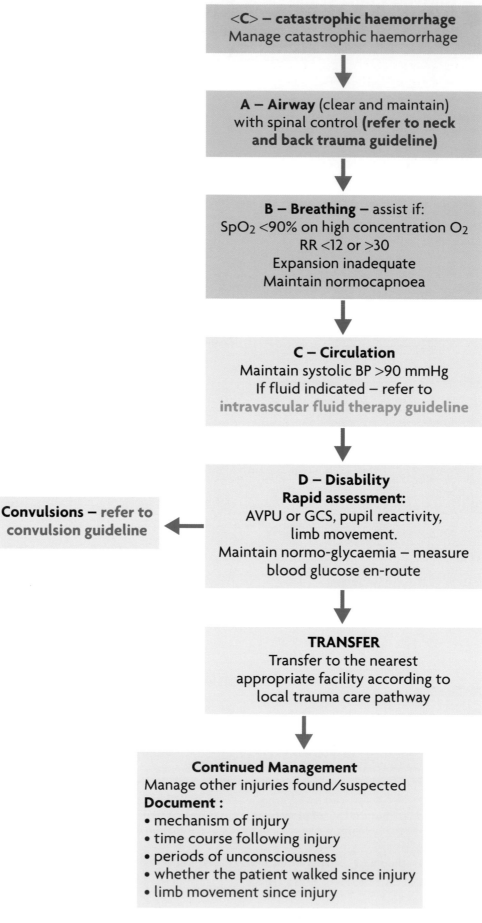

<C> – catastrophic haemorrhage
Manage catastrophic haemorrhage

A – Airway (clear and maintain)
with spinal control **(refer to neck
and back trauma guideline)**

B – Breathing – assist if:
SpO_2 <90% on high concentration O_2
RR <12 or >30
Expansion inadequate
Maintain normocapnoea

C – Circulation
Maintain systolic BP >90 mmHg
If fluid indicated – refer to
intravascular fluid therapy guideline

**Convulsions – refer to
convulsion guideline**

D – Disability
Rapid assessment:
AVPU or GCS, pupil reactivity,
limb movement.
Maintain normo-glycaemia – measure
blood glucose en-route

TRANSFER
Transfer to the nearest
appropriate facility according to
local trauma care pathway

Continued Management
Manage other injuries found/suspected
Document :
• mechanism of injury
• time course following injury
• periods of unconsciousness
• whether the patient walked since injury
• limb movement since injury

Figure 4.7 – Significant head injury algorithm.

SECTION
4 Trauma

Limb Trauma [29, 49, 521–548]

1. Introduction

- There is one fundamental rule to apply to limb trauma cases and that is **NOT** to let limb injuries, however dramatic in appearance, distract the clinician from less visible but life-threatening problems such as airway obstruction, compromised breathing, poor perfusion and spinal injury.

- Patients with limb trauma are likely to be in considerable pain and distress; therefore consider pain management as soon as clinically possible after arriving on scene (**refer to pain management guidelines**).

Table 4.14 – TYPES OF LIMB INJURY

Greenstick fracture
One side of the bone breaks, the other side bends – common accidental injury in children.

Transverse fracture
A fracture across the bone that occurs due to direct blow or force on the end of the bone e.g. a fall on the hand may break the forearm bones or the distal humerus.

Spiral or oblique fracture
A fracture around the bone or at an angle across it, due to a twisting force.

Compound fracture (open)
A fracture in which the bone is broken into multiple (more than two) pieces.

Comminuted fracture
A fracture that comprises small fragmented ends.

Closed fracture
A fracture that is contained i.e. skin is unbroken.

Dislocations
Dislocations are very painful and commonly affect the digits, elbow, shoulder, patella and occasionally the hip (high energy).

Compartment syndrome
A complication of limb fractures arising from increased pressure in muscular compartments due to contained haemorrhage. This can lead to ischaemia, with potentially catastrophic consequences for the limb.

Degloving
Degloving can accompany limb fractures and be to the superficial fascia or full depth down to the bone.

Amputations/partial amputations
Amputations most frequently involve digits, but can involve part or whole limbs. Amputations may still result in a viable limb, providing there is minimal crushing damage and survival of some vascular and nerve structures.

Neck of femur fractures
Such fractures commonly occur in the elderly and are one of the most common limb injuries encountered in the prehospital environment. Typical patients present with shortening and external rotation of the leg on the injured side, with pain in the hip and referred pain in the knee. The circumstances of the injury must be taken into account – often the elderly person has been on the floor for some time, which increases the possibility of hypothermia, dehydration, pressure sores and chest infection, so careful monitoring of vital signs is essential.

2. Pathophysiology

- The pathophysiology differs depending on the nature of the injury – refer to Table 4.14.

- Blood loss from femoral shaft fractures can be considerable, involving loss of 500–2000 millilitres in volume. If the fracture is open, blood loss is increased.

- Nerves and blood vessels are placed at risk from sharp bony fragments, especially in very displaced fractures, hence the need to return fractured limbs to normal alignment as rapidly as possible. Fractures around the elbow and knee are especially likely to injure arteries and nerves.

- The five 'P's of ischaemia are shown in Table 4.15.

Table 4.15 – 'P's OF ISCHAEMIA

Sign	Symptom
Pain	Out of proportion to the apparent injury; often in the muscle, which may not ease with splinting/analgesia.
Pallor	Due to compromised blood flow to limb.
Paralysis	Loss of movement.
Paraesthesia	Changes in sensation.
Pulselessness	The loss of peripheral pulses is a grave late sign caused by swelling which can lead to the complete occlusion of circulation.
Perishing cold	The limb is cold to the touch.

3. Incidence

- Limb trauma is a common injury in high energy impacts. Causes can include but are not limited to falls, sports, traffic, occupational and intentional causes, and can occur at any age.

- In older people injuries can occur from relatively minor trauma e.g. falls from a standing height can lead to femoral fractures.

4. Severity and Outcome

- The severity and outcome differ depending on the nature of the injury. However, limb trauma can have serious consequences, for example, infection following an open fracture can affect the future viability and long-term function of the limb.

Splinting

- Splinting will contribute to 'circulation' care by considerably reducing further blood loss and pain en-route to hospital.

- **Traction splint** – is a device for applying longitudinal traction to the femur, using the pelvis and the ankle as static points. Correct splintage technique using a traction splint reduces:
  - pain
  - haemorrhage and damage to blood vessels and nerves

Limb Trauma

- bone fragment movement and the risk of a closed fracture becoming an open fracture
- the risk of fat embolisation (brain and lungs)
- muscle spasm by pulling thigh to a natural cylindrical shape
- blood loss by compression of bleeding sites.

● Traction splints such as the Sager, Trac 3, Donway splints, Kendrick are easy to apply and some now have quantifiable traction, measured on a scale in pounds. The correct amount of traction is best judged by the injured leg being the same length as the uninjured limb.

5. Assessment and Management
For the assessment and management of limb trauma refer to Table 4.17.

Table 4.16 – SPLINTING

Injury	Splintage type
Fractured neck of femur	Padding between legs. Figure of eight bandage around ankles. Broad bandage: two above, two below the knee.
Fractured shaft of femur	Traction splint. NB Fractures of the ankle, tibia, fibula, knee or pelvis on the same side as the femoral fracture may limit use of a traction splint, Trust guidelines should be followed.
Fracture or fracture dislocation around the knee	Long leg box splint. Vacuum splint. Traction splint without the application of traction.
Patella dislocation	Companion strapping (one leg to the other). Support on pillow. Contoured vacuum splint. If the leg is gently straightened the patella often spontaneously relocates, if resistance is felt, the leg should be splinted in the position of comfort.
Tibia/fibula shaft fracture	Long leg box splint. Long vacuum splint.
Ankle fracture	Short leg box splint. Short vacuum splint.
Foot fractures	Short box splint. Short vacuum splint.
Clavicle Humerus Radius Ulna	Self-splintage may be adequate and less painful than a sling. Sling. Vacuum splints may be well suited to immobilising forearm fractures. Short box splint.

KEY POINTS

Limb Trauma

- Ensure <C>ABCs are assessed and managed; consider C-spine immobilisation.
- DO NOT become distracted, by the appearance of limb trauma, from assessing less visible but life-threatening problems, such as airway obstruction, compromised breathing, poor perfusion and spinal injury.
- Transfer to nearest appropriate hospital as per local trauma care pathway; provide an alert/information call.
- Limb trauma can cause life-threatening haemorrhage.
- Assess for intact circulation and nerve function distal to the fracture site.
- Any dislocation that threatens the neurovascular status of a limb must be treated with urgency.
- Splintage is fundamental to prevention of further blood loss and can reduce pain.
- Limb trauma can cause considerable pain and distress – consider pain management as soon as clinically possible after arriving on scene.
- In cases of life-threatening trauma commence a time critical transfer and perform any splinting en-route if possible.

Methodology
For details of the methodology used in the development of this guideline refer to the guideline webpage.

Table 4.17 – ASSESSMENT and MANAGEMENT of:

Limb Trauma

ASSESSMENT	MANAGEMENT

● Assess **<C>ABCD**	Control any external catastrophic haemorrhage – **refer to trauma emergencies overview**.
	● If any of the following **TIME CRITICAL** features are present:
	  – major **ABC** problems
	  – haemodynamic compromise – **refer to intravascular fluid management guideline**
	  – altered level of consciousness – **refer to altered level of consciousness guideline**
	  – neck and back injuries – **refer to neck and back trauma guideline**
	  – threatened limb – loss of neurovascular function e.g. as a result of a dislocation which requires prompt realignment, then:
	● Start correcting **A** and **B** problems.
	● Mid shaft femoral fracture – apply a traction splint if this can be applied quickly without delaying transfer, otherwise apply manual traction where sufficient personnel are available – once applied it should not be released.
	● Undertake a **TIME CRITICAL** transfer to nearest appropriate hospital as per local trauma care pathway.
	● Provide an alert/information call.
	● Continue patient management en-route.

● External haemorrhage	Control any external haemorrhage – **refer to trauma emergencies overview**.

● Specifically assess	● Ascertain the mechanism of injury and any factors indicating the forces involved e.g. the pattern of fractures may indicate mechanism of injury:
	  – fractures of the heel in a fall from a height may be accompanied by pelvic and spinal crush fractures (**refer to pelvic trauma and neck and back trauma guidelines**)
	  – 'dashboard' injury to the knee may be accompanied by a fracture or dislocation of the hip
	  – humeral fractures from a side impact are associated with chest injuries (**refer to thoracic trauma guidelines**)
	  – tibial fractures are rarely isolated injuries and often associated with high energy trauma and other life-threatening injuries.
	● All four limbs for injury to long bones and joints – in suspected fracture – expose site(s) to assess swelling and deformity.
	● Assess neurovascular function – MSC × 4: motor, sensation and circulation, distal to the fracture site. Assess foot pulses; palpate dorsalis pedis as capillary refill time can be misleading.
	● Assess general skin colour.
	● Assess age of patient – consider greenstick fractures in children, and fractures of wrist and hip in the elderly.
	● For accompanying illnesses:
	  – some cancers can involve bones (e.g. breast, lung and prostate) and result in fractures from minor injuries
	  – osteoporosis in elderly females makes fractures more likely.
	NB Where possible avoid unnecessary pain stimulus.

● Oxygen	● Administer high levels of supplemental oxygen (aim for SpO$_2$ 94–98%) **refer to oxygen guideline**.
● Splintage	In prehospital care it is difficult to differentiate between ligament sprain and a fracture; therefore **ASSUME** a fracture and immobilise. ● Remove jewellery from the affected limbs before swelling occurs. ● Check and record the presence/absence of pulses, and muscle function distal to injury. ● Consider realignment of grossly deformed limbs, to a position, as close to normal anatomic alignment as possible. Where deformity is minor and both distal sensation and circulation are intact, then realignment may not be necessary. ● If the pulse disappears during realignment then reposition limb slowly to previous site until pulse returns. ● Apply splintage, refer to Table 4.16. NB Vacuum splints are used if limbs need to be immobilised in an abnormal alignment. Rigid splints may need to be padded to conform to anatomy.

4 SECTION Trauma

Table 4.17 – ASSESSMENT and MANAGEMENT of:

Limb Trauma *continued*

ASSESSMENT	MANAGEMENT
• Compound fracture	• Irrigate grossly contaminated wounds with saline. • Apply a moist field dressing. • Any gross displacement from normal alignment must, where possible, be corrected, and splints applied (refer to Table 4.16). NB Document the nature of the contamination as contaminates may be drawn inside following realignment.
• Amputations, partial amputations and degloving	• Irrigate grossly contaminated wounds with saline. • Immobilise a partially amputated limb in a position of normal anatomical alignment. • Where possible dress the injured limb to prevent further contamination. • Apply a moist field dressing. NB Reimplantation following amputation or partial amputation may be possible; in order that the amputated parts are maintained and transported in the best condition possible: • Remove any gross contamination. • Cover the part(s) with a moist field dressing. • Secure in a sealed plastic bag. • Place the bag on ice – do not place body parts in direct contact with ice as this can cause tissue damage; the aim is to keep the temperature low but not freezing.
Neck of femur fractures	• Assess for shortening and external rotation of the leg on the injured side, with pain in the hip and referred pain in the knee. • Ascertain whether the patient has been on the floor for some time, assess for signs of hypothermia, dehydration, pressure sores and chest infection (refer to relevant guidelines). • Monitor vital signs. • Immobilise by strapping the injured leg to the normal one with foam padding between the limbs – extra padding with blankets and strapping around the hips and pelvis can be used to provide additional support whilst moving the patient (refer to Table 4.16).
• Compartment Syndrome	Consider the need for rapid transfer to nearest appropriate hospital as per local trauma care pathway as the patient may require immediate surgery elevate limb and consider pain relief en route.
• Pain management	• Pain management is an important intervention – if indicated **refer to pain management guidelines**.
• Fluid	• If fluid resuscitation is indicated – **refer to intravascular fluid therapy guideline**. • DO NOT delay on scene for fluid replacement if peripheral pulses are present.
• Non-accidental injury	When assessing an injury in a child, consider the possibility of non-accidental injury – **refer to safeguarding children guideline**.

• Transfer to further care	• Transfer to nearest appropriate hospital as per local trauma care pathway.
	• Continue patient management en-route.
	• Provide an alert/information call.
	• **At hospital inform staff of:**
	  – any skin wound relating to a fracture
	  – an underlying fracture(s) that was initially open.
	• Complete documentation.

Neck and Back Trauma

1. Introduction

- There are a number of injuries that can lead to Spinal Cord Injury (SCI) (see below).
- Effective management from the time of injury is important to ensure good outcomes. This guideline provides guidance for the assessment and management of neck and back trauma including indicators to guidance for related conditions.

2. Pathophysiology

- The spinal cord runs in the spinal canal down to the level of the second lumbar vertebra in adults.
- The amount of space in the spinal canal in the upper neck is relatively large, and risk of secondary injury in this area can be reduced if adequate immobilisation is applied. In the thoracic area, the cord is wide, and the spinal canal relatively narrow and injury in this area is more likely to completely disrupt and damage the spinal cord.
- Spinal shock is a state of complete loss of motor function and often sensory function found sometimes after SCI. This immediate reaction may go on for some considerable time, and some recovery may well be possible.
- Neurogenic shock is the state of poor tissue perfusion caused by sympathetic tone loss after spinal cord injury.

3. Incidence

- SCI most commonly affects young and fit people and will continue to affect them to a varying degree for the rest of their lives.
- Road traffic collisions, falls and sporting injuries are the most common causes of SCI – as a group, motorcyclists occupy more spinal injury unit beds than any other group involved in road traffic collisions. Roll over road traffic collisions where occupants are not wearing seatbelts, and the head comes into contact with the vehicle body and pedestrians struck by vehicles are likely to suffer SCI. Ejection from a vehicle increases the risk of injury significantly.

Risk Factors

Road traffic collisions (RTC):

- Rollover RTC.
- Non-wearing of seatbelts.
- Ejection from vehicle.
- Struck by a vehicle.

Sporting injuries:

- Diving into shallow water.
- Horse riding.
- Rugby.
- Gymnastics and trampolining.

Falls:

- Older people.
- Rheumatoid arthritis.
- Certain sporting accidents, especially diving into shallow water, horse riding, rugby, gymnastics and trampolining have a higher than average risk of SCI.

Rapid deceleration injury such as gliding and light aircraft accidents also increase the risk of SCI.

- Older people and those with rheumatoid arthritis are prone to odontoid peg fractures, that may be difficult to detect clinically. Such injuries can occur from relatively minor trauma e.g. falls from a standing height.

4. Severity and Outcome

- Injury most frequently occurs at junctions of mobile and fixed sections of the spine. Hence fractures are more commonly seen in the lower cervical vertebrae where the cervical and thoracic spine meets (C5, 6,7/T1 area) and the thoracolumbar junction (T12/L1) (Figure 4.8). Of patients with one identified spinal fracture, 10–15% will be found to have another.
- In the extreme, SCI may prove immediately fatal where the upper cervical cord is damaged, paralysing the diaphragm and respiratory muscles.
- Partial cord damage, however, may solely affect individual sensory or motor nerve tracts producing varying long-term disability. It is important to note that there is an increasing percentage of cases where the cord damage is only partial and some considerable recovery is possible, providing the condition is recognised and managed appropriately.

5. Immobilisation

- All patients with the possibility of spinal injury should have manual immobilisation commenced at the earliest time, whilst initial assessment is undertaken.
- If immobilisation is indicated then the whole spine must be immobilised.

Only **two** methods are acceptable:

1. Manual immobilisation whilst the back is supported.
2. Collar, head blocks and back support.

NB There are several acceptable means of back support and the optimal method will vary according to circumstances. The following techniques may be used:

1. Patient lying supine:

- Use a scoop stretcher and head immobilisation. This can be achieved with a minimal amount of log rolling, and is preferable.
- Log roll patient with manual immobilisation of the neck to enable long extrication board to be used. Log rolling can result in lateral movement throughout the spinal column as well as disrupting clots and caution is advised.
- Directly lift patient using a spinal lift if there are adequately trained personnel on scene or use a scoop stretcher then insert a vacuum mattress underneath patient.
- Patients should be transported on the scoop stretcher unless there is a prolonged journey time where a vacuum mattress should be utilised.

2. Patient lying prone:

- Log roll patient with manual immobilisation of the neck to enable scoop stretcher to be used. This can be achieved with a minimal amount of log rolling as is preferable.

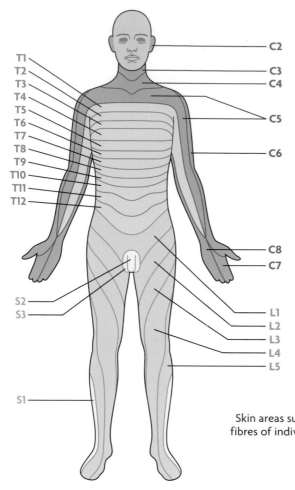
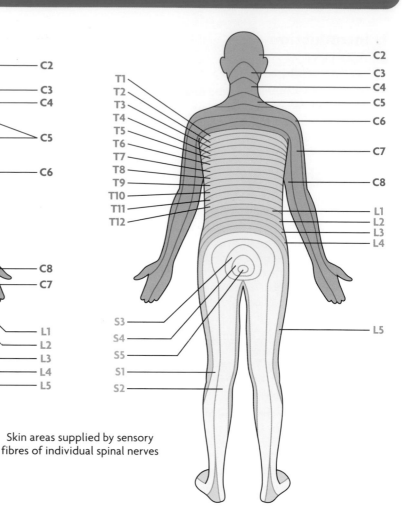

Skin areas supplied by sensory
fibres of individual spinal nerves

Figure 4.8 – Spinal nerves.

- 2-stage log roll on to a vacuum mattress.

3. Patient requiring extrication:

- Extrication devices should be used if there is any risk of rotational movement.
- Rearward extrication on an extrication board.
- Slide extrication invariably involves some rotational component and therefore has higher risks in many circumstances.

The techniques for use of devices are described in Pre-hospital Trauma Life Support (PHTLS) and other manuals.

5.1 Cautions/precautions
Vomiting

- Vomiting and consequent aspiration are serious consequences of immobilisation. Ambulance clinicians must always have a plan of action in case vomiting should occur.
- The collar will usually need to be removed and manual in-line immobilisation instituted. This may include:
  - suction
  - head-down tilt of the immobilisation device
  - rolling onto side on the immobilisation device.

Restless/combatative patients

- There are many reasons for the patient to be restless and it is important to rule out reversible causes e.g. hypoxia, pain, fear.

- If, despite appropriate measures the patient remains restless, then immobilisation techniques may need to be modified. A struggling patient is more likely to increase any injury, so a compromise between full immobilisation and degree of agitation/movement is appropriate.
- The use of restraint can increase forces on the injured spine and therefore a 'best possible' approach should be adopted.

Head injury

- Patients with a head injury may have raised intracranial pressure which restraint can increase; therefore, a 'best possible' approach should be adopted.

Special cases

- Some older patients, and those with cervical spine abnormalities e.g. ankylosing spondylitis, may not be able to breathe adequately when positioned absolutely flat or tolerate a collar. Therefore a 'best possible' approach should be adopted which may include manual in-line immobilisation or maintenance of the pre-existing spinal deformity e.g. ankylosing spondilytis where putting the position is unsafe.

Immobilisation – evidence for how to immobilise

A recent Cochrane review found no randomised controlled trials comparing out of hospital spinal immobilisation techniques:

SECTION **4** Trauma

- Soft collars do not limit movement and should not be used.
- There is variable difference between the various types of semi-rigid collars.
- Addition of side supports and tapes increases immobilisation.
- Combining collar with extrication board improves immobilisation.
- The application of devices is more important than the variation of devices.
- Neutral position needs slight flexion of the neck and the occiput should be raised by two centimetres in an adult. Extrication devices are better than extrication boards at reducing rotational movement.
- Patients should spend no longer than 30 minutes on a rigid extrication board, but padding can extend this time.
- Vacuum mattress is more comfortable, and gives better immobilisation.
- Vacuum mattresses cannot be used for extrication and are vulnerable to damage.
- Log-rolling is not without risk and use of the scoop stretcher may be safer for lifting patients.
- Long extrication/spinal board should only be used as an extrication device. Usually patients should be immobilised using a scoop. Once on a scoop they should remain on a scoop unless they are placed on a vacuum mattress when there is a prolonged journey time.

Emergency extrication

- If there is an immediate threat to life, for example, fire or airway obstruction that cannot be resolved in-situ, then the ambulance clinicians must decide on the relative risks of spinal immobilisation and the other factors.
- Rapid extrication techniques with manual immobilisation of the cervical spine are appropriate in these circumstances; this includes side extrication.

5.2 Immobilisation – when not to apply immobilisation

- Penetrating injury to the head has not been shown to be an indication for spinal immobilisation, and even penetrating injuries of the neck only rarely need selective immobilisation.
- A small prospective prehospital study indicated that the presence of **ALL** the following criteria can exclude significant spinal injury:
  - normal mental status with ability to appreciate pain
  - no neurological deficit
  - no spinal pain or tenderness
  - no evidence of intoxication
  - no evidence of distracting injury e.g. extremity fracture.
- The few patients missed with SCI are often at the extremes of age. Such criteria can be reproducibly used in the prehospital environment. Mechanism of injury was not shown to be an independent predictor of injury.

- Use of such guidelines can significantly reduce the use of unnecessary immobilisation.
- Some patients may sustain thoracic or lumbar injuries, in addition to, or in isolation from cervical spine injuries. If you suspect thoracic or lumbar injuries whether the cervical spine has been cleared, then full spinal immobilisation should be undertaken whenever possible.

5.3 Immobilisation – hazards

The value of routine prehospital spinal immobilisation remains uncertain and any benefits may be outweighed by the risks of rigid collar immobilisation, including:

1. airway difficulties
2. increased intracranial pressure
3. increased risk of aspiration
4. restricted ventilation
5. dysphagia
6. skin ulceration
7. can induce pain, even in those with no injury.

5.4 Sequence for immobilisation

- All patients should be initially immobilised if the mechanism of injury suggests the possibility of SCI.

Blunt trauma

- Following assessment it is possible to remove the immobilisation if **ALL** the criteria are met (refer to the immobilisation algorithm Figure 4.9).
- Spinal pain does not include tenderness isolated to the muscles of the side of the neck.

Penetrating trauma

- Those with isolated penetrating injuries to limbs or the head do not require immobilisation.
- Those with truncal or neck trauma should be immobilised if there is new neurology and/or the trajectory of the penetrating wound could pass near or through the spinal column.

5.5 Children

- None of the studies have been validated in children. It is recommended that these guidelines are interpreted with caution in children although there is some evidence to support similar principles.
- In children it is difficult to assess the neutral position but a padded board, head blocks, straps and collar appear to be the optimal method.

6. Assessment and Management

For assessment and management of neck and back trauma refer to Table 4.18 and Figure 4.8.

Methodology

For details of the methodology used in the update of this guideline refer to the guideline webpage.

Table 4.18 – ASSESSMENT and MANAGEMENT of:

Neck and Back Trauma

ASSESSMENT	MANAGEMENT
● Assess **<C>ABCD** whilst controlling the spine	● Control any external catastrophic haemorrhage – **refer to trauma emergencies overview guideline**. ● All patients with the possibility of spinal injury should have manual immobilisation commenced at the earliest time, whilst initial assessment is undertaken.
● Evaluate whether the patient is **TIME CRITICAL** or **NON-TIME CRITICAL**	● Follow criteria in trauma emergencies overview. ● If the patient is **TIME CRITICAL**: – control the airway – immobilise the spine – transfer to the nearest suitable receiving hospital – provide a hospital alert/information message – continue patient management en-route (see below).
● Assess oxygen saturation (refer to oxygen guideline)	● Adults – administer high levels of supplemental oxygen and aim for target saturation within the range of 94–98% – except for patients with COPD. ● Children – administer high levels of supplemental oxygen.
● Determine mechanism of injury – forces causing injury include	● Hyperflexion. ● Hyperextension. ● Rotation. ● Compression. ● One or more of these.
● Specific symptoms of SCI	The patient may complain of: ● Neck or back pain. ● Loss of sensation in the limbs. ● Loss of movement in the limbs. ● Sensation of burning in the trunk or limbs. ● Sensation of electric shock in the trunk or limbs.
● Rapidly assess to determine presence and estimate level of spinal cord injury	The following signs may indicate injury: ● Diaphragmatic or abdominal breathing. ● Hypotension (BP often <80–90 mmHg) with bradycardia. ● Warm peripheries or vasodilatation in presence of low blood pressure. ● Flaccid (floppy) muscles with absent reflexes. ● Priapism – partial or full erection of the penis. **In a conscious patient** – assess sensory and motor function. ● Use light touch and response to pain. ● Examine upper limbs and hands. ● Examine lower limbs and feet. ● Examine both sides. ● Undertake the examination in the **MID-AXILLARY** line **NOT** the **MID-CLAVICULAR** line as **C2**, **C3**, and **C4** all supply sensation to the nipple line; use the forehead as the reference point to guide what is normal sensation. NB Always presume SCI in the unconscious trauma victim.
● If the patient is non-time critical, perform a more thorough assessment with a brief secondary survey	
● Assess for neurogenic shock	Diagnosis is difficult in prehospital care – the aim is to: ● Maintain blood pressure of approximately 90 mmHg systolic. ● Obtain IV access. ● Determine need for fluid replacement but **DO NOT** delay on scene (refer to intravascular fluid therapy guideline). ● In neurogenic shock, a few degrees of head-down tilt may improve the circulation, but remember that in cases of abdominal breathing, this manoeuvre may further worsen respiration and ventilation. This position is also unsuitable for a patient who has, or may have, a head injury. ● If bradycardia is present consider atropine (refer to atropine guideline) – but it is important to rule out other causes, e.g. hypoxia, severe hypovolaemia.
● Assess the need for assisted ventilation	● **Refer to airway management guideline**.

Table 4.18 – ASSESSMENT and MANAGEMENT of:

Neck and Back Trauma *continued*

• Steroids	• Evidence is conflicting on the use of early high dose steroids in acute spinal cord injury. If benefit exists then steroids need to be given within 8 hours of injury and therefore can be delayed until arrival at hospital.
• At hospital	• In addition to the usual information given at the time of hand-over it is important to inform the hospital staff of the duration period of immobilisation. • Assist in the early removal from the extrication board. • Complete documentation.
	ADDITIONAL INFORMATION Transportation of spinal patients: • Driving should balance the advantages of smooth driving and time to arrival at hospital. No immobilisation technique eliminates movement from vehicle swaying and jarring. The technique of loosening the collar is not supported by evidence. • There is no evidence to show advantage of direct transport to a spinal injury centre. • Patients can tolerate 30-minutes on a long extrication board. The receiving ED should be told how long the patient has already been on the board so they can make an appropriate judgement on the timing of its removal. The duration of time on the extrication board should be recorded on the clinical record. The extrication board should be removed as soon as possible on arrival in hospital. • If a journey time of greater than 30-minutes is anticipated, the patient should be transferredfrom the extrication board using an orthopaedic ('scoop') stretcher to a vacuum mattress. It may be appropriate to immobilise the patient using a vacuum mattress in the first instance in non-extrication situations. • If there is a clear paralysing injury to the spinal cord then the benefits of the back board may be limited, while the risk of pressure sores may be very high. In these circumstances, the use of a vacuum mattress is often preferred. • However, as half of cases of spinal injuries have other serious injuries, any unnecessary delay at scene or in transit should be avoided.

KEY POINTS

Neck and Back Trauma

- **Immobilise the spine until it is positively cleared.**
- **Immobilise the spine of all unconscious blunt trauma victims**
- **If the neck is immobilised the thoracic and lumbar spine also need immobilisation.**
- **Standard immobilisation is by means of collar, headblocks, tapes and scoop or long board where patients require extrication.**
- **Aspiration of vomit, pressure sores and raised intracranial pressure are major complications of immobilisation.**

4 Trauma
SECTION

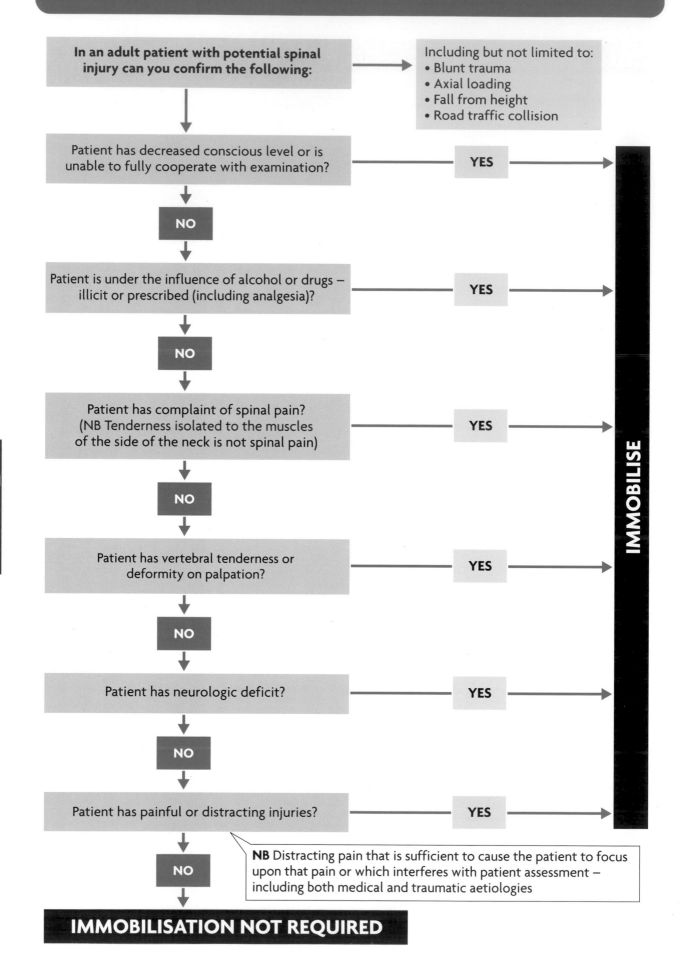

Figure 4.9 – Immobilisation algorithm.

1. Introduction

Major pelvic injuries are predominantly observed where there is a high-energy transfer to the patient such as might occur following road traffic collision, pedestrian accident, fall from height, or crush injury.

Less serious pelvic injuries may also occur following low-energy transfer events, particularly in the elderly (such as a simple fall), amongst patients with degenerative bone disease or receiving radiotherapy, and rarely as a direct consequence of seizure activity.

The majority of pelvic injuries do not result in major disruption of the pelvic ring, but rather involve fractures of the pubic ramus or acetabulum. Presentation of these injuries is very similar to neck of femur fractures; therefore please **refer to the limb trauma guideline** for management of these less serious pelvic injuries.

Mechanism of injury
- High energy transfer
- Fall from height
- Crush injury

Risk Factors
- Advancing age
- Degenerative bone disease
- Radiotherapy

2. Incidence

Pelvic fractures represent 3–6% of all fractures in adults and occur in up to 20% of all polytrauma cases. They display a bimodal distribution of age with most injuries occurring in the age ranges 15–30 and over 60 years; up to 75% of all pelvic injuries occur in men.

Unstable pelvic fracture is estimated to occur in up to 20% of pelvic fractures; a further 22% of pelvic fractures will remain stable despite significant damage to the pelvic ring. The remaining 58% of pelvic fractures are less serious retaining both haemodynamic and structural stability.

The incidence of pelvic fracture resulting from blunt trauma ranges from 5% to 11.9%; with obese patients more likely to sustain a pelvic fracture from blunt trauma than non-obese patients. Pelvic fracture associated with penetrating trauma is far less frequent. Open pelvic fractures are rare and account for only 2.7–4% of all pelvic fractures.

3. Severity and Outcome

Major pelvic injuries can be devastating and are often associated with a number of complications that may require extensive rehabilitation. Pelvic trauma deaths frequently occur as a result of associated injuries and complications rather than the pelvic injury itself.

Haemorrhage is the cause of death in 40% of all pelvic trauma victims and the leading cause of death (60% of fatal cases) in unstable pelvic fracture. Bleeding is usually retroperitoneal; the volume of blood loss correlates with the degree and type of pelvic disruption.

Reported mortality rates range from 6.4% to 30% depending on the type of pelvic fracture, haemodynamic status, and the nature of concomitant injuries and their complications.

The mortality rate among haemodynamically stable patients is around 10%, whereas the mortality rate amongst haemodynamically unstable patients approaches 20–30% but has been reported to be as high as 50% in cases of unstable open fracture; combined mortality approaches 16%.

4. Pathophysiology

4.1 Skeletal Anatomy

Increasing pelvic volume allows for increased haemorrhage; conversely, reducing pelvic volume reduces potential for bleeding by realignment of broken bone ends.

4.2 Classification of Injury

As with other fractures, pelvic fractures may be classified as open or closed, and benefit from being further described as either haemodynamically stable or unstable. Patients who are haemodynamically unstable are at greater risk of death and would benefit greatly from a suitable prehospital alert message.

Pelvic ring disruptions (as identified by in-hospital imaging) can be subdivided into four classes by mechanism of injury: antero-posterior compression (APC), lateral compression (LC), vertical shear (VS), and combined mechanical injury (CMI), a combination of the aforementioned classes.

4.3 Vascular Injury

The arteries most frequently injured are the iliolumbar arteries, the superior gluteal, and the internal pudendal because of their proximity to the bone, the sacro-iliac joint and the inferior ligaments of the pelvis. Bleeding from the venous network after a pelvic fracture is more frequent than arterial bleeding because the walls of the veins are more fragile than arteries. Blood may pool in the retroperitoneal space and haemostasis may occur spontaneously in closed fractures, especially if there is no concomitant arterial haemorrhage.

4.4 Other Injuries

The incidence of urogenital injury ranges from 23% to 57%. Urethral and vaginal injuries are the most common injuries. Vaginal lacerations result from either penetration of a bony fragment or from indirect forces from diastasis of the symphysis pubis. Injuries to the cervix, uterus and ovaries are rare. Bladder rupture occurs in up to 10% of pelvic fractures.

The incidence of rectal injury ranges from 17% to 64% dependent upon type of fracture. Bowel entrapment is rare.

Pelvic injury is commonly associated with concomitant intra-thoracic and or intra-abdominal injury.

Major Pelvic Trauma

Table 4.19 – ASSESSMENT and MANAGEMENT of:

Major Pelvic Trauma

ASSESSMENT

- Assess: **<C> ABCD; <C> catastrophic haemorrhage**
  - Airway
  - Breathing
  - Disability (mini neurological examination).
- Evaluate whether patient is **TIME CRITICAL** or **NON-TIME CRITICAL** following criteria as per trauma emergencies guideline. If patient is **TIME CRITICAL, correct A and B problems, stabilise the pelvis on scene, and rapidly transport to nearest suitable receiving hospital. Provide an alert/information call.** En-route, continue patient management of pelvic trauma (see below).
- In **NON-TIME CRITICAL** patients perform a more thorough patient assessment with a brief Secondary Survey.

Specifically Consider

- Pelvic fracture should be considered based upon the mechanism of injury.
- Clinical assessment of the pelvis includes observation for physical injury such as bruising, bleeding, deformity or swelling to the pelvis. Shortening of a lower limb may be present (see also **limb trauma guideline**).
- Assessment by compression or distraction (e.g. springing) of the pelvis is unreliable and may both dislodge clots and exacerbate any injury and should not be performed. Any patient with a relevant mechanism of injury and concomitant hypotension **MUST** be managed as having a **time critical pelvic injury** until proven otherwise.
- Reduction and stabilisation of the pelvic ring should occur as soon as is practicable whilst still on scene, as stabilisation helps to reduce blood loss by realigning fracture surfaces, thereby limiting active bleeding and additionally helping to stabilise clots. Reduction of the pelvis may have a tamponade effect, particularly for venous bleeding; however there is little evidence to support this belief.
- Log rolling of the patient with possible pelvic fracture should be avoided as this may exacerbate any pelvic injury; where possible utilise an orthopaedic scoop stretcher to lift patients off the ground and limit movement to a 15° tilt.

MANAGEMENT

- Control any external catastrophic haemorrhage – **refer to trauma emergencies overview**.

Oxygen Therapy

- Major pelvic injury falls into the category of critical illness and requires high levels of supplemental oxygen regardless of initial oxygen saturation reading (SpO$_2$). Maintain high flow oxygen (15 litres per minute) until vital signs are normal; thereafter reduce flow rate, titrating to maintain oxygen saturations (SpO$_2$) in the 94–98% range (refer to oxygen guideline).

Pelvic Stabilisation

There is currently no evidence to suggest that any particular pelvic immobilisation device or approach is superior in terms of outcome in pelvic trauma and a number of methods have been reported. Effective stabilisation of the pelvic ring should be instigated at the earliest possible opportunity, preferably before moving the patient, and may be achieved by:

- Use of an appropriate pelvic splint.
- Apply the pelvic splint directly to skin, if this can be done easily with minimal handling.
- Expert consensus suggests the use of an appropriate pelvic splint is preferable to improvised immobilisation techniques. In all methods, circumferential pressure is applied over the greater trochanters and not the iliac crests. Care must be exercised so as to ensure that the pelvis is not reduced beyond its normal anatomical position.
- Pressure sores and soft tissue injuries may occur when immobilisation devices are incorrectly fitted.

Fluid Therapy

- There is little evidence to support the routine use of IV fluids in adult trauma patients; refer to the intravascular fluid therapy guideline.

Pain Management

- Patients' pain should be managed appropriately (**refer to pain management guidelines**); analgesia in the form of entonox (refer to entonox drug guidelines for administration and information) or morphine sulphate may be appropriate (refer to morphine drug guidelines for dosages and information).

5. Referral Pathway

5.1 The following cases should ALWAYS be transferred to further care:

- Any patient with hypotension and potential pelvic injury **MUST** be treated as a **TIME CRITICAL** pelvic injury until proven otherwise.
- Any patient with sufficient mechanism of injury to cause a pelvic injury.

5.2 The following cases MAY be considered suitable/safe to be left at home:

- None.

6. Special Considerations for Children
(See also paediatric trauma guideline.)

- Pelvic fractures represent 1–3% of all fractures in children, thus there is a lower incidence compared with adults.
- In children, pelvic injuries have a lower mortality accounting for 3.6–5.7% of trauma deaths, with fewer deaths occurring as a direct result of pelvic haemorrhage; blood loss is more likely to be from solid visceral injury than the pelvis.
- Different injury patterns – multi-system injuries in 60%; greater incidence of diaphragmatic injury.
- Principles of management are the same, with the exception of fluid and oxygen therapy (**refer to fluid therapy and oxygen guidelines**).
- Clinical findings in small children can be unreliable.

7. Audit Information

- Incidence of suspected/actual pelvic fracture.
- Incidence of concomitant hypotension.
- Frequency of pelvic immobilisation when pelvic fracture suspected.
- Method of pelvic immobilisation.

Methodology

For details of the methodology used in the development of this guideline refer to the guideline webpage.

KEY POINTS

Pelvic Trauma

- **Pelvic fracture should be considered based upon mechanism of injury.**
- **The majority of pelvic fractures are stable pubic ramus or acetablar fractures.**
- **Any patient with hypotension and potentially relevant mechanism of injury MUST be considered to have a TIME CRITICAL pelvic injury.**
- **'Springing' or distraction of the pelvis must not be undertaken.**
- **Pelvic stabilisation should be implemented as soon as is practicable whilst still on scene.**
- **Consider appropriate pain management.**
- **The use of a scoop stretcher is recommended to avoid log rolling the patient unless extrication is required.**

1. Introduction

- In prehospital care, the most common problem associated with severe thoracic injuries is hypoxia, either from impaired ventilation or secondary to hypovolaemia from massive bleeding into the chest (haemothorax) or major vessel disruption (e.g. ruptured thoracic aorta).

2. Incidence

- Severe thoracic injuries are one of the most common causes of death from trauma accounting for approximately 25% of such deaths.

3. Severity and Outcome

- Despite the very high percentage of serious thoracic injuries, the vast majority of them can be managed in hospital with chest drainage and resuscitation and only 10–15% require surgical intervention.

4. Pathophysiology

- The mechanism of injury is an important guide to the likelihood of significant thoracic injuries. Injuries to the chest wall usually arise from direct contact, for example, intrusion of wreckage in a road traffic collision or blunt trauma arising from direct blow. Seat belt injuries fall into this category and may cause fractures of sternum, ribs and clavicle.

- If the force is sufficient, the deformity and the damage to the chest wall structures may induce tearing and contusion to the underlying lung and other structures. This may produce a combination of severe pain on breathing (pleuritic pain) and a damaged lung, both of which will significantly reduce the ability to ventilate adequately. This combination is a common cause of **hypoxia**.

- Blunt trauma to the sternum may cause myocardial contusion which may result in cardiac rhythm disturbances (ECG rhythm disturbances).

- Penetrating trauma may well damage the heart, the lungs and great vessels both in isolation or combination. It must be remembered that **penetrating wounds to the upper abdomen and neck may well have caused injuries within the chest remote from the entry wound**. Conversely, penetrating wounds to the chest may well involve the liver, kidneys and spleen.

- The lung may be damaged with bleeding causing a haemothorax or an air-leak causing a pneumothorax. Penetrating or occasionally a blunt injury may result in cardiac injuries. Blood can leak into the non-elastic surrounding pericardial sac and build up pressure to an extent that the heart is incapable of refilling to pump blood into circulation. This is known as **cardiac tamponade** and can be fatal if not rapidly relieved at hospital (see additional information in Table 4.21).

- Rapid deceleration injuries may result in sheering forces sufficient to rupture great vessels such as the aorta, caused by compressing the vessels between the sternum and spine.

- The six major thoracic injuries encountered in the prehospital setting include:
  i) a tension pneumothorax,
  ii) massive haemothorax (following, uncontrolled haemorrhage into the chest cavity
  iii) open chest wounds,
  iv) flail chest,
  v) cardiac tamponade
  vi) air embolism.

5. Assessment/Management

For the assessment and management of thoracic trauma refer to Table 4.20 and 4.21.

Methodology

For details of the methodology used in the development of this guideline refer to the guideline webpage.

KEY POINTS

Thoracic Trauma

- **Thoracic injury is commonly associated with hypoxia, either from impaired ventilation or secondary to hypovolaemia from massive bleeding into the chest (haemathorax) or major vessel disruption.**

- **Count respiratory rate and look for asymmetrical chest movement.**

- **Pulse oximetry MUST BE used as this will assist in recognising hypoxia.**

- **The mechanism of injury is an important guide to the likelihood of significant thoracic injury.**

- **Blunt trauma to the sternum may induce myocardial contusion which may result in ECG rhythm disturbances.**

- **ECG monitoring.**

- **Impaling objects should be adequately secured. If the object is pulsating do not completely immobilise, but allow the object to pulsate.**

- **Do not probe or explore penetrating injuries.**

Table 4.20 – ASSESSMENT and MANAGEMENT of:

Thoracic Trauma

ASSESSMENT	MANAGEMENT

● Assess **<C>ABCD**	● Control any external catastrophic haemorrhage – **refer to trauma emergencies overview guideline**.
	● If any of the following **TIME CRITICAL** features are present:
	  – major ABCD problems
	  – penetrating chest injury
	  – flail chest
	  – tension pneumothorax
	  – air embolism
	  – cardiac tamponade
	  – surgical emphysema
	  – blast injury to the lungs, then:
	● Correct **A** and **B** problems.
	● Undertake a **TIME CRITICAL** transfer to the nearest appropriate receiving hospital.[a]
	● Provide an alert/information call.
	● Continue patient management en-route.

● If the patient is **NON-TIME CRITICAL** undertake a brief secondary survey	

● Specifically consider:
  – tension pneumothorax
  – open chest wounds
  – flail chest
  – surgical emphysema
  – cardiac tamponade
  – air embolism
  – impaling objects.
	Refer to Table 4.21 for the assessment and management of these conditions/situations.

● Monitor SpO_2 and assess for signs of hypoxia – NB Normal readings **DO NOT** exclude hypoxia	● Administer high levels of supplemental oxygen until the vital signs are normal then aim for a target saturation within the range of 94–98% (**refer to oxygen guideline**).
● Monitor heart rate and rhythm	● Attach ECG monitor.
● Assess breathing adequacy, respiratory rate, effort and volume, and equality of air entry	Consider assisted ventilation at a rate of 12-20 respirations per minute, if any of the following are present: ● SpO_2 <90% on high levels of supplemental oxygen. ● Respiratory rate is <12 or >30 breaths per minute. ● Inadequate chest expansion. NB Exercise caution as any positive pressure ventilation may increase the size of a pneumothorax.
● Consider the need for IV fluids	● Refer to the fluid therapy guideline – **DO NOT** delay on scene. ● Obtain IV access.
● Assess patient's level of pain	**Refer to the pain management guideline**. NB Avoid **entonox** in a patient with chest injury as there is a significant risk of enlarging a pneumothorax. NB Adequate morphine analgesia may improve ventilation by allowing better chest wall movement, but high doses may induce respiratory depression. Careful titration of doses is therefore required (**refer to morphine drug guideline for dosage and information**). ● Transfer to further care. ● Provide an alert/information call. ● Continue patient management en-route.
Assessment (children) ● Assess as above	Management (children) Manage as above but consider: ● Children can have severe internal chest injuries with minimal or no external evidence of chest injuries.

[a]Patients should normally be transported in a semi recumbent or upright posture, however this may often not be possible due to other injuries present or suspected.

Thoracic Trauma

Table 4.20 – ASSESSMENT and MANAGEMENT of:

Thoracic Trauma *continued*

ASSESSMENT	MANAGEMENT
Assessment (children) *continued*	Management (children) *continued* ● Children show signs of shock late due to good compensatory mechanisms. ● Always consider multiple injuries in children with rib fractures as this suggests a significant mechanism of injury and isolated chest injuries are rare in children. ● Consider non-accidental injury.
	ADDITIONAL INFORMATION ● Chest trauma is treated with difficulty in the field and prolonged treatment before transportation is **NOT** indicated if significant chest injury is suspected. ● Penetrating trauma – in particular where lung or cardiac wounds are suspected, patients must be transferred to further care immediately to the nearest appropriate receiving hospital, with resuscitation en-route and an alert/information call. **Open chest wounds** – seal the wound with a non-occlusive dressing. ● Specifically consider the need for thoracic surgery intervention. ● **Impaling objects** – handle carefully, secure the object with dressing and if the object is pulsating do not completely immobilise it but allow the object to pulsate. NB Be vigilant – the patient may try to remove the object and this could be used as a weapon. ● Remember any stab or bullet wound to the chest, abdomen or back may penetrate the heart. ● Patients with significant chest trauma may often insist on sitting upright and this especially common in patients with diaphragmatic injury who may get extremely breathless when lying down. In this instance a decision will have to be made as to whether a patient is best managed sitting upright or whether spinal immobilisation should be continued. ● In the rare incident of gunshot/stab injury to personnel wearing protection vests e.g. ballistic and stab, these may protect from penetrating injury. However, serious underlying blunt trauma (e.g. pulmonary contusion) may be caused to the thorax. ● **NEVER UNDERESTIMATE THESE INJURIES**. There is a strong link between serious chest wall injury and thoracic spine injury. Maintain a high index of suspicion.

Table 4.21 – ASSESSMENT and MANAGEMENT of:

Specific Thoracic Trauma

Flail Chest

Flail chest is usually the result of a significant blunt chest injury, causing two or more rib fractures in two or more places. A sternal flail can also occur where the ribs or costal cartilages are fractured on both sides of the chest. This results in a flail segment that moves independently of the rest of the chest during respiration leading to inadequate ventilation. The ensuing pulmonary insufficiency is caused by three patho-physiological processes:

1. The negative pressure required for effective ventilation is disrupted due to the paradoxical motion of the flail segment.
2. The underlying pulmonary contusion which causes haemorrhage and oedema of the lung.
3. The pain associated with the multiple rib fractures will result in a degree of hypoventilation.
● Small flailed segments may not be detectable.
● Large flail segments may impair ventilation considerably as a result of pain.

ASSESSMENT	MANAGEMENT
● Assess for signs of a flail chest	● Flail segments should not be immobilised and efforts to maintain ventilation are the priority. NB Traditionally, the patient has been turned onto the affected side for transportation, but this **CANNOT** be achieved on a long board.
● Assess patient's level of pain	● Consider the need for analgesia – if indicated **refer to the pain management guidelines**.
	● Undertake a **TIME CRITICAL** transfer to the nearest appropriate receiving hospital. ● Provide an alert/information call. ● Continue patient management en-route.

SECTION **4** Trauma

Table 4.21 – ASSESSMENT and MANAGEMENT of:

Specific Thoracic Trauma *continued*

Tension pneumothorax

- This is a rare respiratory emergency which may require immediate action at the scene or en-route to further care. A tension pneumothorax occurs when a damaged area of lung leaks air out into the pleural space on each inspiration, but does not permit the air to exit from the chest via the lung on expiration.
- This progressively builds up air under tension on the affected side collapsing that lung and putting increasing pressure on the heart and great vessels and the opposite lung. Decreased venous return is significantly affected by the kinking of the vessels, especially the inferior vena cava, as the mediastinum is pushed towards the contralateral side. Coughing and shouting can make a situation worse. If this air is not released externally, the heart will be unable to fill and the other lung will no longer be able to ventilate inducing cardiac arrest.
- Tension pneumothorax is most related to penetrating trauma but can arise spontaneously from blunt or crushing injuries to the chest and as the result of a blast wave. This will present rapidly with an increase in breathlessness and extreme respiratory distress (respiratory rate often >30 breaths per minute). Subsequently the patient may deteriorate and the breathing rate may rapidly slow to <10 breaths per minute before the patient arrests.
- **Signs and symptoms:** the chest on the affected side may appear to be moving poorly or not at all; at the same time, the affected chest wall may appear to be over-expanded (hyperexpansion); air entry will be greatly reduced or absent on the affected side. In the absence of shock, the neck veins may become distended. Later, the trachea and apex beat of the heart may become displaced away from the side of the pneumothorax and cyanosis and breathlessness may appear. Hyperresonance may be present. Occasionally, the patient will only present with rapidly deteriorating respiratory distress. The patient may appear shocked as a result of decreased cardiac output. They are usually tachycardic and hypotensive.
- Ventilation of a patient with a chest injury is a common cause of tension pneumothorax in the prehospital setting. Forcing oxygenated air down into the lung under positive pressure will progressively expand a small, undetected simple pneumothorax into a tension pneumothorax. This will take some minutes and may well be several minutes after ventilation has commenced. It is usually noticed by increasing back pressure during ventilation; either by the bag becoming harder to squeeze or the ventilator alarms sounding.

ASSESSMENT	MANAGEMENT
• Assess breathing adequacy, respiratory rate and volume, and equality of air entry **FEEL, LOOK, AUSCULTATE and PERCUSS** • View both sides of the chest and check they are moving; auscultate to ensure air entry is present and percuss on both sides	• If a tension pneumothorax is confirmed, decompress rapidly by needle thoracocentesis.
• Closely monitor the patient to ensure the procedure was successful	• If the procedure was unsuccessful repeat the thoracocentesis. Consider the use of a thicker needle in patients with a thicker chest wall, following Trust guidelines.
	• Undertake a **TIME CRITICAL** transfer to the nearest appropriate receiving hospital. • Provide an alert/information call. NB Needle thoracocentesis may not always decompress pneumothoraces in large patients. In such cases, a thoracostomy with or without a chest drain may need to be performed. This needs to be done either in hospital or by appropriately skilled practitioners e.g. BASICS or HEMS doctors on scene or in hospital.

Air embolism

Air embolism – is a rare fatal complication of penetrating injury involving the central chest. It can also occur if an IV line is left open.

ASSESSMENT	MANAGEMENT
• Assess for signs of air embolism – If a conscious patient becomes unconscious or develops neurological signs in the absence of a head injury, the possibility of an air embolism must be raised	• The patient should be transported in the head down position. • Undertake a **TIME CRITICAL** transfer to the nearest appropriate receiving hospital. • Provide an alert/information call.

Table 4.21 – ASSESSMENT and MANAGEMENT of:

Specific Thoracic Trauma *continued*

Cardiac tamponade

The heart is enclosed in a tough, non-elastic membrane, called the pericardium. A potential space exists between the pericardium and the heart itself. If a penetrating wound injures the heart, the blood may flow under pressure into the

pericardial space. As the pericardium cannot expand, a leak of as little as 20–30 mls of blood can cause compression of the heart! This decreases cardiac output and causes tachycardia and hypotension. Further compression reduces cardiac output and cardiac arrest may occur.

ASSESSMENT	MANAGEMENT
● Assess for signs of cardiac tamponade ● Signs of hypovolaemic shock, tachycardia and hypotension, accompanied by blunt or penetrating chest trauma may be an indication of cardiac tamponade ● Note presence of distended neck veins and muffled heart sounds when with a stethoscope	● Cardiac tamponade is a **TIME CRITICAL LIFE-THREATENING** condition that requires rapid surgical intervention in an open chest operation to evacuate the compressing blood. ● **DO NOT** delay on scene inserting cannulae or commencing fluid therapy.
● Transfer	● Undertake a **TIME CRITICAL** transfer to the nearest appropriate receiving hospital. ● Provide an alert/information call.
● Re-assess ABC	NB Pericardiocentesis is not recommended in the prehospital setting as it is rarely successful and has significant complications and delays definitive care.

Surgical emphysema

Surgical emphysema – produces swelling of the chest wall, neck and face with a cracking feeling under the fingers when the skin is pressed. This indicates an air leak from within the chest, either from a pneumothorax, a ruptured large airway or a fractured larynx.

Normally it requires no specific treatment but it does indicate potentially **SERIOUS** underlying chest trauma. Sometimes the

surgical emphysema might be extensive and cause the patient to swell up. Where the emphysema is progressively increasing, look for a possible underlying tension pneumothorax.

In some cases, surgical emphysema may become so severe as to tighten the overlying skin and restrict chest movement. A tension pneumothorax must be excluded as above. If there is no improvement, the patient must be transferred to hospital as soon as possible.

ASSESSMENT	MANAGEMENT
● Assess for signs of surgical emphysema swelling of the chest wall, neck and face with a cracking feeling under the fingers when the skin is pressed	
● Consider possible underlying tension pneumothorax	● Refer to tension pneumothorax for guidance.
	● Undertake a **TIME CRITICAL** transfer to the nearest appropriate receiving hospital. ● Provide an alert/information call.

Blast injury

Blast injury – is caused by three mechanisms:

1. Rupture of air-filled organs
2. Missiled debris
3. Contact injury.

NB Although rare in survivors, strongly suspect a blast lung injury if the patient is suffering from tympanic injury. However the absence of a tympanic injury **DOES NOT** exclude lung injury.

NB Being shielded from blast debris **DOES NOT** exclude lung injury.

ASSESSMENT	MANAGEMENT
● Assess for blast injury	● Prehospital management is supportive.
	● Undertake a **TIME CRITICAL** transfer to the nearest appropriate receiving hospital. ● Provide an alert/information call.

Trauma in Pregnancy [329, 870, 873–877]

1. Introduction

- The management of obstetric patients with major injuries requires a special approach.
- Mechanism of injury may indicate possible trauma to enlarged internal organs and structures especially trauma occurring in the third trimester. For example, trauma to the gravid uterus during domestic violence can be linked to placental abruption.
- It is important to remember that resuscitation of the mother facilitates resuscitation of the fetus.

2. Incidence

- In the UK 5% of maternal deaths are as a result of trauma with a high proportion related to domestic violence and road traffic collisions.

Mechanism of injury
- Domestic violence.
- High energy transfer.
- Fall from height.

3. Severity and Outcome

- Managing an obstetric patient with major trauma is rare; both blunt and penetrating trauma causing catastrophic haemorrhage, and significant burns are the likely causes.

4. Pathophysiology

- There are a number of physiological and anatomical changes during pregnancy that may influence the management of the obstetric patient (**refer to obstectric and gynaecology overview guideline**).

Methodology

For details of the methodology used in the development of this clinical practice guideline refer to the guideline webpage.

Table 4.22 – ASSESSMENT and MANAGEMENT of:

Trauma in pregnancy

ASSESSMENT	MANAGEMENT
• Quickly scan the patient and scene as you approach. • Undertake a primary survey **<C>ABCDEF** – specifically assess for: • Abdominal pain – should be presumed to be significant and may be associated with internal unseen blood loss. • Vaginal blood loss. • Abruption may occur three–four days after the initial incident. • Stage of the pregnancy. • Any problems with the pregnancy. • Fetal movements (refer to obstetric and gynaecology overview guideline). • Whether the mother has her pregnancy record card available.	• Control external catastrophic haemorrhage using direct and indirect pressure or tourniquets where indicated – **refer to trauma emergencies overview**. • Open, maintain and protect the airway in accordance with the patient's clinical need. • Administer high levels of supplemental oxygen and aim for a target saturation within the range of 94–98% (refer to oxygen guideline). Provide assisted ventilation as indicated (**refer to airway management guideline**). • Manually displace the uterus to the left or tilt the patient to the left (15–30 degrees) (**refer to obstetric and gynaecology emergencies overview**). • Provide cervical spine protection as necessary (**refer to neck and back trauma guideline**). • Manage thoracic injuries (**refer to thoracic trauma guideline**). NB The management of thoracic injuries are the same as for the non-obstetric patient. • Insert a **large bore** IV cannula – do not delay transfer. • Administer intravascular fluids as indicated to maintain a systolic blood pressure of 90 mmHg (refer to intravascular fluid therapy guideline).
• Undertake a secondary survey **CABCDEF**.	
• Assess patient's level of pain.	• Pain management (**refer to adult pain management guidelines**) NB Administer morphine cautiously if the patient is hypotensive. • Apply splints as appropriate e.g. pelvis (**refer to pelvic trauma guideline**), long bone fractures (**refer to limb trauma guideline**).
• Assess blood glucose.	• Measure blood glucose en-route.
	• Nil by mouth.
• Assess for burns and scalds.	• For the management of burns treat as non-obstetric patient (**refer to the burns and scalds guideline** / refer to intravascular fluid therapy guideline).

KEY POINTS

Trauma in Pregnancy

- Main principle of treatment is that resuscitation of the mother facilitates resuscitation of the fetus.

- Compression of the inferior vena cava by the pregnant uterus (>20 weeks) is a serious potential complication; tilt the patient 15–30 degrees to the left side or manually displace the uterus.

- Signs of shock appear very late and hypotension is an extremely late sign. Any signs of hypovolaemia during pregnancy are likely to indicate a 35% (class III) blood loss and must be treated aggressively.

- All trauma is significant.

- If the mother is found in cardiac arrest or develops cardiac/respiratory arrest en-route, commence life support and alert the hospital so that an obstetrician can be on standby in the ED for emergency caesarean section.

- Abruption may occur three–four days after the initial incident.

Burns and Scalds (Adults) [49, 745–821]

1. Introduction

- Burns arise in a number of accident situations, and may have a variety of presentations (Table 4.23), accompanying injuries or pre-existing medical problems associated with the burn injury. Scalds, flame or thermal burns, chemical and electrical burns will all produce a different burn pattern, and inhalation of smoke or toxic chemicals from the fire may cause serious accompanying complications.

- A number of burn patients will also be seriously injured following falls from a height in fires, or injuries sustained as a result of road traffic collision where a vehicle ignites after a collision or crash.

- Explosions will often induce flash burns, and other serious injuries due to the effect of the blast wave or flying debris.

- Inhalation of superheated smoke, steam or gases in a fire, will induce major airway swelling and respiratory obstruction – refer to Table 4.24 for signs of airway burns. The likelihood of an airway injury increases with the presence of multiple risk factors or signs.

- Non-accidental injury should always be considered when burns have occurred in vulnerable adults including the elderly, in particular where the mechanism of injury described does not match the injury sustained, or there is inconsistency in the history (**refer to safeguarding adults guideline**).

Table 4.23 – BURNS/SCALDS

Electrical
Search for entry and exit sites. Assess ECG rhythm. The extent of burn damage in electrical burns is often impossible to assess fully at the time of injury (refer to guidelines).

Thermal
The skin contact time and temperature of the source determines the depth of the burn. Scalds with boiling water are frequently of short duration as the water flows off the skin rapidly. Record the type of clothing, e.g. wool retains the hot water. Those resulting from hot fat and other liquids that remain on the skin may cause significantly deeper and more serious burns. Also the time to cold water and removal of clothing is of significant impact.

Chemical
It is vital to note the nature of the chemical. Alkalis in particular may cause deep, penetrating burns, sometimes with little initial discomfort. Certain chemicals such as phenol or hydrofluoric acid can cause poisoning by absorption through the skin and therefore must be irrigated with COPIOUS amounts of water for a minimum of 15 minutes (this should be continued until definitive care is available if patient condition and water supply allows (**refer to CBRNE guideline**).

Table 4.24 – SIGNS/INCREASED RISK OF AIRWAY BURNS

Signs
- Facial or neck burns.
- Soot in the nasal and oral cavities.
- Coughing up blackened sputum.
- Cough and hoarseness.
- Difficulty with breathing and swallowing.
- Blistering around the mouth and tongue.
- Scorched hair, eyebrows or facial hair.
- Stridor or altered breath sounds such as wheezing.
- Loss of consciousness.
- Fires/blasts in enclosed spaces.

- Preceding long-term illness, especially chronic bronchitis and emphysema, will seriously worsen the outcome from airway burns.

- Remember that a burn injury may be preceded by a medical condition causing a collapse (e.g. elderly patient with a stroke collapsing against a radiator).

- Burns can be very painful (**refer to pain management in adults guideline**).

2. Burn Severity

- Refer to Wallace's Rule of Nines or the Lund and Browder chart to assess TBSA.

- For small or large burns (<15% or > 85%) it is acceptable to use the patient's palmar surface including the fingers as a size estimate. This equates to approximately 1% total body surface area (TBSA).

- Be aware of the risk of underestimating the size of burns with patients with large breasts or the obese patient. These factors can significantly affect the proportion of total body surface area using standardised charts.

- Use all of the burn area, but do not consider areas of erythema as this is often transient in the initial phases of a burn. Do not try to differentiate between levels of burn (superficial, partial thickness, full thickness etc.) as it is impractical to estimate the depth of burns in the initial hours following injury.

- Only a rough estimate is required; an accurate measure is not possible in the early stages; however, the size of a burn may well influence referral and management pathways.

3. Assessment and Management

- For the assessment and management of burns and scalds in adults refer to Table 4.25.

Burns and Scalds (Adults)

Table 4.25 – ASSESSMENT and MANAGEMENT of:

Burns and Scalds in Adults

ASSESSMENT	MANAGEMENT
● Ensure scene safety for rescuer and patient	**If safe to do so, stop the burning process:** ● Remove from the burn source. ● Brush off dry chemical.
● Assess **ABCD**	● If any of the following **TIME CRITICAL** features present: — major ABCD problems — airway burns (soot or oedema around the mouth and nose) — history of hot air or gas inhalation; these patients may initially appear well but can deteriorate very rapidly and need complex airway intervention — respiratory distress — evidence of circumferential (completely encircling) burns of the chest, neck, limb — significant facial burns — burns >15% total body surface area (TBSA) — presence of other major injuries, then: ● Start correcting A and B and undertake a **TIME CRITICAL** transfer to nearest appropriate hospital according to local care pathways. ● Continue patient management en-route. ● Provide an alert/information call.
● Specifically assess:	● Airway patency as early intervention may be required with inhalational burns; if intubation is impossible, needle cricothyroidotomy is the management of choice. ● Breathing for rate, depth and any breathing difficulty – **refer to airway management guideline**. ● Evidence of trauma – for neck and back trauma **refer to neck and back trauma guideline**. ● Co-existing or precipitating medical conditions.
● Oxygen	● Administer supplemental **oxygen** via a non-rebreathing mask – SpO_2 readings may be false due to carboxyhaemoglobin.
● Cool/irrigate the burn	● Irrigate with copious amounts of water (minimum 15 minutes chemical burns; maximum of 20 mins for all other burns to avoid hypothermia) – as soon as is practicable, this can still be effective up to 3 hours after the injury. ● Cut off burning, or smouldering clothing, providing it is not adhering to the skin. ● Remove any constricting jewellery including rings. ● **DO NOT** use ice or ice water as this can worsen the burn injury. ● Use saline if no other irrigant available. ● Gel based dressings may be used but water treatment is preferred. ● Alkali burns require prolonged irrigation – continue until definitive care.
● Assess burn size	● Rule of Nines or Lund and Browder Chart. ● Patient's palmar surface including adducted fingers. ● Consider obesity and large breasts when estimating burn size.
● Dress the burn	● Use small sheets of clingfilm – do not wrap around limbs but layer the film. ● In the absence of clingfilm use a wet non-adherent dressing. NB Do not apply creams/ointments; they interfere with the assessment process.
● Fluid resuscitation	If indicated refer to intravascular fluid therapy guideline.
● Wheezing	If the patient is wheezing as a result of smoke inhalation: ● Administer nebulised **salbutamol** (refer to salbutamol guideline) 6–8 litres of O_2 per minute.
● Assess the need for analgesia	If indicated: **refer to pain management guideline in adults**. NB Cooling and application of dressings frequently eases pain.
● Documentation	● How the patient was burned. ● Time the burn occurred and how long patient was exposed to source of burning. ● Temperature of the source of burning (e.g. boiling water, hot fat etc.). ● Whether first aid was undertaken? ● Time and volume of infusions.
● Transfer to further care	● Consider receiving service; refer to local guidance. ● Complete documentation.

Table 4.25 – ASSESSMENT and MANAGEMENT of:

Burns and Scalds in Adults *continued*

ASSESSMENT	MANAGEMENT
● **Alkali burns** to the skin and eye(s)[a]	● Irrigate with water and continue en-route to hospital – it may take hours of irrigation to neutralise the alkali – this also applies to eyes which require copious and continual irrigation ideally with water or saline in the absence of a water source.
● **Acid/chemical burns** to the skin and eye(s)[a]	● Irrigate copiously ideally with water or saline if no water source available. NB Specific treatment agents may be available in industrial settings with on-site medical/ first aid.
● **Chemical burns**	● **DO NOT** wrap in clingfilm. ● Cover with wet dressings (**refer to CBRNE guideline**).
● **Circumferencial burns**	● Encircling completely a limb or digit. Full thickness burns, may be 'limb threatening', and require early in-hospital incision/release of the burn area along the length of the burnt area of the limb (surgical escharotomy).

[a] When irrigating the eyes ensure that the fluid runs away from the contralateral eye to avoid contamination.

Methodology

For details of the methodology used in the development of this guideline refer to the guideline webpage.

KEY POINTS

Burns and Scalds in Adults

- **Airway status can deteriorate rapidly and may need complex interventions available at the emergency departments.**
- **Stopping the burning process is essential.**
- **The time from burning is an essential piece of information.**
- **Pain relief is important.**
- **Consider non-accidental injury in vulnerable adults including the elderly.**

1. Introduction

- Burns and scalds are relatively common in children and can arise from a number of accidental situations. They have a variety of presentations (Table 4.26) and children may present with accompanying injuries or pre-existing medical problems associated with the burn injury. Scalds, flame or thermal burns, chemical and electrical burns will all produce a different burn pattern, and inhalation of smoke or toxic chemicals from the fire may cause serious accompanying complications.

- A number of burn cases will also be seriously injured following falls from a height in fires, or injuries sustained as a result of road traffic collision where a vehicle ignites after an accident.

- Explosions will often induce flash burns, and other serious injuries due to the effect of the blast wave or flying debris.

- Inhalation of superheated smoke, steam or gases in a fire, will induce major airway swelling and may lead to fatal airway obstruction – refer to Table 4.27 for signs of airway burns. The likelihood of an airway injury increases with the presence of multiple risk factors or signs.

- Non-accidental injury should always be borne in mind when burns have occurred in small children, in particular where the mechanism of injury described does not match the injury sustained, or there is inconsistency in the history (**refer to safeguarding children guideline**).

Table 4.26 – BURNS/SCALDS

Electrical
Search for entry and exit sites.
Assess ECG rhythm.
The extent of burn damage in electrical burns is often impossible to assess fully at the time of injury.

Thermal
The skin contact time and temperature of the burning fluid determines the depth of the burn.
Scalds with boiling water are frequently of extremely short duration as the water flows off the skin rapidly.
Record the type of clothing, e.g. wool retains the hot water.
Scalds resulting from hot fat and other liquids that remain on the skin may cause significantly deeper and more serious burns.
Times of contact, the application of cold water and the removal of clothing determine tissue damage.

Chemical
It is vital to note the nature of the chemical. Alkalis cause deep, penetrating burns, sometimes with little initial discomfort. Certain chemicals such as phenol or hydrofluoric acid can cause poisoning by absorption through the skin and therefore must be irrigated with **copious** amounts of water for a minimum of 15 minutes (this should be continued until definitive care if patient condition and water supply allows).

Table 4.27 – SIGNS/INCREASED RISK OF AIRWAY BURNS

Signs
- Facial or neck burns.
- Soot in the nasal and oral cavities.
- Coughing up blackened sputum.
- Cough and hoarseness.
- Difficulty with breathing and swallowing.
- Blistering around the mouth and tongue.
- Scorched hair, eyebrows or facial hair.
- Stridor or altered breath sounds such as wheezing.
- Loss of consciousness.
- Fires/blasts in enclosed spaces.

- Preceding long-term illness, especially respiratory disease, will seriously worsen outcome.

- Burns can be very painful (**refer to pain management in children guideline**).

2. Burn Severity

Calculation of Burn Area

- The Rule of Nines does not work in children under the age of 14 because of different body proportions.

- Local guidance or charts such as the Lund and Browder Paediatric Chart should be used; a rough guide is to assume that the size of the palmar surface of the child's hand, including the digits equates to approximately 1% of the total body surface area (TBSA) of the child.

- Use all of the burn area, but do not consider areas of erythema as this is often transient in the initial phases of a burn injury. Attempts to differentiate burn depths (e.g. superficial, partial thickness, full thickness etc.) in the initial hours following injury are not helpful.

3. Assessment and Management

For the assessment and management of burns and scalds in children refer to Table 4.28.

SECTION
4
Trauma

Table 4.28 – ASSESSMENT and MANAGEMENT of:

Burns and Scalds in Children

ASSESSMENT	MANAGEMENT
● Ensure scene safety for rescuer and patient	**If safe to do so, stop the burning process.** ● Remove from the burn source. ● Brush off dry chemical.

● Assess **ABCD**	● Identify **TIME CRITICAL** features such as:
	  – major ABCD problems
	  – airway burns (soot or oedema around the mouth and nose)
	  – history of hot air or gas inhalation; these patients may initially appear well but can deteriorate very rapidly and need complex airway intervention
	  – respiratory distress
	  – evidence of circumferential (completely encircling) burns of the chest, neck, limb
	  – significant facial burns
	  – burns >10% total body surface area (TBSA)
	  – presence of other major injuries e.g. possible C-spine injury in explosions, then:
	● Start correcting **A** and **B** and undertake a **TIME CRITICAL** transfer to nearest appropriate hospital according to local care pathways.
	● Continue patient management en-route.
	● Provide an alert/information call.

● Specifically assess:	● Airway patency as early intervention may be required with inhalational burns; if intubation is impossible, needle cricothyroidotomy is the management of choice. ● Breathing for rate, depth and any breathing difficulty – **refer to airway and breathing management guideline**. ● Evidence of trauma – for neck and back trauma **refer to neck and back trauma guideline**. ● Co-existing or precipitating medical conditions.
● Oxygen	● Administer supplemental oxygen via a non-rebreathing mask – SpO_2 readings may be false due to carboxyhaemoglobin.
● Cool/irrigate the burn	● Irrigate with copious amounts of water (chemical burns: minimum 15 minutes); all other burns: 20 minutes but **NO LONGER as this may cause hypothermia**. This can still be beneficial up to 3 hours after the injury. ● Cut off burning, or smouldering clothing, providing it is not adhering to the skin. ● **DO NOT** use ice or ice water as this can worsen the burn injury and exagerate hypothermia. ● Use saline if no other irrigant available. ● Gel based dressings may be used but water treatment is preferred. ● Alkali burns require prolonged irrigation – continue until definitive care.
● Assess burn size	● Lund and Browder Paediatric Chart. ● Child's palmar surface including adducted fingers. ● NB Consider obesity when estimating burn size.
● Dress the burn	● Use small sheets of clingfilm – do not wrap around limbs but layer the film. ● In the absence of clingfilm use a wet non-adherent dressing. NB Do not apply creams/ointments as they compromise assessment.
● Assess the need for fluid resuscitation	Large burns (>10%) require intravenouse fluids refer to intravascular fluid therapy in children guideline. ● If IV access is required, obtain on a non-affected limb, where possible.
● Wheezing	If the patient is wheezing as a result of smoke inhalation: ● Administer nebulised salbutamol (refer to salbutamol guideline) 6–8 litres of O_2 per minute.
● Assess the need for child's pain score	If indicated: ● Obtain IV access. ● Refer to pain management guideline in children. NB Cooling and application of dressings frequently eases pain.
● Documentation	● How the patient was burned. ● Time the burn occurred and how long patient was exposed to source of burning. ● Temperature of the source of burning (e.g. boiling water, hot fat etc.). ● What treatments have been undertaken. ● Time and volume of infusions.
● Transfer to further care	● Consider receiving service; refer to local guidance.

Burns and Scalds (Children)

Table 4.28 – ASSESSMENT and MANAGEMENT of:

Burns and Scalds in Children *continued*

ASSESSMENT	MANAGEMENT
● **Chemical burns**	● Cover in clingfilm; **DO NOT** wrap in clingfilm. ● Cover with wet dressings (**refer to CBRNE guideline**).
● **Alkali burns** to the skin and eye(s)[a]	● Irrigate with water and continue en-route to hospital. It may take hours of irrigation to neutralise the alkali. ● Alkali burns to the eyes require copious and continual irrigation ideally with water (saline can be used in the absence of a water source).
● **Acid/chemical burns** to the skin and eye(s)[a]	● Irrigate copiously ideally with water or saline if no water source available. NB Specific treatment agents may be available on site e.g. medical kit or first aid boxes.
● **Circumferential burns**	● Encircling completely a limb or digit. Full thickness burns, may be 'limb threatening', and require early in-hospital incision/release of the burn area along the length of the burnt area of the limb (a surgical escharotomy).

[a] When irrigating the eyes ensure that the fluid runs away from the contralateral eye to avoid contamination.

Methodology

For details of the methodology used in the development of this guideline refer to the guideline webpage.

KEY POINTS

Burns and Scalds in Children

- **Warm the child and cool the burn.**
- **Consider the possibility of other injuries including inhalational injury, spinal injury.**
- **Give early adequate analgesia.**
- **Large burns (>10%) require intravenous fluids** (see intravascular fluid therapy in children guideline).
- **Consider non-accidental injury when burns have occurred in small children; in particular where the mechanism of injury does not match the injury sustained, or there is inconsistency in the history.**

1. Introduction

- Electrical injury is potentially life-threatening.
- In adults incidents generally occur in the workplace, involving high voltage electricity (415 volts).
- In children incidents generally occur in the home and involve lower voltage electricity (240 volts).
- Electrical injury may also result from a lightning strike which may deliver up to 300kV.

2. Incidence

- In the UK, approximately 1000 people at work are injured following contact with an electrical supply; of these 25 will die from their injuries (HSE).
- Electrical injuries resulting from a lightning strike lead to approximately 1,000 deaths per annum worldwide.

3. Severity and Outcome

- Electrical injury can cause serious multi-system damage leading to morbidity and mortality. This is caused by electric shock and tissue damage from the thermal effects along the current pathway.

The nature and extent of injury depends on:

- The voltage and whether it is alternating (AC) or direct (DC).
- The magnitude of the current.
- Resistance to current flow.
- Duration of exposure to the current.
- The pathway of the current – current traversing the myocardium is more likely to be fatal and hand-to-hand travel is more dangerous than hand-to-foot or foot-to-foot.

4. Pathophysiology

Injury occurs when electricity passes through the body causing:

- **Cardiac** arrhythmias e.g. ventricular fibrillation; cardio-respiratory arrest can arise from the direct effects of the current on cell membranes and smooth muscle as it traverses the myocardium. Myocardial ischaemia can occur due to spasm of the coronary artery.

- **Burns** to the skin at the point of contact (entry and exit) and in deeper tissues, including viscera, muscles and nerves as thermal energy traverses the body and tends to follow neurovascular bundles. Unusual burn patterns my be left on the body following a lightning strike.
- **Trauma** including joint dislocation, fractures and compartment syndrome can arise from sustained tetanic muscle contraction, falling or being thrown.
- **Muscular paralysis** may occur from contact with high voltage electricity affecting the central respiratory control system or respiratory muscles.
- **Pregnancy** can be affected depending on the magnitude and duration of contact with the current.

5. Assessment and Management

For the assessment and management of electrical injuries refer to Table 4.29 and Figure 4.10.

Methodology

For details of the methodology used in the development of this guideline refer to the guideline webpage.

KEY POINTS

Electrical Injuries

- **Scene safety.**
- **Manage cardiac/respiratory arrest.**
- **Consider trauma.**
- **Severe tissue damage may be present despite apparently minor injury.**
- **Exposure to domestic voltage may not require hospitalisation.**

Electrical Injuries

Table 4.29 – ASSESSMENT and MANAGEMENT of:

Electrical Injuries

ASSESSMENT	MANAGEMENT
⚠ Ensure scene safety for rescuer and patient	⚠ **DO NOT** approach the patient until the electricity supply is cut off and you are certain it is safe to approach.
	NOTE: Attach defibrillator pad at the earliest opportunity and keep defibrillator with the patient until hand-over to hospital staff.
● Assess **ABCD**	● If any of the following **TIME CRITICAL** features present: – major **ABCD** problems – cardio-respiratory arrest – **refer to advanced life support guideline** – facial/airway burns – **refer to airway management guideline** – cardiac arrhythmia – **refer to cardiac rhythm disturbance guideline** – significant trauma – **refer to appropriate trauma guideline** – extensive burns – **refer to burns and scalds guideline** then: ● Start correcting A and B and undertake a **TIME CRITICAL** transfer to nearest receiving hospital or specialist burns unit if appropriate. ● Continue patient management en-route. ● Provide an alert/information call.
● Burn process	● Remove smouldering clothing and shoes to prevent further thermal injury – **refer to burns and scalds guideline**.
● Specifically assess:	● Airway patency as early intervention may be required. ● Breathing for rate, depth and any breathing difficulty – **refer to airway management guideline**. ● Heart rate/rhythm – undertake a 12-lead ECG: – arrhythmias are unlikely to develop in cases of contact with domestic low voltage sources once the patient is isolated from the current – in cases of contact with high voltage sources arrhythmias may develop later. ● Evidence of trauma e.g. neck and back, burns – **refer to appropriate trauma guideline**. ● Magnitude of the current i.e. domestic low voltage (≤240 volts)/industrial high voltage (>480 volts).
● Oxygen	● Administer supplemental oxygen and aim for a target saturation within the range of 94–98%.
● Fluid	● If fluid resuscitation indicated – refer to intravascular fluid therapy guideline.
● Assess the need for pain relief	● If pain relief indicated – **refer to pain management guideline**.
● Transfer to further care	● **ALL** patients exposed to high voltage current. ● Patients exposed to a domestic or low voltage electrical source, who are asymptomatic, with no injuries and have normal initial 12-lead ECG may not require hospital assessment.

SECTION **4** Trauma

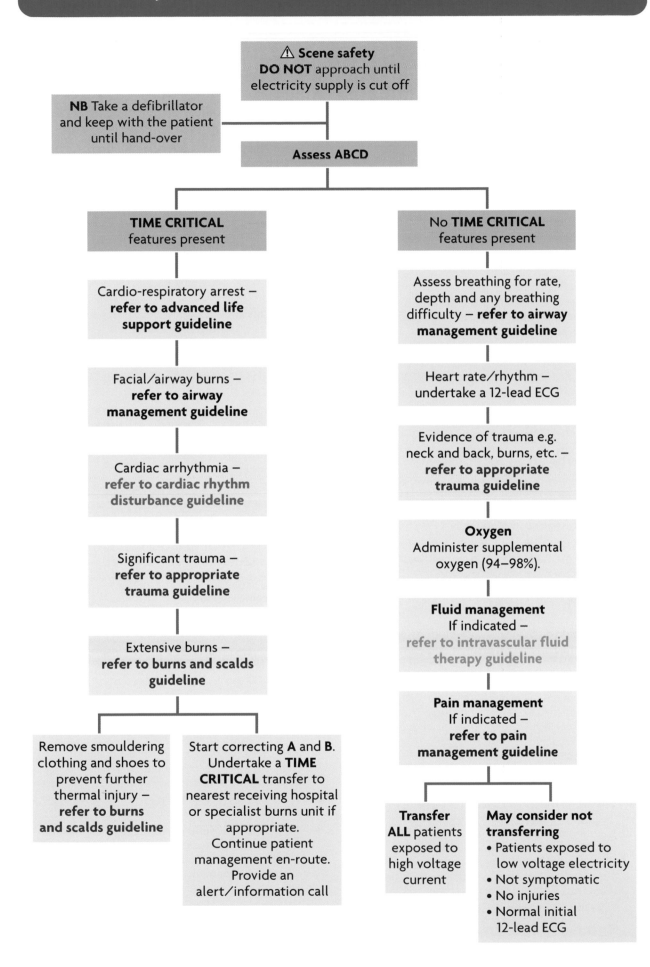

Figure 4.10 – Assessment and management of electrical injuries algorithm.

Immersion and Drowning [60, 835–868]

1. Introduction

- Drowning is a common cause of accidental death.
- **Drowning** refers to the 'process resulting in primary respiratory impairment from submersion/immersion in a liquid medium'. Thus the person is prevented from breathing air due to liquid medium at the entrance of the airway. NB Drowning does not infer that the patient has died.
- **Immersion** refers to being covered in a liquid medium and the main problems will be hypothermia and cardiovascular collapse from the hydrostatic pressure of the surrounding water on the lower limbs.
- **Submersion** refers to the entire body, including the airway being under the liquid medium and the main problems are asphyxia and hypoxia.
- **Exacerbating factors** – intoxication from alcohol or drugs may often accompany incidents. Occasionally, an immersion incident may be precipitated by a medical cause such as a convulsion.

2. Incidence

- Worldwide there are approximately 450,000 deaths per year with 205 deaths from accidental drowning occurring in England and Wales in 2009; with many more near-drownings. A high percentage of deaths will involve young males and children.

3. Severity and Outcome

- The extent of hypoxia and hypothermia, resulting from duration of immersion and/or submersion and/or the temperature of the liquid medium will determine severity and outcome.
- Concomitant trauma may result; for example, 0.5% of patients may suffer neck and/or head injury; diving into shallow water is a common cause.

4. Pathophysiology

- Following submersion, the patient will initially try to hold their breath. They may develop laryngospasm as water irritates the vocal cords or may aspirate large quantities of water. Both processes result in rapid hypoxia and hypercapnia.
- If rescue is not made, the patient will aspirate water into their lungs, exacerbating hypoxia. The patient will become bradycardic and sustain a cardiac arrest; thus correction of hypoxaemia is critical to obtaining a return of spontaneous circulation. In 10–15% of cases, the laryngeal spasm is so intense, none of the liquid medium enters the lungs.
- Changes in haemodynamics after immersion (the 'hydrostatic squeeze effect') make positional hypotension likely. If the patient is raised vertically from the water their blood pressure will fall – 'after-drop' – may lead to cardio-vascular collapse. Therefore it is recommended that rescuers must always attempt to maintain the patient flat and avoid vertical removal from water.

5. Rescue and Resuscitation

- ⚠ Safety first – **DO NOT** put yourself in danger. Carry out a dynamic risk assessment and undertake measures to preserve your own safety and that of other rescuers.
- Establish the number of patients involved.
- History is often incomplete at the scene, both relating to the incident and the patient.

5.1 Aquatic rescue

- When the patient is rescued, attempt to maintain the patient flat and avoid vertical removal from water.
- If neck and back trauma is suspected, wait until the patient has been rescued before attempting to apply spinal immobilisation, but limit neck flexion and extension.

5.2 Airway and breathing

- Alleviate hypoxaemia as soon as possible, as adequate ventilation and oxygenation may restore cardiac activity.
- In patients in cardiac arrest clear airway and commence CPR as soon as the patient is rescued.
- Administer supplemental oxygen, preferably via bag-valve-mask. Apply pulse oximeter. If the patient does not respond to oxygen therapy consider assisted ventilation.
- Mechanical drainage of water from the lungs should not be carried out. The lungs can be ventilated even with large volumes of water inside them, although ventilation may be difficult due to reduced lung compliance.
- Approximately 80% of patients will aspirate water into their stomach. There is a high risk of regurgitation of the stomach contents, especially if the patient has ingested alcohol/drugs – have suction at hand. Tilting to drain aspirated water simply empties water from the stomach into the pharynx, risking further airway contamination.

5.3 Chest compression

- Commence chest compressions when the patient is on a firm surface (it's usually impossible to perform CPR in a boat) and commence CPR appropriate to patient's age.
- Apply ECG monitoring to aid diagnosis.

5.4 Hypothermia

- If the patient's core body temperature is <30°C, limit defibrillation attempts to 3.
- In the presence of hypothermia, drugs are less effective; withhold intravenous drugs until the patient's body temperature reaches ≥30°C. When at this temperature, double the dose interval until the patient's temperature reaches 35°C.
- If the patient is hypothermic, the heart rate may be extremely slow and external cardiac compression may be required – **refer to cardiac rhythm disturbance guideline**. NB Bradycardia often responds to improved ventilation.

5.5 Intravascular fluid therapy

- Following prolonged immersion patients may become hypovolaemic – if fluid resuscitation indicated **refer to intravascular fluid therapy guideline**.

Table 4.30 – ASSESSMENT and MANAGEMENT of:

Immersion Incident

⚠ Safety First – DO NOT put yourself in danger – carry out a dynamic risk assessment and undertake measures to preserve your own safety, and where possible that of the patient, bystanders and other rescuers.

- Take a defibrillator at the earliest opportunity.
- Ascertain how many patients are involved. NB Information may be incomplete at the scene.
- Note the environment – in certain circumstances hair may become entangled in a drain/filter e.g. pools/hot tubs.

- If the patient has been submerged (entire body, including the airway under the liquid medium) for >90 minutes? Refer to ROLE guideline. In all other cases commence management as set out below.

NB The duration of hypoxia is the most important factor in determining outcome. Oxygenate and restore circulation at the earliest opportunity.

ASSESSMENT	MANAGEMENT

● Assess <C>ABCDE	● If any of the following **TIME CRITICAL** features present:
	  – major **<C>ABCDE** problems – **refer to trauma emergencies overview**
	  – pulseless and apnoeic – **refer to relevant resuscitation guideline**
	  – major life-threatening trauma – **refer to relevant trauma guideline**
	  – neck and back injuries – **refer to neck and back trauma guideline**, then:
	● Start correcting **A** and **B** and undertake a **TIME CRITICAL** transfer to nearest receiving hospital.
	● Administer high levels of supplemental oxygen – refer to oxygen guideline.
	● Prevent further heat loss/consider warming the patient – **refer to hypothermia guideline**.
	● Continue patient management en-route.
	● Provide an alert/information call.

● Airway	● Clear airway. ● There is a high risk of regurgitation of the stomach contents, especially if the patient has ingested alcohol/drugs – have suction at hand.

● Ventilation	● Adequate ventilation and oxygenation may restore cardiac activity. Consider assisted ventilation if:
	  – SpO_2 is <90% with oxygen therapy
	  – respiratory rate <12 or >30 breaths per minute
	  – expansion is inadequate.
	NB Ventilation may be difficult due to reduced lung compliance if water has been inhaled – **refer to airway and breathing management guideline**.

● Oxygen	● Administer supplemental oxygen – refer to oxygen guideline.
	● Apply pulse oximeter – NB the measurement maybe unreliable in patients with cold peripheries.
	  – **children** – administer high levels of supplemental oxygen
	  – **adults** – aim for a target saturation within the range of 94–98%.

● Heart rate	● In the presence of hypothermia the heart rate may be extremely slow and external cardiac compression may be required – **refer to cardiac rhythm disturbance guideline**. NB Bradycardia often responds to improved ventilation and oxygenation.
● Concomitant injuries	● Consider concomitant injuries. ● Consider neck and back injuries – **refer to neck and back trauma guideline**. ● Treat associated injuries – refer to specific guideline(s).
● ECG	● Undertake a 12-lead ECG.
● Fluid	● In cases of prolonged immersion patients may become hypovolaemic – if fluid resuscitation indicated refer to intravascular fluid therapy guideline.
● Pain	● If pain management indicated **refer to pain management guideline**.
● Position	● If possible, the patient should be removed from the water and managed in a horizontal position, especially in rescue involving a helicopter or large vessel, where the patient is lifted more than a few metres – however in **TIME CRITICAL** conditions speed of removal from the water takes precedence over method of removal.

4 SECTION Trauma

Table 4.30 – ASSESSMENT and MANAGEMENT of:

Immersion Incident *continued*

ASSESSMENT	MANAGEMENT
● Transfer to further care	● Transfer all patients to further care. ● If neck and back injury not suspected transfer in the recovery position. ● If the patient is immobilised prepare for side-tilt. ● Prevent further heat loss/consider warming the patient – **refer to hypothermia guideline**. ● Provide an alert/information call. ● Continue patient management en-route.
● Discontinuation of resuscitative efforts	● **Refer to ROLE guideline**.

5.6 Discontinuing resuscitative efforts

If the patient has been submerged for 90 minutes. In all other cases for guidance on discontinuation of resuscitative efforts refer to Recognition Of Life Extinct (**ROLE**).

5.7 Survival and submersion

Research has shown that there is little accurate data on which factors predict survival, following submersion. Submersion time is a significant factor but there is little accurate data. In order to obtain more accurate data on the factors associated with good outcomes following submersion, data will be collected on a number of parameters, such as:

● Time of the incident.

● Time the patient was rescued.

● Time of first effective CPR.

● Duration of submersion.

● Water temperature.

● Type (salt, fresh, contaminated).

● Precipitating factors e.g. intoxication from alcohol or drugs, convulsion etc.

As it is often difficult to obtain accurate time information from witnesses, for the purpose of deciding whether to commence resuscitation the submersion time is measured from the time of initial call to ambulance control centre. For full details refer to Appendix.

6. Assessment and Management

For the assessment and management of the immersion incident refer to Table 4.30.

Methodology

For details of the methodology used in the development of this guideline refer to the guideline webpage.

KEY POINTS

The Immersion Incident

● **Ensure own personal safety.**

● **Successful resuscitations have occurred after prolonged submersion/immersion.**

● **Hypothermia is a condition often associated with the immersion incident.**

● **Special considerations in cardiac arrest treatment in the presence of hypothermia.**

● **Severe complications may develop several hours after submersion/immersion.**

SECTION **4** Trauma

5

Obstetrics and Gynaecology

Obstetrics and Gynaecology

1. Introduction

- Any female of childbearing age **MAY** be pregnant, and, unless there is a history of hysterectomy, even the slightest doubt must make one consider if any abdominal pain or vaginal bleeding may be pregnancy related.

- There are three fundamental rules which must be followed at all times when dealing with the pregnant patient:

  - the maternal well-being is essential to the survival of the fetus and thus resuscitation of the mother must always be the priority

  - compression of the inferior vena cava by the pregnant uterus (beyond 20 weeks) is a serious potential complication and suitable positioning or manual displacement must be employed (see displacement below)

  - signs of shock appear very late during pregnancy and hypotension is an extremely late sign. Any signs of hypovolaemia during pregnancy are likely to indicate a 35% (class III) blood loss and must be treated aggressively. **ESTABLISH LARGE BORE IV CANNULATION EARLY**.

If the mother is in cardiac arrest it is important to undertake a **TIME CRITICAL** transfer immediately to the nearest suitable receiving hospital and provide an alert/information call to ask for an **OBSTETRICIAN ON STANDBY IN THE EMERGENCY DEPARTMENT** for an emergency caesarean section – delivering the fetus **MAY** facilitate maternal resuscitation. NB Effective resuscitation of the mother will provide effective resuscitation of the fetus.

2. Pathophysiology

Pregnancy is timed from the FIRST day of the last period, and from that date lasts up to 42 weeks. The pregnancy is divided into **first** (1–12 weeks), **second** (13–23+6) and **third** (24+) trimesters. These terms are used on shared care antenatal records i.e. the patient's personal maternity plan.

There are a multitude of physiological and anatomical changes during pregnancy that may influence the management of the obstetric patient. These changes include:

- An increase in cardiac output by 20–30% in the first 10 weeks of pregnancy.

- An increase in average maternal heart rate by 10–15 beats per minute.

- A decrease in systolic and diastolic blood pressure by an average of 10–15 mmHg.

- Uterine pressure may cause compression of the inferior vena cava, reducing venous return, and lowering cardiac output, by up to 40%, for patients in the supine position; this in turn will reduce blood pressure.

- An increase in breathing rate and effort and a decrease in vital capacity, as the fetus enlarges and the diaphragm becomes splinted.

- An increase in blood volume (↑45%) and the numbers of red cells; but not in proportion, so the patient becomes **relatively anaemic**. Due to the increase in blood volume the obstetric patient is able to tolerate greater blood or plasma loss before showing signs of hypovolaemia. This compensation is at the expense of shunting blood away from the uterus and placenta and therefore fetus.

- An increase in the acidity of the stomach contents, due to a delay in gastric emptying, caused by progesterone-like effects of the placental hormones.

- Relaxation of the cardiac sphincter makes regurgitation of the stomach contents more likely.

- Oedema of the larynx.

- Enlargement of the breasts.

3. Procedures

- In medical cases the patient can either position themselves to avoid compression of the vena cava or the uterus can be manually displaced to the left (Figure 5.1). In trauma cases the patient should be tilted 15–30° to the left, preferably using a scoop stretcher or long-spine board and head blocks (**refer to trauma in pregnancy guideline**).

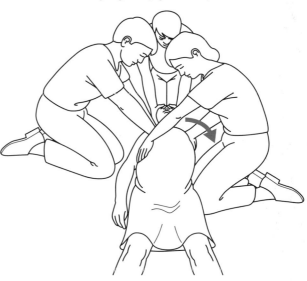

Figure 5.1 – Manual tilt.

4. Assessment

4.1 Quickly assess the patient and scene as you approach

4.2 Primary survey

- It is important to remember there are two patients: neither the mother nor a newly born baby should be overlooked whilst assessing and caring for the other. Both may be at risk, or one may need more urgent attention than the other – it is unlikely to be possible to determine which until a primary survey has been completed on both patients.

- The aim of the primary survey is to identify the existence of life-threatening problems, to enable management to be commenced as rapidly as possible and to reach an early determination of the priority for transportation. The primary survey should be modified in the presence of actual or suspected trauma (**refer to trauma in pregnancy guideline**).

Circulation/massive external haemorrhage

Is there a significant volume of blood visible without the need to disturb the patient's clothing?

- On the floor?
- Is the patient's clothing soaked?
- Are there a number of blood-soaked pads in evidence?

Airway

- Is the patient able to talk? (yes = airway open).
- Is the patient making unusual sounds? (gurgling = fluid in the airway).
- Requiring suction (snoring = tongue/swelling/foreign body obstruction).
- If the patient is unresponsive, open the airway and look in – suction for fluids, manually remove solid obstructions.

Breathing

- Document respiratory rate and effort (are accessory muscles being used?).
- Obtain oxygen saturations as soon as possible.
- Auscultate for added sounds (wheeze bronchospasm; coarse sounds = pulmonary oedema).
- Assess for the presence of cyanosis.
- Give oxygen based on clinical findings (not routinely).

Circulation

- Document radial pulse rate and volume (capillary refill time [CRT] may be used if neither the radial nor carotid pulses can be palpated).
- Assess skin colour and temperature (to touch) (pallor, or cold or damp skin = an adrenergic reaction to shock).
- Assess for bleeding – check underwear, pads, the surface the patient is sitting on, and briefly examine the vaginal opening with the patient's consent and considering their privacy. Ask the patient about bleeding during this problem – if they have discarded pads, how saturated were they? How many pads have they used in what time period?
- Check for visible blood loss again and feel under any clothing or bed linen the patient is sitting or lying on, as this can absorb significant volumes of blood. Look at your gloved hands to see if they are stained with blood. Check the vaginal opening for evidence of bleeding (soaked pads or underwear, wounds).
- Check the abdominal area for evidence of internal bleeding (tenderness, guarding, firm woody uterus,).
- Document blood pressure measurement – the systolic is most valuable if you suspect shock.

Disability

- Perform an AVPU assessment of conscious level (is the patient Alert, responding only to Voice, responding only to Pain, or Unresponsive?).
- Document the patient's posture (normal, convulsing [state whether focal or generalised], abnormal flexion, abnormal extension).

- Document pupil size and reaction (PEaRL – Pupils Equal and Reacting to Light).

Expose/environment/evaluate

- If you haven't already done so, briefly examine the vaginal opening:
  - is there any evidence of bleeding? Can you see a presenting part of the baby?
  - is there a prolapsed loop of cord? Have the waters broken?
  - does the perineum bulge with each contraction?
  - if the baby has been delivered, is there a significant perineal tear? Can you see part of the uterus?
- Is the room warm – is a newborn at risk of hypothermia? Are the surroundings as clean as you can make them if you are going to deliver on-site? Are there other children present (indicates previous pregnancy with live birth)?
- Make an early evaluation about how time critical the patient's problem is. If the patient is time critical, decide immediately whether you need to transport the patient urgently to hospital, with a hopsital obstetric pre-alert, or whether it is more prudent to treat them at the scene – remember to call for skilled obstetric help if this is the case.

Fundus

- Make a quick assessment of fundal height: a fundus at the level of the umbilicus equates to a gestation of approximately 22 weeks. By definition, fundal height below the umbilicus suggests that if the fetus is delivered it is unlikely to survive.

4.3 Obstetric secondary survey

If any critical problems are identified during the primary survey the secondary survey should only be undertaken when any ABCDE problems have been addressed and transportation to definitive care has commenced (if this is possible). In many cases where critical problems are identifed it will not be possible or appropriate to undertake a secondary survey in the prehospital phase of care.

Methodology

For details of the methodology used in the development of this guideline refer to the guidelines development webpage. Refer to methodology section.

Table 5.1

Glossary

ABBREVIATION	TERM
LMP	Last menstrual period.
EDD	Estimated date of delivery – the timing of the pregnancy is written in the notes as 12/40, i.e. 12 weeks have elapsed out of the 40 weeks pregnancy.
T	Term or expected end of pregnancy, therefore T+3 in the notes is 3 days over the EDD.
CEPH	Cephalic (head).
BR	Breech.
G	Gravida, the number of times a woman has been pregnant.
P	Parity, the number of times a woman has given birth.
Colposcopy	An outpatient test where the cervix is inspected when a smear has been abnormal. Treatment such as cone biopsy for the abnormal smear may have been undertaken. Heavy colposcopy bleeding affects very few women in this situation.

KEY POINTS

Obstetrics and Gynaecology Emergencies Overview

- Any female of childbearing age MAY be pregnant.
- Due to the increase in blood volume the obstetric patient is able to tolerate greater blood or plasma loss before showing signs of hypovolaemia.
- Any signs of hypovolaemia during pregnancy are likely to indicate a 35% (class III) blood loss and must be treated aggressively – ESTABLISH LARGE BORE IV CANNULATION EARLY.

SECTION 5 Obstetrics & Gynaecology

Birth Imminent: Normal Delivery and Delivery Complications [329, 870, 875, 876, 879–886]

1. Introduction

The best clinical management for a mother who is experiencing an abnormal labour or delivery is to be transferred to further care without delay.

When there is a midwife on scene it is their responsibility to manage the delivery, and crews should work under their direction. If the midwife is not present, the decision on whether to move the mother should be based on the principle that any situation which deviates from a normal uncomplicated delivery should result in the mother being transported immediately to hospital.

In this situation the crew must alert the hospital via control en-route. Ambulance clinicians should make an early assessment of the need for additional assistance from an additional ambulance and ensure that the request is made as soon as possible.

The most important feature of managing an obstetric incident is a rapid and accurate assessment of the mother to ascertain whether there is anything abnormal taking place.

The following maternal assessment process **MUST** be followed in order to decide whether to:

- **STAY ON SCENE AND REQUEST A MIDWIFE** (if not already present).
- **TRANSFER TO FURTHER CARE IMMEDIATELY**.

In maternity cases where delivery is not imminent and there are no complications (refer to maternal assessment flowchart) the mother may be transported to the unit into which she is booked.

The assessment should be repeated en-route and if any complications occur, the condition should be treated appropriately, and the woman's destination revised if necessary. If the mother is booked into a unit that is not within a reasonable distance or travelling time, crews should base their judgements on the maternal assessment, and take the mother to the most appropriate unit.

Table 5.2 – ASSESSMENT and MANAGEMENT of:

Normal Delivery

ASSESSMENT	MANAGEMENT
• Quickly assess the patient and scene as you approach. • Undertake a primary survey **<C>ABCDEF**.	• If any time critical features are present correct **<C>ABC** and transport to nearest suitable receiving hospital (**refer to medical emergencies guideline**). • Provide an alert/information call.
• Ascertain the period of gestation. • Ask to see the patient-held record for indications of multiple births, breech presentation, obstetric complications.	
Assess for: – show – waters broken – contractions – and/or bleeding. (**refer to obstetric and gynaecology overview for guidance**)	If **NONE** of these indications are present **AND** there is no other medical/traumatic condition discuss the mother's management with the **BOOKED OBSTETRIC UNIT** – informing of: • Mother's name. • Mother's age and date of birth. • Hospital registration number. • Name of lead clinician. • History of this pregnancy. • Estimated date of delivery (EDD). • Previous obstetric history.
If **ANY** of the above indications are present assess: • Contraction interval. • The urge to push or bear down. • Crowning/top of the baby's head/breech presentation visible at the vulva.	• Undertake a visual inspection if there are regular contractions (1–2 minute intervals) and an urge to push or bear down.
• If delivery is imminent i.e. regular contractions (1–2 minute intervals) and an urge to push or bear down and or crowning /top of the baby's head/breech presentation visible at the vulva.	• Remain on scene, request a midwife, an additional ambulance with a paramedic if not present and prepare for delivery (see below).

Table 5.2 – ASSESSMENT and MANAGEMENT of:

Normal Delivery *continued*

ASSESSMENT	MANAGEMENT
Second stage of labour (10 cm cervical dilatation – delivery).	• Reassure the mother, tell her what you are doing and include her partner if present. • Prepare delivery area: – **incontinence pads** – cover the ambulance stretcher or delivery area – **maternity pack** – open and set out – **towels** – enough to dry and wrap the baby – **blanket(s)** – cover the mother for warmth and modesty – **heat** – turn the heat up in the delivery area (aim for 25°C). • Support the mother in a semi-recumbent (or other comfortable) position with padding under her buttocks – discourage her from lying flat on her back because of the risk of supine hypotension.
• Continue assessing the mother's level of pain.	• Encourage the mother to continue taking entonox to relieve pain/discomfort. • **CAUTION – morphine** should only be administered in exceptional circumstances due to the risk of neonatal respiratory depression. • As the baby's head is delivering, help the mother to avoid pushing by telling her to concentrate on panting or breathing out in little puffs – entonox may help. • Instruct the mother to pant or puff, allowing the head to advance slowly with the contraction. Consider applying gentle pressure to the top of the baby's head as it advances through the vaginal entrance to prevent very rapid delivery of the head. • Check to see if the umbilical cord is around the baby's neck. If it is, gently attempt to loop it over the head. If it is too tight, it is better to deliver the rest of the baby with the cord left in place. A tight cord will not prevent the baby delivering. • Hold the baby as it is born and lift it towards the mother's abdomen. • Wipe any obvious large collections of mucous from the baby's mouth and nose.
• Undertake an initial ABCD assessment of the baby – include head, trunk, axilla and groin.	• Newborns are at risk of hypothermia. • **CAUTION** – premature babies lose heat even faster than full term babies • Quickly and thoroughly dry the baby using a warm towel while you make your initial assessment. • Remove the now wet towel and wrap the baby in dry towelling to minimise heat losses.
• Assess the baby's airway.	• If the baby is crying they have a clear airway. • If the baby is not breathing, confirm that the airway is open – the head is ideally placed in the 'neutral' position – i.e. not the extended 'sniffing position' used in older children and adults.

Figure reproduced with the kind permission of the Resuscitation Council (UK).

• **SUCTION IS NOT USUALLY NECESSARY** – if required, use the suction unit on half speed with a CH12–14 catheter and then only within the oral cavity.
• If the baby is not breathing **refer to newborn life support guideline**.

• Once the baby is breathing adequately, cyanosis will gradually improve over several minute – if the cyanosis is not clearing, enrich the atmosphere near the baby's face with low flow of oxygen.

• **Refer to care of the newborn guideline.**

5 Obstetrics & Gynaecology SECTION

Table 5.2 – ASSESSMENT and MANAGEMENT of:

Normal Delivery *continued*

ASSESSMENT	MANAGEMENT
Cutting the cord ● Assess whether the cord has stopped pulsating.	1. Wait until the cord has stopped pulsating; apply two cord clamps securely 3 cm apart and about 15 cm from the umbilicus. Cut the cord between the two clamps. **CAUTION:** ensure the newborn's fingers and genitals are clear of the scissors. 2. Ensure the baby remains wrapped and keep the baby warm. 3. Place the baby with its mother in a position where the mother can feed if she wants to (breast feeding will also encourage delivery of the placenta). 4. Reassure the mother. 5. Await the midwife and third stage (delivery of the placenta and membranes). 6. If delivery has occurred en-route proceed to the nearest obstetric unit. It is not necessary to await delivery of the placenta before continuing with the transfer. 7. Provide an alert/information call.
Third stage of labour (delivery of the placenta and membranes) – may take 15–20 minutes.	● Assist the mother in expelling the placenta naturally by encouraging her to adopt a squatting, upright position, but only if there has been no delay in delivery of the placenta and **NOT IF THERE IS ANY SIGNIFICANT BLEEDING**. ● Do not pull the cord during delivery of the placenta as this could rupture the cord, making delivery of the placenta difficult and cause excessive bleeding or inversion of uterus. ● Deliver the placenta straight into a bowl or plastic bag. Keep it, together with any blood and membranes, for inspection by a doctor or midwife. NB If the placenta has not been delivered within 20 minutes after delivery insert a **LARGE BORE** cannula, as patients are at increased risk of haemorrhage and may require intravascular fluid and medication.
● Assess how much blood has accompanied the delivery of the placenta and membranes – this should not exceed 200–300 mls.	● If bleeding continues after delivery of the placenta, palpate the abdomen and feel for the top of the uterus (fundus) usually at the level of the umbilicus and massage gently with a cupped hand in a circular motion. ● The fundus will become firm as massage is applied and this may be quite uncomfortable so entonox (**refer to the entonox drug guideline for administration and information**) can be offered.
● Assess blood loss – if bleeding is severe.	● Obtain IV access – insert **LARGE BORE** cannulae. ● Administer fluid replacement (**refer to fluid therapy guideline**) ● Administer syntometrine if available (**refer to syntometrine guideline**). ● If syntometrine is **NOT** available or the patient is hypertensive (≥140/90) administer misoprostol (**refer to misoprostol guideline**).
● Assess and monitor respiration rate, pulse and blood pressure.	● Administer O_2 to aim for a target saturation within the range of 94–98%.
	A number of complications may arise during pregnancy and/or labour. Refer to Table 5.3 for the assessment and management of: 1. Pre-term delivery 2. Maternal seizures 3. Prolapsed umbilical cord 4. Post-partum haemorrhage 5. Continuous severe/sudden abdominal/back pain/placental abruption 6. Multiple births – delayed delivery of second or subsequent baby 7. Malpresentation 8. Shoulder dystocia.

Birth Imminent: Normal Delivery and Delivery Complications

Table 5.3 – ASSESSMENT and MANAGEMENT of:

Delivery complications
1. Preterm delivery – delivery before the completion of 37 weeks

ASSESSMENT	MANAGEMENT
● Ascertain the period of gestation.	● **<22 weeks gestation** – transfer the mother and baby to the **NEAREST GYNAECOLOGY UNIT or follow local protocols.**. ● **22–37 weeks gestation** – every effort should be made to transport the mother to a **CONSULTANT-LED UNIT** without delay as the baby will need specialist care once delivered.
● Re-assess the mother constantly en-route.	● Manage as circumstances change. ● Should delivery take place en-route assess the baby and take appropriate action. Convey mother and baby to the **NEAREST ED or CONSULTANT-LED UNIT**[a] depending on local arrangements. ● Provide an alert/information call to the receiving hospital.
	● If transfer to further care is not possible because the birth is so advanced, request a midwife plus an additional ambulance and inform control (**refer to birth imminent guideline**). ● Once the baby is born, utilise the additional ambulance to transport the infant **IMMEDIATELY** to the **NEAREST ED or OBSTETRIC UNIT**[a] depending on local arrangements. ● The infant should be transported even if the midwife has not yet arrived. ● Provide an alert/information call to the hospital, giving an ETA and description of the baby's condition. ● The mother should then be transferred to the **OBSTETRIC UNIT** of the **same hospital as the baby**.

2. Maternal seizures

ASSESSMENT	MANAGEMENT
● Quickly assess the patient and scene as you approach.	● Correct A and B problems and transfer to **CONSULTANT-LED UNIT**. ● If the patient is convulsing **refer to convulsion guideline**.
● Undertake a primary survey **<C>ABCDEF**. ● Assess for **TIME CRITICAL** features.	
	● Refer to pregnancy-induced hypertension (including pre-eclampsia).

3. Prolapsed umbilical cord

ASSESSMENT	MANAGEMENT

The descent of the umbilical cord into the lower uterine segment. This is a TIME CRITICAL EMERGENCY requiring immediate intervention, rapid removal and transfer to an CONSULTANT-LED UNIT.	● Use two fingers to replace the cord **GENTLY** in the vagina. Only make **ONE** attempt to replace the cord.
	● Handle the cord as little as possible to prevent spasm.
	● If it is not possible to replace the cord easily in the vagina (particularly if a large loop has prolapsed):
	  – use dry padding to prevent further prolapse (this will keep the cord warm and moist within the vagina and prevent cord spasm)
	  – position the mother on her side with padding placed under her hips to raise the pelvis and reduce pressure on the cord.

	● Determine the best means of removal – ideally the ambulance stretcher should be used, but where necessary and expedient the mother may be helped to walk to the nearest point of access for the ambulance stretcher. Use of the service carrying chair should be avoided if at all possible and if used should only be to convey the mother to the nearest point of access for the stretcher. ● Administer entonox to help prevent the urge to push, which increases pressure on the cord.
	● Transfer to the nearest **CONSULTANT-LED UNIT** with the mother positioned on her side, with padding under the pelvis to reduce pressure on the cord. ● Provide an alert/information call. ● Alert the hospital that the mother has a prolapsed cord.

[a] When placing the alert call ask what the arrangements are for units receiving distressed neonates where this is not the Obstetric Unit.

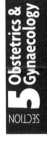

5 Obstetrics & Gynaecology SECTION

Table 5.3 – ASSESSMENT and MANAGEMENT of:

Delivery complications
4. Post-partum haemorrhage (PPH)[b]

ASSESSMENT	MANAGEMENT
	NOTE – If severe haemorrhage occurs following delivery (post-partum) follow one of the two treatment regimens below en-route to further care if possible.
Primary PPH: blood loss of 500 ml or more within 24 hours of delivery. **Massive PPH: blood loss of 50% of the blood volume within 3 hours of delivery.**	**1. IF THE PLACENTA HAS DELIVERED:** ● Palpate the abdomen and feel for the top of the uterus (fundus) usually at the level of the umbilicus and massage gently with a cupped hand in a circular motion. ● The fundus will become firm as massage is applied and this may be quite uncomfortable and entonox can be offered (refer to the entonox drug guideline for administration and information). ● Administer a bolus of syntometrine (refer to syntometrine guideline) – if **syntometrine** or other oxytocics are unavailable, have been ineffective at reducing haemorrhage after 15 minutes or the patient is hypertensive (BP >140/90) administer **misoprostol** (refer to misoprostol guideline).
	2. IF THE PLACENTA HAS NOT DELIVERED: ● In the presence of haemorrhage, **DO NOT** massage the top of the uterus (fundus) when the placenta is undelivered. This may provoke **partial separation** of the placenta and cause further haemorrhage. ● Administer a bolus of **syntometrine** (refer to syntometrine guideline) – if **syntometrine** or other oxytocics are unavailable, have been ineffective at reducing haemorrhage after 15 minutes or if the patient is hypertensive (BP >140/90), administer **misoprostol** (refer to misoprostol guideline). NB Administration of **syntometrine** or **misprostol** may cause the placenta to separate and deliver. If the placenta delivers ensure there is no further bleeding. If bleeding continues after the placenta is delivered – commence massage of uterine fundus (**see 1 above**).
● Assess blood loss – if bleeding is >500 mls. ● Re-assess prior to further fluid replacement. ● If bleeding continues check for bleeding from tears at the vaginal entrance.	● Obtain IV access – insert a **LARGE BORE** cannula. ● Administer fluid replacement (refer to intravascular fluid therapy guideline). ● Apply direct pressure to a tear using a gauze or maternity pad. ● If not in transit transfer the mother and baby to the **NEAREST OBSTETRIC UNIT** immediately. Provide an alert/information call. Include details as to whether the placenta has been delivered or is still in-situ.

5. Continuous severe abdominal pain/placental abruption[c]

ASSESSMENT	MANAGEMENT
● Quickly assess the patient and scene as you approach. NB In the presence of severe/sudden continuous abdominal/back pain consider abruption.. ● Undertake a primary survey **<C>ABCDEF** ● Assess for **TIME CRITICAL** features.	● Correct A and B problems and transfer to the **CONSULTANT-LED UNIT WITHOUT DELAY**.
● Assess for signs of shock. **A separation of a normally sited placenta from the uterine wall.**	● Obtain IV access – insert a **LARGE BORE** cannula. ● If fluid therapy indicated refer to intravascular fluid therapy guideline. ● Encourage the mother to lie on her side or sit when in transit, whichever position is the more comfortable for her. ● Provide an alert/information call. ● Commence the appropriate resuscitation regimen as soon as possible.

[b] The commonest cause of severe haemorrhage immediately after delivery is uterine atony (i.e. poor uterine contraction).

[c] Major placental abruption is when a large part of the placenta detaches from the uterine wall. Bleeding occurs under the placenta causing significant abdominal, back and/or epigastric pain. There may be no visible vaginal bleeding ('concealed'abruption). Alternatively there may be a variable amount of vaginal bleeding ('concealed' abruption). Despite little or no visible bleeding, there may be signs of hypovolaemic shock.

Table 5.3 – ASSESSMENT and MANAGEMENT of:

Delivery complications
6. Multiple births – delayed delivery of second or subsequent baby[d]

ASSESSMENT	MANAGEMENT
NOTE – with a twin delivery, the mother is at increased risk of immediate post-partum haemorrhage due to poor uterine tone (**refer to 4 above**). **It is now very unusual for a mother expecting a multiple birth to deliver outside hospital. However, twin pregnancies are at much higher risk of delivering preterm (i.e. before 37 weeks) – the babies may therefore need resuscitation.**	If delivery is **NOT** in progress: ● Transfer mother to the **CONSULTANT-LED UNIT** without delay. ● Constantly re-assess en-route and take appropriate action if the circumstances change.
	If delivery **IS** in progress or occurs en-route: ● Request back up following local guidelines (as not every area can request a midwife). ● Follow the normal delivery process and management of the newborn for each baby.
	● Once the first baby has been born and assessed transfer mother and baby to the **NEAREST OBSTETRIC UNIT IMMEDIATELY** if delivery of the second baby is not imminent. If there are any complications, transfer to a **CONSULTANT-LED UNIT** – it is not necessary to await the arrival of the midwife. ● Provide an alert/information call.
	● If the delivery of the second baby occurs en-route, park the ambulance and make a request via control for an **ADDITIONAL AMBULANCE**. ● Once the second baby has been delivered, utilise both vehicles to transfer mother and babies to the nearest consultant-led obstetric unit. ● Provide an alert/information call.
Assess if any/either baby requires resuscitation.	● Follow the appropriate newborn resuscitation guideline.

7. Malpresentation[e]

ASSESSMENT	MANAGEMENT
Breech birth is where the feet or buttocks present first during delivery rather than the baby's head. **NB Cord prolapse is more common with a breech presentation (refer to 3 – prolapsed umbilical cord).**	**Breech Birth** – If delivery is **NOT** in progress: ● Transfer mother to the **BOOKED OBSTETRIC UNIT** without delay. ● Constantly re-assess en-route and take appropriate action if the circumstances change.
	Breech Birth – If delivery IS in progress treat as for a normal delivery except: ● If the mother is on the bed or sofa etc., encourage her to move to the edge. This will enable gravity to help deliver the baby. The mother's legs should be supported (this may look like the McRobert's Position – page 262). ● Do not touch the baby or the umbilical cord until the body is free of the birth canal and the nape of the neck is visible. The only exception is when the baby's back rotates to face the mother's anus (the umbilicus should always face the anus). Gently hold the baby by its pelvis and rotate the baby's back – the baby's umbilicus must face the mother's anus (take care **NOT** to squeeze the infant's abdomen which could damage internal organs). ● Do not clamp or cut the cord until the **HEAD** is free of the birth canal. ● Once the body of the baby is born and the nape of the neck is visible, gently lift the baby by its feet to facilitate delivery of the head. This should be undertaken as the head is delivering and so as not to over-extend the baby's neck. Care should be taken not to pull the baby. ● Once the baby is born treat as for a normal delivery. Breech babies are more likely to be covered in meconium and may require resuscitation. If the baby requires resuscitation, follow the appropriate newborn resuscitation guideline.
	Any presenting body part other than the head, buttocks or feet (e.g. one foot or a hand/arm) ● Transfer the mother **immediately** to a **CONSULTANT-LED OBSTETRIC UNIT**. ● Provide an alert/information call.

[d] It is now very unusual for a mother expecting a multiple birth to deliver outside hospital. However, twin pregnancies are at much higher risk of delivering preterm (i.e. before 37 weeks) – the babies may therefore need resuscitation.

[e] Breech birth is where the feet or buttocks present first during delivery rather than the baby's head. Cord prolapse is more common with a breech presentation (refer to 3 – prolapsed umbilical cord). Follow local guidelines.

Table 5.3 – ASSESSMENT and MANAGEMENT of:

Delivery complications
8. Shoulder dystocia[f]

ASSESSMENT

An arrest of spontaneous delivery; when delivery of the baby's shoulders is delayed because the baby's anterior shoulder is stuck behind the symphysis pubis.

MANAGEMENT
- **DO NOT** pull, twist or bend the baby's head.
- **DO NOT** press on the uterine fundus.
- **DO NOT** cut the cord before the baby is delivered.
- If the shoulders are not delivered within two contractions following the birth of the head a further attempt can be made to deliver the shoulders using the McRobert's manoeuvre (see below).

McRobert's Manoeuvre (increases the pelvic diameters/alters the angle of the pelvis)

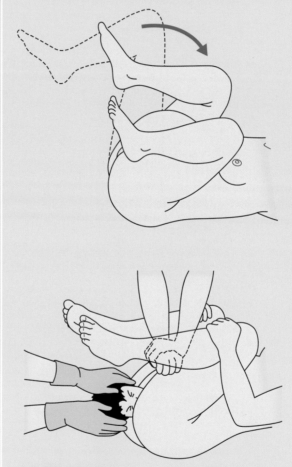

1. Ask the mother to lie flat with only one pillow under her head.
2. Bring the mother's knees up towards her chest and outwards slightly.
3. Now attempt to deliver the shoulders with gentle traction downwards.
4. **If after two attempts the shoulders have not delivered, attempt suprapubic pressure.**

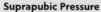

Suprapubic Pressure
1. Identify the side where the fetal back lies. This will often be the opposite side to the direction the baby is facing. NB The mother should be flat with a maximum of one pillow under her head.
2. Ask the assistant to:
   - Stand on the side of the baby's back (if the baby is facing left, stand on the mother's right or vice versa).
   - Use their hands in CPR grip and place the heel of their hand two finger breadths above the symphysis pubis behind the baby's shoulder.
   - Apply moderate pressure on the baby's shoulder pushing downwards and away from them.
   - This will hopefully dislodge and rotate the shoulder from behind the symphysis pubis.
3. Now attempt to deliver the shoulders with gentle traction downwards while the assistant applies suprapubic pressure.
4. **If after two attempts the shoulders have not delivered, apply intermittent pressure.**

[f] This is when delivery of the baby's shoulders is delayed. The baby's anterior shoulder is stuck behind the symphysis pubis.

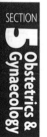

SECTION **5** Obstetrics & Gynaecology

Birth Imminent: Normal Delivery and Delivery Complications

Table 5.3 – ASSESSMENT and MANAGEMENT of:

Delivery complications
8. Shoulder dystocia^f *continued*

ASSESSMENT	MANAGEMENT
	Intermittent Pressure
	1. Encourage the mother to empty her bladder.
	2. Ask the assistant to apply intermittent pressure on the shoulder by rocking gently backwards and forwards.
	3. Try two further attempts to deliver while the assistant applies rocking suprapubic pressure.
	4. **If after two attempts the shoulders have not delivered, place the mother in the all-fours position.**

All-Fours Position
1. Position the mother on her hands and knees with her hips well flexed, bottom elevated and her head is as low as possible.
2. Apply gentle traction downwards towards the floor to try and deliver the shoulder nearer the maternal back first.
3. **If after two attempts, if the shoulders have not delivered:**
   - Undertake a **TIME CRITICAL** transfer to a **CONSULTANT-LED UNIT**.
   - Administer high levels of supplemental oxygen.
   - In this situation do not await the arrival of the midwife.
   - Provide an alert/information call.
   - Ideally, the mother should be removed from scene using the ambulance stretcher. However, if necessary, the mother may be helped to walk a **SHORT** distance to the nearest point of access for the stretcher, but crews should be prepared to deliver the baby as this may precipitate birth. Once on the stretcher and during transportation the mother should be placed on her side with padding placed under her hips to raise the pelvis.

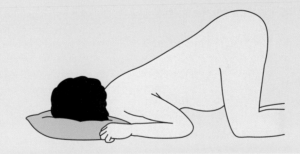

Methodology

For details of the methodology used in the development of this guideline refer to the guideline webpage.

SECTION 5 Obstetrics & Gynaecology

KEY POINTS

Birth Imminent: Normal Delivery and Delivery Complications

- **For a patient experiencing an abnormal labour or delivery, transfer to further care without delay.**
- **Undertake a rapid assessment of the patient to ascertain whether there is anything abnormal taking place.**
- **If the mother presents with an obvious medical or traumatic condition that puts her life in imminent danger treat appropriately.**
- **The period of gestation is important in informing the appropriate course of action.**
- **Severe vaginal bleeding, prolapsed cord, continuous severe abdominal/epigastric pain and presentation of part of the baby other than the head (e.g. an arm or leg) warrant IMMEDIATE transfer to the CONSULTANT-LED UNIT.**
- **Do not allow the baby to become cold during transfer.**

1. Introduction

- Ambulance personnel may become involved in the care of the newborn as some deliveries occur at home, or on the way to hospital. Hence it is important to be aware of the differences in physiology of the newborn baby. The newborn baby has emerged from dependence on the protective uterine environment to independent life. Physiology is changing within the first few hours to weeks after birth. Hence what may apply to infants and children may not necessarily be applicable to newborn babies. Additionally, different management issues arise in premature babies.

- Some babies may deliver at home and a proportion of these may need to be transported to hospital because of unexpected problems.

A newborn baby or mother will need to be transferred to hospital for the reasons listed below.

Reasons in the baby

- Any baby that required resuscitation.
- Birth asphyxia (pale floppy apnoeic baby or APGAR score below 5).
- Meconium staining or aspiration.
- Baby of a diabetic mother.
- Small for dates/growth-retarded baby.
- Prematurity (gestation <36 weeks).
- Any baby that required naloxone at birth.
- Major congenital abnormalities, even if the baby appears well at birth.
- Red flags ⚑ suggesting a high risk of early onset neonatal bacterial infection.

Reasons in the the mother

- Severe maternal blood loss from either antepartum or post-partum haemorrhage.
- Retained products of conception.
- Maternal drugs (especially opiates).
- Suspected or confirmed invasive bacterial infection within 24 hours of birth.

2. Pathophysiology

Birth Asphyxia

- Birth asphyxia can occur for various reasons including cord prolapse, the cord being tightly wrapped around the neck, significant placental or umbilical bleeds, or prolonged second stage of labour.

- Birth asphyxia has a poor outlook and is often associated with neurological deficits and cerebral palsy. A low APGAR score at 10 minutes suggests a high possibility of long-term neurological problems.

- Recent studies have shown that in babies born at >36 weeks gestation with birth asphyxia, moderate hypothermia results in a better neurological outcome. The multicentre CoolCap, ICE and TOBY trials showed that cooling to 33.5°C within 6 hours of birth for 72 hours was associated with a decreased death rate, less neurodevelopmental disability and less cerebral palsy in survivors. This controlled

cooling was done without adverse effects being seen in the babies. A meta-analysis of all the neonatal cooling trials strongly supports the use of therapeutic hypothermia in newborn infants with hypoxic ischaemic encephalopathy to reduce the risk of death and neurological impairment at 18 months.

- Researchers are currently studying the benefits of controlled therapeutic cooling using special blankets or suits during interhospital transfers when taking asphyxiated babies to tertiary neonatal units. The transfer of these babies between neonatal intensive care units is, however, the only situation when babies can be transferred without ensuring the ambulance is well heated, and it will be made clear by the medical staff if this is required. Unless the specific equipment is available and requested by hospital staff then the ambulance should be as warm as possible for transfer.

Hypothermia

- Babies have a large body surface area relative to their weight, and heat loss occurs easily by convection. Premature babies are at particular risk. A wet baby will also lose heat by evaporation, especially if in a draught. Babies lose heat as a result of their proportionately large heads when compared to their bodies. Bonnets, towels and blankets can be used to significantly reduce these heat losses. Transfer the baby in a POD if this is available.

- The body temperature of the baby should be kept at about 36–37°C. The ambulance should therefore be kept well heated to prevent cooling during the transfer to hospital. Accidental hypothermia, especially in the premature baby, can be harmful. A cold baby has increased oxygen consumption, and is at risk of hypoglycaemia and acidosis. It is therefore important that the baby is kept warm during the transfer in the ambulance, to prevent hypoglycaemia and these complications.

Hypoglycaemia

- The newborn baby has a relatively immature liver with limited glycogen stores and so low blood sugars are not an uncommon problem.

- Hypoglycaemia is a blood glucose concentration of <2.2 mmol/l in term babies and <1.7 mmol/l in pre-term neonates. Glucose is the main energy source for the fetus and neonate, and the newborn brain depends almost exclusively on glucose for energy metabolism.

- Hypoglycaemia can therefore lead to seizures and brain injury. Severe and prolonged hypoglycaemia may result in long-term neurological damage. It is therefore important to prevent and treat a low blood sugar level as soon as it is detected.

- Signs and symptoms of hypoglycaemia include:
  - jitteriness
  - irritability
  - lethargy
  - apnoeic episodes
  - seizures.

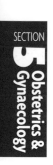

SECTION **5** Obstetrics & Gynaecology

Care of the Newborn

NB Many hypoglycaemic babies are asymptomatic, hence the importance of routine blood glucose checks in babies at risk. Babies at risk of hypoglycaemia include:

- premature babies
- small for gestational age babies
- baby of a diabetic mother due to high circulating insulin levels
- birth asphyxia
- hypothermia
- infection
- delayed feeding.

After birth, give a feed as soon as possible (or at least within the first hour). Failing this, intravenous glucose may be needed, depending on i) the baby's condition and ii) the blood glucose level. The newborn baby's liver has very limited glycogen stores, so hypoglycaemia cannot be treated using intramuscular glucagon (glucagon works by stimulating the liver to convert glycogen into glucose). A baby found to have a persistently low blood glucose level must be transported to hospital for further investigation and management.

Neonatal jaundice

- Jaundice refers to the yellow colouration of the skin and sclera caused by a raised bilirubin level. About 60% of term and 80% of preterm babies develop jaundice in the first week of life. Physiological jaundice occurs around day 2–7, although 10% of breast fed babies are still jaundiced at 1 month of age. Physiological jaundice is due to increased breakdown of haemoglobin in red blood cells to bilirubin, and the immature liver is unable to handle the conversion of bilirubin to a form that can be excreted in the gut. Jaundice is harmless unless the bilirubin level is very high, when this can cross the blood-brain barrier.
- Unconjugated bilirubin is potentially toxic to brain tissue causing kernicterus and brain damage. Different treatment thresholds are recommended for different gestations and age, (see graphs published by National Institute for Health and Clinical Excellence). Jaundice is treated with phototherapy or exchange transfusion depending on the level of bilirubin and the cause. Early jaundice (occurring before day 2) or prolonged jaundice (after day 14) may be due to other pathological causes or underlying diseases and requires investigation. Babies with early jaundice occurring <2 days of age must be referred for an urgent medical review.

Preterm delivery

- Prematurity is defined as <36 weeks gestation. Premature infants are more likely to need help with ventilation. Spontaneous breathing will be inadequate for babies born at <32 weeks gestation. Additionally they are likely to be deficient in surfactant. (Surfactant reduces alveolar surface tension and keeps the lung alveoli open during expiration.) They are therefore likely to need a higher inflation pressure with bag and mask ventilation than term infants to open up their lungs. They are also likely to need surfactant replacement and/or ventilatory support, and require immediate hospital transfer even if apparently well; they are also at particular risk of hypothermia.

- The other complications of prematurity include hypothermia, hypoglycaemia and a higher risk of infection. Preterm infants <32 weeks gestation are also at risk of intracranial bleeds.
- Improving neonatal intensive care has seen better outcomes for babies born preterm (especially in babies born after 28 weeks gestation). However the EPICure study following up babies born in the UK at the limits of viability before 26 weeks gestation show a high mortality and morbidity. Overall survival was only 39% and survivors commonly have severe disabilities. Hypothermia was one of the factors associated with death.

Congenital abnormalities

- The outcome of babies born with congenital abnormalities varies but is improving with advancement in medical therapies and interventions. The abnormality may have been detected on previous antenatal scans or may have been undiagnosed until birth. Hence all babies who are known to have a congenital abnormality should be transferred to hospital where the abnormality can be assessed and treated, even when the baby appears to be normal at birth.
- Babies with abdominal wall defects should be transferred with food grade clingfilm covering the defect to reduce fluid and heat losses.

  NB Do not wrap the clingfilm circumferentially around the newborn's body as this will inhibit breathing.

Early onset neonatal infection

- Early onset neonatal bacterial infection can be life-threatening and it is important that it is recognised and treated early. The following **red flags** suggest a high risk of early onset neonatal bacterial infection:

  - systemic antibiotic treatment given to the mother for confirmed or suspected invasive bacteria
  - seizures in the baby
  - signs for shock in the baby
  - need for mechanical ventilation in a term baby
  - suspected or confirmed infection in a co-twin.

3. Assessment and Management

- For the assessment and management of the newborn see below and refer to Table 5.5.

APGAR score

- The condition of the baby at birth is assessed using the APGAR score. Dr Virginia Apgar first devised these scores to assess the effect of obstetric anaesthesia on the baby, but it has been used universally to assess the condition of the baby after birth. APGAR is an easy to use mnemonic to remember what needs to be assessed:

A appearance (skin colour)

P pulse rate

G grimace (response to stimulation)

A activity or tone (whether active or floppy)

R respiratory rate.

- A healthy term baby normally takes the first breath or cries within 1 minute after the umbilical cord is clamped. The newborn's condition should be assessed at 1 and 5 minutes after birth (see Table 5.5). This helps inform resuscitation decisions. (NB Resuscitation should not be delayed whilst calculating the APGAR score (see Table 5.4).) The baby's condition can be assessed quickly just from their colour, heart rate and breathing effort.

- A pink baby with a lusty cry and a heart rate >100/min will need no further treatment, and just needs to be dried, and given to the mother to hold. Most babies fall into this category and only require drying, warming, and some gentle stimulation.

- A blue baby with a heart rate >80/min, who has some tone and some response to stimulation may begin to breathe spontaneously after a short wait (not >1 minute) if given some gentle stimulation and 'blow by' oxygen.

- A pale, floppy and apnoeic baby with a heart rate <80/min will need bag and mask ventilation, followed by cardiac compression if the heart rate does not improve or breathing does not start (**refer to newborn life support guidelines**) and undertake **TIME CRITICAL** transfer.

- Use gentle suctioning of the mouth and nose with a soft suction catheter to remove excess secretions. Avoid deep pharyngeal suctioning as this can cause bradycardia (from vagal stimulation) or laryngospasm.

- If there has been either meconium staining of the liquor or baby, or evidence of meconium aspiration, the baby will need to be transferred to hospital quickly, as this indicates foetal distress and possible foetal hypoxia. Meconium aspiration can lead to respiratory distress and the need for ventilatory support. The baby may additionally have associated complications from birth asphyxia.

Methodology

For details of the methodology used in the development of this guideline refer to the guideline webpage.

KEY POINTS

Care of the Newborn

- **The need for resuscitation can be made from a quick assessment of the baby's condition at birth.**

- **Keep the baby warm and dry.**

- **Treat hypoglycaemia as soon as it is detected to prevent seizures or long-term neurological damage.**

- **Preterm babies require further management in hospital.**

- **All babies with congenital abnormalities should be transferred to hospital for assessment.**

- **Be aware of red flags in mother or baby which might suggest a high risk of early onset neonatal bacterial infection**

Table 5.4 – APGAR Score

Score	0	1	2
Appearance	blue or pale all over	blue at extremities body pink	body and extremities pink
Pulse rate	absent	<100	≥100
Grimace or response to stimulation	no response to stimulation	grimace/feeble cry when stimulated	cry or pull away when stimulated
Activity or muscle tone	none	some flexion	flexed arms and legs that resist extension
Respiration	absent	weak, irregular, gasping	strong, lusty cry

Care of the Newborn

Table 5.5 – ASSESSMENT and MANAGEMENT of:

The Newborn

ASSESSMENT	MANAGEMENT
● Assess **ABCD**.	● If any of the following **TIME CRITICAL** features present: – major **ABCD** problems – birth asphyxia – major congenital abnormalities – prematurity – hypoglycaemia. ● Start correcting **A** and **B** problems. ● Undertake a **TIME CRITICAL** transfer to a hospital where there is a neonatal unit. ● Continue patient management en-route. ● Provide an alert/information call.
● Assess need for resuscitation at birth.	● Use a quick assessment observing: – the colour – heart rate and – respiratory effort. ● If time permits, perform an APGAR score at 1 and 5 minutes after birth. ● Preterm babies require ongoing hospital care and should be transferred as soon as possible to a hospital with a neonatal unit.
● Birth asphyxia.	● If resuscitation required at birth or there is evidence of asphyxia, transfer to a hospital with a neonatal unit for ongoing care. ● Consider controlled cooling of the baby during the transfer as there is evidence from clinical trials of improved neurological outcome.
● Suspected hypoglycaemia.	● Check blood sugar level from a heel prick. ● If hypoglycaemia confirmed, treatment is **TIME CRITICAL** to prevent seizures and brain damage. ● Consider early feed. ● IM glucagon will **NOT** work due to poor glycogen stores in the newborn. ● If transferring the baby to hospital keep baby warm during the transfer unless there has been evidence of birth asphyxia (**see above**).
● Assess temperature.	● Heat loss occurs readily because of the large body surface area. ● Ensure the newborn baby is dried after birth, as heat loss also occurs by evaporation if the baby is wet.
● Transfer to further care.	

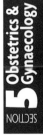

Haemorrhage During Pregnancy (including miscarriage and ectopic pregnancy) [60, 329, 872, 874, 875, 877]

1. Introduction

- This guidance is for the assessment and management of patients with bleeding during early and late pregnancy (including miscarriage and ectopic pregnancy). For post-partum haemorrhage **refer to birth imminent: normal delivery and delivery complications guideline**. For complications associated with abortion **refer to vaginal bleeding: gynaecological causes (including abortion) guideline**.

Haemorrhage may be:

- **Revealed** with evident vaginal loss of blood (e.g. miscarriage and placenta praevia).

- **Concealed** where bleeding occurs within the abdomen or uterus. This presents with little or no external loss, but pain and signs of hypovolaemic shock (e.g. ruptured ectopic pregnancy and placental abruption). **REMEMBER**, pregnant women may appear well even with a large amount of concealed blood loss. Tachycardia may not appear until 30% or more of the circulating volume has been depleted.

Haemorrhage during pregnancy is broadly divided into two types:

1. **Haemorrhage occurring in early pregnancy (≤22 weeks).**

2. **Haemorrhage occurring in late pregnancy (>22 weeks).**

Section 1 – Haemorrhage occurring in early pregnancy (≤22 weeks) may indicate miscarriage or ectopic pregnancy

1. Incidence

- Miscarriage is more common in the first 12 weeks.

2. Pathophysiology

- **Miscarriage (previously known as spontaneous abortion)** is the loss of pregnancy before 23 completed weeks; commonly seen at 6–14 weeks of gestation but can occur after 14 weeks.

- This occurs when some products of conception are partly passed through the cervix and become trapped, leading to blood loss. The level of shock is often out of proportion to the amount of blood loss.

> **Risk Factors – Miscarriage**
> - Previous history of miscarriage.
> - Previously identified potential miscarriage at scan.
> - Smoker.
> - Obesity.

Symptoms:

- Bleeding – light or heavy, often with clots and or jelly-like tissue.

- Pain – central, crampy, suprapubic, or backache.

- Signs of pregnancy may be subsiding e.g. nausea or breast tenderness.

- Significant symptoms (including hypotension) without obvious external blood loss may indicate 'cervical shock' due to retained miscarriage tissue stuck in the cervix. Symptomatic bradycardia may arise due to vagal stimulation.

- **Ectopic pregnancy/ruptured ectopic pregnancy** usually presents at around 6–8 weeks gestation, so usually only one period has been missed.

Symptoms characteristic of a ruptured ectopic pregnancy:

- Acute lower abdominal pain.

- Slight bleeding or brownish vaginal discharge.

- Signs of blood loss within the abdomen with tachycardia and skin coolness.

Other suspicious symptoms:

- Unexplained fainting.

- Shoulder-tip pain.

- Unusual bowel symptoms.

> **Risk Factors – Ectopic pregnancy**
> - An intra-uterine contraceptive device fitted.
> - A previous ectopic pregnancy.
> - Tubal surgery.
> - Sterilisation or reversal of sterilisation.
> - Endometriosis.
> - Pelvic inflammatory disease.

Section 2 – Haemorrhage occurring in late pregnancy – antepartum haemorrhage or prepartum (>22weeks) may indicate placenta praevia or placental abruption

1. Incidence

Placenta praevia occurs in 1 in 200 pregnancies and usually presents at 24–32 weeks with small episodes of painless bleeding.

2. Pathophysiology

- **Placenta praevia:** the placenta develops low down in the uterus and completely or partially covers the cervical canal; this can lead to severe haemorrhage during the pregnancy i.e. painless bleed or when labour begins.

- **Placental abruption** is any vaginal bleeding in late pregnancy or during labour which is accompanied by severe/sudden continuous abdominal/back pain; signs of shock may be due to placental abruption.

  Bleeding occurs between the placenta and the wall of the uterus, detaching an area of the placenta from the uterine wall. It can be associated with severe pregnancy-induced hypertension (PIH). Placental abruption causes continuous severe/sudden abdominal/back pain, tightening of the uterus, signs

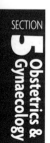

Haemorrhage During Pregnancy (including miscarriage and ectopic pregnancy)

of hypovolaemic shock and puts the baby at immediate risk. There may be some external blood loss, but more commonly the haemorrhage is concealed behind the placenta. Where there is a combination of revealed (external) blood loss and concealed haemorrhage, this can be particularly dangerous, as it can lead to an underestimation of the amount of total blood lost. The woman's abdomen will be tender when felt and the uterus will feel rigid or 'woody' with no signs of relaxation.

NOTE:

- **OVERALL, ABRUPTION IS OFTEN MORE OMINOUS THAN BLEEDING FROM PLACENTA PRAEVIA** because the true amount of bleeding is concealed. It is also associated with Disseminated Intravascular Coagulation (DIC) which can worsen the tendency to bleed.
- It can be very difficult to differentiate between **placenta praevia and placental abruption**.

Table 5.6 – ASSESSMENT and MANAGEMENT of:

Haemorrhage during Pregnancy

ASSESSMENT	MANAGEMENT
<ul><li>Quickly assess the patient and scene as you approach.</li><li>Undertake a primary survey **<C>ABCDEF**.</li><li>Assess for **TIME CRITICAL** features.</li></ul>	<ul><li>If any time critical features are present correct **<C>ABC** and transport to nearest suitable receiving hospital (**refer to medical emergencies guideline**).</li><li>Provide an alert/information call.</li></ul>
<ul><li>Monitor SpO$_2$.</li></ul>	<ul><li>If **oxygen** (O$_2$) <94% administer O$_2$ to aim for a target saturation within the range of 94–98%.</li></ul>
<ul><li>Assess volume of blood loss.[a, b]</li></ul>	<ul><li>Obtain IV access – insert **LARGE BORE** cannulae.</li></ul>
<ul><li>In the event of **LIFE-THREATENING HAEMORRHAGE** AND a confirmed diagnosis of miscarriage e.g. where a patient has gone home with medical management and starts to bleed.</li></ul>	<ul><li>Administer syntometrine if available (**refer to syntometrine guideline**).</li><li>If syntometrine is **NOT** available or the patient is hypertensive (≥140/90) administer misoprostol (**refer to misoprostol guideline**).</li></ul>**CAUTION: DO NOT** administer **syntometrine** or **misoprostol** with a fetus in situ.
<ul><li>Assess for signs of shock e.g. tachycardia >100 bpm, SBP <90 mmHg with cool sweaty skin.</li><li>Undertake a capillary refill test.</li></ul>**NOTE** – hypovolaemia is manifested late in pregnant women; the patient may be very unwell and the fetus may be compromised, therefore **ADMINISTER** fluid replacement early (**refer to intravascular therapy guideline**).	<ul><li>If >20 weeks the gravid uterus may compress the inferior vena cava in a patient who is supine, therefore, it is important to ensure adequate venous return before determining the need for fluid resuscitation; this can be achieved by placing the patient in left lateral tilt, or manually displacing of the uterus.</li><li>Administer 250ml of **sodium chloride 0.9%** IV to maintain SBP of 90 mmHg (**refer to intravascular therapy guideline**).</li><li>Re-assess vital signs prior to further fluid therapy.</li><li>Take any blood-soaked pads to hospital.</li></ul>NB Symptoms of hypovolaemic shock occur very late in otherwise fit young women; tachycardia may not appear until 30% of circulating volume has been lost by which stage the patient is very unwell.
Ask **'When did you last feel the baby move?'**	<ul><li>Be particularly tactful, so as not to cause alarm, as anxiety in the mother will only exacerbate the situation.</li></ul>
<ul><li>If no **TIME CRITICAL** features, perform a more thorough patient assessment with secondary survey including fetal assessment (**refer to obstetrics and gynaecology overview**).</li><li>Check the patient-carried notes for scan results confirming a 'low-lying' placenta.</li></ul>	
<ul><li>Assess patient's level of pain.</li></ul>	Titrate pain relief against pain (**refer to pain management guideline**): – **Paracetamol** – **Entonox** – **Morphine: NOTE** administer cautiously if the patient is hypotensive.
	<ul><li>Nil by mouth.</li></ul>
	<ul><li>Symptomatic bradycardia due to vagal stimulation can be treated with atropine (**refer to atropine and cardiac rhythm disturbance guidelines**).</li></ul>
	<ul><li>Adjust patient's position as required.</li></ul>
	<ul><li>Transfer to further care.</li></ul>

[a] Large sanitary towel can absorb 50 ml of blood.

[b] Blood loss will appear greater if mixed with amniotic fluid.

Haemorrhage During Pregnancy (including miscarriage and ectopic pregnancy)

Methodology

For details of the methodology used in the development of this guideline refer to guideline website.

KEY POINTS

Haemorrhage During Pregnancy (including miscarriage and ectopic pregnancy)

- Haemorrhage during pregnancy is broadly divided into two categories, occurring in early and late pregnancy.
- Haemorrhage may be revealed (evident vaginal blood loss) or concealed (little or no loss).
- Pregnant women may appear well even when a large amount of blood has been lost.
- Obtain venous access with large bore cannulae.
- Tachycardia may not appear until 30% of circulating volume has been lost. In otherwise fit young women, symptoms of hypovolaemic shock occur very late, by which stage the patient is very unwell.

SECTION 1 – Pregnancy-induced hypertension and severe pre-eclampsia

1. Introduction

- Pregnancy-induced hypertension (PIH) is a generic term used to define a significant rise in blood pressure after 22 weeks, in the absence of proteinuria or other features of pre-eclampsia.

- Remember that treating and resuscitating the mother is also assisting the baby.

2. Incidence

- Hypertension from all causes is a common medical problem affecting 10–15% of all pregnancies.

- Approximately 15% of women who present with pregnancy-induced hypertension will develop pre-eclampsia.

3. Severity and Outcome

- PIH is usually mild (i.e. blood pressure (BP) 140/90 mmHg) and there is only a 10% risk of developing pre-eclampsia with mild rises in BP beyond 37 weeks.

- Earlier onset of PIH (i.e. 20–24 weeks) results in a 40% risk of developing pre-eclampsia. If PIH is uncomplicated by pre-eclampsia, then maternal and fetal outcomes are good; however, pre-eclampsia accounted for 13.6% of maternal deaths related to pregnancy causes.

4. Pathophysiology

Pre-eclampsia

- Pre-eclampsia is PIH associated with proteinuria. It commonly occurs beyond 24–28 weeks gestation, but can occur as early as 22 weeks.

- Although the underlying pathophysiology is not fully understood, pre-eclampsia is primarily a placental disorder associated with poor placental perfusion which often results in a fetus which is growth-restricted (i.e. smaller than expected because of the poor placental blood flow).

- In the UK the diagnosis of pre-eclampsia includes an increase in BP above 140/90 mmHg, oedema and detection of protein in the patient's urine.

- Pre-eclampsia is usually diagnosed at routine antenatal visits and may require admission to hospital and early delivery.

- The disease may be of mild, moderate or severe degree.

Severe pre-eclampsia

- May present in a patient with known mild pre-eclampsia or may present with little prior warning.

Symptoms of severe pre-eclampsia:

- The BP is significantly raised (i.e. 160/110 mmHg) with proteinuria and often one or more of the following symptoms:
  - headache – severe and frontal
  - visual disturbances
  - epigastric pain – often mistaken for heartburn
  - right-sided upper abdominal pain – due to stretching of the liver capsule
  - muscle twitching or tremor
  - nausea
  - vomiting
  - confusion
  - rapidly progressive oedema.

Risk Factors – Pre-eclampsia
- Primiparity or first child with a new partner.
- Previous severe pre-eclampsia.
- Essential hypertension.
- Diabetes.
- Obesity.
- Twins or higher multiples.
- Renal disease.
- Advanced maternal age (over 40 years).
- Young maternal age (less than 16 years).
- Pre-existing cardiovascular disease.

Severe pre-eclampsia is:

- a 'multi-organ' disease; although hypertension is a cardinal feature, other complications include:
  - intracranial haemorrhage
  - stroke
  - renal failure
  - liver failure
  - abnormal blood clotting e.g. disseminated intravascular coagulation (DIC).

5. Assessment and Management

- For the assessment and management of mild/moderate pre-eclampsia refer to Table 5.7.

- For the assessment and management of severe pre-eclampsia refer to Table 5.8.

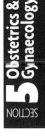

SECTION 5 Obstetrics & Gynaecology

Pregnancy-Induced Hypertension (including eclampsia)

Table 5.7 – ASSESSMENT and MANAGEMENT of:

Mild/Moderate Pre-eclampsia

Definition – raised blood pressure >140/90 mmHg, detection of proteinurina, and sometimes oedema.

ASSESSMENT	MANAGEMENT
● Undertake a quick scan assessment. ● Undertake a primary survey **ABCDEF**. ● Assess for **TIME CRITICAL** features (see definition and symptoms of severe pre-eclampsia below).	● If any time critical features are present correct A and B and transport to nearest suitable receiving hospital (**refer to medical emergencies guideline**). ● Provide an alert/information call.
● If no **TIME CRITICAL** features perform a more thorough patient assessment with secondary survey including fetal assessment (**refer to obstetric and gynaecology overview for guidance**).	
● Measure blood pressure.	Transfer to further care: ● If pregnancy >22 weeks and systolic blood pressure is ≥140/90 mmHg discuss management directly with the **BOOKED OBSTETRIC UNIT** or **MIDWIFE**.

Table 5.8 – ASSESSMENT and MANAGEMENT

Severe Pre-eclampsia

Definition and symptoms – raised blood pressure >160/110 mmHg, detection of proteinurina, and with one or more of the following: headache (severe and frontal), visual disturbances, epigastric pain, right-sided upper abdominal pain, muscle twitching or tremor, nausea, vomiting, confusion, rapidly progressive oedema.

ASSESSMENT	MANAGEMENT
● Undertake a quick scan assessment. ● Undertake a primary survey **ABCDEF**. ● Assess for signs of severe pre-eclampsia (see definition and symptoms above). Signs of severe pre-eclampsia are **TIME CRITICAL FEATURES**.	● If any time critical features are present correct A and B problems (**refer to medical emergencies guideline**) and transfer to a consultant-led obstetric unit. NB Caution with 'lights and sirens' as strobe lights and noise may precipitate convulsions. ● If the patient is convulsing **refer to convulsion guideline**. ● Provide an alert/information call. ● If the convulsion is **NOT** self-limiting transfer to consultant-led obstetric unit.
● Monitor SpO$_2$ (94–98%).	● Attach pulse oximeter; if O$_2$ <94% administer O$_2$ to aim for a target saturation within the range of 94–98%.
	● Obtain IV access – insert a **LARGE BORE** cannula en-route. ● **DO NOT** administer intravenous fluid boluses because of the risk of provoking pulmonary oedema.
● Measure blood glucose level.	**Refer to glycaemic emergencies guideline.**

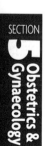

SECTION 2 – Eclampsia

1. Introduction

● Eclampsia is generalised tonic/clonic 'grand mal' convulsion and identical to an epileptic convulsion.

● Many patients will have had pre-existing pre-eclampsia (of mild, moderate or severe degree), but cases of eclampsia can present acutely with no prior warning – **ONE-THIRD** of cases present for the **FIRST TIME** post-delivery (usually in the first 48 hours). **THE BP MAY ONLY BE MILDLY ELEVATED AT PRESENTATION** (i.e. 140/80–90 mmHg).

● A convulsion is usually 'self-limiting' and will end after 2–3 minutes and can present for up to 6 weeks post partum (**refer to convulsion guideline**).

2. Incidence

● Eclampsia occurs in approximately 2.7:10,000 deliveries, usually beyond 24 weeks.

Pregnancy-Induced Hypertension (including eclampsia)

3. Severity and Outcome

- Eclampsia is one of the most dangerous complications of pregnancy and is a significant cause of maternal mortality with a mortality rate of 2% in the UK.
- Convulsions are usually self-limiting, but may be severe and repeated.
- Other complications associated with eclampsia include renal failure, hepatic failure and DIC.

4. Pathophysiology

- The hypoxia caused during a tonic/clonic convulsion may lead to significant fetal compromise and even death.

5. Assessment and Management

- For the assessment and management mild/moderate eclampsia and eclamptic convulsion refer to Table 5.9.

Risk Factors – Eclampsia
- Known pre-eclampsia.
- Primiparity or first child with a new partner.
- Previous severe pre-eclampsia.
- Essential hypertension.
- Diabetes.
- Obesity.
- Twins or higher multiples.
- Renal disease.
- Advanced maternal age (over 40 years).
- Young maternal age (less than 16 years).

Table 5.9 – ASSESSMENT and MANAGEMENT of:

Eclampsia

Definition – Eclampsia is generalised tonic/clonic 'grand mal' convulsion and identical to an epileptic convulsion.

ASSESSMENT	MANAGEMENT
• Undertake a primary survey **ABCDEF**. • Assess for **TIME CRITICAL** features such as recurrent convulsions.	• Correct A and B and transport to a consultant-led obstetric unit (**refer to medical emergencies guideline**). • Obtain IV (**LARGE BORE** cannulae) or IO access. **DO NOT** administer fluid boluses because of the risk of provoking pulmonary oedema. • Provide an alert/ information call.
• If no **TIME CRITICAL** features perform a more thorough patient assessment with secondary survey including fetal assessment (**refer to obstetric and gynaecology overview for guidance**).	NOTE: epileptic patients may suffer tonic/clonic convulsions: • If >22 weeks gestation with a history of hypertension or pre-eclampsia treat as for eclampsia – refer to Table 5.4 and 5.5. • If there is no history of hypertension or pre-eclampsia and blood pressure is normal treat as for epilepsy (**refer to convulsion guideline**). • Position the patient in 15–30 degree **LEFT LATERAL TILT** or left lateral (recovery) position.
• Monitor SpO$_2$ (94–98%).	• Attach pulse oximeter; if O$_2$ <94% administer O$_2$ to aim for a target saturation within the range of 94–98%.
• Continuous or recurrent convulsion.	• If the patient convulses for longer than 2–3 minutes or has a second or subsequent convulsion administer diazepam IV/PR titrated against effect (refer to diazepam guideline for dosages and information). NOTE: in hospital, IV magnesium sulphate will be given and it is better to avoid multiple drugs if possible.

Methodology

For details of the methodology used in the development of this guideline refer to the guideline webpage.

KEY POINTS

Pregnancy-Induced Hypertension (including eclampsia)

- Pregnancy-induced hypertension commonly occurs beyond 24–28 weeks but can occur as early as 22 weeks.

- Can present up to 6 weeks post delivery.

- Diagnosis includes an increase in blood pressure above 140/90 mmHg, oedema and detection of protein in the patient's urine.

- Eclampsia is one of the most dangerous complications of pregnancy.

- Eclampsia patients present with generalised tonic/clonic convulsions which are usually self-limiting.

- Only administer diazepam if the convulsions are prolonged or recurrent.

- Severe pre-eclampsia and eclampsia are TIME CRITICAL EMERGENCIES for both mother and unborn child.

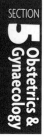

SECTION

5

Obstetrics & Gynaecology

Vaginal Bleeding: Gynaecological Causes [870, 872, 873]

1. Introduction

- A number of conditions can cause vaginal bleeding that is different from normal menstruation. Such conditions may result in a call to the ambulance service, including:
  - excessive menstrual period

    normal or excessive menstrual period associated with severe abdominal pain
  - surgical or medical therapeutic abortion (may occur up to 10 days after treatment)
  - following gynaecological surgery (e.g. hysterectomy) (may occur up to 10 days after surgery)
  - colposcopy (may occur up to 10 days after a colposcopy)
  - gynaecological cancers, either before diagnosis or after treatment (i.e. cervix, uterus or vagina).
- This guideline provides guidance for the assessment and management of gynaecological vaginal bleeding. For causes of bleeding in early or late pregnancy, **refer to haemorrhage during early/late pregnancy (including miscarriage and ectopic pregnancy) guideline**.

2. Incidence

- Women over 50 years are more at risk of cancers of the uterus and cervix.

3. Severity and Outcome

- The majority of causes of vaginal bleeding do not compromise the circulation, but blood loss can be alarming.

4. Pathophysiology

- Various pathophysiology.

Methodology

For details of the methodology used to develop this guideline refer to the guideline webpage.

Table 5.10 – ASSESSMENT and MANAGEMENT

Vaginal Bleeding

ASSESSMENT	MANAGEMENT
• Quickly scan the patient and scene as you approach. • Undertake a primary survey **ABCD**. • Evaluate whether the patient has any **TIME CRITICAL** features or any signs of hypovolaemic shock.	• If any **TIME CRITICAL** features are present correct **A** and **B** and transport to nearest suitable receiving hospital (**refer to medical emergencies guidance**). • Provide an alert/information call.
• Assess blood loss – ask about clots, blood-soaked clothes bed sheets, number of soaked tampons/towels/pads. NB Blood under the feet or between toes implies significant bleeding.	• Obtain IV access – insert a **LARGE BORE** cannula. • If there is visible external blood loss >500mls **refer to intravascular fluid therapy guideline**.
• If no **TIME CRITICAL** features, perform a more thorough patient assessment with brief secondary survey for lower abdominal tenderness or guarding.	
• Measure temperature.	
• Check the patient's age: – >50 years – more at risk of cancers of the uterus/cervix – <50 years may be pregnant.	
• Monitor SpO$_2$ (94–98%).	• If oxygen (O$_2$) <94% administer O$_2$ to aim for a target saturation within the range of 94–98%.
• Assess patient's level of pain.	Titrate pain relief against pain (**refer to pain management guideline**): – Paracetamol – Entonox – Morphine NB administer cautiously if the patient is hypotensive.
• Assess patient's comfort.	• Nil by mouth.
	• Adjust patient's position as required.
	• Transfer to further care.

Vaginal Bleeding: Gynaecological Causes

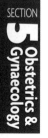

SECTION **5** Obstetrics & Gynaecology

6

Drugs

Drugs

1. Introduction

- The guidelines contained in this section are the current medicines that can be administered by registered paramedics[a].

- The Medicines Act 1968 governs what paramedics can administer and this is regulated by The Medicines and Healthcare products Regulatory Agency (MHRA).

- Where a Prescription-Only Medicines (POMs) exemption exists the MHRA has agreed a Patient Group Direction (PGD) is no longer required for paramedics to administer drugs where a JRCALC drug protocol is issued. Currently POMs exemptions have not been issued for intravenous paracetamol, ondansetron, and tranexamic acid, therefore a PGD is required. A POMs exemption is not required for dexamethasone as the intravenous preparation is administered orally.

- The drugs administered by ambulance clinicians fall into two categories:

1. **Non-prescription drugs** e.g. aspirin
2. **Prescription-only medicines (POMs)** e.g. morphine. POMs can only be prescribed by a qualified doctor (or dentist) and non-medical prescribers but exemptions exist under Part III of Schedule 5 to the Prescription Only Medicines (Human Use) Order 1997 allows suitably trained paramedics to administer these drugs in specified circumstances.

1.1 Safety aspects

- Always check the following:
  - the drug type
  - the drug strength
  - whether the packaging is intact
  - the clarity of fluid
  - the expiry date.

1.2 Prescribing terms

In the case of prescription medicines, a variety of abbreviations are used, some of which are described – refer to Table 6.2

NB Internationally recognised units and symbols should be used where possible.

Table 6.2 – COMMON ABBREVIATIONS

Abbreviation	Translation
ac	ante cibum (before food)
approx	approximately
bd	twice daily
CD	preparation subject to prescription requirements control – The Misuse of Drugs Act
ec	enteric-coated (termed gastro-resistant in British Pharmacopoeia)
f/c	film-coated
IM	intramuscular
IV	intravenous
m/r	modified-release
MAOI	monoamine-oxidase inhibitors
max	maximum
NSAID	non-steroidal anti-inflammatory drug
o. d	omni die (every day)
o. m	omni mane (every morning)
o. n	omni nocte (every night)
p. c	post cibum (after food)
PGD	patient group direction
POM	prescription only medicine
pr	per rectum (rectally)
prn	when required
q.d.s	quater die sumendus (to be taken four times daily)
q.q.h	quarta quaque hora (every four hours)
s/c	sugar-coated
SSRI	selective serotonin re-uptake inhibitor
SOS	when required
SR	slow release
stat	immediately
t.d.s	ter die sumendus (to be taken three times daily)
t.i.d	ter in die (three times daily)
top	topical

Table 6.1 – DOCUMENTATION

Note the following:	✔	✗
Avoid unnecessary use of decimal points	3 mg	3.0 mg
Quantities of 1 gram or more should be written as	1 g	–
Quantities less than 1 gram should be written in milligrams	500 mg	0.5 g
Quantities less than 1 mg should be written in micrograms	100 micrograms	0.1 mg
When decimals are unavoidable a zero should be written in front of the decimal point where there is no other figure	0.5 mL	not .5 mL
Use of the decimal point is acceptable to express a range	0.5 to 1 g	–
'Micrograms' and 'nanograms' should not be abbreviated nor should 'units'	–	–
The term 'millilitre' is used	ml or ml	cubic centimetre, c.c., or cm^3

[a]Paramedic is defined as being on the register of paramedics maintained by the Health and Care Professions Council pursuant to paragraph 11 of Schedule 2 to the Health Professions Order 2001.

Drugs Overview

1.3 Drug routes

- Drug routes are classified as **parenteral** and **non-parenteral**:
  - **Parenteral routes** are those where a physical breach of the skin or mucous membrane is made, for example, by injection
  - Non-parenteral routes are those where the drug is absorbed passively, for example, via the gastrointestinal tract, mucous membranes or skin.
- Drugs can be administered via a number of routes – refer to Table 6.3. It is important that the most appropriate route is selected – refer to Table 6.4, taking into account the patient's condition and the urgency of the situation.
- Drugs and their possible routes of administration are listed in Table 6.4. In cases of parenteral administration, where at all possible, intravenous (IV) cannulation should be attempted, except for children in cardiac arrest where intra-osseous cannulation is the preferred method. NB If a vein cannot be found it is not necessary to attempt IV cannulation. With intramuscular and subcutaneous routes, absorption may be erratic or incomplete if the patient is hypovolaemic or clinically unstable.

Table 6.3 – DRUG ROUTES

Parenteral Routes

Intramuscular – Injection of the drug into muscle, which is then absorbed into the blood. Absorption may be decreased in poor perfusion states.

Intra-osseous – A rigid needle inserted directly into the bone marrow. Resuscitation drugs and fluid replacement may be administered by this route. Absorption is as quick as by the intravenous route.

Intravenous – Direct introduction of the drug into the cardiovascular system that normally delivers the drug to the target organs very quickly.

Subcutaneous – Injection of the drug into subcutaneous tissue. This usually has a slower rate of absorption than from intramuscular injection and may be decreased in poor perfusion states.

Non-Parenteral Routes

Inhaled – Gaseous drugs that are absorbed via the lungs.

Nebulisation – Liquid drugs agitated in a stream of gas such as oxygen to create fine droplets that are absorbed rapidly from the lungs.

Oral – The drug is swallowed and is absorbed into the blood from the gut. In serious trauma or illness, absorption may be delayed.

Rectal – The drug is absorbed from the wall of the rectum. This route is used for patients who are having seizures and who cannot be cannulated without risk to themselves or ambulance personnel. Effects usually occur 5–15 minutes after administration.

Sub-lingual – Tablet or aerosol spray is absorbed from the mucous membrane beneath the tongue. Effects usually occur within 2–3 minutes.

Transdermal – Absorption of a drug through the skin.

Buccal – Absorption via the mucous membrane.

Intranasal – Aerosol spray absorbed from the mucous membrane.

KEY POINTS

Drugs Overview

- **Check the drug type, strength, whether the packaging is intact, the clarity of fluid and the expiry date.**
- **Select the most appropriate route taking into account the patient's condition and the urgency of the situation.**
- **Only administer drugs via the routes you have been trained for.**
- **The drug codes are provided for INFORMATION ONLY.**
- **Complete documentation.**

SECTION 6 Drugs

Drugs Overview

Table 6.4 – SUGGESTED DRUG ROUTES

Drug/Route	IV	IO	IM	SC	Oral	Sub-lingual	Buccal	Intranasal	Rectal	Inhaled	Nebulised	Transdermal	Flush
Adrenaline	✔	✔	✔	✔	N/A	N/A	N/A	N/A	N/A	N/A	N/A	N/A	N/A
Amiodarone	✔	✔	N/A	N/A	N/A	N/A	N/A	N/A	N/A	N/A	N/A	N/A	N/A
Aspirin	N/A	N/A	N/A	N/A	✔	N/A	N/A	N/A	N/A	N/A	N/A	N/A	N/A
Atropine	✔	✔	✔	N/A	N/A	N/A	N/A	N/A	N/A	N/A	N/A	N/A	N/A
Atropine (CBRNE)	N/A	N/A	✔	N/A	N/A	N/A	N/A	N/A	N/A	N/A	N/A	N/A	N/A
Benzylpenicillin	✔	✔	N/A	N/A	N/A	N/A	N/A	N/A	N/A	N/A	N/A	N/A	N/A
Chlorphenamine	✔	✔	✔	N/A	✔	N/A	N/A	N/A	N/A	N/A	N/A	N/A	N/A
Ciprofloxacin (CBRNE)	N/A	N/A	N/A	N/A	✔	N/A	N/A	N/A	N/A	N/A	N/A	N/A	N/A
Clopidogrel	N/A	N/A	N/A	N/A	✔	N/A	N/A	N/A	N/A	N/A	N/A	N/A	N/A
Dexamethasone	✔	✔	✔	N/A	✔	N/A	N/A	N/A	N/A	N/A	N/A	N/A	N/A
Diazepam	✔	✔	N/A	N/A	N/A	N/A	N/A	N/A	✔	N/A	N/A	N/A	N/A
Dicobalt (CBRNE)	✔	✔	N/A	N/A	N/A	N/A	N/A	N/A	N/A	N/A	N/A	N/A	N/A
Doxycycline (CBRNE)	N/A	N/A	N/A	N/A	✔	N/A	N/A	N/A	N/A	N/A	N/A	N/A	N/A
Entonox/Nitronox	N/A	N/A	N/A	N/A	N/A	N/A	N/A	N/A	N/A	✔	N/A	N/A	N/A
Furosemide	✔	✔	N/A	N/A	N/A	N/A	N/A	N/A	N/A	N/A	N/A	N/A	N/A
Glucagon	N/A	N/A	✔	N/A	N/A	N/A	N/A	N/A	N/A	N/A	N/A	N/A	N/A
Glucose 10%	✔	✔	N/A	N/A	N/A	N/A	N/A	N/A	N/A	N/A	N/A	N/A	N/A
Glucose 40% Gel	N/A	N/A	N/A	N/A	N/A	N/A	✔	N/A	N/A	N/A	N/A	N/A	N/A
Glyceryl Trinitrate	N/A	N/A	N/A	N/A	N/A	✔	✔	N/A	N/A	N/A	N/A	N/A	N/A
Heparin	✔	✔	N/A	N/A	N/A	N/A	N/A	N/A	N/A	N/A	N/A	N/A	N/A
Hydrocortisone	✔	✔	✔	N/A	N/A	N/A	N/A	N/A	N/A	N/A	N/A	N/A	N/A
Ibuprofen	N/A	N/A	N/A	N/A	✔	N/A	N/A	N/A	N/A	N/A	N/A	N/A	N/A
Ipratropium Bromide	N/A	N/A	N/A	N/A	N/A	N/A	N/A	N/A	N/A	N/A	✔	N/A	N/A
Ketamine	✔	✔	✔	N/A	N/A	N/A	N/A	N/A	N/A	N/A	N/A	N/A	N/A
Metoclopramide	✔	✔	✔	N/A	N/A	N/A	N/A	N/A	N/A	N/A	N/A	N/A	N/A
Patient's own Midazolam	N/A	N/A	N/A	N/A	N/A	N/A	✔	✔	N/A	N/A	N/A	N/A	N/A
Misoprostol	N/A	N/A	N/A	N/A	✔	N/A	N/A	N/A	✔	N/A	N/A	N/A	N/A
Morphine Sulphate	✔	✔	✔	✔	✔	N/A	N/A	N/A	N/A	N/A	N/A	N/A	N/A
Naloxone Hydrochloride	✔	✔	✔	✔	N/A	N/A	N/A	✔	N/A	N/A	N/A	N/A	N/A
Obidoxime (CBRNE)	✔	✔	N/A	N/A	N/A	N/A	N/A	N/A	N/A	N/A	N/A	N/A	N/A
Ondansetron	✔	✔	✔	N/A	N/A	N/A	N/A	N/A	N/A	N/A	N/A	N/A	N/A
Oxygen	N/A	N/A	N/A	N/A	N/A	N/A	N/A	N/A	N/A	✔	N/A	N/A	N/A
Paracetamol	✔	✔	N/A	N/A	✔	N/A	N/A	N/A	N/A	N/A	N/A	N/A	N/A
Potassium Iodate (CBRNE)	N/A	N/A	N/A	N/A	✔	N/A	N/A	N/A	N/A	N/A	N/A	N/A	N/A
Pralidoxime Mesylate (CBRNE)	✔	✔	N/A	N/A	N/A	N/A	N/A	N/A	N/A	N/A	N/A	N/A	N/A
Reteplase	✔	N/A	N/A	N/A	N/A	N/A	N/A	N/A	N/A	N/A	N/A	N/A	N/A
Salbutamol	N/A	N/A	N/A	N/A	N/A	N/A	N/A	N/A	N/A	✔	✔	N/A	N/A
0.9% Sodium Chloride	✔	✔	N/A	N/A	N/A	N/A	N/A	N/A	N/A	N/A	N/A	N/A	✔
Sodium Lactate	✔	✔	N/A	N/A	N/A	N/A	N/A	N/A	N/A	N/A	N/A	N/A	N/A
Syntometrine	N/A	N/A	✔	N/A	N/A	N/A	N/A	N/A	N/A	N/A	N/A	N/A	N/A
Tenecteplase	✔	N/A	N/A	N/A	N/A	N/A	N/A	N/A	N/A	N/A	N/A	N/A	N/A
Tetracaine	N/A	N/A	N/A	N/A	N/A	N/A	N/A	N/A	N/A	N/A	N/A	✔	N/A
Tranexamic Acid	✔	N/A	N/A	N/A	N/A	N/A	N/A	N/A	N/A	N/A	N/A	N/A	N/A

Drugs Overview

1.4 Drug Codes

The drug codes listed in Table 6.5 are provided for **INFORMATION ONLY** and represent drugs that may be commonly encountered in the emergency/urgent care environment. **ONLY** the drugs listed in the guidelines are for use by registered paramedics; the remaining drugs are for use by physicians or under patient group directions by paramedics who have undertaken extended training.

Table 6.5 – JRCALC DRUG CODES

Drug	Code	Drug	Code
Adenosine	**ADE**	Erythromycin	**ERY**
Adrenaline (Epinephrine) 1:1,000	**ADM**	Etomidate	**ETO**
Adrenaline (Epinephrine) 1:10,000	**ADX**	Flucloxacillin	**FCX**
Alteplase	**APL**	Flumazenil	**FLZ**
Aminophylline	**AMN**	Fluorescein Sodium	**FLR**
Amiodarone	**AMO**	Furosemide	**FRM**
Amoxicillin	**AMX**	Fusidic Acid Eye Preparation	**FUA**
Aspirin	**ASP**	Glucagon	**GLU**
Atracurium	**ATC**	Glucose 10%	**GLX**
Atropine	**ATR**	Glucose 40% Gel	**GLG**
Benzylpenicillin	**BPN**	Glucose 5%	**GLX**
Cefalexin	**CEF**	Glucose 50%	**GLL**
Cefotaxime	**CFT**	Glycerol Suppositories	**GLS**
Ceftriaxone	**CFX**	Glyceryl Trinitrate (GTN)	**GTN**
Cetirizine	**CTZ**	Haloperidol	**HPD**
Chloramphenicol Eye Preparation	**CPL**	Heparin (Standard Unfractionated)	**HEP**
Chlorphenamine	**CPH**	Hydrocortisone	**HYC**
Chlorpromazine	**CHZ**	Ibuprofen	**IBP**
Ciprofloxacin	**CXN**	Ipratropium Bromide	**IPR**
Clarithromycin	**CMY**	Ketamine	**KET**
Clopidogrel	**CLO**	Levonorgestrel	**LVG**
Clotrimazole	**CZL**	Lidocaine	**LID**
Co-amoxiclav	**CXV**	Lidocaine Gel (Mucocutaneous Anaesthesia)	**LDU**
Codeine	**COD**	Lorazepam	**LRZ**
Codeine-Paracetamol Combination	**CPC**	Methylprednisolone	**MTP**
Co-dydramol	**CDY**	Metoclopramide	**MTC**
Colloid Gel Solution	**COL**	Metronidazole	**MTZ**
Cyclimorph	**CYM**	Midazolam	**MDZ**
Cyclizine	**CYZ**	Midazolam (Patient's Own Midazolam)	**MDZ**
Dexamethasone	**DEX**	Misoprostol	**MIS**
Dextrose 5%	**GLV**	Morphine Sulphate	**MOR**
Diamorphine	**DMO**	Naloxone Hydrochloride	**NLX**
Diazepam	**DZP**	Naproxen	**NPN**
Diclofenac	**DCF**	Nitrofurantoin	**NFT**
Dicobalt Edetate	**DCO**	Nystatin	**NST**
Dihydrocodeine	**DHC**	Obidoxime Chloride	**ODC**
Domperidone	**DMP**	Ondansetron	**ODT**
Doxycycline	**DXN**	Oral Rehydration Salts	**ORS**
Enoxaparin (Low Molecular Weight Heparin)	**ENP**	Oseltamivir	**OSV**
Entonox/Nitronox	**NOO**	Otosporin Ear Drops	**OTS**
Ergometrine Maleate	**ERG**	Oxybuprocaine Benoxinate	**OBP**

Table 6.5 – JRCALC DRUG CODES *continued*

Drug	Code	Drug	Code
Oxygen	**OXG**	0.9% Sodium Chloride	**SCP**
Oxytetracycline	**OXL**	Sodium Lactate, Compound	**SLC**
Oxytocin	**OXT**	Sodium Thiopentone	**STP**
Paracetamol	**PAR**	Suxamethonium	**SUX**
Penicillin V	**PNV**	Syntometrine	**SYN**
Pethidine	**PTH**	Tenecteplase	**TNK**
Potassium iodate	**PIO**	Terbutaline	**TER**
Pralidoxime Mesylate	**PDM**	Tetanus Immunoglobulin	**TIG**
Prednisolone	**PRD**	Tetanus/Low Dose Diphtheria Vaccine	**TTD**
Prochlorperazine	**PCZ**	Tetracaine (Amethocaine)	**TTC**
Procyclidine	**PCY**	Tramadol	**TRM**
Propofol	**PPL**	Tranexamic Acid	**TXA**
Reteplase	**RPA**	Trimethoprim	**TMP**
Rocuronium	**RCR**	Vecuronium	**VEC**
Salbutamol	**SLB**	Water For Injection	**WFI**

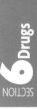

Presentation

Pre-filled syringe or ampoule containing 1 milligram of adrenaline (epinephrine) in 1 ml (1:1,000) ADM.

Pre-filled syringe containing 1 milligram of adrenaline (epinephrine) in 10 ml (1:10,000) ADX.

Indications

Cardiac arrest.

Anaphylaxis.

Life-threatening asthma with failing ventilation and continued deterioration despite nebuliser therapy.

Actions

Adrenaline is a sympathomimetic that stimulates both alpha- and beta-adrenergic receptors. As a result myocardial and cerebral blood flow is enhanced during CPR and CPR becomes more effective due to increased peripheral resistance which improves perfusion pressures.

Reverses allergic manifestations of acute anaphylaxis.

Relieves bronchospasm in acute severe asthma.

Contra-indications

Do not give repeated doses of adrenaline in hypothermic patients.

Cautions

Severe hypertension may occur in patients on beta-blockers and half doses should be administered unless there is profound hypotension.

For patients taking tricyclic antidepressants (e.g. amitriptyline, imipramine) half doses of adrenaline should be administered for anaphylaxis.

Dosage and Administration

1. **Cardiac arrest:**

● **Shockable rhythms:** administer adrenaline after the 3rd shock and then after alternate shocks i.e. 5th, 7th etc.

● **Non-shockable rhythms:** administer adrenaline immediately IV access is achieved then alternate loops.

Route: Intravenous/intra-osseous — **administer as a rapid bolus**.

AGE	INITIAL DOSE	REPEAT DOSE	DOSE INTERVAL	CONCENTRATION	VOLUME	MAXIMUM DOSE
Adult	1 milligram	1 milligram	3–5 minutes	1 milligram in 10 ml (1:10,000)	10 ml	No limit
11 years	350 micrograms	350 micrograms	3–5 minutes	1 milligram in 10 ml (1:10,000)	3.5 ml	No limit
10 years	320 micrograms	320 micrograms	3–5 minutes	1 milligram in 10 ml (1:10,000)	3.2 ml	No limit
9 years	300 micrograms	300 micrograms	3–5 minutes	1 milligram in 10 ml (1:10,000)	3 ml	No limit
8 years	260 micrograms	260 micrograms	3–5 minutes	1 milligram in 10 ml (1:10,000)	2.6 ml	No limit
7 years	230 micrograms	230 micrograms	3–5 minutes	1 milligram in 10 ml (1:10,000)	2.3 ml	No limit
6 years	210 micrograms	210 micrograms	3–5 minutes	1 milligram in 10 ml (1:10,000)	2.1 ml	No limit
5 years	190 micrograms	190 micrograms	3–5 minutes	1 milligram in 10 ml (1:10,000)	1.9 ml	No limit
4 years	160 micrograms	160 micrograms	3–5 minutes	1 milligram in 10 ml (1:10,000)	1.6 ml	No limit
3 years	140 micrograms	140 micrograms	3–5 minutes	1 milligram in 10 ml (1:10,000)	1.4 ml	No limit
2 years	120 micrograms	120 micrograms	3–5 minutes	1 milligram in 10 ml (1:10,000)	1.2 ml	No limit
18 months	110 micrograms	110 micrograms	3–5 minutes	1 milligram in 10 ml (1:10,000)	1.1 ml	No limit
12 months	100 micrograms	100 micrograms	3–5 minutes	1 milligram in 10 ml (1:10,000)	1 ml	No limit
9 months	90 micrograms	90 micrograms	3–5 minutes	1 milligram in 10 ml (1:10,000)	0.9 ml	No limit
6 months	80 micrograms	80 micrograms	3–5 minutes	1 milligram in 10 ml (1:10,000)	0.8 ml	No limit
3 months	60 micrograms	60 micrograms	3–5 minutes	1 milligram in 10 ml (1:10,000)	0.6 ml	No limit
1 month	50 micrograms	50 micrograms	3–5 minutes	1 milligram in 10 ml (1:10,000)	0.5 ml	No limit
Birth	35 micrograms	35 micrograms	3–5 minutes	1 milligram in 10 ml (1:10,000)	0.35 ml	No limit

2. **Anaphylaxis** and **life-threatening asthma** (NB In cases of anaphylaxis in patients taking tricyclic antidepressants (e.g. amitriptyline, imipramine) administer half doses).

Route: Intramuscular – antero-lateral aspect of thigh or upper arm.

AGE	INITIAL DOSE	REPEAT DOSE	DOSE INTERVAL	CONCENTRATION	VOLUME	MAXIMUM DOSE
Adult	500 micrograms	500 micrograms	5 minutes	1 milligram in 1 ml (1:1,000)	0.5 ml	No limit
11 years	300 micrograms	300 micrograms	5 minutes	1 milligram in 1 ml (1:1,000)	0.3 ml	No limit
10 years	300 micrograms	300 micrograms	5 minutes	1 milligram in 1 ml (1:1,000)	0.3 ml	No limit
9 years	300 micrograms	300 micrograms	5 minutes	1 milligram in 1 ml (1:1,000)	0.3 ml	No limit
8 years	300 micrograms	300 micrograms	5 minutes	1 milligram in 1 ml (1:1,000)	0.3 ml	No limit
7 years	300 micrograms	300 micrograms	5 minutes	1 milligram in 1 ml (1:1,000)	0.3 ml	No limit
6 years	300 micrograms	300 micrograms	5 minutes	1 milligram in 1 ml (1:1,000)	0.3 ml	No limit
5 years	150 micrograms	150 micrograms	5 minutes	1 milligram in 1 ml (1:1,000)	0.15 ml	No limit
4 years	150 micrograms	150 micrograms	5 minutes	1 milligram in 1 ml (1:1,000)	0.15 ml	No limit
3 years	150 micrograms	150 micrograms	5 minutes	1 milligram in 1 ml (1:1,000)	0.15 ml	No limit
2 years	150 micrograms	150 micrograms	5 minutes	1 milligram in 1 ml (1:1,000)	0.15 ml	No limit
18 months	150 micrograms	150 micrograms	5 minutes	1 milligram in 1 ml (1:1,000)	0.15 ml	No limit
12 months	150 micrograms	150 micrograms	5 minutes	1 milligram in 1 ml (1:1,000)	0.15 ml	No limit
9 months	150 micrograms	150 micrograms	5 minutes	1 milligram in 1 ml (1:1,000)	0.15 ml	No limit
6 months	150 micrograms	150 micrograms	5 minutes	1 milligram in 1 ml (1:1,000)	0.15 ml	No limit
3 months	150 micrograms	150 micrograms	5 minutes	1 milligram in 1 ml (1:1,000)	0.15 ml	No limit
1 months	150 micrograms	150 micrograms	5 minutes	1 milligram in 1 ml (1:1,000)	0.15 ml	No limit
Birth	150 micrograms	150 micrograms	5 minutes	1 milligram in 1 ml (1:1,000)	0.15 ml	No limit

Drugs – A

SECTION 6

Presentation

Pre-filled syringe containing 300 milligrams amiodarone in 10 ml.

Indications

Cardiac arrest

- **Shockable rhythms:** if unresponsive to defibrillation administer amiodarone after the 3rd shock and an additional bolus depending on age to unresponsive VF or pulseless VT following the 5th shock.

Actions

Antiarrhythmic; lengthens cardiac action potential and therefore effective refractory period. Prolongs QT interval on ECG.

Blocks sodium and potassium channels in cardiac muscle.

Acts to stabilise and reduce electrical irritability of cardiac muscle.

Contra-indications

No contra-indications in the context of the treatment of cardiac arrest.

Side Effects

Bradycardia.

Vasodilatation causing hypotension, flushing.

Bronchospasm.

Arrhythmias – Torsades de pointes.

Dosage and Administration

- Administer into large vein as extravasation can cause burns.
- Follow administration with a 0.9% sodium chloride flush – **refer to sodium chloride guideline.**
- Cardiac arrest – Shockable rhythms: if unresponsive to defibrillation administer amiodarone after the 3rd shock.

Route: intravenous/intra-osseous – administer as a rapid bolus.

AGE	INITIAL DOSE	REPEAT DOSE	DOSE INTERVAL	CONCENTRATION	VOLUME	MAXIMUM DOSE
Adult	300 milligrams	150 mg	After 5th shock	300 milligrams in 10 ml	10 ml	450 milligrams
11 years	180 milligrams	180 mg	After 5th shock	300 milligrams in 10 ml	6 ml	360 milligrams
10 years	160 milligrams	160 mg	After 5th shock	300 milligrams in 10 ml	5.3 ml	320 milligrams
9 years	150 milligrams	150 mg	After 5th shock	300 milligrams in 10 ml	5 ml	300 milligrams
8 years	130 milligrams	130 mg	After 5th shock	300 milligrams in 10 ml	4.3 ml	260 milligrams
7 years	120 milligrams	120 mg	After 5th shock	300 milligrams in 10 ml	4 ml	240 milligrams
6 years	100 milligrams	100 mg	After 5th shock	300 milligrams in 10 ml	3.3 ml	200 milligrams
5 years	100 milligrams	100 mg	After 5th shock	300 milligrams in 10 ml	3.3 ml	200 milligrams
4 years	80 milligrams	80 mg	After 5th shock	300 milligrams in 10 ml	2.7 ml	160 milligrams
3 years	70 milligrams	70 mg	After 5th shock	300 milligrams in 10 ml	2.3 ml	140 milligrams
2 years	60 milligrams	60 mg	After 5th shock	300 milligrams in 10 ml	2 ml	120 milligrams
18 months	55 milligrams	55 mg	After 5th shock	300 milligrams in 10 ml	1.8 ml	110 milligrams
12 months	50 milligrams	50 mg	After 5th shock	300 milligrams in 10 ml	1.7 ml	100 milligrams
9 months	45 milligrams	45 mg	After 5th shock	300 milligrams in 10 ml	1.5 ml	90 milligrams
6 months	40 milligrams	40 mg	After 5th shock	300 milligrams in 10 ml	1.3 ml	80 milligrams
3 months	30 milligrams	30 mg	After 5th shock	300 milligrams in 10 ml	1 ml	60 milligrams
1 month	25 milligrams	25 mg	After 5th shock	300 milligrams in 10 ml	0.8 ml	50 milligrams
Birth	18 milligrams	18 mg	After 5th shock	300 milligrams in 10 ml	0.6 ml	36 milligrams

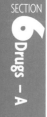

SECTION

6

Drugs – A

286

Drugs

2013

Page **1** of **1**

Aspirin [898]   ASP

Presentation

300 milligram aspirin (acetylsalicylic acid) in tablet form (dispersible).

Indications

Adults with:

- Clinical or ECG evidence suggestive of myocardial infarction or ischaemia.

Actions

Has an anti-platelet action which reduces clot formation.

Analgesic, anti-pyretic and anti-inflammatory.

Contra-indications

- Known aspirin allergy or sensitivity.
- Children under 16 years (see additional information).
- Active gastrointestinal bleeding.
- Haemophilia or other known clotting disorders.
- Severe hepatic disease.

Cautions

As the likely benefits of a single 300 milligram aspirin outweigh the potential risks, aspirin may be given to patients with:

- Asthma
- Pregnancy
- Kidney or liver failure
- Gastric or duodenal ulcer
- Current treatment with anticoagulants.

Side Effects

- Gastric bleeding.
- Wheezing in some asthmatics.

Additional Information

In suspected myocardial infarction a 300 milligram aspirin tablet should be given regardless of any previous aspirin taken that day.

Clopidogrel may be indicated in acute ST segment elevation myocardial infarction – **refer to clopidogrel guideline**.

Aspirin is contra-indicated in children under the age of 16 years as it may precipitate Reye's Syndrome. This syndrome is very rare and occurs in young children, damaging the liver and brain. It has a mortality rate of 50%.

Dosage and Administration

Route: Oral – chewed or dissolved in water.

AGE	INITIAL DOSE	REPEAT DOSE	DOSE INTERVAL	CONCENTRATION	VOLUME	MAXIMUM DOSE
Adults	300 milligrams	NONE	N/A	300 milligrams in 2 ml	1 tablet	300 milligrams

Presentation

Pre-filled syringe containing 1 milligram atropine in 10 ml.

Pre-filled syringe containing 1 milligram atropine in 5 ml.

Pre-filled syringe containing 3 milligrams atropine in 10 ml.

An ampoule containing 600 micrograms in 1 ml.

Indications

Symptomatic bradycardia in the presence of **ANY** of these adverse signs:

- Absolute bradycardia (pulse <40 beats per minute).
- Systolic blood pressure below expected for age (**refer to page for age guideline** for age related blood pressure readings in children).
- Paroxysmal ventricular arrhythmias requiring suppression.
- Inadequate perfusion causing, confusion etc.

NB Hypoxia is the most common cause of bradycardia in children, therefore interventions to support ABC and oxygen therapy should be the first-line therapy.

Contra-indications

Should **NOT** be given to treat bradycardia in suspected hypothermia.

Actions

May reverse effects of vagal overdrive.

May increase heart rate by blocking vagal activity in sinus bradycardia, second or third degree heart block.

Enhances A-V conduction.

Side Effects

Dry mouth, visual blurring and pupil dilation.

Confusion and occasional hallucinations.

Tachycardia.

In the elderly retention of urine may occur.

Do not use small (<100 micrograms) doses as they may cause paradoxical bradycardia.

Additional Information

May induce tachycardia when used after myocardial infarction, which will increase myocardial oxygen demand and worsen ischaemia. Hence, bradycardia in a patient with an MI should **ONLY** be treated if the low heart rate is causing problems with perfusion, such as hypotension.

Dosage and Administration

SYMPTOMATIC BRADYCARDIA

NB BRADYCARDIA in children is most commonly caused by **HYPOXIA**, requiring immediate ABC care, **NOT** drug therapy; therefore **ONLY** administer atropine in cases of bradycardia caused by vagal stimulation (e.g. suction).

Route: Intravenous/intra-osseous **administer as a rapid bolus**.

AGE	INITIAL DOSE	REPEAT DOSE	DOSE INTERVAL	CONCENTRATION	VOLUME	MAXIMUM DOSE
≥12 years	600 micrograms*	600 micrograms*	3–5 minutes	600 micrograms per ml	1 ml	3 milligrams
11 years	500 micrograms	NONE	N/A	600 micrograms per ml	0.8 ml	500 micrograms
10 years	500 micrograms	NONE	N/A	600 micrograms per ml	0.8 ml	500 micrograms
9 years	500 micrograms	NONE	N/A	600 micrograms per ml	0.8 ml	500 micrograms
8 years	500 micrograms	NONE	N/A	600 micrograms per ml	0.8 ml	500 micrograms
7 years	400 micrograms	NONE	N/A	600 micrograms per ml	0.7 ml	400 micrograms
6 years	400 micrograms	NONE	N/A	600 micrograms per ml	0.7 ml	400 micrograms
5 years	300 micrograms	NONE	N/A	600 micrograms per ml	0.5 ml	300 micrograms
4 years	300 micrograms	NONE	N/A	600 micrograms per ml	0.5 ml	300 micrograms
3 years	240 micrograms	NONE	N/A	600 micrograms per ml	0.4 ml	240 micrograms
2 years	240 micrograms	NONE	N/A	600 micrograms per ml	0.4 ml	240 micrograms
18 months	200 micrograms	NONE	N/A	600 micrograms per ml	0.3 ml	200 micrograms
12 months	200 micrograms	NONE	N/A	600 micrograms per ml	0.3 ml	200 micrograms
9 months	120 micrograms	NONE	N/A	600 micrograms per ml	0.2 ml	120 micrograms
6 months	120 micrograms	NONE	N/A	600 micrograms per ml	0.2 ml	120 micrograms
3 months	120 micrograms	NONE	N/A	600 micrograms per ml	0.2 ml	120 micrograms
1 month	100 micrograms	NONE	N/A	600 micrograms per ml	0.17 ml	100 micrograms
Birth	100 micrograms	NONE	N/A	600 micrograms per ml	0.17 ml	100 micrograms

*The adult dosage can be given as 500 or 600 micrograms to a maximum of 3 milligrams depending on presentation available.

SECTION
6
Drugs – A

Atropine

Route. Intravenous/Intra-osseous **administer as a rapid bolus**.

AGE	INITIAL DOSE	REPEAT DOSE	DOSE INTERVAL	CONCENTRATION	VOLUME	MAXIMUM DOSE
≥12 years	600 micrograms*	600 micrograms*	3–5 minutes	300 micrograms per ml	2 ml	3 milligrams
11 years	500 micrograms	NONE	N/A	300 micrograms per ml	1.7 ml	500 micrograms
10 years	500 micrograms	NONE	N/A	300 micrograms per ml	1.7 ml	500 micrograms
9 years	500 micrograms	NONE	N/A	300 micrograms per ml	1.7 ml	500 micrograms
8 years	500 micrograms	NONE	N/A	300 micrograms per ml	1.7 ml	500 micrograms
7 years	400 micrograms	NONE	N/A	300 micrograms per ml	1.3 ml	400 micrograms
6 years	400 micrograms	NONE	N/A	300 micrograms per ml	1.3 ml	400 micrograms
5 years	300 micrograms	NONE	N/A	300 micrograms per ml	1 ml	300 micrograms
4 years	300 micrograms	NONE	N/A	300 micrograms per ml	1 ml	300 micrograms
3 years	240 micrograms	NONE	N/A	300 micrograms per ml	0.8 ml	240 micrograms
2 years	240 micrograms	NONE	N/A	300 micrograms per ml	0.8 ml	240 micrograms
18 months	200 micrograms	NONE	N/A	300 micrograms per ml	0.7 ml	200 micrograms
12 months	200 micrograms	NONE	N/A	300 micrograms per ml	0.7 ml	200 micrograms
9 months	120 micrograms	NONE	N/A	300 micrograms per ml	0.4 ml	120 micrograms
6 months	120 micrograms	NONE	N/A	300 micrograms per ml	0.4 ml	120 micrograms
3 months	120 micrograms	NONE	N/A	300 micrograms per ml	0.4 ml	120 micrograms
1 month	100 micrograms	NONE	N/A	300 micrograms per ml	0.3 ml	100 micrograms
Birth	100 micrograms	NONE	N/A	300 micrograms per ml	0.3 ml	100 micrograms

Route: Intravenous/intra-osseous **administer as a rapid bolus**.

AGE	INITIAL DOSE	REPEAT DOSE	DOSE INTERVAL	CONCENTRATION	VOLUME	MAXIMUM DOSE
≥12 years	600 micrograms*	600 micrograms*	3–5 minutes	200 micrograms per ml	3 ml	3 milligrams
11 years	500 micrograms	NONE	N/A	200 micrograms per ml	2.5 ml	500 micrograms
10 years	500 micrograms	NONE	N/A	200 micrograms per ml	2.5 ml	500 micrograms
9 years	500 micrograms	NONE	N/A	200 micrograms per ml	2.5 ml	500 micrograms
8 years	500 micrograms	NONE	N/A	200 micrograms per ml	2.5 ml	500 micrograms
7 years	400 micrograms	NONE	N/A	200 micrograms per ml	2 ml	400 micrograms
6 years	400 micrograms	NONE	N/A	200 micrograms per ml	2 ml	400 micrograms
5 years	300 micrograms	NONE	N/A	200 micrograms per ml	1.5 ml	300 micrograms
4 years	300 micrograms	NONE	N/A	200 micrograms per ml	1.5 ml	300 micrograms
3 years	240 micrograms	NONE	N/A	200 micrograms per ml	1.2 ml	240 micrograms
2 years	240 micrograms	NONE	N/A	200 micrograms per ml	1.2 ml	240 micrograms
18 months	200 micrograms	NONE	N/A	200 micrograms per ml	1 ml	200 micrograms
12 months	200 micrograms	NONE	N/A	200 micrograms per ml	1 ml	200 micrograms
9 months	120 micrograms	NONE	N/A	200 micrograms per ml	0.6 ml	120 micrograms
6 months	120 micrograms	NONE	N/A	200 micrograms per ml	0.6 ml	120 micrograms
3 months	120 micrograms	NONE	N/A	200 micrograms per ml	0.6 ml	120 micrograms
1 month	100 micrograms	NONE	N/A	200 micrograms per ml	0.5 ml	100 micrograms
Birth	100 micrograms	NONE	N/A	200 micrograms per ml	0.5 ml	100 micrograms

*The adult dosage can be given as 500 or 600 micrograms to a maximum of 3 milligrams depending on presentation available.

Drugs – A

SECTION 6

Atropine

Route: Intravenous/Intra-osseous **administer as a rapid bolus**.

AGE	INITIAL DOSE	REPEAT DOSE	DOSE INTERVAL	CONCENTRATION	VOLUME	MAXIMUM DOSE
≥12 years	600 micrograms*	600 micrograms*	3–5 minutes	100 micrograms per ml	6 ml	3 milligrams
11 years	500 micrograms	NONE	N/A	100 micrograms per ml	5 ml	500 micrograms
10 years	500 micrograms	NONE	N/A	100 micrograms per ml	5 ml	500 micrograms
9 years	500 micrograms	NONE	N/A	100 micrograms per ml	5 ml	500 micrograms
8 years	500 micrograms	NONE	N/A	100 micrograms per ml	5 ml	500 micrograms
7 years	400 micrograms	NONE	N/A	100 micrograms per ml	4 ml	400 micrograms
6 years	400 micrograms	NONE	N/A	100 micrograms per ml	4 ml	400 micrograms
5 years	300 micrograms	NONE	N/A	100 micrograms per ml	3 ml	300 micrograms
4 years	300 micrograms	NONE	N/A	100 micrograms per ml	3 ml	300 micrograms
3 years	240 micrograms	NONE	N/A	100 micrograms per ml	2.4 ml	240 micrograms
2 years	240 micrograms	NONE	N/A	100 micrograms per ml	2.4 ml	240 micrograms
18 months	200 micrograms	NONE	N/A	100 micrograms per ml	2 ml	200 micrograms
12 months	200 micrograms	NONE	N/A	100 micrograms per ml	2 ml	200 micrograms
9 months	120 micrograms	NONE	N/A	100 micrograms per ml	1.2 ml	120 micrograms
6 months	120 micrograms	NONE	N/A	100 micrograms per ml	1.2 ml	120 micrograms
3 months	120 micrograms	NONE	N/A	100 micrograms per ml	1.2 ml	120 micrograms
1 month	100 micrograms	NONE	N/A	100 micrograms per ml	1 ml	100 micrograms
Birth	100 micrograms	NONE	N/A	100 micrograms per ml	1 ml	100 micrograms

*The adult dosage can be given as 500 or 600 micrograms to a maximum of 3 milligrams depending on presentation available.

Benzylpenicillin (Penicillin G) [901, 902]

Presentation

Ampoule containing 600 milligrams of benzylpenicillin as powder.

Administered intravenously or intramuscularly.

NB Different concentrations and volumes of administration (refer to administration and dosage tables).

Indications

Suspected meningococcal disease in the presence of:

i) a non-blanching rash (the classical, haemorrhagic, non-blanching rash (may be petechial or purpuric) – seen in approximately 40% of infected children)

and

ii) signs/symptoms suggestive of meningococcal septicaemia (refer to meningococcal meningitis and septicaemia guideline for signs/symptoms).

Action

Antibiotic: broad-spectrum.

Contra-indications

Known severe penicillin allergy (more than a simple rash alone).

Additional Information

● Meningococcal septicaemia is commonest in children and young adults.

● It may be rapidly progressive and fatal.

● Early administration of benzylpenicillin improves outcome.

Dosage and Administration

Administer en-route to hospital (unless already administered).

NB IV/IO and IM concentrations are different and have different volumes of administration.

Route: Intravenous/Intra-osseous – by slow injection.

AGE	INITIAL DOSE	REPEAT DOSE	DOSE INTERVAL	CONCENTRATION	VOLUME	MAXIMUM DOSE
Adult	1.2 grams	NONE	N/A	1.2 grams dissolved in 19.2 ml water for injection	20 ml	1.2 grams
11 years	1.2 grams	NONE	N/A	1.2 grams dissolved in 19.2 ml water for injection	20 ml	1.2 grams
10 years	1.2 grams	NONE	N/A	1.2 grams dissolved in 19.2 ml water for injection	20 ml	1.2 grams
9 years	600 milligrams	NONE	N/A	600 milligrams dissolved in 9.6 ml water for injection	10 ml	600 milligrams
8 years	600 milligrams	NONE	N/A	600 milligrams dissolved in 9.6 ml water for injection	10 ml	600 milligrams
7 years	600 milligrams	NONE	N/A	600 milligrams dissolved in 9.6 ml water for injection	10 ml	600 milligrams
6 years	600 milligrams	NONE	N/A	600 milligrams dissolved in 9.6 ml water for injection	10 ml	600 milligrams
5 years	600 milligrams	NONE	N/A	600 milligrams dissolved in 9.6 ml water for injection	10 ml	600 milligrams
4 years	600 milligrams	NONE	N/A	600 milligrams dissolved in 9.6 ml water for injection	10 ml	600 milligrams
3 years	600 milligrams	NONE	N/A	600 milligrams dissolved in 9.6 ml water for injection	10 ml	600 milligrams
2 years	600 milligrams	NONE	N/A	600 milligrams dissolved in 9.6 ml water for injection	10 ml	600 milligrams
18 months	600 milligrams	NONE	N/A	600 milligrams dissolved in 9.6 ml water for injection	10 ml	600 milligrams
12 months	600 milligrams	NONE	N/A	600 milligrams dissolved in 9.6 ml water for injection	10 ml	600 milligrams
9 months	300 milligrams	NONE	N/A	600 milligrams dissolved in 9.6 ml water for injection	5 ml	300 milligrams
6 months	300 milligrams	NONE	N/A	600 milligrams dissolved in 9.6 ml water for injection	5 ml	300 milligrams
3 months	300 milligrams	NONE	N/A	600 milligrams dissolved in 9.6 ml water for injection	5 ml	300 milligrams
1 month	300 milligrams	NONE	N/A	600 milligrams dissolved in 9.6 ml water for injection	5 ml	300 milligrams
Birth	300 milligrams	NONE	N/A	600 milligrams dissolved in 9.6 ml water for injection	5 ml	300 milligrams

Benzylpenicillin (Penicillin G) BPN

Route: Intramuscular (antero-lateral aspect of thigh or upper arm – preferably in a well perfused area) if rapid intravascular access cannot be obtained.

AGE	INITIAL DOSE	REPEAT DOSE	DOSE INTERVAL	CONCENTRATION	VOLUME	MAXIMUM DOSE
Adult	1.2 grams	NONE	N/A	1.2 grams dissolved in 3.2 ml water for injection	4 ml	1.2 grams
11 years	1.2 grams	NONE	N/A	1.2 grams dissolved in 3.2 ml water for injection	4 ml	1.2 grams
10 years	1.2 grams	NONE	N/A	1.2 grams dissolved in 3.2 ml water for injection	4 ml	1.2 grams
9 years	600 milligrams	NONE	N/A	600 milligrams dissolved in 1.6 ml water for injection	2 ml	600 milligrams
8 years	600 milligrams	NONE	N/A	600 milligrams dissolved in 1.6 ml water for injection	2 ml	600 milligrams
7 years	600 milligrams	NONE	N/A	600 milligrams dissolved in 1.6 ml water for injection	2 ml	600 milligrams
6 years	600 milligrams	NONE	N/A	600 milligrams dissolved in 1.6 ml water for injection	2 ml	600 milligrams
5 years	600 milligrams	NONE	N/A	600 milligrams dissolved in 1.6 ml water for injection	2 ml	600 milligrams
4 years	600 milligrams	NONE	N/A	600 milligrams dissolved in 1.6 ml water for injection	2 ml	600 milligrams
3 years	600 milligrams	NONE	N/A	600 milligrams dissolved in 1.6 ml water for injection	2 ml	600 milligrams
2 years	600 milligrams	NONE	N/A	600 milligrams dissolved in 1.6 ml water for injection	2 ml	600 milligrams
18 months	600 milligrams	NONE	N/A	600 milligrams dissolved in 1.6 ml water for injection	2 ml	600 milligrams
12 months	600 milligrams	NONE	N/A	600 milligrams dissolved in 1.6 ml water for injection	2 ml	600 milligrams
9 months	300 milligrams	NONE	N/A	600 milligrams dissolved in 1.6 ml water for injection	1 ml	300 milligrams
6 months	300 milligrams	NONE	N/A	600 milligrams dissolved in 1.6 ml water for injection	1 ml	300 milligrams
3 months	300 milligrams	NONE	N/A	600 milligrams dissolved in 1.6 ml water for injection	1 ml	300 milligrams
1 month	300 milligrams	NONE	N/A	600 milligrams dissolved in 1.6 ml water for injection	1 ml	300 milligrams
Birth	300 milligrams	NONE	N/A	600 milligrams dissolved in 1.6 ml water for injection	1 ml	300 milligrams

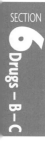

Chlorphenamine (Piriton) [903, 904]

Presentation

Ampoule containing 10 milligrams of chlorphenamine malleate in 1 ml.

Tablet containing 4 milligrams of chlorphenamine malleate.

Oral solution containing 2 milligrams of chlorphenamine malleate in 5 ml.

Indications

Severe anaphylactic reactions (when indicated, should follow initial treatment with IM adrenaline).

Symptomatic allergic reactions falling short of anaphylaxis but causing patient distress e.g. severe itching.

Actions

An antihistamine that blocks the effect of histamine released during a hypersensitivity (allergic) reaction.

Also has anticholinergic properties.

Contra-indications

Known hypersensitivity.

Children less than 1 year of age.

Cautions

Hypotension.

Epilepsy.

Glaucoma.

Hepatic disease.

Prostatic disease.

Side Effects

Sedation.

Dry mouth.

Headache.

Blurred vision.

Psychomotor impairment.

Gastrointestinal disturbance.

Transient hypotension.

Convulsions (rare).

The elderly are more likely to suffer side effects.

Warn anyone receiving chlorphenamine against driving or undertaking any other complex psychomotor task, due to the sedative and psychomotor side effects.

Dosage and Administration

Route: Intravenous – **SLOWLY** over 1 minute/intramuscular.

AGE	INITIAL DOSE	REPEAT DOSE	DOSE INTERVAL	CONCENTRATION	VOLUME	MAXIMUM DOSE
Adult	10 milligrams	NONE	N/A	10 milligrams in 1 ml	1 ml	10 milligrams
11 years	5–10 milligrams	NONE	N/A	10 milligrams in 1 ml	0.5 ml–1 ml	5–10 milligrams
10 years	5–10 milligrams	NONE	N/A	10 milligrams in 1 ml	0.5 ml–1 ml	5–10 milligrams
9 years	5–10 milligrams	NONE	N/A	10 milligrams in 1 ml	0.5 ml–1 ml	5–10 milligrams
8 years	5–10 milligrams	NONE	N/A	10 milligrams in 1 ml	0.5 ml–1 ml	5–10 milligrams
7 years	5–10 milligrams	NONE	N/A	10 milligrams in 1 ml	0.5 ml–1 ml	5–10 milligrams
6 years	5–10 milligrams	NONE	N/A	10 milligrams in 1 ml	0.5 ml–1 ml	5–10 milligrams
5 years	2.5 milligrams	NONE	N/A	10 milligrams in 1 ml	0.25 ml	2.5 milligrams
4 years	2.5 milligrams	NONE	N/A	10 milligrams in 1 ml	0.25 ml	2.5 milligrams
3 years	2.5 milligrams	NONE	N/A	10 milligrams in 1 ml	0.25 ml	2.5 milligrams
2 years	2.5 milligrams	NONE	N/A	10 milligrams in 1 ml	0.25 ml	2.5 milligrams
18 months	2.5 milligrams	NONE	N/A	10 milligrams in 1 ml	0.25 ml	2.5 milligrams
12 months	2.5 milligrams	NONE	N/A	10 milligrams in 1 ml	0.25 ml	2.5 milligrams
9 months	N/A	N/A	N/A	N/A	N/A	N/A
6 months	N/A	N/A	N/A	N/A	N/A	N/A
3 months	N/A	N/A	N/A	N/A	N/A	N/A
1 month	N/A	N/A	N/A	N/A	N/A	N/A
Birth	N/A	N/A	N/A	N/A	N/A	N/A

Drugs – B – C

SECTION 6

Chlorphenamine (Piriton)

Route: Oral (tablet).

AGE	INITIAL DOSE	REPEAT DOSE	DOSE INTERVAL	CONCENTRATION	VOLUME	MAXIMUM DOSE
Adult	4 milligrams	NONE	N/A	4 milligrams per tablet	1 tablet	4 milligrams
11 years	2 milligrams	NONE	N/A	4 milligrams per tablet	½ of one tablet	2 milligrams
10 years	2 milligrams	NONE	N/A	4 milligrams per tablet	½ of one tablet	2 milligrams
9 years	2 milligrams	NONE	N/A	4 milligrams per tablet	½ of one tablet	2 milligrams
8 years	2 milligrams	NONE	N/A	4 milligrams per tablet	½ of one tablet	2 milligrams
7 years	2 milligrams	NONE	N/A	4 milligrams per tablet	½ of one tablet	2 milligrams
6 years	2 milligrams	NONE	N/A	4 milligrams per tablet	½ of one tablet	2 milligrams
5 years	1 milligram	NONE	N/A	4 milligrams per tablet	¼ of one tablet	1 milligram
4 years	1 milligram	NONE	N/A	4 milligrams per tablet	¼ of one tablet	1 milligram
3 years	1 milligram	NONE	N/A	4 milligrams per tablet	¼ of one tablet	1 milligram
2 years	1 milligram	NONE	N/A	4 milligrams per tablet	¼ of one tablet	1 milligram
18 months	1 milligram	NONE	N/A	4 milligrams per tablet	¼ of one tablet	1 milligram
12 months	1 milligram	NONE	N/A	4 milligrams per tablet	¼ of one tablet	1 milligram
9 months	N/A	N/A	N/A	N/A	N/A	N/A
6 months	N/A	N/A	N/A		N/A	N/A
3 months	N/A	N/A	N/A	N/A	N/A	N/A
1 month	N/A	N/A	N/A		N/A	N/A
Birth	N/A	N/A	N/A	N/A	N/A	N/A

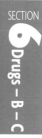

Chlorphenamine (Piriton)

Route: Oral (solution).

AGE	INITIAL DOSE	REPEAT DOSE	DOSE INTERVAL	CONCENTRATION	VOLUME	MAXIMUM DOSE
Adult	4 milligrams	NONE	N/A	2 milligrams in 5 ml	10 ml	4 milligrams
11 years	2 milligrams	NONE	N/A	2 milligrams in 5 ml	5 ml	2 milligrams
10 years	2 milligrams	NONE	N/A	2 milligrams in 5 ml	5 ml	2 milligrams
9 years	2 milligrams	NONE	N/A	2 milligrams in 5 ml	5 ml	2 milligrams
8 years	2 milligrams	NONE	N/A	2 milligrams in 5 ml	5 ml	2 milligrams
7 years	2 milligrams	NONE	N/A	2 milligrams in 5 ml	5 ml	2 milligrams
6 years	2 milligrams	NONE	N/A	2 milligrams in 5 ml	5 ml	2 milligrams
5 years	1 milligram	NONE	N/A	2 milligrams in 5 ml	2.5 ml	1 milligram
4 years	1 milligram	NONE	N/A	2 milligrams in 5 ml	2.5 ml	1 milligram
3 years	1 milligram	NONE	N/A	2 milligrams in 5 ml	2.5 ml	1 milligram
2 years	1 milligram	NONE	N/A	2 milligrams in 5 ml	2.5 ml	1 milligram
18 months	1 milligram	NONE	N/A	2 milligrams in 5 ml	2.5 ml	1 milligram
12 months	1 milligram	NONE	N/A	2 milligrams in 5 ml	2.5 ml	1 milligram
9 months	N/A	N/A	N/A	N/A	N/A	N/A
6 months	N/A	N/A	N/A	N/A	N/A	N/A
3 months	N/A	N/A	N/A	N/A	N/A	N/A
1 month	N/A	N/A	N/A	N/A	N/A	N/A
Birth	N/A	N/A	N/A	N/A	N/A	N/A

Clopidogrel [905]

CLO

Presentation

Tablet containing clopidogrel:

- 75 milligrams
- 300 milligrams.

Indications

Acute ST segment elevation myocardial infarction (STEMI)

- In patients not already taking clopidogrel.
- Receiving thrombolytic treatment.
- Anticipated thrombolytic treatment.
- Anticipated primary percutaneous coronary intervention (PPCI).

Actions

Inhibits platelet aggregation.

Contra-indications

- Known allergy or sensitivity to clopidogrel.
- Severe liver impairment.
- Active pathological bleeding such as peptic ulcer or intracranial haemorrhage.
- Breastfeeding.

Cautions

As the likely benefits of a single dose of clopidogrel outweigh the potential risks, clopidogrel may be administered in:

- Pregnancy
- Patients taking non-steroidal anti-inflammatory drugs (NSAIDs)
- Patients with renal impairment.

Side Effects

- Dyspepsia.
- Abdominal pain.
- Diarrhoea.
- Bleeding (gastrointestinal and intracranial) – the occurrence of severe bleeding is similar to that observed with the administration of aspirin.

Dosage and Administration

Adults aged 18–75 years with acute ST-elevation myocardial infarction (STEMI) receiving thrombolysis or anticipated primary PCI, as per locally agreed STEMI care pathways.

NOTE: To be administered in conjunction with aspirin unless there is a known aspirin allergy or sensitivity (refer to aspirin protocol for administration and dosage).

Route: Oral.

Patient care pathway: Thrombolysis.

AGE	INITIAL DOSE	REPEAT DOSE	DOSE INTERVAL	CONCENTRATION	VOLUME	MAXIMUM DOSE
Adult	300 milligrams	NONE	N/A	300 milligrams per tablet	1 tablet	300 milligrams
Adult	300 milligrams	NONE	N/A	75 milligrams per tablet	4 tablets	300 milligrams

Patient care pathway: Primary percutaneous coronary intervention.

AGE	INITIAL DOSE	REPEAT DOSE	DOSE INTERVAL	CONCENTRATION	VOLUME	MAXIMUM DOSE
Adult	600 milligrams	NONE	N/A	300 milligrams per tablet	2 tablets	600 milligrams
Adult	600 milligrams	NONE	N/A	75 milligrams per tablet	8 tablets	600 milligrams

SECTION 6 Drugs – B – C

Dexamethasone [906, 907]

Presentation

Ampoules of **intravenous** preparation 4 mg/ml.

Indications

Moderate/severe croup.

Actions

Corticosteroid – reduces subglottic inflammation.

Contra-indications

Previously diagnosed hypertension.

Systemic infection/sepsis.

Cautions

Upper airway compromise can be worsened by any procedure distressing the child – including the administration of medication and measuring blood pressure.

Side Effects

None.

Additional Information

Additional doses given acutely do not have additional benefits.

Dosage and Administration

Route: Oral. — The intravenous preparation is administered ORALLY.

AGE	INITIAL DOSE	REPEAT DOSE	DOSE INTERVAL	CONCENTRATION	VOLUME	MAXIMUM DOSE
11 years	N/A	N/A	N/A	N/A	N/A	N/A
10 years	N/A	N/A	N/A	N/A	N/A	N/A
9 years	N/A	N/A	N/A	N/A	N/A	N/A
8 years	N/A	N/A	N/A	N/A	N/A	N/A
7 years	N/A	N/A	N/A	N/A	N/A	N/A
6 years	4 milligrams	NONE	N/A	4 milligrams per ml	1 ml	4 milligrams
5 years	4 milligrams	NONE	N/A	4 milligrams per ml	1 ml	4 milligrams
4 years	4 milligrams	NONE	N/A	4 milligrams per ml	1 ml	4 milligrams
3 years	4 milligrams	NONE	N/A	4 milligrams per ml	1 ml	4 milligrams
2 years	4 milligrams	NONE	N/A	4 milligrams per ml	1 ml	4 milligrams
18 months	4 milligrams	NONE	N/A	4 milligrams per ml	1 ml	4 milligrams
12 months	2 milligrams	NONE	N/A	4 milligrams per ml	0.5 ml	2 milligrams
9 months	2 milligrams	NONE	N/A	4 milligrams per ml	0.5 ml	2 milligrams
6 months	2 milligrams	NONE	N/A	4 milligrams per ml	0.5 ml	2 milligrams
3 months	2 milligrams	NONE	N/A	4 milligrams per ml	0.5 ml	2 milligrams
1 month	2 milligrams	NONE	N/A	4 milligrams per ml	0.5 ml	2 milligrams
Birth	N/A	N/A	N/A	N/A	N/A	N/A

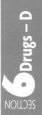

Presentation

Ampoule containing 10 milligrams diazepam in an oil-in-water emulsion making up 2 ml.

Rectal tube containing 2.5 milligrams, 5 milligrams or 10 milligrams diazepam.

Indications

Fits longer than 5 minutes and **STILL FITTING**.

Repeated fits – not secondary to an uncorrected hypoxia or hypoglycaemic episode.

Status epilepticus.

Eclamptic fits (initiate treatment if fit lasts >2–3 minutes or if it is recurrent).

Symptomatic cocaine toxicity (severe hypertension, chest pain or fitting).

Actions

Central nervous system depressant, acts as an anticonvulsant and sedative.

Cautions

Respiratory depression.

Should be used with caution if alcohol, antidepressants or other CNS depressants have been taken as side effects are more likely.

Recent doses by carers/relatives should be taken into account when calculating the maximum cumulative dose.

Contra-indications

None.

Side Effects

Respiratory depression may occur, especially in the presence of alcohol, which enhances the depressive side effect of diazepam. In addition, opioid drugs also enhance the cardiac and respiratory depressive effect of diazepam.

Hypotension may occur. This may be significant if the patient has to be moved from a horizontal position to allow for extrication from an address. Caution should therefore be exercised and consideration given to either removing the patient flat or, if fitting has stopped and it is considered safe, allowing a 10 minute recovery period prior to removal.

Drowsiness and light-headedness, confusion and unsteadiness.

Occasionally amnesia may occur.

Additional Information

The intravenous route is preferred for terminating fits and thus, where IV access can be gained rapidly, this should be the first choice. Early consideration should be given to using the PR route when IV access cannot be rapidly and safely obtained, **which is particularly likely in the case of children**. In small children the PR route should be considered the first choice treatment and IV access sought subsequently.

NB If a **SINGLE** dose of diazepam has been administered via the PR route and IV access is subsequently available, a **SINGLE** dose of IV diazepam may be administered where required.

The earlier the drug is given the more likely the patient is to respond, which is why the rectal route is preferred in children, while the IV route is sought.

Diazepam should only be used if the patient has been fitting for >5 minutes (and is still fitting), or if fits recur in rapid succession without time for full recovery in between. There is no value in giving this drug 'preventatively' if the fit has ceased. **In any clearly sick or ill child, there must be no delay at the scene** while administering the drug, and if it is essential to give diazepam, this should be done en-route to hospital.

Care must be taken when inserting the rectal tube and this should be inserted no more than 2.5 cm in children and 4–5 cm in adults. (All tubes have an insertion marker on nozzle.)

SECTION

6

Drugs – D

298

Drugs

2013

Page **1** of **4**

Dosage and Administration

Route: Intravenous/intra-osseous – administer **SLOWLY** titrated to response.

AGE	INITIAL DOSE	REPEAT DOSE	DOSE INTERVAL	CONCENTRATION	VOLUME	MAXIMUM DOSE
Adult	10 milligrams	10 milligrams	5 minutes	10 milligrams in 2 ml	2 ml	20 milligrams
11 years	10 milligrams	NONE	N/A	10 milligrams in 2 ml	2 ml	10 milligrams
10 years	10 milligrams	NONE	N/A	10 milligrams in 2 ml	2 ml	10 milligrams
9 years	9 milligrams	NONE	N/A	10 milligrams in 2 ml	1.8 ml	9 milligrams
8 years	8 milligrams	NONE	N/A	10 milligrams in 2 ml	1.6 ml	8 milligrams
7 years	7 milligrams	NONE	N/A	10 milligrams in 2 ml	1.4 ml	7 milligrams
6 years	6.5 milligrams	NONE	N/A	10 milligrams in 2 ml	1.3 ml	6.5 milligrams
5 years	6 milligrams	NONE	N/A	10 milligrams in 2 ml	1.2 ml	6 milligrams
4 years	5 milligrams	NONE	N/A	10 milligrams in 2 ml	1 ml	5 milligrams
3 years	4.5 milligrams	NONE	N/A	10 milligrams in 2 ml	0.9 ml	4.5 milligrams
2 years	3.5 milligrams	NONE	N/A	10 milligrams in 2 ml	0.7 ml	3.5 milligrams
18 months	3.5 milligrams	NONE	N/A	10 milligrams in 2 ml	0.7 ml	3.5 milligrams
12 months	3 milligrams	NONE	N/A	10 milligrams in 2 ml	0.6 ml	3 milligrams
9 months	2.5 milligrams	NONE	N/A	10 milligrams in 2 ml	0.5 ml	2.5 milligrams
6 months	2.5 milligrams	NONE	N/A	10 milligrams in 2 ml	0.5 ml	2.5 milligrams
3 months	2 milligrams	NONE	N/A	10 milligrams in 2 ml	0.4 ml	2 milligrams
1 month	1.5 milligrams	NONE	N/A	10 milligrams in 2 ml	0.3 ml	1.5 milligrams
Birth	1 milligram	NONE	N/A	10 milligrams in 2 ml	0.2 ml	1 milligram

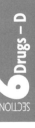

Diazepam

DZP

Route: Rectal (smaller dose).

AGE	INITIAL DOSE	REPEAT DOSE	DOSE TERVAL	CONCENTRATION	RECTAL TUBE	MAXIMUM DOSE
>12 years – Adult	10 milligrams	NONE	N/A	10 milligrams in 2.5 ml	1 × 10 milligram Tube	10 milligrams
11 years	5 milligrams	NONE	N/A	5 milligrams in 2.5 ml	1 × 5 milligram Tube	5 milligrams
10 years	5 milligrams	NONE	N/A	5 milligrams in 2.5 ml	1 × 5 milligram Tube	5 milligrams
9 years	5 milligrams	NONE	N/A	5 milligrams in 2.5 ml	1 × 5 milligram Tube	5 milligrams
8 years	5 milligrams	NONE	N/A	5 milligrams in 2.5 ml	1 × 5 milligram Tube	5 milligrams
7years	5 milligrams	NONE	N/A	5 milligrams in 2.5 ml	1 × 5 milligram Tube	5 milligrams
6 years	5 milligrams	NONE	N/A	5 milligrams in 2.5 ml	1 × 5 milligram Tube	5 milligrams
5 years	5 milligrams	NONE	N/A	5 milligrams in 2.5 ml	1 × 5 milligram Tube	5 milligrams
4 years	5 milligrams	NONE	N/A	5 milligrams in 2.5 ml	1 × 5 milligram Tube	5 milligrams
3 years	5 milligrams	NONE	N/A	5 milligrams in 2.5 ml	1 × 5 milligram Tube	5 milligrams
2 years	5 milligrams	NONE	N/A	5 milligrams in 2.5 ml	1 × 5 milligram Tube	5 milligrams
18 months	5 milligrams	NONE	N/A	5 milligrams in 2.5 ml	1 × 5 milligram Tube	5 milligrams
12 months	5 milligrams	NONE	N/A	5 milligrams in 2.5 ml	1 × 5 milligram Tube	5 milligrams
9 months	5 milligrams	NONE	N/A	5 milligrams in 2.5 ml	1 × 5 milligram Tube	5 milligrams
6 months	5 milligrams	NONE	N/A	5 milligrams in 2.5 ml	1 × 5 milligram Tube	5 milligrams
3 months	5 milligrams	NONE	N/A	5 milligrams in 2.5 ml	1 × 5 milligram Tube	5 milligrams
1 month	5 milligrams	NONE	N/A	5 milligrams in 2.5 ml	1 × 5 milligram Tube	5 milligrams
Birth	1.25 milligrams	NONE	N/A	2.5 milligrams in 1.25 ml	½ × 2.5 milligram Tube	1.25 milligrams

NB If a **SINGLE** dose of diazepam has been given by the PR route and IV access is subsequently available, a **SINGLE** dose of IV diazepam may be given where required.

SECTION **6** Drugs – D

Diazepam

Route: Rectal (larger dose).

AGE	INITIAL DOSE	REPEAT DOSE	DOSE INTERVAL	CONCENTRATION	RECTAL TUBE	MAXIMUM DOSE
>12 years – Adult	20 milligrams	NONE	N/A	10 milligrams in 2.5 ml	2 × 10 milligram Tube	20 milligrams
11 years	10 milligrams	NONE	N/A	10 milligrams in 2.5 ml	1 × 10 milligram Tube	10 milligrams
10 years	10 milligrams	NONE	N/A	10 milligrams in 2.5 ml	1 × 10 milligram Tube	10 milligrams
9 years	10 milligrams	NONE	N/A	10 milligrams in 2.5 ml	1 × 10 milligram Tube	10 milligrams
8 years	10 milligrams	NONE	N/A	10 milligrams in 2.5 ml	1 × 10 milligram Tube	10 milligrams
7 years	10 milligrams	NONE	N/A	10 milligrams in 2.5 ml	1 × 10 milligram Tube	10 milligrams
6 years	10 milligrams	NONE	N/A	10 milligrams in 2.5 ml	1 × 10 milligram Tube	10 milligrams
5 years	10 milligrams	NONE	N/A	10 milligrams in 2.5 ml	1 × 10 milligram Tube	10 milligrams
4 years	10 milligrams	NONE	N/A	10 milligrams in 2.5 ml	1 × 10 milligram Tube	10 milligrams
3 years	10 milligrams	NONE	N/A	10 milligrams in 2.5 ml	1 × 10 milligram Tube	10 milligrams
2 years	10 milligrams	NONE	N/A	10 milligrams in 2.5 ml	1 × 10 milligram Tube	10 milligrams
12 months	5 milligrams	None	N/A	5 milligrams in 2.5 ml	1 x 5 milligram Tube	5 milligrams
9 months	5 milligrams	None	N/A	5 milligrams in 2.5 ml	1 x 5 milligram Tube	5 milligrams
6 months	5 milligrams	None	N/A	5 milligrams in 2.5 ml	1 x 5 milligram Tube	5 milligrams
3 months	5 milligrams	None	N/A	5 milligrams in 2.5 ml	1 x 5 milligram Tube	5 milligrams
1 months	5 milligrams	None	N/A	5 milligrams in 2.5 ml	1 x 5 milligram Tube	5 milligrams
Birth	2.5 milligrams	NONE	N/A	2.5 milligrams in 1.25 ml	1 × 2.5 milligram Tube	2.5 milligrams

NB If a **SINGLE** dose of diazepam has been given by the PR route and IV access is subsequently available, a **SINGLE** dose of IV diazepam may be given where required.

Drugs – D

SECTION 6

Presentation

Entonox is a combination of nitrous oxide 50% and oxygen 50%. It is stored in medical cylinders that have a blue body with white shoulders.

Indications

Moderate to severe pain.

Labour pains.

Actions

Inhaled analgesic agent.

Contra-indications

- Severe head injuries with impaired consciousness.
- Decompression sickness (the bends) where entonox can cause nitrogen bubbles within the blood stream to expand, aggravating the problem further. Consider anyone that has been diving within the previous 24 hours to be at risk.
- Violently disturbed psychiatric patients.

Cautions

Any patient at risk of having a pneumothorax, pneumomediastinum and/or a pneumoperitoneum e.g. polytrauma, penetrating torso injury.

Side Effects

Minimal side effects.

Additional Information

Administration of entonox should be in conjunction with pain score monitoring.

Entonox's advantages include:

- Rapid analgesic effect with minimal side effects.
- No cardio-respiratory depression.
- Self-administered.
- Analgesic effect rapidly wears off.
- The 50% oxygen concentration is valuable in many medical and trauma conditions.
- Entonox can be administered whilst preparing to deliver other analgesics.

The usual precautions must be followed with regard to caring for the Entonox equipment and the cylinder MUST be inverted several times to mix the gases when temperatures are low.

Dosage and Administration

Adults:

- Entonox should be self-administered via a facemask or mouthpiece, after suitable instruction. It takes about **3–5 minutes** to be effective, but it may be **5–10 minutes** before maximum effect is achieved.

Children:

- Entonox is effective in children provided they are capable of following the administration instructions and can activate the demand valve.

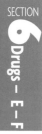

SECTION

6

Drugs – E – F

Presentation

Ampoules containing furosemide 50 milligrams/5 ml.

Ampoules containing furosemide 40 milligrams/2 ml.

Pre-filled syringe containing furosemide 80 milligrams.

Indications

Pulmonary oedema secondary to left ventricular failure.

Actions

Furosemide is a potent diuretic with a rapid onset (within 30 minutes) and short duration.

Contra-indications

Pre-comatose state secondary to liver cirrhosis.

Severe renal failure with anuria.

Children under 18 years old.

Cautions

Hypokalaemia (low potassium) could induce arrhythmias.

Pregnancy.

Hypotensive patient.

Side Effects

Hypotension.

Gastro-intestinal disturbances.

Additional Information

Nitrates are the first-line treatment for acute pulmonary oedema. Use furosemide secondary to nitrates in the treatment of acute pulmonary oedema where transfer times to hospital are prolonged.

Dosage and Administration

Route: Intravenous – administer **SLOWLY OVER** 2 minutes.

AGE	INITIAL DOSE	REPEAT DOSE	DOSE INTERVAL	CONCENTRATION	VOLUME	MAXIMUM DOSE
Adult	50 milligrams	NONE	N/A	50 milligrams/5 ml	5 ml	50 milligrams
Adult	40 milligrams	NONE	N/A	20 milligrams/2 ml	4 ml	40 milligrams
Adult	40 milligrams	NONE	N/A	80 milligrams/8 ml (pre-filled syringe)	4 ml	40 milligrams

Presentation

Glucagon injection, 1 milligram of powder in vial for reconstitution with water for injection.

Indications

- Hypoglycaemia (blood glucose <4.0 millimoles per litre), especially in known diabetics.
- Clinically suspected hypoglycaemia where oral glucose administration is not possible.
- The unconscious patient, where hypoglycaemia is considered a likely cause.

Actions

Glucagon is a hormone that induces the conversion of glycogen to glucose in the liver, thereby raising blood glucose levels.

Contra-indications

- Low glycogen stores (e.g. recent use of glucagon).
- Hypoglycaemic seizures – glucose 10% IV is the preferred intervention.

Cautions

Avoid intramuscular administration of any drug when a patient is likely to require thrombolysis.

Side Effects

- Nausea, vomiting.
- Diarrhoea.
- Acute hypersensitivity reaction (rare).
- Hypokalaemia.
- Hypotension.

Additional Information

- Glucagon should NOT be given by IV injection because of increased vomiting associated with IV use.
- Confirm effectiveness by checking blood glucose 5–10 minutes after administration (i.e. blood sugar >5.0 millimoles per litre).
- When treating hypoglycaemia, use all available clinical information to help decide between glucagon IM, oral glucose gel (40%), or glucose 10% IV (see advice below):
  - glucagon is relatively ineffective once body glycogen stores have been exhausted (especially hypoglycaemic, non-diabetic children). In such patients, use oral glucose gel smeared round the mouth or glucose 10% IV as first-line treatments
  - the newborn baby's liver has very limited glycogen stores, so hypoglycaemia may not be effectively treated using intramuscular glucagon (glucagon works by stimulating the liver to convert glycogen into glucose)
  - glucagon may also be ineffective in some instances of alcohol-induced hypoglycaemia
  - consider oral glucose gel or glucose 10% IV as possible alternatives
  - hypoglycaemic patients who fit should **preferably** be given glucose 10% IV.

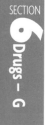

Glucagon (Glucagen)

Dosage and Administration

Route: Intramuscular – antero-lateral aspect of thigh or upper arm.

AGE	INITIAL DOSE	REPEAT DOSE	DOSE INTERVAL	CONCENTRATION	VOLUME	MAXIMUM DOSE
Adult	1 milligram	NONE	N/A	1 milligram per vial	1 vial	1 milligram
11 years	1 milligram	NONE	N/A	1 milligram per vial	1 vial	1 milligram
10 years	1 milligram	NONE	N/A	1 milligram per vial	1 vial	1 milligram
9 years	1 milligram	NONE	N/A	1 milligram per vial	1 vial	1 milligram
8 years	1 milligram	NONE	N/A	1 milligram per vial	1 vial	1 milligram
7 years	500 micrograms	NONE	N/A	1 milligram per vial	0.5 vial	500 micrograms
6 years	500 micrograms	NONE	N/A	1 milligram per vial	0.5 vial	500 micrograms
5 years	500 micrograms	NONE	N/A	1 milligram per vial	0.5 vial	500 micrograms
4 years	500 micrograms	NONE	N/A	1 milligram per vial	0.5 vial	500 micrograms
3 years	500 micrograms	NONE	N/A	1 milligram per vial	0.5 vial	500 micrograms
2 years	500 micrograms	NONE	N/A	1 milligram per vial	0.5 vial	500 micrograms
18 months	500 micrograms	NONE	N/A	1 milligram per vial	0.5 vial	500 micrograms
12 months	500 micrograms	NONE	N/A	1 milligram per vial	0.5 vial	500 micrograms
6 months	500 micrograms	NONE	N/A	1 milligram per vial	0.5 vial	500 micrograms
3 months	500 micrograms	NONE	N/A	1 milligram per vial	0.5 vial	500 micrograms
1 month	500 micrograms	NONE	N/A	1 milligram per vial	0.5 vial	500 micrograms
Birth	100 micrograms	NONE	N/A	1 milligram per vial	0.1 vial	100 micrograms

NB If no response within 10 minutes, administer intravenous glucose – **refer to glucose 10% guideline**.

Drugs – G

SECTION 6

Page **2** of **2**   2013   **Drugs**   305

Glucose 10% [913]

Presentation

500 ml pack of 10% glucose solution (50 grams).

Indications

Hypoglycaemia (blood glucose <4.0 millimoles per litre), especially in known diabetics.

Clinically suspected hypoglycaemia where oral glucose administration is not possible.

The unconscious patient, where hypoglycaemia is considered a likely cause.

Actions

Reversal of hypoglycaemia.

Cautions

Administer via a large gauge cannula into a large vein – a 10% concentration of glucose solution is an irritant to veins (especially in extravasation).

Additional Information

When treating hypoglycaemia, use all available clinical information to help decide between glucose 10% IV, glucose gel 40% oral gel, or glucagon IM.

Side Effects

None.

Contra-indications

None.

Dosage and Administration

- If the patient has shown no response, the dose may be repeated after 5 minutes.
- If the patient has shown a **PARTIAL** response then a further infusion may be necessary, titrated to response to restore a normal GCS.
- If after the second dose there has been **NO** response, pre-alert and transport rapidly to further care. Consider an alternative diagnosis or the likelihood of a third dose en-route benefiting the patient.

Route: Intravenous infusion.

AGE	INITIAL DOSE	REPEAT DOSE	DOSE INTERVAL	CONCENTRATION	VOLUME	MAXIMUM DOSE
Adult	10 grams	10 grams	5 minutes	50 grams in 500 ml	100 ml	30 grams
11 years	7 grams	7 grams	5 minutes	50 grams in 500 ml	70 ml	21 grams
10 years	6.5 grams	6.5 grams	5 minutes	50 grams in 500 ml	65 ml	19.5 grams
9 years	6 grams	6 grams	5 minutes	50 grams in 500 ml	60 ml	18 grams
8 years	5 grams	5 grams	5 minutes	50 grams in 500 ml	50 ml	15 grams
7 years	5 grams	5 grams	5 minutes	50 grams in 500 ml	50 ml	15 grams
6 years	4 grams	4 grams	5 minutes	50 grams in 500 ml	40 ml	12 grams
5 years	4 grams	4 grams	5 minutes	50 grams in 500 ml	40 ml	12 grams
4 years	3 grams	3 grams	5 minutes	50 grams in 500 ml	30 ml	9 grams
3 years	3 grams	3 grams	5 minutes	50 grams in 500 ml	30 ml	9 grams
2 years	2.5 grams	2.5 grams	5 minutes	50 grams in 500 ml	25 ml	7.5 grams
18 months	2 grams	2 grams	5 minutes	50 grams in 500 ml	20 ml	6 grams
12 months	2 grams	2 grams	5 minutes	50 grams in 500 ml	20 ml	6 grams
9 months	2 grams	2 grams	5 minutes	50 grams in 500 ml	20 ml	6 grams
6 months	1.5 grams	1.5 grams	5 minutes	50 grams in 500 ml	15 ml	4.5 grams
3 months	1 gram	1 gram	5 minutes	50 grams in 500 ml	10 ml	3 grams
1 month	1 gram	1 gram	5 minutes	50 grams in 500 ml	10 ml	3 grams
Birth[a]	0.9 grams	0.9 grams	5 minutes	50 grams in 500 ml	9 ml	2.7 grams

[a] **NB** Neonatal doses are intentionally smaller than those used in older children.

Presentation

Plastic tube containing 25g glucose 40% oral gel.

Indications

Known or suspected hypoglycaemia in a conscious patient where there is no risk of choking or aspiration.

Actions

Rapid increase in blood glucose levels via buccal absorption.

Cautions

Altered consciousness – risk of choking or aspiration (in such circumstances glucose gel can be administered by soaking a gauze swab and placing it between the patient's lip and gum to aid absorption).

Side Effects

None.

Additional Information

Can be repeated as necessary in the hypoglycaemic patient.

Treatment failure should prompt the use of an alternative such as glucagon IM or glucose 10% IV.

(refer to glucagon guideline or glucose 10% guideline).

Contra-indications

None.

Dosage and Administration

Route: Buccal – Measure blood glucose level after each dose.

AGE	INITIAL DOSE	REPEAT DOSE	DOSE INTERVAL	CONCENTRATION	VOLUME	MAXIMUM DOSE[a]
Adults	10 grams	10 grams	5 minutes	10 grams in 25 grams of gel	1 tube	No limit
Children ≥12 years	10 grams	10 grams	5 minutes	10 grams in 25 grams of gel	1 tube	No limit
Children <12 years	An appropriate amount should be given, considering the child's age – NB Protect the airway.					

NB Assess more frequently in children who require a smaller dose for a response.

[a]Consider IM glucagon or IV glucose 10% if no clinical improvement.

Drugs – G

SECTION 6

Glyceryl Trinitrate (GTN, Suscard) [914]

GTN

Presentation

Metered dose spray containing 400 micrograms glyceryl trinitrate per dose.

Tablets containing glyceryl trinitrate 2, 3 or 5 milligrams for buccal administration (depends on local ordering).

Indications

Cardiac chest pain due to angina or myocardial infarction.

Acute cardiogenic pulmonary oedema.

Actions

A potent vasodilator drug resulting in:

- Dilatation of coronary arteries/relief of coronary spasm.
- Dilatation of systemic veins resulting in lower pre-load.
- Reduced blood pressure.

Contra-indications

Hypotension (actual or estimated systolic blood pressure <90 mmHg).

Hypovolaemia.

Head trauma.

Cerebral haemorrhage.

Sildenafil (Viagra) and other related drugs – glyceryl trinitrate must not be given to patients who have taken sildenafil or related drugs within the previous 24 hours. Profound hypotension may occur.

Unconscious patients.

Dosage and Administration

The oral mucosa must be moist for GTN absorption, moisten if necessary.

Route: Buccal/sub-lingual (spray under the patient's tongue and close mouth).

AGE	INITIAL DOSE	REPEAT DOSE[a]	DOSE INTERVAL	CONCENTRATION	TABLETS	MAXIMUM DOSE[a]
Adult	1–2 spray	1–2 spray	5–10 minutes	400 micrograms per dose spray	400–800 micrograms	No limit
Adult	2 milligrams	2 milligrams	5–10 minutes	2 milligrams per tablet	1 tablet	No limit
Adult	3 milligrams	3 milligrams	5–10 minutes	3 milligrams per tablet	1 tablet	No limit
Adult	5 milligrams	5 milligrams	5–10 minutes	5 milligrams per tablet	1 tablet	No limit

[a]**The effect of the first dose should be assessed over 5 minutes**; further doses can be administered provided the systolic blood pressure is >90 mmHg. Remove the tablet if side effects occur, for example, hypotension.

Presentation

An ampoule of unfractionated heparin containing 5,000 units/ml.

Indications

ST Elevation Myocardial Infarction (STEMI) where heparin is required as adjunctive therapy with reteplase or tenecteplase to reduce the risk of re-infarction.

It is extremely important that the initial bolus dose is given at the earliest opportunity prior to administration of thrombolytic agents and a heparin infusion is commenced immediately on arrival at hospital.

A further intravenous bolus dose of 1,000 units heparin may be required if a heparin infusion **HAS NOT** commenced within 45 minutes of the original bolus of thrombolytic agent.

Recent trials have suggested that low molecular weight heparin may be useful in patients under 75 years of age (older patients have much higher bleeding risk with this treatment). Research is ongoing and local protocols should be followed.

Actions

Anticoagulant.

Side Effects

Haemorrhage – major or minor.

Contra-indications

- **Haemophilia and other haemorrhagic disorders.**
- Thrombocytopenia.
- Recent cerebral haemorrhage.
- Severe hypertension.
- Severe liver disease.
- Oesophageal varices.
- Peptic ulcer.
- Major trauma.
- Recent surgery to eye or nervous system.
- Acute bacterial endocarditis.
- Spinal or epidural anaesthesia.

Additional Information

Analysis of MINAP data suggests inadequate anticoagulation following prehospital thrombolytic treatment is associated with increased risks of re-infarction.

AT HOSPITAL it is essential that the care of the patient is handed over as soon as possible to a member of hospital staff qualified to administer the second bolus (if not already given) and commence a heparin infusion.

Dosage and Administration

Heparin dosage when administered with **RETEPLASE**.

Route: Intravenous single bolus unfractionated heparin.

AGE	INITIAL DOSE	REPEAT DOSE	DOSE INTERVAL	CONCENTRATION	VOLUME	MAXIMUM DOSE
≥18	5,000 units	*See footnote	N/A	5,000 units/ml	1 ml	5,000 units

Heparin dosage when administered with **TENECTEPLASE**.

Route: Intravenous single bolus unfractionated heparin.

AGE	WEIGHT	INITIAL DOSE	REPEAT DOSE	DOSE INTERVAL	CONCENTRATION	VOLUME	MAXIMUM DOSE
≥18	<67 kg	4,000 units	*See footnote	N/A	5,000 units/ml	0.8 ml	4,000 units
≥18	≥67 kg	5,000 units	*See footnote	N/A	5,000 units/ml	1 ml	5,000 units

*A further intravenous bolus dose of 1,000 units heparin may be required if a heparin infusion **HAS NOT** commenced within 45 minutes of the original bolus of thrombolytic agent.

Drugs – H – I

SECTION 6

Presentation

An ampoule containing 100 milligrams hydrocortisone as either sodium succinate or sodium phosphate in 1 ml.

An ampoule containing 100 milligrams hydrocortisone sodium succinate for reconstitution with up to 2 ml of water.

Indications

Severe or life-threatening asthma – where call to hospital time is >30 minutes.

Anaphylaxis.

Adrenal crisis (including Addisonian crisis) – sudden severe deficiency of steroids (occurs in patients on long-term steroid therapy for whatever reason) producing circulatory collapse with or without hypoglycaemia. Administer hydrocortisone to:

1. Patients in an established adrenal crisis.
2. Steroid-dependent patients who have become unwell to prevent them having an adrenal crisis – if in doubt, it is better to administer hydrocortisone.

Actions

Glucocorticoid drug that reduces inflammation and suppresses the immune response.

Contra-indications

Known allergy (which will be to the sodium succinate or sodium phosphate rather than the hydrocortisone itself).

Cautions

None relevant to a single dose.

Avoid intramuscular administration if patient likely to require thrombolysis.

Side Effects

Sodium phosphate may cause burning or itching sensation in the groin if administered too quickly.

Dosage and Administration

1. **Asthma and adrenal crisis**. NB If there is any doubt about previous steroid administration, it is better to administer hydrocortisone.

Route: Intravenous (**SLOW** injection over a minimum of 2 minutes to avoid side effects)/intra-osseous OR intramuscular (when IV access is impossible).

AGE	INITIAL DOSE	REPEAT DOSE	DOSE INTERVAL	CONCENTRATION	VOLUME	MAXIMUM DOSE
Adult	100 milligrams	NONE	N/A	100 milligrams in 1 ml	1 ml	100 milligrams
11 years	100 milligrams	NONE	N/A	100 milligrams in 1 ml	1 ml	100 milligrams
10 years	100 milligrams	NONE	N/A	100 milligrams in 1 ml	1 ml	100 milligrams
9 years	100 milligrams	NONE	N/A	100 milligrams in 1 ml	1 ml	100 milligrams
8 years	100 milligrams	NONE	N/A	100 milligrams in 1 ml	1 ml	100 milligrams
7 years	100 milligrams	NONE	N/A	100 milligrams in 1 ml	1 ml	100 milligrams
6 years	100 milligrams	NONE	N/A	100 milligrams in 1 ml	1 ml	100 milligrams
5 years	50 milligrams	NONE	N/A	100 milligrams in 1 ml	0.5 ml	50 milligrams
4 years	50 milligrams	NONE	N/A	100 milligrams in 1 ml	0.5 ml	50 milligrams
3 years	50 milligrams	NONE	N/A	100 milligrams in 1 ml	0.5 ml	50 milligrams
2 years	50 milligrams	NONE	N/A	100 milligrams in 1 ml	0.5 ml	50 milligrams
18 months	50 milligrams	NONE	N/A	100 milligrams in 1 ml	0.5 ml	50 milligrams
12 months	50 milligrams	NONE	N/A	100 milligrams in 1 ml	0.5 ml	50 milligrams
9 months	50 milligrams	NONE	N/A	100 milligrams in 1 ml	0.5 ml	50 milligrams
6 months	50 milligrams	NONE	N/A	100 milligrams in 1 ml	0.5 ml	50 milligrams
3 months	25 milligrams	NONE	N/A	100 milligrams in 1 ml	0.25 ml	25 milligrams
1 month	25 milligrams	NONE	N/A	100 milligrams in 1 ml	0.25 ml	25 milligrams
Birth	10 milligrams	NONE	N/A	100 milligrams in 1 ml	0.1 ml	10 milligrams

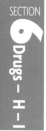

310

Drugs

2013

Page **1** of 4

SECTION
6
Drugs – H – I

Hydrocortisone

Route: Intravenous (**SLOW** injection over a minimum of 2 minutes to avoid side effects)/intra-osseous OR intramuscular (when IV access is impossible).

AGE	INITIAL DOSE	REPEAT DOSE	DOSE INTERVAL	CONCENTRATION	VOLUME	MAXIMUM DOSE
Adult	100 milligrams	NONE	N/A	100 milligrams in 2 ml	2 ml	100 milligrams
11 years	100 milligrams	NONE	N/A	100 milligrams in 2 ml	2 ml	100 milligrams
10 years	100 milligrams	NONE	N/A	100 milligrams in 2 ml	2 ml	100 milligrams
9 years	100 milligrams	NONE	N/A	100 milligrams in 2 ml	2 ml	100 milligrams
8 years	100 milligrams	NONE	N/A	100 milligrams in 2 ml	2 ml	100 milligrams
7 years	100 milligrams	NONE	N/A	100 milligrams in 2 ml	2 ml	100 milligrams
6 years	100 milligrams	NONE	N/A	100 milligrams in 2 ml	2 ml	100 milligrams
5 years	50 milligrams	NONE	N/A	100 milligrams in 2 ml	1 ml	50 milligrams
4 years	50 milligrams	NONE	N/A	100 milligrams in 2 ml	1 ml	50 milligrams
3 years	50 milligrams	NONE	N/A	100 milligrams in 2 ml	1 ml	50 milligrams
2 years	50 milligrams	NONE	N/A	100 milligrams in 2 ml	1 ml	50 milligrams
18 months	50 milligrams	NONE	N/A	100 milligrams in 2 ml	1 ml	50 milligrams
12 months	50 milligrams	NONE	N/A	100 milligrams in 2 ml	1 ml	50 milligrams
9 months	50 milligrams	NONE	N/A	100 milligrams in 2 ml	1 ml	50 milligrams
6 months	50 milligrams	NONE	N/A	100 milligrams in 2 ml	1 ml	50 milligrams
3 months	25 milligrams	NONE	N/A	100 milligrams in 2 ml	0.5 ml	25 milligrams
1 month	25 milligrams	NONE	N/A	100 milligrams in 2 ml	0.5 ml	25 milligrams
Birth	10 milligrams	NONE	N/A	100 milligrams in 2 ml	0.2 ml	10 milligrams

Section 6 Drugs – H – I

2. **Anaphylaxis**

Route: Intravenous (**SLOW** injection over a minimum of 2 minutes to avoid side effects)/intra-osseous OR intramuscular (when IV access is impossible).

AGE	INITIAL DOSE	REPEAT DOSE	DOSE INTERVAL	CONCENTRATION	VOLUME	MAXIMUM DOSE
Adult	200 milligrams	NONE	N/A	100 milligrams in 1 ml	2 ml	200 milligrams
11 years	100 milligrams	NONE	N/A	100 milligrams in 1 ml	1 ml	100 milligrams
10 years	100 milligrams	NONE	N/A	100 milligrams in 1 ml	1 ml	100 milligrams
9 years	100 milligrams	NONE	N/A	100 milligrams in 1 ml	1 ml	100 milligrams
8 years	100 milligrams	NONE	N/A	100 milligrams in 1 ml	1 ml	100 milligrams
7 years	100 milligrams	NONE	N/A	100 milligrams in 1 ml	1 ml	100 milligrams
6 years	100 milligrams	NONE	N/A	100 milligrams in 1 ml	1 ml	100 milligrams
5 years	50 milligrams	NONE	N/A	100 milligrams in 1 ml	0.5 ml	50 milligrams
4 years	50 milligrams	NONE	N/A	100 milligrams in 1 ml	0.5 ml	50 milligrams
3 years	50 milligrams	NONE	N/A	100 milligrams in 1 ml	0.5 ml	50 milligrams
2 years	50 milligrams	NONE	N/A	100 milligrams in 1 ml	0.5 ml	50 milligrams
18 months	50 milligrams	NONE	N/A	100 milligrams in 1 ml	0.5 ml	50 milligrams
12 months	50 milligrams	NONE	N/A	100 milligrams in 1 ml	0.5 ml	50 milligrams
9 months	50 milligrams	NONE	N/A	100 milligrams in 1 ml	0.5 ml	50 milligrams
6 months	50 milligrams	NONE	N/A	100 milligrams in 1 ml	0.5 ml	50 milligrams
3 months	25 milligrams	NONE	N/A	100 milligrams in 1 ml	0.25 ml	25 milligrams
1 month	25 milligrams	NONE	N/A	100 milligrams in 1 ml	0.25 ml	25 milligrams
Birth	10 milligrams	NONE	N/A	100 milligrams in 1 ml	0.1 ml	10 milligrams

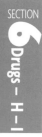

Hydrocortisone

Route: Intravenous (**SLOW** injection over a minimum of 2 minutes to avoid side effects)/intra-osseous OR intramuscular (when IV access is impossible).

AGE	INITIAL DOSE	REPEAT DOSE	DOSE INTERVAL	CONCENTRATION	VOLUME	MAXIMUM DOSE
Adult	200 milligrams	NONE	N/A	100 milligrams in 2 ml	4 ml	200 milligrams
11 years	100 milligrams	NONE	N/A	100 milligrams in 2 ml	2 ml	100 milligrams
10 years	100 milligrams	NONE	N/A	100 milligrams in 2 ml	2 ml	100 milligrams
9 years	100 milligrams	NONE	N/A	100 milligrams in 2 ml	2 ml	100 milligrams
8 years	100 milligrams	NONE	N/A	100 milligrams in 2 ml	2 ml	100 milligrams
7 years	100 milligrams	NONE	N/A	100 milligrams in 2 ml	2 ml	100 milligrams
6 years	100 milligrams	NONE	N/A	100 milligrams in 2 ml	2 ml	100 milligrams
5 years	50 milligrams	NONE	N/A	100 milligrams in 2 ml	1 ml	50 milligrams
4 years	50 milligrams	NONE	N/A	100 milligrams in 2 ml	1 ml	50 milligrams
3 years	50 milligrams	NONE	N/A	100 milligrams in 2 ml	1 ml	50 milligrams
2 years	50 milligrams	NONE	N/A	100 milligrams in 2 ml	1 ml	50 milligrams
18 months	50 milligrams	NONE	N/A	100 milligrams in 2 ml	1 ml	50 milligrams
12 months	50 milligrams	NONE	N/A	100 milligrams in 2 ml	1 ml	50 milligrams
9 months	50 milligrams	NONE	N/A	100 milligrams in 2 ml	1 ml	50 milligrams
6 months	50 milligrams	NONE	N/A	100 milligrams in 2 ml	1 ml	50 milligrams
3 months	25 milligrams	NONE	N/A	100 milligrams in 2 ml	0.5 ml	25 milligrams
1 month	25 milligrams	NONE	N/A	100 milligrams in 2 ml	0.5 ml	25 milligrams
Birth	10 milligrams	NONE	N/A	100 milligrams in 2 ml	0.2 ml	10 milligrams

Presentation

Solution or suspension containing ibuprofen 100 milligrams in 5 ml.

Tablet containing 200 milligrams or 400 milligrams.

Indications

Relief of mild to moderate pain and/or high temperature.

Soft tissue injuries.

Best when used as part of a balanced analgesic regimen.

Actions

Analgesic (relieves pain).

Antipyretic (reduces temperature).

Anti-inflammatory (reduces inflammation).

Contra-indications

Do **NOT** administer if the patient is:

- Dehydrated.
- Hypovolaemic.
- Known to have renal insufficiency.
- Suffering active upper gastrointestinal disturbance e.g. oesophagitis, peptic ulcer, dyspepsia.
- Pregnant.

Avoid giving further non-steroidal anti-inflammatory drugs (NSAIDs) i.e. ibuprofen, if an NSAID containing product (e.g. Diclofenac, Naproxen) has been used within the previous four hours or if the maximum cumulative daily dose has already been given.

Cautions

Asthma: Use cautiously in asthmatic patients due to the possible risk of hypersensitivity and bronchoconstriction. If an asthmatic has not used NSAIDs previously, do not use acutely in the prehospital setting.

Elderly: Exercise caution in older patients (>65 years old) that have not used and tolerated NSAIDs recently.

Side Effects

May cause nausea, vomiting and tinnitus.

SECTION **6** Drugs – H – I

Ibuprofen

Dosage and Administration

Route: Oral.

AGE	INITIAL DOSE	REPEAT DOSE	DOSE INTERVAL	CONCENTRATION	VOLUME	MAXIMUM DOSE
12 years – Adult	400 milligrams	400 milligrams	8 hours	Various	Varies	1.2 grams per 24 hours
11 years	300 milligrams	300 milligrams	8 hours	100 milligrams in 5 ml	15 ml	900 milligrams per 24 hours
10 years	300 milligrams	300 milligrams	8 hours	100 milligrams in 5 ml	15 ml	900 milligrams per 24 hours
9 years	200 milligrams	200 milligrams	8 hours	100 milligrams in 5 ml	10 ml	600 milligrams per 24 hours
8 years	200 milligrams	200 milligrams	8 hours	100 milligrams in 5 ml	10 ml	600 milligrams per 24 hours
7 years	200 milligrams	200 milligrams	8 hours	100 milligrams in 5 ml	10 ml	600 milligrams per 24 hours
6 years	150 milligrams	150 milligrams	8 hours	100 milligrams in 5 ml	7.5 ml	450 milligrams per 24 hours
5 years	150 milligrams	150 milligrams	8 hours	100 milligrams in 5 ml	7.5 ml	450 milligrams per 24 hours
4 years	150 milligrams	150 milligrams	8 hours	100 milligrams in 5 ml	7.5 ml	450 milligrams per 24 hours
3 years	100 milligrams	100 milligrams	8 hours	100 milligrams in 5 ml	5 ml	300 milligrams per 24 hours
2 years	100 milligrams	100 milligrams	8 hours	100 milligrams in 5 ml	5 ml	300 milligrams per 24 hours
18 months	100 milligrams	100 milligrams	8 hours	100 milligrams in 5 ml	5 ml	300 milligrams per 24 hours
12 months	100 milligrams	100 milligrams	8 hours	100 milligrams in 5 ml	5 ml	300 milligrams per 24 hours
9 months	50 milligrams	50 milligrams	8 hours	100 milligrams in 5 ml	2.5 ml	150 milligrams per 24 hours
6 months	50 milligrams	50 milligrams	8 hours	100 milligrams in 5 ml	2.5 ml	150 milligrams per 24 hours
3 months	50 milligrams	50 milligrams	8 hours	100 milligrams in 5 ml	2.5 ml	150 milligrams per 24 hours
1 month	N/A	N/A	N/A	N/A	N/A	N/A
Birth	N/A	N/A	N/A	N/A	N/A	N/A

NB

- Ibuprofen can be given in addition to paracetamol – both drugs may be safely administered in full dosages as they are metabolised differently and work synergistically.
- Given up to 3 times a day, preferably following food.

Ipratropium Bromide (Atrovent) [920, 921]

Presentation

Nebules containing ipratropium bromide 250 micrograms in 1 ml or 500 micrograms in 2 ml.

Indications

Acute severe or life-threatening asthma.

Acute asthma unresponsive to salbutamol.

Exacerbation of chronic obstructive pulmonary disease (COPD), unresponsive to salbutamol.

Actions

1. Ipratropium bromide is an antimuscarinic bronchodilator drug. It may provide short-term relief in acute asthma, but beta2 agonists (such as salbutamol) generally work more quickly.
2. Ipratropium is considered of greater benefit in:
   a. children suffering acute asthma
   b. adults suffering with COPD.

Contra-Indications

None in the emergency situation.

Cautions

Ipratropium should be used with care in patients with:
- Glaucoma (protect the eyes from mist).
- Pregnancy and breastfeeding.
- Prostatic hyperplasia.

If COPD is a possibility limit nebulisation to six minutes.

Side Effects

Headache.

Nausea and vomiting.

Dry mouth (common).

Difficulty in passing urine and/or constipation.

Tachycardia/arrhythmia.

Paroxysmal tightness of the chest.

Allergic reaction.

Dosage and Administration

- **In life-threatening or acute severe asthma:** undertake a **TIME CRITICAL** transfer to the **NEAREST SUITABLE RECEIVING HOSPITAL** and provide nebulisation en-route.
- If COPD is a possibility limit nebulisation to six minutes.

Route: Nebuliser with 6–8 litres per minute oxygen (**refer to oxygen guideline**).

AGE	INITIAL DOSE	REPEAT DOSE	DOSE INTERVAL	CONCENTRATION	VOLUME	MAXIMUM DOSE
Adult	500 micrograms	NONE	N/A	250 micrograms in 1 ml	2 ml	500 micrograms
11 years	250 micrograms	NONE	N/A	250 micrograms in 1 ml	1 ml	250 micrograms
10 years	250 micrograms	NONE	N/A	250 micrograms in 1 ml	1 ml	250 micrograms
9 years	250 micrograms	NONE	N/A	250 micrograms in 1 ml	1 ml	250 micrograms
8 years	250 micrograms	NONE	N/A	250 micrograms in 1 ml	1 ml	250 micrograms
7 years	250 micrograms	NONE	N/A	250 micrograms in 1 ml	1 ml	250 micrograms
6 years	250 micrograms	NONE	N/A	250 micrograms in 1 ml	1 ml	250 micrograms
5 years	250 micrograms	NONE	N/A	250 micrograms in 1 ml	1 ml	250 micrograms
4 years	250 micrograms	NONE	N/A	250 micrograms in 1 ml	1 ml	250 micrograms
3 years	250 micrograms	NONE	N/A	250 micrograms in 1 ml	1 ml	250 micrograms
2 years	250 micrograms	NONE	N/A	250 micrograms in 1 ml	1 ml	250 micrograms
18 months	250 micrograms	NONE	N/A	250 micrograms in 1 ml	1 ml	250 micrograms
12 months	125–250 micrograms	NONE	N/A	250 micrograms in 1 ml	0.5 ml–1 ml	125–250 micrograms
9 months	125–250 micrograms	NONE	N/A	250 micrograms in 1 ml	0.5 ml–1 ml	125–250 micrograms
6 months	125–250 micrograms	NONE	N/A	250 micrograms in 1 ml	0.5 ml–1 ml	125–250 micrograms
3 months	125–250 micrograms	NONE	N/A	250 micrograms in 1 ml	0.5 ml–1 ml	125–250 micrograms
1 month	125–250 micrograms	NONE	N/A	250 micrograms in 1 ml	0.5 ml–1 ml	125–250 micrograms
Birth	N/A	N/A	N/A	N/A	N/A	N/A

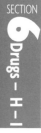

Ipratropium Bromide (Atrovent)

IPR

Route: Nebuliser with 6–8 litres per minute oxygen (**refer to oxygen guideline**).

AGE	INITIAL DOSE	REPEAT DOSE	DOSE INTERVAL	CONCENTRATION	VOLUME	MAXIMUM DOSE
Adult	500 micrograms	NONE	N/A	500 micrograms in 2 ml	2 ml	500 micrograms
11 years	250 micrograms	NONE	N/A	500 micrograms in 2 ml	1 ml	250 micrograms
10 years	250 micrograms	NONE	N/A	500 micrograms in 2 ml	1 ml	250 micrograms
9 years	250 micrograms	NONE	N/A	500 micrograms in 2 ml	1 ml	250 micrograms
8 years	250 micrograms	NONE	N/A	500 micrograms in 2 ml	1 ml	250 micrograms
7 years	250 micrograms	NONE	N/A	500 micrograms in 2 ml	1 ml	250 micrograms
6 years	250 micrograms	NONE	N/A	500 micrograms in 2 ml	1 ml	250 micrograms
5 years	250 micrograms	NONE	N/A	500 micrograms in 2 ml	1 ml	250 micrograms
4 years	250 micrograms	NONE	N/A	500 micrograms in 2 ml	1 ml	250 micrograms
3 years	250 micrograms	NONE	N/A	500 micrograms in 2 ml	1 ml	250 micrograms
2 years	250 micrograms	NONE	N/A	500 micrograms in 2 ml	1 ml	250 micrograms
18 months	250 micrograms	NONE	N/A	500 micrograms in 2 ml	1 ml	250 micrograms
12 months	125–250 micrograms	NONE	N/A	500 micrograms in 2 ml	0.5 ml–1 ml	125–250 micrograms
9 months	125–250 micrograms	NONE	N/A	500 micrograms in 2 ml	0.5 ml–1 ml	125–250 micrograms
6 months	125–250 micrograms	NONE	N/A	500 micrograms in 2 ml	0.5 ml–1 ml	125–250 micrograms
3 months	125–250 micrograms	NONE	N/A	500 micrograms in 2 ml	0.5 ml–1 ml	125–250 micrograms
1 month	125–250 micrograms	NONE	N/A	500 micrograms in 2 ml	0.5 ml–1 ml	125–250 micrograms
Birth	N/A	N/A	N/A	N/A	N/A	N/A

Presentation

Ampoule containing metoclopramide 10 milligrams in 2 ml.

Indications

The treatment of nausea or vomiting in adults aged 20 and over.

Prevention and treatment of nausea and vomiting following administration of morphine sulphate.

Actions

An anti-emetic which acts centrally as well as on the gastrointestinal tract.

Contra-indications

- Age less than 20 years.
- Renal failure.
- Phaeochromocytoma.
- Gastrointestinal obstruction.
- Perforation/haemorrhage/3–4 days after GI surgery.

Cautions

If patient is likely to require thrombolysis then intramuscular administration of any drug should be avoided.

Avoid in cases of drug overdose.

Side Effects

Severe extra-pyramidal effects are more common in children and young adults.

- Drowsiness and restlessness.
- Cardiac conduction abnormalities following IV administration.
- Diarrhoea.
- Rash.

Additional Information

Metoclopramide should always be given in a separate syringe to morphine sulphate. The drugs must not be mixed.

Dosage and Administration

Route: Intravenous – administer over 2 minutes.

AGE	INITIAL DOSE	REPEAT DOSE	DOSE INTERVAL	CONCENTRATION	VOLUME	MAXIMUM DOSE
Adult	10 milligrams	NONE	N/A	10 milligrams in 2 ml	2 ml	10 milligrams

NB Monitor pulse, blood pressure, respiratory rate and cardiac rhythm before, during and after administration.

Presentation

Presented in a glass bottle containing 5 ml of midazolam, 10 milligrams per 1ml and supplied with four 1 ml syringes to draw up the dose.

Indications

Buccal Midazolam can be used as an anticonvulsant for grand-mal **convulsions** lasting **more than 5 minutes**, as they may not stop spontaneously.

Ambulance paramedics and technicians can administer the patient's own prescribed midazolam provided they are competent to administer buccal medication and are familiar with midazolam's indications, actions and side effects. Those that are not familiar with the use of this medication should use rectal (PR) or intravenous (IV) diazepam instead.

NB If the child continues fitting **10 minutes after their first dose of anticonvulsant**, they should receive intravenous **diazepam** for any further anticonvulsant treatment. If it is not possible to gain vascular access for the second dose of medication, no further drug treatment should be used, even if this means that the child continues to fit i.e. do not give a second dose of buccal or rectal medication

Where a grand-mal convulsion continues ten minutes after the second anticonvulsant, senior medical advice should be sought.

Contra-indications

None.

Dosage and Administration

Route: buccal (administered by carers).

Dosage – individual tailored dose as per the patient's individualised treatment plan.

Administration

The required dose is drawn up and half the dose is administered quickly to each side of the lower buccal cavity (between the cheek and gum).

NB Due to the time taken to cannulate and administer intravenous diazepam and the time it takes for rectal diazepam to act a second dose of midazolam is preferable. If a grand-mal convulsion continues ten minutes after the second dose, senior medical advice should be sought.

Actions

Midazolam has a sedative action similar to that of diazepam but of shorter duration. The onset of action usually occurs within five minutes, but is dependent on the route of administration. In 80% of episodes convulsions have stopped after ten minutes.

Side Effects

The side effects of buccal midazolam are similar in effect to IV administration, although, the timings may differ:

- Respiratory depression.
- Hypotension.
- Drowsiness.
- Muscle weakness.
- Slurred speech.
- Occasionally agitation, restlessness and disorientation may occur.

Additional Information

- **Midazolam is a benzodiazepine drug, which is now being administered by carers to treat convulsions as an alternative to rectal diazepam.**
- Some patients may have a Patient Specific Direction (PSD) drawn up by their specialist, customised to the specific nature of their convulsions. This is especially true of patients with learning disabilities living in residential care homes. Whenever possible check with the carers for the existence of a PSD for the patient, as this will normally give further guidance on treatment and when the patient should be further assessed.

Misoprostol [872, 876, 884–886]

MIS

Presentation

Tablet containing misoprostol:

● 200 micrograms.

Indications

Postpartum haemorrhage within 24 hours of delivery of the infant where bleeding from the uterus is uncontrollable by uterine massage.

Miscarriage with life-threatening bleeding and a confirmed diagnosis e.g. where a patient has gone home with medical management and starts to bleed.

Both syntometrine and ergometrine are contra-indicated in hypertension (BP >140/90); in this case misoprostol (or preferably syntocinon if available) should be administered instead.

In all other circumstances misoprostol should only be used if syntometrine or other oxytocics are unavailable or if they have been ineffective at reducing haemorrhage after 15 mins.

Actions

Stimulates contraction of the uterus.

Onset of action 7–10 minutes.

Contra-indications

● Known hypersensitivity to misoprostol.
● Active labour.
● Possible multiple pregnancy/known or suspected fetus in utero.

Side Effects

● Abdominal pain.
● Nausea and vomiting.
● Diarrhoea.
● Pyrexia.
● Shivering.

Additional Information

Syntometrine and misoprostol reduce bleeding from a pregnant uterus through different pathways; therefore if one drug has not been effective after 15 mins, the other may be administered in addition.

Dosage and Administration

● Administer orally unless the patient is unable to swallow.
● The vaginal route is not appropriate in postpartum haemorrhage.

Route: Oral.

AGE	INITIAL DOSE	REPEAT DOSE	DOSE INTERVAL	CONCENTRATION	TABLETS	MAXIMUM DOSE
Adult	600 micrograms	**None**	N/A	200 micrograms per tablet	3 tablets	600 micrograms

Route: Rectal. — **NB** At the time of publication there is no rectal preparation of misoprostol – therefore the same tablets can be administered orally or rectally.

AGE	INITIAL DOSE	REPEAT DOSE	DOSE INTERVAL	CONCENTRATION	TABLETS	MAXIMUM DOSE
Adult	1 mg	**None**	N/A	200 micrograms per tablet	5 tablets	1 mg

SECTION 6 Drugs – M

Presentation

Parenteral – ampoules containing morphine sulphate 10 milligrams in 1 ml.

Oral – vials containing morphine sulphate 10 milligrams in 5 ml.

Indications

Pain associated with suspected myocardial infarction (analgesic of first choice).

Severe pain as a component of a balanced analgesia regimen.

The decision about which analgesia and which route should be guided by clinical judgement (**refer to adult and child pain management guidelines**).

Actions

Morphine is a strong opioid analgesic. It is particularly useful for treating continuous, severe musculoskeletal and soft tissue pain.

Morphine produces sedation, euphoria and analgesia; it may both depress respiration and induce hypotension.

Histamine is released following morphine administration and this may contribute to its vasodilatory effects. This may also account for the urticaria and bronchoconstriction that are sometimes seen.

Contra-indications

Do **NOT** administer morphine in the following circumstances:

- Children under 1 year of age.
- Respiratory depression (adult <10 breaths per minute, child <20 breaths per minute).
- Hypotension (actual, not estimated, systolic blood pressure <90 mmHg in adults, <80 mmHg in school children, <70 mmHg in pre-school children).
- Head injury with significantly impaired level of consciousness (e.g. below P on the AVPU scale or below 9 on the GCS).
- Known hypersensitivity to morphine.

Cautions

Known severe renal or hepatic impairment – smaller doses may be used carefully and titrated to effect.

Use with **extreme** caution (minimal doses) during pregnancy. **NOTE:** Not to be used for labour pain where entonox is the analgesic of choice.

Use morphine **WITH GREAT CAUTION** in patients with chest injuries, particularly those with any respiratory difficulty, although if respiration is inhibited by pain, analgesia may actually improve respiratory status.

Any patients with other respiratory problems e.g. asthma, COPD.

Head injury. Agitation following head injury may be due to acute brain injury, hypoxia or pain. The decision to administer analgesia to an agitated head injured patient is a clinical one. It is vital that if such a patient receives opioids they are closely monitored since opioids can cause disproportionate respiratory depression, which

may ultimately lead to an elevated intracranial pressure through a raised arterial pCO_2.

Acute alcohol intoxication. All opioid drugs potentiate the central nervous system depressant effects of alcohol and they should therefore be used with great caution in patients who have consumed significant quantities of alcohol.

Medications. Prescribed antidepressants, sedatives or major tranquillisers may potentiate the respiratory and cardiovascular depressant effects of morphine.

Side Effects

- Respiratory depression.
- Cardiovascular depression.
- Nausea and vomiting.
- Drowsiness.
- Pupillary constriction.

Additional Information

Morphine is a Class A controlled drug under Schedule 2 of the Misuse of Drugs Regulations 1985, and must be stored and its prescription and administration documented in accordance with these regulations.

Morphine is not licensed for use in children but its use has been approved by the Medicines and Healthcare products Regulatory Agency (MHRA) for 'off label' use. This means that it can legally be administered under these guidelines by paramedics.

Unused morphine in open vials or syringes must be discarded in the presence of a witness.

Special Precautions

Naloxone can be used to reverse morphine related respiratory or cardiovascular depression. It should be carefully titrated after assessment and appropriate management of ABC for that particular patient and situation (**refer to naloxone guideline**).

Morphine frequently induces nausea or vomiting which may be potentiated by the movement of the ambulance. Titrating to the lowest dose to achieve analgesia will reduce the risk of vomiting. The use of an anti-emetics should also be considered whenever administering any opioid analgesic (**refer to ondansetron and metoclopramide guidelines**).

Dosage and Administration

Administration must be in conjunction with pain score monitoring (**refer to pain management guidelines**).

Intravenous morphine takes a minimum of 2–3 minutes before starting to take effect, reaching its peak between 10–20 minutes.

The absorption of intramuscular, subcutaneous or oral morphine is variable particularly in patients with major trauma, shock and cardiac conditions; these routes should preferably be avoided if the circumstances favour intravenous or intra-osseous administration.

Morphine **should be** diluted with sodium chloride 0.9% to make a concentration of 10 milligrams in 10 ml (1 milligram in 1 ml) unless it is being administered by the intramuscular or subcutaneous route when it should not be diluted.

ADULTS – If pain is not reduced to a tolerable level after 10 milligrams of IV/IO morphine, then further **2 milligram** doses may be administered by slow IV/IO injection every 5 minutes to **20 milligrams maximum**. The patient should be closely observed throughout the remaining treatment and transfer. Care should be taken with elderly patients who may be more susceptible to complications and in whom smaller doses of morphine may be adequate.

CHILDREN – The doses and volumes given below are for the initial and maximum doses. Administer **0.1 ml/kg** (equal to **0.1 milligrams/kg**) as an initial slow IV injection over 2 minutes. If pain is not reduced to a tolerable level after 5 minutes then a further dose of up to **0.1 milligrams/kg**, titrated to response, may be repeated (**maximum dose 0.2 milligrams/kg**).

NOTE: Peak effect of each dose may not occur until 10–20 minutes after administration.

Route: Intravenous/intra-osseous – administer by slow IV injection (rate of approximately 2 milligram per minute up to appropriate dose for age). Observe the patient for at least 5 minutes after completion of initial dose before repeating the dose if required.

AGE	INITIAL DOSE	REPEAT DOSE	DOSE INTERVAL	DILUTED CONCENTRATION	VOLUME	MAXIMUM DOSE
Adult	10 milligrams	10 milligrams	5 minutes	10 milligrams in 10 ml	10 ml	20 milligrams
11 years	3.5 milligrams	3.5 milligrams	5 minutes	10 milligrams in 10 ml	3.5 ml	7 milligrams
10 years	3 milligrams	3 milligrams	5 minutes	10 milligrams in 10 ml	3 ml	6 milligrams
9 years	3 milligrams	3 milligrams	5 minutes	10 milligrams in 10 ml	3 ml	6 milligrams
8 years	2.5 milligrams	2.5 milligrams	5 minutes	10 milligrams in 10 ml	2.5 ml	5 milligrams
7 years	2.5 milligrams	2.5 milligrams	5 minutes	10 milligrams in 10 ml	2.5 ml	5 milligrams
6 years	2 milligrams	2 milligrams	5 minutes	10 milligrams in 10 ml	2 ml	4 milligrams
5 years	2 milligrams	2 milligrams	5 minutes	10 milligrams in 10 ml	2 ml	4 milligrams
4 years	1.5 milligrams	1.5 milligrams	5 minutes	10 milligrams in 10 ml	1.5 ml	3 milligrams
3 years	1.5 milligrams	1.5 milligrams	5 minutes	10 milligrams in 10 ml	1.5 ml	3 milligrams
2 years	1 milligram	1 milligram	5 minutes	10 milligrams in 10 ml	1 ml	2 milligrams
18 months	1 milligram	1 milligram	5 minutes	10 milligrams in 10 ml	1 ml	2 milligrams
12 months	1 milligram	1 milligram	5 minutes	10 milligrams in 10 ml	1 ml	2 milligrams
9 months	N/A	N/A	N/A	N/A	N/A	N/A
6 months	N/A	N/A	N/A	N/A	N/A	N/A
3 months	N/A	N/A	N/A	N/A	N/A	N/A
1 month	N/A	N/A	N/A	N/A	N/A	N/A
Birth	N/A	N/A	N/A	N/A	N/A	N/A

Route: Oral.

AGE	INITIAL DOSE	REPEAT DOSE	DOSE INTERVAL	CONCENTRATION	VOLUME	MAXIMUM DOSE
Adult	20 milligrams	20 milligrams	60 minutes	10 milligrams in 5 ml	10 ml	40 milligrams
11 years	7 milligrams	NONE	N/A	10 milligrams in 5 ml	3.5 ml	7 milligrams
10 years	6 milligrams	NONE	N/A	10 milligrams in 5 ml	3 ml	6 milligrams
9 years	6 milligrams	NONE	N/A	10 milligrams in 5 ml	3 ml	6 milligrams
8 years	5 milligrams	NONE	N/A	10 milligrams in 5 ml	2.5 ml	5 milligrams
7 years	5 milligrams	NONE	N/A	10 milligrams in 5 ml	2.5 ml	5 milligrams
6 years	4 milligrams	NONE	N/A	10 milligrams in 5 ml	2 ml	4 milligrams
5 years	4 milligrams	NONE	N/A	10 milligrams in 5 ml	2 ml	4 milligrams
4 years	3 milligrams	NONE	N/A	10 milligrams in 5 ml	1.5 ml	3 milligrams
3 years	3 milligrams	NONE	N/A	10 milligrams in 5 ml	1.5 ml	3 milligrams
2 years	2 milligrams	NONE	N/A	10 milligrams in 5 ml	1 ml	2 milligrams
18 months	2 milligrams	NONE	N/A	10 milligrams in 5 ml	1 ml	2 milligrams
12 months	2 milligrams	NONE	N/A	10 milligrams in 5 ml	1 ml	2 milligrams
9 months	N/A	N/A	N/A	N/A	N/A	N/A
6 months	N/A	N/A	N/A	N/A	N/A	N/A
3 months	N/A	N/A	N/A	N/A	N/A	N/A
1 month	N/A	N/A	N/A	N/A	N/A	N/A
Birth	N/A	N/A	N/A	N/A	N/A	N/A

NB Only administer via the oral route in patients with major trauma, shock or cardiac conditions if the IV/IO routes are not accessible.

Route: Intramuscular/subcutaneous.

AGE	INITIAL DOSE	REPEAT DOSE	DOSE INTERVAL	CONCENTRATION	VOLUME	MAXIMUM DOSE
Adult	10 milligrams	10 milligrams	60 minutes	10 milligrams in 1 ml	1 ml	20 milligrams
11 years	3.5 milligrams	3.5 milligrams	60 minutes	10 milligrams in 1 ml	0.35 ml	7 milligrams
10 years	3 milligrams	3 milligrams	60 minutes	10 milligrams in 1 ml	0.30 ml	6 milligrams
9 years	3 milligrams	3 milligrams	60 minutes	10 milligrams in 1 ml	0.30 ml	6 milligrams
8 years	2.5 milligrams	2.5 milligrams	60 minutes	10 milligrams in 1 ml	0.25 ml	5 milligrams
7 years	2.5 milligrams	2.5 milligrams	60 minutes	10 milligrams in 1 ml	0.25 ml	5 milligrams
6 years	2 milligrams	2 milligrams	60 minutes	10 milligrams in 1 ml	0.20 ml	4 milligrams
5 years	2 milligrams	2 milligrams	60 minutes	10 milligrams in 1 ml	0.20 ml	4 milligrams
4 years	1.5 milligrams	1.5 milligrams	60 minutes	10 milligrams in 1 ml	0.15 ml	3 milligrams
3 years	1.5 milligrams	1.5 milligrams	60 minutes	10 milligrams in 1 ml	0.15 ml	3 milligrams
2 years	1 milligram	1 milligram	60 minutes	10 milligrams in 1 ml	0.10 ml	2 milligrams
18 months	1 milligram	1 milligram	60 minutes	10 milligrams in 1 ml	0.10 ml	2 milligrams
12 months	1 milligram	1 milligram	60 minutes	10 milligrams in 1 ml	0.10 ml	2 milligrams
9 months	N/A	N/A	N/A	N/A	N/A	N/A
6 months	N/A	N/A	N/A	N/A	N/A	N/A
3 months	N/A	N/A	N/A	N/A	N/A	N/A
1 months	N/A	N/A	N/A	N/A	N/A	N/A
Birth	N/A	N/A	N/A	N/A	N/A	N/A

NB Only administer via the intramuscular or subcutaneous route in patients with major trauma, shock or cardiac conditions if the IV/IO routes are not accessible.

SECTION **6** Drugs – M

Presentation

Naloxone hydrochloride 400 micrograms per 1 ml ampoule.

Indications

Opioid overdose producing respiratory, cardiovascular and central nervous system depression.

Overdose of either an opioid analgesic, e.g. dextropropoxyphene, codeine, or a compound analgesic (see table 6.6) e.g. co-codamol (combination of codeine and paracetamol).

Unconsciousness, associated with respiratory depression of unknown cause, where opioid overdose is a possibility, **refer to altered level of consciousness guideline**.

Reversal of respiratory and central nervous system depression in a neonate following maternal opioid use during labour.

Actions

Antagonism of the effects (including respiratory depression) of opioid drugs.

Contra-indications

Neonates born to opioid addicted mothers – produces serious withdrawal effects. Emphasis should be on bag-valve-mask ventilation and oxygenation – as with all patients.

Side Effects

In patients who are physically dependent on opiates, naloxone may precipitate violent withdrawal symptoms, including cardiac dysrrhythmias. It is better, in these cases, to titrate the dose of naloxone as described (see dosing charts below), to effectively reverse the cardiac and respiratory depression, but still leave the patient in a 'groggy' state with regular re-assessment of ventilation and circulation.

Additional information

When indicated, naloxone should be administered via the intravenous route.

If IV access is impossible, naloxone may be administered intramuscularly, **undiluted** (into the outer aspect of the thigh or upper arm), but absorption may be unpredictable.

Opioid induced respiratory and cardiovascular depression can be fatal.

When used, naloxone's effects are **short lived** and once its effects have worn off respiratory and cardiovascular depression can recur with fatal consequences. **All** cases of opioid overdose should be transported to hospital, even if the initial response to naloxone has been good. If the patient refuses hospitalisation, consider, if the patient consents, a loading dose of **800 micrograms IM** to minimise the risk described above.

Table 6.6 – Examples of prescription opioid drugs

Buprenorphine	Temgesic
Codeine	Used in combination in Codis, Diarrest, Migraleve, Paracodol, Phensedyl, Solpadeine, Solpadol, Syndol, Terpoin, Tylex, Veganin
Dextromoramide	Palfium
Dipipanone	Dicanol
Dextropropoxyphene	Used in combination in Distalgesic/co-proxamol
Diamorphine	'Heroin'
Dihydrocodeine	Co-dydramol, DF 118
Meptazinol	Meptid
Methadone	Physeptone, Methadose
Morphine	Oramorph, Sevredol, MST Continus, SRM Rhotard
Oxycodone	Oxycontin
Pentazocine	Fortral
Pethidine	Pamergan
Phenazocine	Narphen

NB This list is not comprehensive; other opioid drugs are available.

Drugs–N–O

SECTION 6

Dosage and Administration

Respiratory arrest/extreme respiratory depression.

- If there is no response after the initial dose, repeat every 3 minutes, up to the maximum dose, until an effect is noted. NB The half-life of naloxone is short.
- Known or potentially aggressive adults suffering respiratory depression: Dilute up to 800 micrograms (2 ml) of naloxone into 8 ml of water for injections or sodium chloride 0.9% to a total volume of 10 ml and administer **SLOWLY**, titrating to response, 1 ml at a time.

Route: Intravenous/intra-osseous – administer **SLOWLY** 1 ml at a time. Titrated to response relieving respiratory depression but maintain patient in 'groggy' state.

AGE	INITIAL DOSE	REPEAT DOSE	DOSE INTERVAL	CONCENTRATION	VOLUME	MAXIMUM DOSE
12 years–adult	400 micrograms	400 micrograms	3 minutes	400 micrograms in 1 ml	1 ml	4400 micrograms
11 years	350 micrograms	350 micrograms	3 minutes	400 micrograms in 1 ml	0.9 ml	3850 micrograms
10 years	320 micrograms	320 micrograms	3 minutes	400 micrograms in 1 ml	0.8 ml	3520 micrograms
9 years	280 micrograms	280 micrograms	3 minutes	400 micrograms in 1 ml	0.7 ml	3080 micrograms
8 years	280 micrograms	280 micrograms	3 minutes	400 micrograms in 1 ml	0.7 ml	3080 micrograms
7 years	240 micrograms	240 micrograms	3 minutes	400 micrograms in 1 ml	0.6 ml	2640 micrograms
6 years	200 micrograms	200 micrograms	3 minutes	400 micrograms in 1 ml	0.5 ml	2200 micrograms
5 years	200 micrograms	200 micrograms	3 minutes	400 micrograms in 1 ml	0.5 ml	2200 micrograms
4 years	160 micrograms	160 micrograms	3 minutes	400 micrograms in 1 ml	0.4 ml	1760 micrograms
3 years	160 micrograms	160 micrograms	3 minutes	400 micrograms in 1 ml	0.4 ml	1760 micrograms
2 years	120 micrograms	120 micrograms	3 minutes	400 micrograms in 1 ml	0.3 ml	1320 micrograms
18 months	120 micrograms	120 micrograms	3 minutes	400 micrograms in 1 ml	0.3 ml	1320 micrograms
12 months	100 micrograms	100 micrograms	3 minutes	400 micrograms in 1 ml	0.25 ml	1100 micrograms
9 months	80 micrograms	80 micrograms	3 minutes	400 micrograms in 1 ml	0.2 ml	880 micrograms
6 months	80 micrograms	80 micrograms	3 minutes	400 micrograms in 1 ml	0.2 ml	880 micrograms
3 months	60 micrograms	60 micrograms	3 minutes	400 micrograms in 1 ml	0.15 ml	660 micrograms
1 month	40 micrograms	40 micrograms	3 minutes	400 micrograms in 1 ml	0.1 ml	440 micrograms
Birth	40 micrograms	40 micrograms	3 minutes	400 micrograms in 1 ml	0.1 ml	440 micrograms

Respiratory arrest/extreme respiratory depression where the IV/IO route is unavailable or the ambulance clinician is not trained to administer drugs via the IV/IO route.

- If there is no response after the initial dose, repeat every 3 minutes, up to the maximum dose, until an effect is noted. NB The half-life of naloxone is short.
- **For adults when administering naloxone via the intramuscular route:** Administering large volumes intramuscularly could lead to poor absorption and/or tissue damage; therefore divide the dose where necessary and practicable. Vary the site of injection for repeated doses; appropriate sites include: buttock (gluteus maximus), thigh (vastus lateralis), lateral hip (gluteus medius) and upper arm (deltoid).

Route: Intramuscular – initial dose.

AGE	INITIAL DOSE	REPEAT DOSE	DOSE INTERVAL	CONCENTRATION	VOLUME	MAXIMUM DOSE
12 years–adult	400 micrograms	See over	3 minutes	400 micrograms in 1ml	1 ml	See below
11 years	350 micrograms	See over	3 minutes	400 micrograms in 1 ml	0.9 ml	See below
10 years	320 micrograms	See over	3 minutes	400 micrograms in 1 ml	0.8 ml	See below
9 years	280 micrograms	See over	3 minutes	400 micrograms in 1 ml	0.7 ml	See below
8 years	280 micrograms	See over	3 minutes	400 micrograms in 1 ml	0.7 ml	See below
7 years	240 micrograms	See over	3 minutes	400 micrograms in 1 ml	0.6 ml	See below
6 years	200 micrograms	See over	3 minutes	400 micrograms in 1 ml	0.5 ml	See below
5 years	200 micrograms	See over	3 minutes	400 micrograms in 1 ml	0.5 ml	See below
4 years	160 micrograms	See over	3 minutes	400 micrograms in 1 ml	0.4 ml	See below
3 years	160 micrograms	See over	3 minutes	400 micrograms in 1 ml	0.4 ml	See below
2 years	120 micrograms	See over	3 minutes	400 micrograms in 1 ml	0.3 ml	See below
18 months	120 micrograms	See over	3 minutes	400 micrograms in 1 ml	0.3 ml	See below
12 months	100 micrograms	See over	3 minutes	400 micrograms in 1 ml	0.25 ml	See below
9 months	80 micrograms	See over	3 minutes	400 micrograms in 1 ml	0.2 ml	See below
6 months	80 micrograms	See over	3 minutes	400 micrograms in 1 ml	0.2 ml	See below
3 months	60 micrograms	See over	3 minutes	400 micrograms in 1 ml	0.15 ml	See below
1 month	40 micrograms	See over	3 minutes	400 micrograms in 1 ml	0.1 ml	See below
Birth	40 micrograms	See over	3 minutes	100 micrograms in 1 ml	0.5 ml	See below

Drugs–N–O

6 SECTION

Route: Intramuscular – repeat dose.

AGE	INITIAL DOSE	REPEAT DOSE	DOSE INTERVAL	CONCENTRATION	VOLUME	MAXIMUM DOSE
12 years–adult	See previous	400 micrograms	3 minutes	400 micrograms in 1 ml	1 ml	4400 micrograms
11 years	See previous	400 micrograms	3 minutes	400 micrograms in 1 ml	1 ml	750 micrograms
10 years	See previous	400 micrograms	3 minutes	400 micrograms in 1 ml	1 ml	720 micrograms
9 years	See previous	400 micrograms	3 minutes	400 micrograms in 1 ml	1 ml	680 micrograms
8 years	See previous	400 micrograms	3 minutes	400 micrograms in 1 ml	1 ml	680 micrograms
7 years	See previous	400 micrograms	3 minutes	400 micrograms in 1 ml	1 ml	640 micrograms
6 years	See previous	400 micrograms	3 minutes	400 micrograms in 1 ml	1 ml	600 micrograms
5 years	See previous	400 micrograms	3 minutes	400 micrograms in 1 ml	1 ml	600 micrograms
4 years	See previous	400 micrograms	3 minutes	400 micrograms in 1 ml	1 ml	560 micrograms
3 years	See previous	400 micrograms	3 minutes	400 micrograms in 1 ml	1 ml	560 micrograms
2 years	See previous	400 micrograms	3 minutes	400 micrograms in 1 ml	1 ml	520 micrograms
18 months	See previous	400 micrograms	3 minutes	400 micrograms in 1 ml	1 ml	520 micrograms
12 months	See previous	400 micrograms	3 minutes	400 micrograms in 1 ml	1 ml	500 micrograms
9 months	See previous	400 micrograms	3 minutes	400 micrograms in 1 ml	1 ml	480 micrograms
6 months	See previous	400 micrograms	3 minutes	400 micrograms in 1 ml	1 ml	480 micrograms
3 months	See previous	400 micrograms	3 minutes	400 micrograms in 1 ml	1 ml	460 micrograms
1 month	See previous	400 micrograms	3 minutes	400 micrograms in 1 ml	1 ml	440 micrograms
Birth	See previous	400 micrograms	3 minutes	400 micrograms in 1 ml	1 ml	440 micrograms

Reversal of respiratory and central nervous system depression in a neonate following maternal opioid use during labour.

● Administer a single dose only.

Route: Intramuscular.

AGE	INITIAL DOSE	REPEAT DOSE	DOSE INTERVAL	CONCENTRATION	VOLUME	MAXIMUM DOSE
Birth	200 micrograms	NONE	N/A	400 micrograms in 1 ml	0.5 ml	200 micrograms

NB In the event of IV access being unavailable for the administration of naloxone in children it is advised that the initial IM dose be given dependent on age and, if required, a single subsequent IM dose of 400 micrograms to be given once only. If IV access becomes available and further doses of naloxone are clinically indicated then revert to the IV dosage table.

Presentation

Ampoule containing 4 milligrams of ondansetron (as hydrochloride) in 2 ml.

Ampoule containing 8 milligrams of ondansetron (as hydrochloride) in 4 ml.

NB Both these preparations share the same concentration (2 milligrams in 1 ml).

Indications

Adults:

● Prevention and treatment of opiate-induced nausea and vomiting e.g. morphine sulphate.

● Treatment of nausea or vomiting.

Children:

● Prevention and treatment of opiate-induced nausea and vomiting e.g. morphine sulphate.

● For travel associated nausea or vomiting.

Actions

An anti-emetic that blocks 5HT receptors both centrally and in the gastrointestinal tract.

Contra-indications

Known sensitivity to ondansetron.

Infants <1 month old.

Cautions

QT interval prolongation (avoid concomitant administration of drugs that prolong QT interval).

Hepatic impairment.

Pregnancy.

Breastfeeding.

Side Effects

Hiccups.

Constipation.

Flushing.

Hypotension.

Chest pain.

Arrhythmias.

Bradycardia.

Headache.

Seizures.

Movement disorders.

Injection site reactions.

Additional Information

Ondansetron should always be given in a separate syringe to morphine sulphate – the drugs must **NOT** be mixed.

Ondansetron should **NOT** be routinely administered in the management of childhood gastroenteritis (**refer to gastroenteritis in children guideline**).

SECTION **6** Drugs–N–O

Dosage and Administration

Note: Two preparations exist (4 mg in 2 ml and 8 mg in 4 ml). They share the same concentration i.e. 2 milligrams in 1 ml.

Route: Intravenous (**SLOW** IV injection over 2 minutes) /intramuscular.

AGE	INITIAL DOSE	REPEAT DOSE	DOSE INTERVAL	CONCENTRATION	VOLUME	MAXIMUM DOSE
12 years – Adult	4 milligrams	NONE	N/A	2 milligrams in 1 ml	2 ml	4 milligrams
11 years	3 milligrams	NONE	N/A	2 milligrams in 1 ml	1.5 ml	3 milligrams
10 years	3 milligrams	NONE	N/A	2 milligrams in 1 ml	1.5 ml	3 milligrams
9 years	3 milligrams	NONE	N/A	2 milligrams in 1 ml	1.5 ml	3 milligrams
8 years	2.5 milligrams	NONE	N/A	2 milligrams in 1 ml	1.3 ml	2.5 milligrams
7 years	2.5 milligrams	NONE	N/A	2 milligrams in 1 ml	1.3 ml	2.5 milligrams
6 years	2 milligrams	NONE	N/A	2 milligrams in 1 ml	1 ml	2 milligrams
5 years	2 milligrams	NONE	N/A	2 milligrams in 1 ml	1 ml	2 milligrams
4 years	1.5 milligrams	NONE	N/A	2 milligrams in 1 ml	0.75 ml	1.5 milligrams
3 years	1.5 milligrams	NONE	N/A	2 milligrams in 1 ml	0.75 ml	1.5 milligrams
2 years	1 milligram	NONE	N/A	2 milligrams in 1 ml	0.5 ml	1 milligram
18 months	1 milligram	NONE	N/A	2 milligrams in 1 ml	0.5 ml	1 milligram
12 months	1 milligram	NONE	N/A	2 milligrams in 1 ml	0.5 ml	1 milligram
9 months	1 milligram	NONE	N/A	2 milligrams in 1 ml	0.5 ml	1 milligram
6 months	1 milligram	NONE	N/A	2 milligrams in 1 ml	0.5 ml	1 milligram
3 months	0.5 milligrams	NONE	N/A	2 milligrams in 1 ml	0.25 ml	0.5 milligrams
1 month	0.5 milligrams	NONE	N/A	2 milligrams in 1 ml	0.25 ml	0.5 milligrams
Birth	N/A	N/A	N/A	N/A	N/A	N/A

NB Monitor pulse, blood pressure, respiratory rate and cardiac rhythm before, during and after administration.

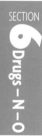

SECTION **6** Drugs – N – O

Presentation

Oxygen (O_2) is a gas provided in compressed form in a cylinder. It is also available in liquid form, in a system adapted for ambulance use. It is fed via a regulator and flow meter to the patient by means of plastic tubing and an oxygen mask/nasal cannulae.

Indications

Children

● Significant illness and/or injury.

Adults

● Critical illnesses requiring high levels of supplemental oxygen (refer to Table 6.1).

● Serious illnesses requiring moderate levels of supplemental oxygen if the patient is hypoxaemic (refer to Table 6.2).

● COPD and other conditions requiring controlled or low-dose oxygen therapy (refer to Table 6.3).

● Conditions for which patients should be monitored closely but oxygen therapy is not required unless the patient is hypoxaemic (refer to Table 6.4).

Actions

Essential for cell metabolism. Adequate tissue oxygenation is essential for normal physiological function.

Oxygen assists in reversing hypoxia, by raising the concentration of inspired oxygen. Hypoxia will, however, only improve if respiratory effort or ventilation and tissue perfusion are adequate.

If ventilation is inadequate or absent, assisting or completely taking over the patient's ventilation is essential to reverse hypoxia.

Contra-indications

Explosive environments.

Cautions

Oxygen increases the fire hazard at the scene of an incident.

Defibrillation – ensure pads firmly applied to reduce spark hazard.

Side Effects

Non-humidified O_2 is drying and irritating to mucous membranes over a period of time.

In patients with COPD there is a risk that even moderately high doses of inspired oxygen can produce increased carbon dioxide levels which may cause respiratory depression and this may lead to respiratory arrest. Refer to Table 6.3 for guidance.

Dosage and Administration

● Measure oxygen saturation (SpO_2) in all patients using pulse oximetry.

● For the administration of **moderate** levels of supplemented oxygen nasal cannulae are recommended in preference to simple face mask as they offer more flexible dose range.

● Patients with tracheostomy or previous laryngectomy may require alternative appliances e.g. tracheostomy masks.

● Entonox may be administered when required.

● Document oxygen administration.

Children

● **ALL** children with significant illness and/or injury should receive **HIGH** levels of supplementary oxygen.

Adults

● Administer the initial oxygen dose until a reliable oxygen saturation reading is obtained.

● If the desired oxygen saturation cannot be maintained with simple face mask change to reservoir mask (non-rebreathe mask).

● For dosage and administration of supplemental oxygen refer to **Tables 6.1–6.3**.

● For conditions where **NO** supplemental oxygen is required unless the patient is hypoxaemic refer to **Table 6.4**.

Table 6.1 – High levels of supplemental oxygen for adults with critical illnesses

Target saturation 94–98%	Administer the initial oxygen dose until the vital signs are normal, then reduce oxygen dose and aim for target saturation within the range of **94–98%** as per the table below.	
Condition	**Initial dose**	**Method of administration**

● Cardiac arrest or resuscitation:
  – basic life support
  – advanced life support
  – foreign body airway obstruction
  – traumatic cardiac arrest
  – maternal resuscitation.
● Carbon monoxide poisoning.
 	
NOTE – Some oxygen saturation monitors cannot differentiate between carboxyhaemoglobin and oxyhaemoglobin owing to carbon monoxide poisoning
	Maximum dose until the vital signs are normal	Bag-valve-mask

● Major trauma:
  – abdominal trauma
  – burns and scalds
  – electrocution
  – head trauma
  – limb trauma
  – neck and back trauma (spinal)
  – pelvic trauma
  – the immersion incident
  – thoracic trauma
  – trauma in pregnancy.
● Anaphylaxis
● Major pulmonary haemorrhage
● Sepsis e.g. meningococcal septicaemia
● Shock
	15 litres per minute	Reservoir mask (non-rebreathe mask)

● Active convulsion ● Hypothermia	Administer 15 litres per minute until a reliable SpO_2 measurement can be obtained and then adjust oxygen flow to aim for target saturation within the range of **94–98%**	Reservoir mask (non-rebreathe mask)

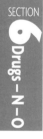

Table 6.2 – Moderate levels of supplemental oxygen for adults with serious illnesses if the patient is hypoxaemic

Target saturation 94–98% — Administer the initial oxygen dose until a reliable SpO_2 measurement is available, then adjust oxygen flow to aim for target saturation within the range of **94–98%** as per the table below.

Condition	Initial dose	Method of administration
• Acute hypoxaemia (cause not yet diagnosed) • Deterioration of lung fibrosis or other interstitial lung disease • Acute asthma • Acute heart failure • Pneumonia • Lung cancer • Postoperative breathlessness • Pulmonary embolism • Pleural effusions • Pneumothorax • Severe anaemia • Sickle cell crisis	**SpO_2 <85%** 10–15 litres per minute	Reservoir mask (non-rebreathe mask)
	SpO_2 ≥85–93% 2–6 litres per minute	Nasal cannulae
	SpO_2 ≥85–93% 5–10 litres per minute	Simple face mask

Table 6.3 – Controlled or low-dose supplemental oxygen for adults with COPD and other conditions requiring controlled or low-dose oxygen therapy

Target saturation 88–92% — Administer the initial oxygen dose until a reliable SpO_2 measurement is available, then adjust oxygen flow to aim for target saturation within the range of **88–92%** or **prespecified range** detailed on the patient's alert card, as per the table below.

Condition	Initial dose	Method of administration
• Chronic obstructive pulmonary disease (COPD) • Exacerbation of cystic fibrosis	4 litres per minute	28% Venturi mask or patient's own mask
	NB If respiratory rate is >30 breaths/min using Venturi mask set flow rate to 50% above the minimum specified for the mask.	
• Chronic neuromuscular disorders • Chest wall disorders • Morbid obesity (body mass index >40 kg/m²)	4 litres per minute	28% Venturi mask or patient's own mask
NB If the oxygen saturation remains below 88% change to simple face mask.	5–10 litres per minute	Simple face mask
NB Critical illness **AND** COPD/or other risk factors for hypercapnia.	If a patient with COPD or other risk factors for hypercapnia sustains or develops critical illness/injury ensure the same target saturations as indicated in Table 6.1.	

SECTION **6** Drugs–N–O

Table 6.4 – No supplemental oxygen required for adults with these conditions unless the patient is hypoxaemic but patients should be monitored closely

Target saturation

94–98%

If hypoxaemic (SpO$_2$ <94%) administer the initial oxygen dose, then adjust oxygen flow to aim for target saturation within the range of **94–98%**, as per the table below.

Condition	Initial dose	Method of administration

• Myocardial infarction and acute coronary syndromes
• Stroke
• Cardiac rhythm disturbance
• Non-traumatic chest pain/discomfort
• Implantable cardioverter defibrillator firing
• Pregnancy and obstetric emergencies:
  – birth imminent
  – haemorrhage during pregnancy
  – pregnancy induced hypertension
  – vaginal bleeding.
• Abdominal pain
• Headache
• Hyperventilation syndrome or dysfunctional breathing
• Most poisonings and drug overdoses (refer to **Table 6.1** for **carbon monoxide poisoning** and special cases below for **paraquat poisoning**)
• Metabolic and renal disorders
• Acute and sub-acute neurological and muscular conditions producing muscle weakness (assess the need for assisted ventilation if **SpO$_2$ <94%**)
• Post convulsion
• Gastrointestinal bleeds
• Glycaemic emergencies
• Heat exhaustion/heat stroke
 	
SPECIAL CASES
• Poisoning with paraquat
	SpO$_2$ <85%
	10–15 litres per minute
	
	SpO$_2$ ≥85–93%
	2–6 litres per minute
	
	SpO$_2$ ≥85–93%
	5–10 litres per minute
		Reservoir mask
		(non-rebreathe mask)
		
		Nasal cannulae
		
		Simple face mask

NOTE – patients with paraquat poisoning may be harmed by supplemental oxygen so avoid oxygen unless the patient is hypoxaemic. Target saturation 88–92%.

Table 6.1 – Critical illnesses in adults requiring HIGH levels of supplemental oxygen

- Cardiac arrest or resuscitation:
  - basic life support
  - advanced life support
  - foreign body airway obstruction
  - traumatic cardiac arrest
  - maternal resuscitation.
- Major trauma:
  - abdominal trauma
  - burns and scalds
  - electrocution
  - head trauma
  - limb trauma
  - neck and back trauma (spinal)
  - pelvic trauma
  - the immersion incident
  - thoracic trauma
  - trauma in pregnancy.
- Active convulsion
- Anaphylaxis
- Carbon monoxide poisoning
- Hypothermia
- Major pulmonary haemorrhage
- Sepsis e.g. meningococcal septicaemia
- Shock

Table 6.2 – Serious illnesses in adults requiring MODERATE levels of supplemental oxygen if hypoxaemic

- Acute hypoxaemia
- Deterioration of lung fibrosis or other interstitial lung disease
- Acute asthma
- Acute heart failure
- Pneumonia
- Lung cancer
- Postoperative breathlessness
- Pulmonary embolism
- Pleural effusions
- Pneumothorax
- Severe anaemia
- Sickle cell crisis

Table 6.3 – COPD and other conditions in adults requiring CONTROLLED OR LOW-DOSE supplemental oxygen

- Chronic Obstructive Pulmonary Disease (COPD)
- Exacerbation of cystic fibrosis
- Chronic neuromuscular disorders
- Chest wall disorders
- Morbid obesity (body mass index >40 kg/m^2)

Table 6.4 – Conditions in adults NOT requiring supplemental oxygen unless the patient is hypoxaemic

- Myocardial infarction and acute coronary syndromes
- Stroke
- Cardiac rhythm disturbance
- Non-traumatic chest pain/discomfort
- Implantable cardioverter defibrillator firing
- Pregnancy and obstetric emergencies:
  - birth imminent
  - haemorrhage during pregnancy
  - pregnancy induced hypertension
  - vaginal bleeding.
- Abdominal pain
- Headache
- Hyperventilation syndrome or dysfunctional breathing
- Most poisonings and drug overdoses (except carbon monoxide poisoning)
- Metabolic and renal disorders
- Acute and sub-acute neurological and muscular conditions producing muscle weakness
- Post convulsion
- Gastrointestinal bleeds
- Glycaemic emergencies
- Heat exhaustion/heat stroke

Special cases:
- Paraquat poisoning

Section 6 — Drugs—N–O

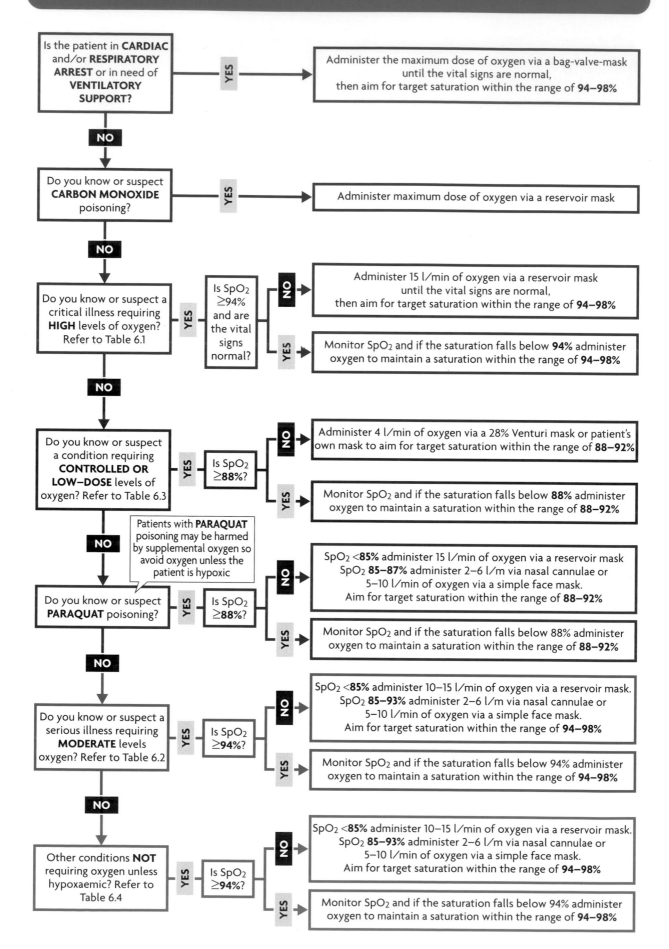

Figure 6.1 – Administration of supplemental oxygen algorithm.

Table 6.1 – Critical illnesses in adults requiring **HIGH** levels of supplemental oxygen

- Cardiac arrest or resuscitation:
  - basic life support
  - advanced life support
  - foreign body airway obstruction
  - traumatic cardiac arrest
  - maternal resuscitation.
- Major trauma:
  - abdominal trauma
  - burns and scalds
  - electrocution
  - head trauma
  - limb trauma
  - neck and back trauma (spinal)
  - pelvic trauma
  - the immersion incident
  - thoracic trauma
  - trauma in pregnancy.
- Active convulsion
- Anaphylaxis
- Carbon monoxide poisoning
- Hypothermia
- Major pulmonary haemorrhage
- Sepsis e.g. meningococcal septicaemia
- Shock

Table 6.2 – Serious illnesses in adults requiring **MODERATE** levels of supplemental oxygen if hypoxaemic

- Acute hypoxaemia
- Deterioration of lung fibrosis or other interstitial lung disease
- Acute asthma
- Acute heart failure
- Pneumonia
- Lung cancer
- Postoperative breathlessness
- Pulmonary embolism
- Pleural effusions
- Pneumothorax
- Severe anaemia
- Sickle cell crisis

Table 6.3 – COPD and other conditions in adults requiring **CONTROLLED OR LOW-DOSE** supplemental oxygen

- Chronic Obstructive Pulmonary Disease (COPD)
- Exacerbation of cystic fibrosis
- Chronic neuromuscular disorders
- Chest wall disorders
- Morbid obesity (body mass index >40 kg/m^2)

Table 6.4 – Conditions in adults **NOT** requiring supplemental oxygen unless the patient is hypoxaemic

- Myocardial infarction and acute coronary syndromes
- Stroke
- Cardiac rhythm disturbance
- Non-traumatic chest pain/discomfort
- Implantable cardioverter defibrillator firing
- Pregnancy and obstetric emergencies:
  - birth imminent
  - haemorrhage during pregnancy
  - pregnancy induced hypertension
  - vaginal bleeding.
- Abdominal pain
- Headache
- Hyperventilation syndrome or dysfunctional breathing
- Most poisonings and drug overdoses (except carbon monoxide poisoning)
- Metabolic and renal disorders
- Acute and sub-acute neurological and muscular conditions producing muscle weakness
- Post convulsion
- Gastrointestinal bleeds
- Glycaemic emergencies
- Heat exhaustion/heat stroke

Special cases:
- Paraquat poisoning

Drugs–N–O

6 SECTION

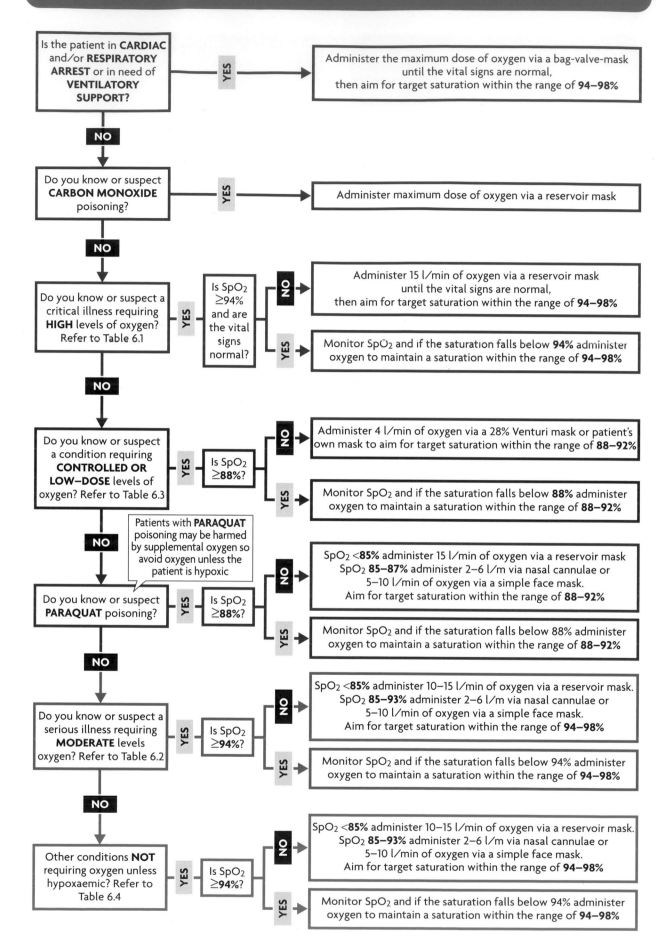

Figure 6.1 – Administration of supplemental oxygen algorithm.

Is the patient in **CARDIAC** and/or **RESPIRATORY ARREST** or in need of **VENTILATORY SUPPORT?**

YES → Administer the maximum dose of oxygen via a bag-valve-mask until the vital signs are normal, then aim for target saturation within the range of **94–98%**

NO

Do you know or suspect **CARBON MONOXIDE** poisoning?

YES → Administer maximum dose of oxygen via a reservoir mask

NO

Do you know or suspect a critical illness requiring **HIGH** levels of oxygen? Refer to Table 6.1

YES → Is SpO_2 ≥94% and are the vital signs normal?

NO → Administer 15 l/min of oxygen via a reservoir mask until the vital signs are normal, then aim for target saturation within the range of **94–98%**

YES → Monitor SpO_2 and if the saturation falls below **94%** administer oxygen to maintain a saturation within the range of **94–98%**

NO

Do you know or suspect a condition requiring **CONTROLLED OR LOW–DOSE** levels of oxygen? Refer to Table 6.3

YES → Is SpO_2 ≥88%?

NO → Administer 4 l/min of oxygen via a 28% Venturi mask or patient's own mask to aim for target saturation within the range of **88–92%**

YES → Monitor SpO_2 and if the saturation falls below **88%** administer oxygen to maintain a saturation within the range of **88–92%**

NO

Patients with **PARAQUAT** poisoning may be harmed by supplemental oxygen so avoid oxygen unless the patient is hypoxic

Do you know or suspect **PARAQUAT** poisoning?

YES → Is SpO_2 ≥88%?

NO → SpO_2 <85% administer 15 l/min of oxygen via a reservoir mask SpO_2 85–87% administer 2–6 l/m via nasal cannulae or 5–10 l/min of oxygen via a simple face mask. Aim for target saturation within the range of **88–92%**

YES → Monitor SpO_2 and if the saturation falls below 88% administer oxygen to maintain a saturation within the range of **88–92%**

NO

Do you know or suspect a serious illness requiring **MODERATE** levels oxygen? Refer to Table 6.2

YES → Is SpO_2 ≥94%?

NO → SpO_2 <85% administer 10–15 l/min of oxygen via a reservoir mask. SpO_2 85–93% administer 2–6 l/m via nasal cannulae or 5–10 l/min of oxygen via a simple face mask. Aim for target saturation within the range of **94–98%**

YES → Monitor SpO_2 and if the saturation falls below 94% administer oxygen to maintain a saturation within the range of **94–98%**

NO

Other conditions **NOT** requiring oxygen unless hypoxaemic? Refer to Table 6.4

YES → Is SpO_2 ≥94%?

NO → SpO_2 <85% administer 10–15 l/min of oxygen via a reservoir mask. SpO_2 85–93% administer 2–6 l/m via nasal cannulae or 5–10 l/min of oxygen via a simple face mask. Aim for target saturation within the range of **94–98%**

YES → Monitor SpO_2 and if the saturation falls below 94% administer oxygen to maintain a saturation within the range of **94–98%**

Paracetamol [931, 932]   PAR

Presentation

Both oral and intravenous preparations are available.

Oral

Paracetamol solutions/suspensions:

- **Infant paracetamol suspension** (120 milligrams in 5 ml), used from 3 months to 5 years.
- **Paracetamol Six Plus Suspension** (250 milligrams in 5 ml), used from 5 years of age upwards.

Paracetamol tablets

- 500 milligram tablets.

Intravenous

- Bottle containing paracetamol 1 gram in 100 ml (10 mg/ml) for intravenous infusion.

Indications

Relief of mild to moderate pain and/or high temperature.

As part of a balanced analgesic regimen for severe pain (IV paracetamol is effective in reducing opioid requirements while improving analgesic efficacy). Only use IV paracetamol for severe pain or if contra-indication to opiates.

Actions

Analgesic (pain relieving) and antipyretic (temperature reducing) drug.

Contra-indications

Known paracetamol allergy.

Do **NOT** give further paracetamol if a paracetamol containing product (e.g. Calpol, Co-codamol) has already been given within the last four hours or if the maximum cumulative daily dose has been given already.

Side Effects

Side effects are extremely rare; occasionally intravenous paracetamol may cause may cause systemic hypotension if administered too rapidly.

Additional Information

A febrile child should not be left at home except where:

- a full assessment has been carried out,

and

- the child has no apparent serious underlying illness,

and

- the child has a defined clinical pathway for re-assessment and follow up, with the full consent of the parent (or carer).

Any IV paracetamol that remains within the giving set can be flushed using 0.9% saline. Take care to ensure that air does not become entrained into the giving set; if there is air in the giving set ensure that it does not run into the patient with further fluids. Ambulance clinicians should stictly adhere to the administration procedure as set out by their Trust to minimise this risk.

Paracetamol

Dosage and Administration

NB Ensure:

1. Paracetamol has not been taken within the previous 4 hours.
2. The correct paracetamol containing solution/suspension for the patient's age is being used i.e. 'infant paracetamol suspension' for age groups 0–5 years: 'paracetamol 6 plus suspension' for ages 6 years and over.

Route: Oral – infant paracetamol suspension.

AGE	INITIAL DOSE	REPEAT DOSE	DOSE INTERVAL	CONCENTRATION	VOLUME	MAXIMUM DOSE
Adult	N/A	N/A	N/A	N/A	N/A	N/A
11 years	N/A	N/A	N/A	N/A	N/A	N/A
10 years	N/A	N/A	N/A	N/A	N/A	N/A
9 years	N/A	N/A	N/A	N/A	N/A	N/A
8 years	N/A	N/A	N/A	N/A	N/A	N/A
7 years	N/A	N/A	N/A	N/A	N/A	N/A
6 years	N/A	N/A	N/A	N/A	N/A	N/A
5 years	240 milligrams	240 milligrams	4–6 hours	120 milligrams in 5 ml	10 ml	960 milligrams in 24 hours
4 years	240 milligrams	240 milligrams	4–6 hours	120 milligrams in 5 ml	10 ml	960 milligrams in 24 hours
3 years	180 milligrams	180 milligrams	4–6 hours	120 milligrams in 5 ml	7.5 ml	720 milligrams in 24 hours
2 years	180 milligrams	180 milligrams	4–6 hours	120 milligrams in 5 ml	7.5 ml	720 milligrams in 24 hours
18 months	120 milligrams	120 milligrams	4–6 hours	120 milligrams in 5 ml	5 ml	480 milligrams in 24 hours
12 months	120 milligrams	120 milligrams	4–6 hours	120 milligrams in 5 ml	5 ml	480 milligrams in 24 hours
9 months	120 milligrams	120 milligrams	4–6 hours	120 milligrams in 5 ml	5 ml	480 milligrams in 24 hours
6 months	120 milligrams	120 milligrams	4–6 hours	120 milligrams in 5 ml	5 ml	480 milligrams in 24 hours
3 months	60 milligrams	60 milligrams	4–6 hours	120 milligrams in 5 ml	2.5 ml	240 milligrams in 24 hours
1 month	N/A	N/A	N/A	N/A	N/A	N/A
Birth	N/A	N/A	N/A	N/A	N/A	N/A

SECTION **6** Drugs – P – R

NB Ensure:

1. Paracetamol has not been taken within the previous 4 hours.
2. The correct paracetamol containing solution/suspension for the patient's age is being used i.e. 'infant paracetamol suspension' for age groups 0–5 years: 'paracetamol 6 plus suspension' for ages 6 years and over.

Route: Oral – Paracetamol Six Plus Suspension.

AGE	INITIAL DOSE	REPEAT DOSE	DOSE INTERVAL	CONCENTRATION	VOLUME	MAXIMUM DOSE
12 years – Adult	1 gram	1 gram	4–6 hours	250 milligrams in 5 ml	20 ml	4 grams in 24 hours
11 years	500 milligrams	500 milligrams	4–6 hours	250 milligrams in 5 ml	10 ml	2 grams in 24 hours
10 years	500 milligrams	500 milligrams	4–6 hours	250 milligrams in 5 ml	10 ml	2 grams in 24 hours
9 years	375 milligrams	375 milligrams	4–6 hours	250 milligrams in 5 ml	7.5 ml	1.5 grams in 24 hours
8 years	375 milligrams	375 milligrams	4–6 hours	250 milligrams in 5 ml	7.5 ml	1.5 grams in 24 hours
7 years	250 milligrams	250 milligrams	4–6 hours	250 milligrams in 5 ml	5 ml	1 gram in 24 hours
6 years	250 milligrams	250 milligrams	4–6 hours	250 milligrams in 5 ml	5 ml	1 gram in 24 hours
5 years	N/A	N/A	N/A	N/A	N/A	N/A
4 years	N/A	N/A	N/A	N/A	N/A	N/A
3 years	N/A	N/A	N/A	N/A	N/A	N/A
2 years	N/A	N/A	N/A	N/A	N/A	N/A
18 months	N/A	N/A	N/A	N/A	N/A	N/A
12 months	N/A	N/A	N/A	N/A	N/A	N/A
9 months	N/A	N/A	N/A	N/A	N/A	N/A
6 months	N/A	N/A	N/A	N/A	N/A	N/A
3 months	N/A	N/A	N/A	N/A	N/A	N/A
1 month	N/A	N/A	N/A	N/A	N/A	N/A
Birth	N/A	N/A	N/A	N/A	N/A	N/A

Route: Oral – tablet.

AGE	INITIAL DOSE	REPEAT DOSE	DOSE INTERVAL	CONCENTRATION	VOLUME	MAXIMUM DOSE
12 years – Adult	1 gram	1 gram	4–6 hours	500 milligrams per tablet	2 TABLETS	4 grams in 24 hours

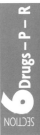

Paracetamol

PAR

NB Ensure:

Paracetamol has not been taken within the previous 4 hours.

Route: Intravenous infusion; typically given over 5–10 minutes.

AGE	INITIAL DOSE	REPEAT DOSE	DOSE INTERVAL	CONCENTRATION	VOLUME	MAXIMUM DOSE
12 years – Adult	1 gram	1 gram	4–6 hours	10 milligrams in 1 ml	100 ml	4 grams in 24 hours
11 years	500 milligrams	500 milligrams	4–6 hours	10 milligrams in 1 ml	50 ml	2 grams in 24 hours
10 years	500 milligrams	500 milligrams	4–6 hours	10 milligrams in 1 ml	50 ml	2 grams in 24 hours
9 years	500 milligrams	500 milligrams	4–6 hours	10 milligrams in 1 ml	50 ml	2 grams in 24 hours
8 years	300 milligrams	300 milligrams	4–6 hours	10 milligrams in 1 ml	30 ml	1.2 grams in 24 hours
7 years	300 milligrams	300 milligrams	4–6 hours	10 milligrams in 1 ml	30 ml	1.2 grams in 24 hours
6 years	300 milligrams	300 milligrams	4–6 hours	10 milligrams in 1 ml	30 ml	1.2 grams in 24 hours
5 years	250 milligrams	250 milligrams	4–6 hours	10 milligrams in 1 ml	25 ml	1 gram in 24 hours
4 years	250 milligrams	250 milligrams	4–6 hours	10 milligrams in 1 ml	25 ml	1 gram in 24 hours
3 years	250 milligrams	250 milligrams	4–6 hours	10 milligrams in 1 ml	25 ml	1 gram in 24 hours
2 years	125 milligrams	125 milligrams	4–6 hours	10 milligrams in 1 ml	12.5 ml	500 milligrams in 24 hours
18 months	125 milligrams	125 milligrams	4–6 hours	10 milligrams in 1 ml	12.5 ml	500 milligrams in 24 hours
12 months	125 milligrams	125 milligrams	4–6 hours	10 milligrams in 1 ml	12.5 ml	500 milligrams in 24 hours
9 months	50 milligrams	50 milligrams	4–6 hours	10 milligrams in 1 ml	5 ml	200 milligrams in 24 hours
6 months	50 milligrams	50 milligrams	4–6 hours	10 milligrams in 1 ml	5 ml	200 milligrams in 24 hours
3 months	N/A	N/A	N/A	N/A	N/A	N/A
1 month	N/A	N/A	N/A	N/A	N/A	N/A
Birth	N/A	N/A	N/A	N/A	N/A	N/A

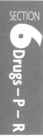
SECTION 6 Drugs – P – R

Presentation

Vials of **reteplase** 10 units for reconstitution with 10 ml water for injection.

NOTE: Whilst the strength of thrombolytics is traditionally expressed in 'units', these units are unique to each particular drug and are **NOT** interchangeable.

Indications

Acute ST segment elevation MI (STEMI) 12 hours of symptom onset where primary percutaneous coronary intervention (PPCI) is **NOT** readily available.

Ensure patient fulfils the criteria for drug administration following the model checklist (below). Variation of these criteria is justifiable at local level with agreement of appropriate key stakeholders (e.g. cardiac network, or in the context of an approved clinical trial).

Contra-indications

See check list.

Actions

Activates the fibrinolytic system, inducing the breaking up of intravascular thrombi and emboli.

Side Effects

Bleeding:

- major – seek medical advice and transport to hospital rapidly
- minor e.g. at injection sites – use local pressure.

Arrhythmias – these are usually benign in the form of transient idioventricular rhythms and usually require no special treatment. Treat ventricular fibrillation (VF) as a complication of myocardial infarction (MI) with standard protocols; bradycardia with atropine as required.

Anaphylaxis – extremely rare (0.1%) with third generation bolus agents.

Hypotension – often responds to laying the patient flat.

Additional Information

PPCI is now the dominant reperfusion treatment and should be used where available; patients with STEMI will be taken direct to a specialist cardiac centre instead of receiving thrombolysis (**refer to acute coronary syndrome guideline**). Local guidelines should be followed.

'Time is muscle!' Do not delay transportation to hospital if difficulties arise whilst setting up the equipment or establishing IV access. Qualified single responders should administer a thrombolytic if indicated while awaiting arrival of an ambulance.

In All Cases

Ensure a defibrillator is immediately available at all times.

Monitor conscious level, pulse, blood pressure and cardiac rhythm during and following injections. Manage complications (associated with the acute MI) as they occur using standard protocols. The main early adverse event associated with thrombolysis is bleeding, which should be managed according to standard protocols.

AT HOSPITAL – emphasise the need to commence a heparin infusion in accordance with local protocols – to reduce the risk of re-infarction.

Thrombolysis Checklist

Is primary PCI available?
- **YES** – undertake a **TIME CRITICAL** transfer to PPCI capable hospital.
- **NO** – ask the patient the questions listed below, to determine whether they are suitable to receive thrombolysis.

Assessment Questions

	Yes	No
Has the patient suffered a haemorrhagic stroke or stroke of unknown origin at any time?	☐	☐
Has the patient suffered a transient ischaemic attack in the preceding 6 months?	☐	☐
Has the patient suffered a central nervous system trauma or neoplasm?	☐	☐
Has the patient had recent trauma, surgery, or head injury within the preceding 3 weeks?	☐	☐
Has the patient suffered from gastrointestinal bleeding (within the last month)?	☐	☐
Has the patient a known bleeding disorder?	☐	☐
Do you suspect aortic dissection?	☐	☐
Has the patient a non-compressible puncture (e.g. liver biopsy, lumbar puncture)?	☐	☐
Is the patient taking oral anticoagulant therapy (e.g. warfarin)?	☐	☐
Is the patient pregnant or within 1 week post-partum?	☐	☐
Is the patient's systolic blood pressure >180 mmHg and/or diastolic blood pressure >110 mmHg?	☐	☐
Is the patient suffering from advanced liver disease?	☐	☐
Is the patient suffering from active peptic ulcer?	☐	☐

If the patient answers **YES TO ANY** of the above questions, thrombolysis **IS NOT** indicated; seek advice.

If the patient answers **NO TO ALL** of the above questions and thrombolysis is indicated, refer to the dosage and administration table.

SECTION

6

Drugs – P – R

342

Drugs

2013

Page **2** of **3**

Dosage and Administration

RETEPLASE

1. Administer a bolus of intravenous injection un-fractionated heparin before the first dose of reteplase (**refer to heparin guideline**). Flush the cannula well with saline **OR** use a separate cannula to administer reteplase as the two agents are physically incompatible.

2. Note the time the first dose is administered.

3. Administer the second dose 30 minutes after the first.

4. **AT HOSPITAL** – It is essential that the care of the patient is handed over as soon as possible to a member of hospital staff qualified to administer the second bolus (if not already given) and commence a heparin infusion.

Route: Intravenous bolus injections separated by 30 minutes.

AGE	INITIAL DOSE	REPEAT DOSE	DOSE INTERVAL	CONCENTRATION	VOLUME	MAXIMUM DOSE
≥18	First dose 10 units	NONE	N/A	10 units in 10 ml	10 ml	10 units
	Second dose 10 units	NONE	N/A	10 units in 10 ml	10 ml	10 units

Drugs – P – R

SECTION 6

Salbutamol [937, 938]

SLB

Presentation

Nebules containing salbutamol 2.5 milligrams/2.5 ml or 5 milligrams/2.5 ml.

Indications

Acute asthma attack where normal inhaler therapy has failed to relieve symptoms.

Expiratory wheezing associated with allergy, anaphylaxis, smoke inhalation or other lower airway cause.

Exacerbation of chronic obstructive pulmonary disease (COPD).

Shortness of breath in patients with severe breathing difficulty due to left ventricular failure (secondary treatment).

Actions

Salbutamol is a selective beta2 adrenoreceptor stimulant drug. This has a relaxant effect on the smooth muscle in the medium and smaller airways, which are in spasm in acute asthma attacks. If given by nebuliser, especially if oxygen powered, its smooth-muscle relaxing action, combined with the airway moistening effect of nebulisation, can relieve the attack rapidly.

Contra-indications

None in the emergency situation.

Cautions

Salbutamol should be used with care in patients with:
- Hypertension.
- Angina.
- Overactive thyroid.
- Late pregnancy (can relax uterus).
- Severe hypertension may occur in patients on beta-blockers and half doses should be used unless there is profound hypotension.

If COPD is a possibility limit nebulisation to six minutes.

Side Effects

Tremor (shaking).

Tachycardia.

Palpitations.

Headache.

Feeling of tension.

Peripheral vasodilatation.

Muscle cramps.

Rash.

Additional Information

In acute severe or life-threatening asthma ipratropium should be given after the first dose of salbutamol. In acute asthma or COPD unresponsive to salbutamol alone, a single dose of ipratropium may be given after salbutamol.

Salbutamol often provides initial relief. In more severe attacks however, the use of steroids by injection or orally and further nebuliser therapy will be required. Do not be lulled into a false sense of security by an initial improvement after salbutamol nebulisation.

SECTION

6 Drugs – S

344

Drugs

2013

Page **1** of **3**

Salbutamol SLB

Dosage and Administration

- **In life-threatening or acute severe asthma:** undertake a **TIME CRITICAL** transfer to the **NEAREST SUITABLE RECEIVING HOSPITAL** and provide nebulisation en-route.
- If COPD is a possibility limit nebulisation to six minutes.
- The pulse rate in children may exceed 140 after significant doses of salbutamol; this is not usually of any clinical significance and should not usually preclude further use of the drug.
- Repeat doses should be discontinued if the side effects are becoming significant (e.g. tremors, tachycardia >140 beats per minute in adults) – this is a clinical decision by the ambulance clinician.

Route: Nebulised with 6–8 litres per minute of oxygen.

AGE	INITIAL DOSE	REPEAT DOSE	DOSE INTERVAL	CONCENTRATION	VOLUME	MAXIMUM DOSE
Adult	5 milligrams	5 milligrams	5 minutes	2.5 milligrams in 2.5 ml	5 ml	No limit
11 years	5 milligrams	5 milligrams	5 minutes	2.5 milligrams in 2.5 ml	5 ml	No limit
10 years	5 milligrams	5 milligrams	5 minutes	2.5 milligrams in 2.5 ml	5 ml	No limit
9 years	5 milligrams	5 milligrams	5 minutes	2.5 milligrams in 2.5 ml	5 ml	No limit
8 years	5 milligrams	5 milligrams	5 minutes	2.5 milligrams in 2.5 ml	5 ml	No limit
7 years	5 milligrams	5 milligrams	5 minutes	2.5 milligrams in 2.5 ml	5 ml	No limit
6 years	5 milligrams	5 milligrams	5 minutes	2.5 milligrams in 2.5 ml	5 ml	No limit
5 years	2.5 milligrams	2.5 milligrams	5 minutes	2.5 milligrams in 2.5 ml	2.5 ml	No limit
4 years	2.5 milligrams	2.5 milligrams	5 minutes	2.5 milligrams in 2.5 ml	2.5 ml	No limit
3 years	2.5 milligrams	2.5 milligrams	5 minutes	2.5 milligrams in 2.5 ml	2.5 ml	No limit
2 years	2.5 milligrams	2.5 milligrams	5 minutes	2.5 milligrams in 2.5 ml	2.5 ml	No limit
18 months	2.5 milligrams	2.5 milligrams	5 minutes	2.5 milligrams in 2.5 ml	2.5 ml	No limit
12 months	2.5 milligrams	2.5 milligrams	5 minutes	2.5 milligrams in 2.5 ml	2.5 ml	No limit
9 months	2.5 milligrams	2.5 milligrams	5 minutes	2.5 milligrams in 2.5 ml	2.5 ml	No limit
6 months	2.5 milligrams	2.5 milligrams	5 minutes	2.5 milligrams in 2.5 ml	2.5 ml	No limit
3 months	2.5 milligrams	2.5 milligrams	5 minutes	2.5 milligrams in 2.5 ml	2.5 ml	No limit
1 month	2.5 milligrams	2.5 milligrams	5 minutes	2.5 milligrams in 2.5 ml	2.5 ml	No limit
Birth	N/A	N/A	N/A	N/A	N/A	N/A

Salbutamol

Route: Nebulised with 6–8 litres per minute of oxygen.

AGE	INITIAL DOSE	REPEAT DOSE	DOSE INTERVAL	CONCENTRATION	VOLUME	MAXIMUM DOSE
Adult	5 milligrams	5 milligrams	5 minutes	5 milligrams in 2.5 ml	2.5 ml	No limit
11 years	5 milligrams	5 milligrams	5 minutes	5 milligrams in 2.5 ml	2.5 ml	No limit
10 years	5 milligrams	5 milligrams	5 minutes	5 milligrams in 2.5 ml	2.5 ml	No limit
9 years	5 milligrams	5 milligrams	5 minutes	5 milligrams in 2.5 ml	2.5 ml	No limit
8 years	5 milligrams	5 milligrams	5 minutes	5 milligrams in 2.5 ml	2.5 ml	No limit
7 years	5 milligrams	5 milligrams	5 minutes	5 milligrams in 2.5 ml	2.5 ml	No limit
6 years	5 milligrams	5 milligrams	5 minutes	5 milligrams in 2.5 ml	2.5 ml	No limit
5 years	2.5 milligrams	2.5 milligrams	5 minutes	5 milligrams in 2.5 ml	1.25 ml	No limit
4 years	2.5 milligrams	2.5 milligrams	5 minutes	5 milligrams in 2.5 ml	1.25 ml	No limit
3 years	2.5 milligrams	2.5 milligrams	5 minutes	5 milligrams in 2.5 ml	1.25 ml	No limit
2 years	2.5 milligrams	2.5 milligrams	5 minutes	5 milligrams in 2.5 ml	1.25 ml	No limit
18 months	2.5 milligrams	2.5 milligrams	5 minutes	5 milligrams in 2.5 ml	1.25 ml	No limit
12 months	2.5 milligrams	2.5 milligrams	5 minutes	5 milligrams in 2.5 ml	1.25 ml	No limit
9 months	2.5 milligrams	2.5 milligrams	5 minutes	5 milligrams in 2.5 ml	1.25 ml	No limit
6 months	2.5 milligrams	2.5 milligrams	5 minutes	5 milligrams in 2.5 ml	1.25 ml	No limit
3 months	2.5 milligrams	2.5 milligrams	5 minutes	5 milligrams in 2.5 ml	1.25 ml	No limit
1 month	2.5 milligrams	2.5 milligrams	5 minutes	5 milligrams in 2.5 ml	1.25 ml	No limit
Birth	N/A	N/A	N/A	N/A	N/A	N/A

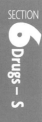

SECTION
6
Drugs – S

0.9% Sodium Chloride

Presentation

100 ml, 250 ml, 500 ml and 1,000 ml packs of sodium chloride intravenous infusion 0.9%.

5 ml and 10 ml ampoules for use as flushes.

5 ml and 10 ml pre-loaded syringes for use as flushes.

Indications

Adult Fluid Therapy
- Medical conditions without haemorrhage.
- Medical conditions with haemorrhage.
- Trauma related haemorrhage.
- Burns.
- Limb crush injury.

Child Fluid Therapy
- Medical conditions.
- Trauma related haemorrhage.
- Burns.

Flush
- As a flush to confirm patency of an intravenous or intraosseous cannula.
- As a flush following drug administration.

Actions

Increases vascular fluid volume which consequently raises cardiac output and improves perfusion.

Contra-indications

None.

Side Effects

Over-infusion may precipitate pulmonary oedema and cause breathlessness.

Additional Information

Fluid replacement in cases of dehydration should occur over hours; rapid fluid replacement is seldom indicated; refer to intravascular fluid therapy guidelines.

Dosage and Administration

Route: Intravenous or Intraosseous for **ALL** conditions.

FLUSH

AGE	INITIAL DOSE	REPEAT DOSE	DOSE INTERVAL	CONCEN-TRATION	VOLUME	MAXIMUM DOSE
Adult	2 ml – 5 ml	2 ml – 5 ml	PRN	0.9%	2 – 5 ml	N/A
Adult	10 ml – 20 ml (if infusing glucose)	10 ml – 20 ml (if infusing glucose)	PRN	0.9%	10 – 20 ml	N/A
5 – 11 years	2 ml – 5 ml	2 ml – 5 ml	PRN	0.9%	2 – 5 ml	N/A
5 – 11 years	5 ml – 10 ml (if infusing glucose)	5 ml – 10 ml (if infusing glucose)	PRN	0.9%	5 – 10 ml	N/A
Birth – <5 years	2 ml	2 ml	PRN	0.9%	2 ml	N/A
Birth – <5 years	2 ml – 5 ml (if infusing glucose)	2 ml – 5ml (if infusing glucose)	PRN	0.9%	2 – 5 ml	N/A

Drugs – S

SECTION 6

ADULT MEDICAL EMERGENCIES

General medical conditions without haemorrhage: Anaphylaxis, hyperglycaemic ketoacidosis, dehydration[a]

AGE	INITIAL DOSE	REPEAT DOSE	DOSE INTERVAL	CONCENTRATION	VOLUME	MAXIMUM DOSE
Adult	250 ml	250 ml	PRN	0.9%	250 ml	2 litres

Sepsis: Clinical signs of infection **AND** systolic BP<90 mmHg **AND** tachypnoea

AGE	INITIAL DOSE	REPEAT DOSE	DOSE INTERVAL	CONCENTRATION	VOLUME	MAXIMUM DOSE
Adult	1 litre	1 litre	30 minutes	0.9%	1 litre	2 litres

Medical conditions with haemorrhage: Systolic BP<90 mmHg and signs of poor perfusion

AGE	INITIAL DOSE	REPEAT DOSE	DOSE INTERVAL	CONCENTRATION	VOLUME	MAXIMUM DOSE
Adult	250 ml	250 ml	PRN	0.9%	250 ml	2 litres

[a] In cases of dehydration fluid replacement should usually occur over hours.

ADULT TRAUMA EMERGENCIES

Blunt trauma, head trauma or penetrating limb trauma: Systolic BP<90 mmHg and signs of poor perfusion

AGE	INITIAL DOSE	REPEAT DOSE	DOSE INTERVAL	CONCENTRATION	VOLUME	MAXIMUM DOSE
Adult	250 ml	250 ml	PRN	0.9%	250 ml	2 litres

Penetrating torso trauma: Systolic BP<60 mmHg and signs of poor perfusion

AGE	INITIAL DOSE	REPEAT DOSE	DOSE INTERVAL	CONCENTRATION	VOLUME	MAXIMUM DOSE
Adult	250 ml	250 ml	PRN	0.9%	250 ml	2 litres

Burns:

- Total body surface area (TBSA): between 15% and 25% and time to hospital is greater than 30 minutes
- TBSA: more than 25%

AGE	INITIAL DOSE	REPEAT DOSE	DOSE INTERVAL	CONCENTRATION	VOLUME	MAXIMUM DOSE
Adult	1 litre	NONE	N/A	0.9%	1 litre	1 litre

Limb crush injury

AGE	INITIAL DOSE	REPEAT DOSE	DOSE INTERVAL	CONCENTRATION	VOLUME	MAXIMUM DOSE
Adult	2 litres	NONE	N/A	0.9%	2 litres	2 litres

NB Manage crush injury of the torso as per blunt trauma.

MEDICAL EMERGENCIES IN CHILDREN (20 ml/kg)
NB Exceptions: cardiac failure, renal failure, diabetic ketoacidosis (see following).

AGE	INITIAL DOSE	REPEAT DOSE	DOSE INTERVAL	CONCENTRATION	VOLUME	MAXIMUM DOSE
11 years	500 ml	500 ml	PRN	0.9%	500 ml	1000 ml
10 years	500 ml	500 ml	PRN	0.9%	500 ml	1000 ml
9 years	500 ml	500 ml	PRN	0.9%	500 ml	1000 ml
8 years	500 ml	500 ml	PRN	0.9%	500 ml	1000 ml
7 years	460 ml	460 ml	PRN	0.9%	460 ml	920 ml
6 years	420 ml	420 ml	PRN	0.9%	420 ml	840 ml
5 years	380 ml	380 ml	PRN	0.9%	380 ml	760 ml
4 years	320 ml	320 ml	PRN	0.9%	320 ml	640 ml
3 years	280 ml	280 ml	PRN	0.9%	280 ml	560 ml
2 years	240 ml	240 ml	PRN	0.9%	240 ml	480 ml
18 months	220 ml	220 ml	PRN	0.9%	220 ml	440 ml
12 months	200 ml	200 ml	PRN	0.9%	200 ml	400 ml
9 months	180 ml	180 ml	PRN	0.9%	180 ml	360 ml
6 months	160 ml	160 ml	PRN	0.9%	160 ml	320 ml
3 months	120 ml	120 ml	PRN	0.9%	120 ml	240 ml
1 month	90 ml	90 ml	PRN	0.9%	90 ml	180 ml
Birth	70 ml	70 ml	PRN	0.9%	70 ml	140 ml

MEDICAL EMERGENCIES IN CHILDREN
Heart failure or renal failure (10 ml/kg)

AGE	INITIAL DOSE	REPEAT DOSE	DOSE INTERVAL	CONCENTRATION	VOLUME	MAXIMUM DOSE
11 years	350 ml	350 ml	PRN	0.9%	350 ml	700 ml
10 years	320 ml	320 ml	PRN	0.9%	320 ml	640 ml
9 years	290 ml	290 ml	PRN	0.9%	290 ml	580 ml
8 years	250 ml	250 ml	PRN	0.9%	250 ml	500 ml
7 years	230 ml	230 ml	PRN	0.9%	230 ml	460 ml
6 years	210 ml	210 ml	PRN	0.9%	210 ml	420 ml
5 years	190 ml	190 ml	PRN	0.9%	190 ml	380 ml
4 years	160 ml	160 ml	PRN	0.9%	160 ml	320 ml
3 years	140 ml	140 ml	PRN	0.9%	140 ml	280 ml
2 years	120 ml	120 ml	PRN	0.9%	120 ml	240 ml
18 months	110 ml	110 ml	PRN	0.9%	110 ml	220 ml
12 months	100 ml	100 ml	PRN	0.9%	100 ml	200 ml
9 months	90 ml	90 ml	PRN	0.9%	90 ml	180 ml
6 months	80 ml	80 ml	PRN	0.9%	80 ml	160 ml
3 months	60 ml	60 ml	PRN	0.9%	60 ml	120 ml
1 month	45 ml	45 ml	PRN	0.9%	45 ml	90 ml
Birth	35 ml	35 ml	PRN	0.9%	35 ml	70 ml

SECTION
6
Drugs – S

MEDICAL EMERGENCIES IN CHILDREN

Diabetic ketoacidosis (10 ml/kg) administer **ONCE** only over 15 minutes.

AGE	INITIAL DOSE	REPEAT DOSE	DOSE INTERVAL	CONCENTRATION	VOLUME	MAXIMUM DOSE
11 years	350 ml	NONE	NA	0.9%	350 ml	350 ml
10 years	320 ml	NONE	NA	0.9%	320 ml	320 ml
9 years	290 ml	NONE	NA	0.9%	290 ml	290 ml
8 years	250 ml	NONE	NA	0.9%	250 ml	250 ml
7 years	230 ml	NONE	NA	0.9%	230 ml	230 ml
6 years	210 ml	NONE	NA	0.9%	210 ml	210 ml
5 years	190 ml	NONE	NA	0.9%	190 ml	190 ml
4 years	160 ml	NONE	NA	0.9%	160 ml	160 ml
3 years	140 ml	NONE	NA	0.9%	140 ml	140 ml
2 years	120 ml	NONE	NA	0.9%	120 ml	120 ml
18 months	110 ml	NONE	NA	0.9%	110 ml	110 ml
12 months	100 ml	NONE	NA	0.9%	100 ml	100 ml
9 months	90 ml	NONE	NA	0.9%	90 ml	90 ml
6 months	80 ml	NONE	NA	0.9%	80 ml	80 ml
3 months	60 ml	NONE	NA	0.9%	60 ml	60 ml
1 month	45 ml	NONE	NA	0.9%	45 ml	45 ml
Birth	35 ml	NONE	NA	0.9%	35 ml	35 ml

TRAUMA EMERGENCIES IN CHILDREN (5 ml/kg)

NB Exceptions: burns.

AGE	INITIAL DOSE	REPEAT DOSE	DOSE INTERVAL	CONCENTRATION	VOLUME	MAXIMUM DOSE
11 years	175 ml	175 ml	PRN	0.9%	175 ml	1000 ml
10 years	160 ml	160 ml	PRN	0.9%	160 ml	1000 ml
9 years	145 ml	145 ml	PRN	0.9%	145 ml	1000 ml
8 years	130 ml	130 ml	PRN	0.9%	130 ml	1000 ml
7 years	115 ml	115 ml	PRN	0.9%	115 ml	920 ml
6 years	105 ml	105 ml	PRN	0.9%	105 ml	840 ml
5 years	95 ml	95 ml	PRN	0.9%	95 ml	760 ml
4 years	80 ml	80 ml	PRN	0.9%	80 ml	640 ml
3 years	70 ml	70 ml	PRN	0.9%	70 ml	560 ml
2 years	60 ml	60 ml	PRN	0.9%	60 ml	480 ml
18 months	55 ml	55 ml	PRN	0.9%	55 ml	440 ml
12 months	50 ml	50 ml	PRN	0.9%	50 ml	400 ml
9 months	45 ml	45 ml	PRN	0.9%	45 ml	360 ml
6 months	40 ml	40 ml	PRN	0.9%	40 ml	320 ml
3 months	30 ml	30 ml	PRN	0.9%	30 ml	240 ml
1 month	20 ml	20 ml	PRN	0.9%	20 ml	180 ml
Birth	20 ml	20 ml	PRN	0.9%	20 ml	140 ml

SECTION

6

Drugs – S

352

Drugs

2013

Page **6** of **7**

Burns (10 ml/kg, given over 1 hour):
- TBSA: between 10% and 20% and time to hospital is greater than 30 minutes
- TBSA: more than 20%

AGE	INITIAL DOSE	REPEAT DOSE	DOSE INTERVAL	CONCENTRATION	VOLUME	MAXIMUM DOSE
11 years	350 ml	NONE	N/A	0.9%	350 ml	350 ml
10 years	320 ml	NONE	N/A	0.9%	320 ml	320 ml
9 years	290 ml	NONE	N/A	0.9%	290 ml	290 ml
8 years	250 ml	NONE	N/A	0.9%	250 ml	250 ml
7 years	230 ml	NONE	N/A	0.9%	230 ml	230 ml
6 years	210 ml	NONE	N/A	0.9%	210 ml	210 ml
5 years	190 ml	NONE	N/A	0.9%	190 ml	190 ml
4 years	160 ml	NONE	N/A	0.9%	160 ml	160 ml
3 years	140 ml	NONE	N/A	0.9%	140 ml	140 ml
2 years	120 ml	NONE	N/A	0.9%	120 ml	120 ml
18 months	110 ml	NONE	N/A	0.9%	110 ml	110 ml
12 months	100 ml	NONE	N/A	0.9%	100 ml	100 ml
9 months	90 ml	NONE	N/A	0.9%	90 ml	90 ml
6 months	80 ml	NONE	N/A	0.9%	80 ml	80 ml
3 months	60 ml	NONE	N/A	0.9%	60 ml	60 ml
1 month	45 ml	NONE	N/A	0.9%	45 ml	45 ml
Birth	35 ml	NONE	N/A	0.9%	35 ml	35 ml

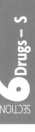

Sodium Lactate Compound (Hartmann's/Ringer's Lactate)

Presentation

250 ml, 500 ml and 1,000 ml packs of compound sodium lactate intravenous infusion (also called Hartmann's solution for injection or Ringer's-Lactate solution for injection).

Indications

Blood and fluid loss, to correct hypovolaemia and improve tissue perfusion if sodium chloride 0.9% is **NOT** available.

Dehydration.

Actions

Increases vascular fluid volume which consequently raises cardiac output and improves perfusion.

Contra-indications

Diabetic hyperglycaemic ketoacidotic coma, and pre-coma. NB Administer 0.9% sodium chloride intravenous infusion.

Neonates.

Cautions

Sodium lactate should not be used in limb crush injury when 0.9% sodium chloride is available.

Renal failure.

Liver failure.

Side Effects

Infusion of an excessive volume may overload the circulation and precipitate heart failure (increased breathlessness, wheezing and distended neck veins). Volume overload is unlikely if the patient is correctly assessed initially and it is very unlikely indeed if patient response is assessed after initial 250 ml infusion and then after each 250 ml of infusion. If there is evidence of this complication, the patient should be transported rapidly to nearest suitable receiving hospital whilst administering high-flow oxygen.

Do not administer further fluid.

Additional Information

Compound sodium lactate intravenous infusion contains mainly sodium, but also small amounts of potassium and lactate. It is useful for initial fluid replacement in cases of blood loss.

The volume of compound sodium lactate intravenous infusion needed is 3 times as great as the volume of blood loss. Sodium lactate has **NO** oxygen carrying capacity.

Dosage and Administration if sodium chloride 0.9% is NOT available.

Route: Intravenous or intra-osseous for **ALL** conditions.

ADULT MEDICAL EMERGENCIES

General medical conditions without haemorrhage: anaphylaxis, dehydration[a]
NB Exception sodium lactate compound is contra-indicated in diabetic ketoacidosis – **refer to sodium chloride 0.9% guideline**.

AGE	INITIAL DOSE	REPEAT DOSE	DOSE INTERVAL	CONCENTRATION	VOLUME	MAXIMUM DOSE
Adult	250 ml	250 ml	PRN	Compound	250 ml	1 litre

Sepsis: Clinical signs of infection **AND** systolic BP<90 mmHg **AND** tachypnoea

AGE	INITIAL DOSE	REPEAT DOSE	DOSE INTERVAL	CONCENTRATION	VOLUME	MAXIMUM DOSE
Adult	1 litre	1 litre	30 minutes	Compound	1 litre	2 litres

[a] In cases of dehydration fluid replacement should usually occur over hours.

ADULT TRAUMA EMERGENCIES

Medical conditions with haemorrhage: Systolic BP<90 mmHg and signs of poor perfusion

AGE	INITIAL DOSE	REPEAT DOSE	DOSE INTERVAL	CONCENTRATION	VOLUME	MAXIMUM DOSE
Adult	250 ml	250 ml	PRN	Compound	250 ml	2 litres

Blunt trauma, head trauma or penetrating limb trauma: Systolic BP<90 mmHg and signs of poor perfusion

AGE	INITIAL DOSE	REPEAT DOSE	DOSE INTERVAL	CONCENTRATION	VOLUME	MAXIMUM DOSE
Adult	250 ml	250 ml	PRN	Compound	250 ml	2 litres

Penetrating torso trauma: Systolic BP<60 mmHg and signs of poor perfusion

AGE	INITIAL DOSE	REPEAT DOSE	DOSE INTERVAL	CONCENTRATION	VOLUME	MAXIMUM DOSE
Adult	250 ml	250 ml	PRN	Compound	250 ml	2 litres

Burns:
- TBSA: between 15% and 25% and time to hospital is greater than 30 minutes.
- TBSA: more than 25%.

AGE	INITIAL DOSE	REPEAT DOSE	DOSE INTERVAL	CONCENTRATION	VOLUME	MAXIMUM DOSE
Adult	1 litre	N/A	N/A	Compound	1 litre	1 litre

Limb crush injury

AGE	INITIAL DOSE	REPEAT DOSE	DOSE INTERVAL	CONCENTRATION	VOLUME	MAXIMUM DOSE
Adult	2 litres	N/A	N/A	Compound	2 litres	2 litres

NB Sodium chloride 0.9% is the fluid of choice in crush injury. NB Manage crush injury of the torso as per blunt trauma.

Sodium Lactate Compound (Hartmann's/Ringer's Lactate)

SLC

MEDICAL EMERGENCIES IN CHILDREN (20 ml/kg) – NB Exceptions heart failure, renal failure, liver failure, diabetic ketoacidosis (sodium lactate compound is contra-indicated in diabetic ketoacidosis – **refer to sodium chloride 0.9% guideline**).

AGE	INITIAL DOSE	REPEAT DOSE	DOSE INTERVAL	CONCENTRATION	VOLUME	MAXIMUM DOSE
11 years	500 ml	500 ml	PRN	Compound	500 ml	1 litre
10 years	500 ml	500 ml	PRN	Compound	500 ml	1 litre
9 years	500 ml	500 ml	PRN	Compound	500 ml	1 litre-
8 years	500 ml	500 ml	PRN	Compound	500 ml	1000 ml
7 years	460 ml	460 ml	PRN	Compound	460 ml	920 ml
6 years	420 ml	420 ml	PRN	Compound	420 ml	840 ml
5 years	380 ml	380 ml	PRN	Compound	380 ml	760 ml
4 years	320 ml	320 ml	PRN	Compound	320 ml	640 ml
3 years	280 ml	280 ml	PRN	Compound	280 ml	560 ml
2 years	240 ml	240 ml	PRN	Compound	240 ml	480 ml
18 months	220 ml	220 ml	PRN	Compound	220 ml	440 ml
12 months	200 ml	200 ml	PRN	Compound	200 ml	400 ml
9 months	180 ml	180 ml	PRN	Compound	180 ml	360 ml
6 months	160 ml	160 ml	PRN	Compound	160 ml	320 ml
3 months	120 ml	120 ml	PRN	Compound	120 ml	240 ml
1 month	90 ml	90 ml	PRN	Compound	90 ml	180 ml
Birth	N/A	N/A	N/A	N/A	N/A	N/A

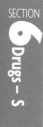

SECTION 6 Drugs – S

MEDICAL EMERGENCIES IN CHILDREN

Heart failure or renal failure (10 ml/kg)

AGE	INITIAL DOSE	REPEAT DOSE	DOSE INTERVAL	CONCENTRATION	VOLUME	MAXIMUM DOSE
11 years	350 ml	350 ml	PRN	Compound	350 ml	700 ml
10 years	320 ml	320 ml	PRN	Compound	320 ml	640 ml
9 years	290 ml	290 ml	PRN	Compound	290 ml	580 ml
8 years	250 ml	250 ml	PRN	Compound	250 ml	500 ml
7 years	230 ml	230 ml	PRN	Compound	230 ml	460 ml
6 years	210 ml	210 ml	PRN	Compound	210 ml	420 ml
5 years	190 ml	190 ml	PRN	Compound	190 ml	380 ml
4 years	160 ml	160 ml	PRN	Compound	160 ml	320 ml
3 years	140 ml	140 ml	PRN	Compound	140 ml	280 ml
2 years	120 ml	120 ml	PRN	Compound	120 ml	240 ml
18 months	110 ml	110 ml	PRN	Compound	110 ml	220 ml
12 months	100 ml	100 ml	PRN	Compound	100 ml	200 ml
9 months	90 ml	90 ml	PRN	Compound	90 ml	180 ml
6 months	80 ml	80 ml	PRN	Compound	80 ml	160 ml
3 months	60 ml	60 ml	PRN	Compound	60 ml	120 ml
1 month	45 ml	45 ml	PRN	Compound	45 ml	90 ml
Birth	N/A	N/A	N/A	N/A	N/A	N/A

Drugs – S

SECTION 6

TRAUMA EMERGENCIES IN CHILDREN (5 ml/kg)

NB Exceptions: burns.

AGE	INITIAL DOSE	REPEAT DOSE	DOSE INTERVAL	CONCENTRATION	VOLUME	MAXIMUM DOSE
11 years	175 ml	175 ml	PRN	Compound	175 ml	1 litre
10 years	160 ml	160 ml	PRN	Compound	160 ml	1 litre
9 years	145 ml	145 ml	PRN	Compound	145 ml	1 litre
8 years	130 ml	130 ml	PRN	Compound	130 ml	1 litre
7 years	115 ml	115 ml	PRN	Compound	115 ml	920 ml
6 years	105 ml	105 ml	PRN	Compound	105 ml	840 ml
5 years	95 ml	95 ml	PRN	Compound	95 ml	760 ml
4 years	80 ml	80 ml	PRN	Compound	80 ml	640 ml
3 years	70 ml	70 ml	PRN	Compound	70 ml	560 ml
2 years	60 ml	60 ml	PRN	Compound	60 ml	480 ml
18 months	55 ml	55 ml	PRN	Compound	55 ml	440 ml
12 months	50 ml	50 ml	PRN	Compound	50 ml	400 ml
9 months	45 ml	45 ml	PRN	Compound	45 ml	360 ml
6 months	40 ml	40 ml	PRN	Compound	40 ml	320 ml
3 months	30 ml	30 ml	PRN	Compound	30 ml	240 ml
1 month	20 ml	20 ml	PRN	Compound	20 ml	180 ml
Birth	N/A	N/A	N/A	N/A	N/A	N/A

Sodium Lactate Compound (Hartmann's/Ringer Lactate)

Burns (10 ml/kg, given over 1 hour):

- TBSA: between 10% and 20% and time to hospital is greater than 30 minutes.
- TBSA: more than 20%.

AGE	INITIAL DOSE	REPEAT DOSE	DOSE INTERVAL	CONCENTRATION	VOLUME	MAXIMUM DOSE
11 years	350 ml	NONE	N/A	Compound	350 ml	350 ml
10 years	320 ml	NONE	N/A	Compound	320 ml	320 ml
9 years	290 ml	NONE	N/A	Compound	290 ml	290 ml
8 years	250 ml	NONE	N/A	Compound	250 ml	250 ml
7 years	230 ml	NONE	N/A	Compound	230 ml	230 ml
6 years	210 ml	NONE	N/A	Compound	210 ml	210 ml
5 years	190 ml	NONE	N/A	Compound	190 ml	190 ml
4 years	160 ml	NONE	N/A	Compound	160 ml	160 ml
3 years	140 ml	NONE	N/A	Compound	140 ml	140 ml
2 years	120 ml	NONE	N/A	Compound	120 ml	120 ml
18 months	110 ml	NONE	N/A	Compound	110 ml	110 ml
12 months	100 ml	NONE	N/A	Compound	100 ml	100 ml
9 months	90 ml	NONE	N/A	Compound	90 ml	90 ml
6 months	80 ml	NONE	N/A	Compound	80 ml	80 ml
3 months	60 ml	NONE	N/A	Compound	60 ml	60 ml
1 month	45 ml	NONE	N/A	Compound	45 ml	45 ml
Birth	N/A	N/A	N/A	N/A	N/A	N/A

Presentation

An ampoule containing ergometrine 500 micrograms and oxytocin 5 units in 1 ml.

Indications

Postpartum haemorrhage within 24 hours of delivery of the infant where bleeding from the uterus is uncontrollable by uterine massage.

Miscarriage with life-threatening bleeding and a confirmed diagnosis e.g. where a patient has gone home with medical management and starts to bleed.

Actions

Stimulates contraction of the uterus.

Onset of action 7–10 minutes.

Contra-indications

- Known hypersensitivity to syntometrine.
- Active labour.
- Severe cardiac, liver or kidney disease.
- Hypertension and severe pre-eclampsia.
- Possible multiple pregnancy/known or suspected fetus in utero.

Side Effects

- Nausea and vomiting.
- Abdominal pain.
- Headache.
- Hypertension and bradycardia.
- Chest pain and, rarely, anaphylactic reactions.

Additional Information

Syntometrine and misoprostol reduce bleeding from a pregnant uterus through different pathways; therefore if one drug has not been effective after 15 mins, the other may be administered in addition.

Dosage and Administration

Route: Intramuscular.

AGE	INITIAL DOSE	REPEAT DOSE	DOSE INTERVAL	CONCENTRATION	VOLUME	MAXIMUM DOSE
Adult	500 micrograms of ergometrine and 5 units of oxytocin.	**None**	N/A	500 micrograms of ergometrine and 5 units of oxytocin in 1 ml.	1 ml	500 micrograms of ergometrine and 5 units of oxytocin.

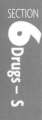

SECTION

6

Drugs – S

Presentation

Vials of **tenecteplase** 10,000 units for reconstitution with 10 ml water for injection, or 8,000 units for reconstitution with 8 ml water for injection.

NOTE: Whilst the strength of thrombolytics is traditionally expressed in 'units' these units are unique to each particular drug and are **NOT** interchangeable.

Indications

Acute ST segment elevation MI (STEMI) within 6 hours of symptom onset where primary percutaneous coronary intervention (PPCI) is **NOT** readily available.

Ensure patient fulfils the criteria for drug administration following the model checklist (below). Variation of these criteria is justifiable at local level with agreement of appropriate key stakeholders (e.g. cardiac network, or in the context of an approved clinical trial).

Contra-indications

See check list.

Actions

Activates the fibrinolytic system, inducing the breaking up of intravascular thrombi and emboli.

Side Effects

Bleeding:
- Major – seek medical advice and transport to hospital rapidly.
- Minor e.g. at injection sites – use local pressure.

Arrhythmias – these are usually benign in the form of transient idioventricular rhythms and usually require no special treatment. Treat ventricular fibrillation (VF) as a complication of myocardial infarction (MI) with standard protocols; bradycardia with atropine as required.

Anaphylaxis – extremely rare (0.1%) with third generation bolus agents.

Hypotension – often responds to laying the patient flat.

Additional Information

PPCI is now the dominant reperfusion treatment and should be used where available; patients with STEMI will be taken direct to a specialist cardiac centre instead of receiving thrombolysis (**refer to acute coronary syndrome guideline**). Local guidelines should be followed.

'Time is muscle!' Do not delay transportation to hospital if difficulties arise whilst setting up the equipment or establishing IV access. Qualified single responders should administer a thrombolytic if indicated while awaiting arrival of an ambulance.

In All Cases

Ensure a defibrillator is immediately available at all times.

Monitor conscious level, pulse, blood pressure and cardiac rhythm during and following injections. Manage complications (associated with the acute MI) as they occur using standard protocols. The main early adverse event associated with thrombolysis is bleeding, which should be managed according to standard guidelines.

AT HOSPITAL – emphasise the need to commence a heparin infusion in accordance with local guidelines – to reduce the risk of re-infarction.

Tenecteplase

Thrombolysis Checklist

Is primary PCI available?

- **YES** – undertake a **TIME CRITICAL** transfer to PPCI capable hospital.
- **NO** – ask the patient the questions listed below, to determine whether they are suitable to receive thrombolysis.

Assessment Questions	Yes	No
Has the patient suffered a haemorrhagic stroke or stroke of unknown origin at any time?	☐	☐
Has the patient suffered a transient ischaemic attack in the preceding 6 months?	☐	☐
Has the patient suffered a central nervous system trauma or neoplasm?	☐	☐
Has the patient had recent trauma, surgery, or head injury within the preceding 3 weeks?	☐	☐
Has the patient suffered from gastrointestinal bleeding (within the last month)?	☐	☐
Has the patient a known bleeding disorder?	☐	☐
Do you suspect aortic dissection?	☐	☐
Has the patient a non-compressible puncture (e.g. liver biopsy, lumbar puncture)?	☐	☐
Is the patient taking oral anticoagulant therapy (e.g. warfarin)?	☐	☐
Is the patient pregnant or within 1 week post-partum?	☐	☐
Is the patient's systolic blood pressure >180 mmHg and/or diastolic blood pressure >110 mmHg?	☐	☐
Is the patient suffering from advanced liver disease?	☐	☐
Is the patient suffering from active peptic ulcer?	☐	☐

If the patient answers **YES TO ANY** of the above questions, thrombolysis **IS NOT** indicated; seek advice.

If the patient answers **NO TO ALL** of the above questions and thrombolysis is indicated, refer to the dosage and administration table.

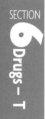

Dosage and Administration

1. Administer a bolus of intravenous injection of un-fractionated heparin before administration of tenecteplase (**refer to heparin guideline**). Flush the cannula well with saline.

2. **AT HOSPITAL** – It is essential that the care of the patient is handed over as soon as possible to a member of hospital staff qualified to administer the second bolus (if not already given) and commence a heparin infusion.

Route: Intravenous single bolus adjusted for patient weight.

AGE	WEIGHT	INITIAL DOSE	REPEAT DOSE	DOSE INTERVAL	CONCENTRATION	VOLUME	MAXIMUM DOSE
≥18	<60 kg (<9st 6lbs)	6000 units	NONE	N/A	1,000 U/ml	6 ml	6,000 units
≥18	60–69 kg (9st 6lbs–10st 13lbs)	7000 units	NONE	N/A	1,000 U/ml	7 ml	7,000 units
≥18	70–79 kg (11st–12st 7lbs)	8000 units	NONE	N/A	1,000 U/ml	8 ml	8,000 units
≥18	80–90 kg (12st 8lbs–14st 2lbs)	9000 units	NONE	N/A	1,000 U/ml	9 ml	9,000 units
≥18	>90 kg (>14st 2lbs)	10,000 units	NONE	N/A	1,000 U/ml	10 ml	10,000 units

Drugs – T

SECTION 6

Tetracaine 4% [942, 943]

Presentation

1 or 1.5 gram tubes of white semi-transparent gel.

Transparent occlusive dressing.

Indications

Where venepuncture may be required in a non-urgent situation, in individuals who are believed to have a fear of, or likely to become upset if undergoing venepuncture (usually children, some vulnerable adults or needle-phobic adults). Venepuncture includes intravenous injection, cannulation and obtaining venous blood.

Time of application should be noted and included in hand-over to the emergency department or other care facility.

Actions

Tetracaine 4% cream is a local anaesthetic agent, that has properties that allow it to penetrate intact skin, thus providing local anaesthesia to the area of skin with which it has been in contact.

Contra-indications

DO NOT apply tetracaine in the following circumstances:

- The application of tetracaine should not take preference over life-saving or any other clinically urgent procedures.
- If the area being considered for anaesthesia will require venepuncture in less than 15 minutes.
- Known allergy to tetracaine cream, or any of its other constituents.
- Known allergy to the brand of transparent occlusive dressing.
- If the patient is allergic to other local anaesthetics.
- If the patient is pregnant or breastfeeding.
- If the patient is less than one month old.
- Avoid applying to open wounds, broken skin, lips, mouth, eyes, ears, anal, or genital region, mucous membranes.

Cautions

Allergy to Elastoplast or other adhesive dressing – discuss risk/benefit with carer.

Side Effects

Expect mild vasodilatation over the treated area.

Occasionally local irritation may occur.

Additional Information

Although the application of tetracaine may not directly improve the quality of care experienced by the patient from the ambulance service, it is in line with good patient care, and its use will benefit the patient's subsequent management.

Tetracaine takes 30–40 minutes after application before the area will become numb and remain numb for 4–6 hours.

Sites of application should be based on local guidelines.

Tetracaine only needs refrigeration if it is unlikely to be used for a considerable time; therefore bulk stores should be kept refrigerated. Generally speaking, it does not require refrigeration in everyday use, however tubes that are not refrigerated or used within 3 months should be discarded.

Special Precautions

Do not leave on for more than an hour.

Do not delay transfer to further care of TIME CRITICAL patients.

Dosage and Administration

- Apply one tube directly over a vein that looks as if it would support cannulation – refer to local care guideline.
- Do not rub the cream in.
- Place an occlusive dressing directly over the 'blob' of cream, taking care to completely surround the cream to ensure it does not leak out.
- Repeat the procedure in one similar, alternative site.
- **REMEMBER** to tell the receiving staff the time of application and location when handing the patient over.

Route: Topical.

AGE	INITIAL DOSE	REPEAT DOSE	DOSE INTERVAL	CONCENTRATION	TABLETS	MAXIMUM DOSE
>1 month	1–1.5 grams	N/A	N/A	4%	1 tube	N/A

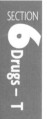

Tranexamic Acid [944–948]

TXA

Presentation
Vial containing 500 mg tranexamic acid in 5ml (100 mg/ ml).

Indications
- Patients with **TIME CRITICAL** injury where significant internal/external haemorrhage is suspected.
- Injured patients fulfilling local Step 1 or Step 2 trauma triage protocol – **refer to Appendix in trauma emergencies overview (adults)**.

Actions
Tranexamic acid is an anti-fibrinolytic which reduces the breakdown of blood clot.

Contra-indications
- Isolated head injury.
- Critical interventions required (if critical interventions leave insufficient time for TXA administration).
- Bleeding now stopped.

Side Effects
Rapid injection might rarely cause hypotension.

Additional Information
- There is good data that this treatment is safe and effective (giving a 9% reduction in the number of deaths in patients in the CRASH2 trial).
- There is no evidence about whether or not tranexamic acid is effective in patients with head injury; however there is no evidence of harm.
- High dose regimes have been associated with convulsions; however, in the low dose regime recommended here, the benefit from giving TXA in trauma outweighs the risk of convulsions.

Dosage and Administration
Route: Intravenous only – **administer SLOWLY over 10 minutes – can be given as 10 aliquots administered 1 minute apart**.

AGE	INITIAL DOSE	REPEAT DOSE	DOSE INTERVAL	CONCENTRATION	VOLUME	MAXIMUM DOSE
>12 years – Adult	1 gram	NONE	N/A	100 mg/ml	10 mls	1 gram
11 years	500 mg	NONE	N/A	100 mg/ml	5 mls	500 mg
10 years	500 mg	NONE	N/A	100 mg/ml	5 mls	500 mg
9 years	450 mg	NONE	N/A	100 mg/ml	4.5 mls	450 mg
8 years	400 mg	NONE	N/A	100 mg/ml	4 mls	400 mg
7 years	350 mg	NONE	N/A	100 mg/ml	3.5 mls	350 mg
6 years	300 mg	NONE	N/A	100 mg/ml	3 mls	300 mg
5 years	300 mg	NONE	N/A	100 mg/ml	3 mls	300 mg
4 years	250 mg	NONE	N/A	100 mg/ml	2.5 mls	250 mg
3 years	200 mg	NONE	N/A	100 mg/ml	2 mls	200 mg
2 years	200 mg	NONE	N/A	100 mg/ml	2 mls	200 mg
18 months	150 mg	NONE	N/A	100 mg/ml	1.5 mls	150 mg
12 months	150 mg	NONE	N/A	100 mg/ml	1.5 mls	150 mg
9 months	150 mg	NONE	N/A	100 mg/ml	1.5 mls	150 mg
6 months	100 mg	NONE	N/A	100 mg/ml	1 ml	100 mg
3 months	100 mg	NONE	N/A	100 mg/ml	1 ml	100 mg
1 month	50 mg	NONE	N/A	100 mg/ml	0.5 ml	50 mg
Birth	50 mg	NONE	N/A	100 mg/ml	0.5 ml	50 mg

Drugs – T

SECTION 6

Intravascular Fluid Therapy (Adults)

1. Introduction [133, 734, 949–954]

- Despite a lack of evidence demonstrating any significant beneficial effects, prehospital fluid therapy has become an established practice.

- There is, however, a significant body of evidence that indicates that routine prehospital intravascular fluid therapy may, in fact, be detrimental.

- Adverse effects may be attributed to prolonged on-scene times delaying time to definitive surgical intervention, thrombus disruption, dilution of clotting factors and other coagulopathies.

2. Pathophysiology [949, 954, 956]

- The objective of fluid therapy is to improve end-organ perfusion and, as a consequence, oxygen delivery.

- By increasing the circulating volume, cardiac output and blood pressure are increased by the Bainbridge Reflex and Frank-Starling Law of the Heart.

- The speed with which a given fluid will produce its effect will largely be determined by how it is distributed throughout the body and how long it remains in the vascular space.

2.1 pH buffering

- Reduced perfusion leads to acidosis as a result of anaerobic metabolism producing lactic acid, phosphoric acids, and unoxidised amino acids.

- This acidosis can depress cardiac function (negative inotropic effect) and cause arrhythmias.

2.2 Oxygen transport

- Crystalloid fluids currently used in the prehospital environment have no oxygen carrying capacity.

- However, the administration of fluids reduces blood viscosity which in turn may lead to improved peripheral blood flow and hence oxygen delivery.

2.3 Haemostasis

- In general, administration of fluid has a detrimental effect on haemostasis and a tendency to increase bleeding.

- The administration of fluid raises intra-vascular pressures and usually causes vasodilation, both of which may precipitate disruption of the primary haemostatic thrombus.

- Furthermore, supplemental administration of fluid reduces blood viscosity and dilutes clotting factors both of which can be detrimental to haemostatic mechanisms.

- Finally, in order to minimise hypothermia-induced coagulopathies, the use of cold fluids should be avoided if possible.

3. Haemorrhagic Emergencies [957–969]

- Haemorrhage may occur as a result of traumatic or medical aetiologies and may be classified as:
  - **apparent** (external) blood loss
  - **concealed** (internal) blood loss.

- Current thinking suggests that fluids should **ONLY** be administered when there are signs of impaired major organ perfusion (Table 6.7).

Table 6.7 – EARLY INDICATORS OF IMPAIRED MAJOR ORGAN PERFUSION

SIGNS	CAUSE
Tachypnoea	↑ Metabolic acidosis
Tachycardia	↓ Cardiac output
Hypotension	↓ Vascular volume
↓ Consciousness	↓ Cerebral perfusion

- Control of external haemorrhage must be achieved before administering fluids.

3.1 Trauma
3.1.1 Penetrating trauma to the trunk

- Penetrating trauma to the trunk carries the risk of significant disruption of major vessels that, due to their location, are not amenable to compression or other methods of haemorrhage control.

- As a consequence of this inability to control further bleeding, the general aim of fluid therapy is to maintain blood pressure at 60 mmHg systolic.

3.1.2 Penetrating trauma to the limbs

- Penetrating trauma to the limbs also carries a risk of significant disruption of major vessels; however, these vessels are both fewer and more amenable to compression or other methods of haemorrhage control.

- As a consequence of this ability to control further bleeding, the general aim of fluid therapy is to maintain blood pressure at 90 mmHg systolic.

3.1.3 Blunt trauma to trunk or limbs

- Blunt trauma to the trunk carries a lower risk of major vessel disruption; consequently, the trigger point for fluid administration is different from penetrating trauma.

- In cases of blunt trauma to the trunk or limbs, the aim of fluid therapy is to maintain blood pressure at 90 mmHg systolic.

3.1.4 Trauma to the head (all types)

- Significant head injury results in raised intracranial pressure (ICP) as cerebral tissues swell within the enclosed skull; to ensure adequate cerebral perfusion pressure (CPP) the body compensates and raises the mean arterial blood pressure (MAP).

CPP = MAP – ICP

- As a result of this compensatory mechanism, significant head injuries are usually associated with hypertension and **NOT** hypotension.

- Hypotension in the setting of significant head injury indicates not only significant blood loss but also **CRITICALLY IMPAIRED CEREBRAL PERFUSION**.

- In order to support cerebral perfusion the administration of fluids may be required.

- In the setting of significant head injury with hypotension, fluid therapy should be titrated to a systolic blood pressure of 90 mmHg.

- Hypertensive head injury does not normally require fluid therapy. Research concerning prehospital hypertonic saline has yet to demonstrate conclusive evidence of beneficial effect.

3.2 Medical conditions

- Principles of fluid therapy in medically-related haemorrhage are fundamentally no different from those of blunt trauma.

- Generally, the aim of fluid therapy is to maintain systolic blood pressure at 90 mmHg.

- Medically-related haemorrhage may also be complicated by vascular disease, coagulopathies or the presence of tumors.

3.3 Fluid therapy following haemorrhage

- **DO NOT** delay at scene to obtain vascular access or to commence fluid replacement; wherever possible obtain vascular access and administer fluid **EN-ROUTE TO HOSPITAL**.

- If the clinician determines that there is a definite need for fluid therapy they should obtain vascular access.

- Clinicians should attempt to gain intravenous access in the first instance; however they may consider intra-osseous access where intravenous access fails or is unlikely to be successful.

- Vascular access devices should be flushed with 5 ml of physiologic saline for injection to confirm patency prior to administering large volumes of fluid.

- Once patent vascular access is confirmed, administer a single bolus of 250 ml of crystalloid (Table 6.8).

- Where the need for intravascular fluid therapy is less certain, clinicians should still obtain vascular access and flush to confirm patency.

- **Do not connect any fluids to the cannula unless intravascular fluid therapy is indicated.**

NB The slow administration of fluids to keep a vein open (TKO/TKVO) should not be practised.

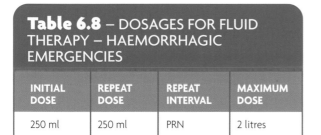

Table 6.8 – DOSAGES FOR FLUID THERAPY – HAEMORRHAGIC EMERGENCIES

INITIAL DOSE	REPEAT DOSE	REPEAT INTERVAL	MAXIMUM DOSE
250 ml	250 ml	PRN	2 litres

- Monitor the physiological response; re-assess perfusion, pulse, respiratory rate and blood pressure wherever possible.

- If these observations improve, suspend any further administration.

- If there is no improvement administer further 250 ml boluses, re-assessing for improvement after each fluid bolus (Table 6.8).

- The maximum cumulative fluid dose is usually 2 litres (Table 6.8).

- If the patient remains hypotensive despite repeated 250 ml boluses **OR** the patient is likely to remain on scene for a considerable time (e.g. due to entrapment), request senior clinical support (according to local procedures).

3.4 Exceptions and special circumstances

3.4.1 Crush injury

- A crush injury is caused by direct compressive force on the body. Crush syndrome is the systemic manifestation of muscle cell damage resulting from pressure or crushing.

- The severity of the injury is related to both the magnitude of the compressing force, and the bulk of muscle affected, but not necessarily the duration for which the force has been applied.

- The pathophysiology of crush syndrome results from the leakiness of the cellular membranes as a consequence of pressure or stretching. Sodium, calcium and water leak through the cellular membrane into the muscle cell, trapping extracellular fluid inside the muscle cells. In addition to the influx of these elements into the cell, the cell releases potassium and other toxic substances such as myoglobin, phosphate and uric acid into the circulation.

- The end result of these events is hypotension, hyperkalaemia (which may precipitate cardiac arrest), hypocalcaemia, metabolic acidosis, compartment syndrome (due to swelling), and acute renal failure (ARF).

- If possible, fluid therapy should commence prior to extrication; however extrication or transport **MUST NOT** be unnecessarily delayed in order to obtain intravenous access or to administer fluid.

- In crush injury of the limbs an initial fluid bolus of 2 litres of sodium chloride 0.9% should be administered (Table 6.9).

- In crush injury of the torso follow blunt trauma fluid therapy practices (see 3.1.3).

- If possible, request senior clinical support to guide further therapy.

Table 6.9 – DOSAGES FOR FLUID THERAPY – CRUSH INJURY OF THE LIMBS

INITIAL DOSE	REPEAT DOSE	REPEAT INTERVAL	MAXIMUM DOSE
2 litres	NONE	N/A	2 litres

3.4.2 Obstetric emergencies

- Clinicians must remember that the gravid uterus may compress the inferior vena cava in a pregnant patient who is supine. Appropriate positioning of the patient i.e. left lateral tilt or manual displacement of the gravid uterus must be considered to ensure adequate venous return before determining that a pregnant patient is in need of fluid resuscitation.

- Due to their increase in blood volume, the obstetric patient is able to tolerate far greater blood loss, up to 50%, before showing signs of hypovolaemia/shock.

- In obstetric patients, the uterus, and thus the fetus, will often become 'underperfused' **PRIOR** to the pregnant women showing outward signs of shock i.e. becoming tachycardic or hypotensive.

- Signs of shock appear very late during pregnancy and hypotension is an extremely late sign.

- Clinicians should take frequent clinical observations and be vigilant for subtle changes that may indicate the onset of shock.

- Fluid replacement should aim to maintain a systolic blood pressure of 90 mmHg in obstetric patients who are bleeding.

4. Non-Haemorrhagic Emergencies [771, 772, 962–967, 970–980]

4.1 Trauma

- The loss of bodily fluids other than blood, as a result of trauma, is rare. Burns injuries are notable exceptions (see exceptions and special circumstances below).

4.2 Medical conditions

- Patients suffering medical emergencies may experience fluid loss as a result of dehydration (e.g. heat related illness, vomiting or diarrhoea) and/or redistribution of fluid from the vascular compartment (e.g. as a result of anaphylaxis).

- The volume of fluids lost to such processes can easily be underestimated.

- Such patients may be significantly dehydrated resulting in reduced fluid volumes in both the vascular and tissue compartments which has usually taken time to develop and will take time to correct.

- Rapid fluid replacement into the vascular compartment can compromise the cardiovascular system particularly where there is pre-existing cardiovascular disease and in the elderly.

- In cases of dehydration, fluid replacement should be aimed at gradual re-hydration over many hours rather than minutes. Oral electrolyte solutions may be an appropriate consideration in some patients e.g. heat illness.

4.3 Fluid therapy

- **DO NOT** delay at scene to obtain vascular access or to provide fluid replacement; wherever possible obtain vascular access and administer fluid **EN-ROUTE TO HOSPITAL**.

- If the clinician determines that there is a definite need for fluid therapy, they should obtain vascular access.

- Clinicians should attempt to gain intravenous access in the first instance; however they may consider intra-osseous access where intravenous access fails or is unlikely to be successful.

- Vascular access devices should be flushed with 5 ml of physiologic saline for injection to confirm patency prior to administering large volumes of fluid.

- Once patent vascular access is confirmed, administer a single bolus of 250 ml of crystalloid (Table 6.10).

- Where the need for intravascular fluid therapy is less certain, clinicians should still obtain vascular access and flush to confirm patency.

- **Do not connect any fluids to the cannula unless intravascular fluid therapy is indicated.**

NB The slow administration of fluids to keep a vein open (TKO/TKVO) should not be practised.

Table 6.10 – DOSAGES FOR FLUID THERAPY

INITIAL DOSE	REPEAT DOSE	REPEAT INTERVAL	MAXIMUM DOSE
250 ml	250 ml	PRN	2 litres

- Monitor the physiological response, re-assess perfusion, pulse, respiratory rate and blood pressure wherever possible.

- If these observations improve, suspend any further administration.

- If there is no improvement, administer further 250 ml boluses, reassessing for improvement after each fluid bolus (Table 6.10).

- The maximum cumulative fluid dose is usually 2 litres (Table 6.10).

- If the patient remains hypotensive despite repeated 250 ml boluses OR the patient is likely to remain on scene for a considerable time (e.g. due to extrication difficulties), request senior clinical support (according to local procedures).

4.4 Exceptions and special circumstances

4.4.1 Burns

Where burn surface area is:

- <15% do not administer fluid.

- ≥15 – <25% and time to hospital is greater than 30 minutes then administer 1 litre sodium chloride 0.9% (Table 6.11).

- ≥25% administer 1 litre sodium chloride 0.9% (Table 6.11).

NB If fluid therapy is indicated **DO NOT** delay transfer to further care but continue fluid therapy en-route – stopping if practicable to insert the cannula.

- Care must be taken to ensure that elderly or heart failure patients are not over-infused.

- In order to minimise the risk of hypothermia, the use of cold fluids should be avoided if possible.

Table 6.11 – DOSAGES FOR FLUID THERAPY – BURNS

INITIAL DOSE	REPEAT DOSE	REPEAT INTERVAL	MAXIMUM DOSE
1 litre over 1 hour	NONE[a]	N/A	1 litre

[a]Seek senior clinical input for prolonged delays

4.4.2 Sepsis

- Sepsis should be suspected in patients who have a history of infection, a systolic blood pressure below 90 mmHg and tachypnoea.

- Patients with sepsis will benefit from early fluid therapy and an appropriate hospital alert/information call.

Intravascular Fluid Therapy (Adults)

- Intravascular fluid should be administered in cases of suspected sepsis (Refer to Tables 6.12 and 6.13).

Table 6.12 – CLINICAL SIGNS OF SEPSIS

- History of infection
- Systolic blood pressure <90 mmHg
- Tachypnoea

- The presence of additional clinical signs helps to confirm the diagnosis (NB not all will be present).

Table 6.13 – ADDITIONAL CLINICAL SIGNS OF SEPSIS

Signs

- Body temperature less than 36°C

  OR

  Body temperature greater than 38°C
- Tachycardia
- Altered mental status
- Mottled skin
- Prolonged capillary refill (>2 seconds)

- Clinicians should administer 1 litre of sodium chloride 0.9%.

Table 6.14 – DOSAGES FOR FLUID THERAPY – SEPSIS

INITIAL DOSE	REPEAT DOSE	REPEAT INTERVAL	MAXIMUM DOSE
1 litre over 30 minutes	Repeat ONCE if still hypotensive	PRN	2 litres

Methodology

For details of the methods used in the development of the Intravascular Fluid Therapy guideline refer to the guideline website.

KEY POINTS

Intravascular Fluid Therapy in Adults

- **Current research shows little evidence to support the routine use of IV fluids in adult acute blood loss.**
- **Current thinking is that fluids should only be administered when major organ perfusion is impaired.**
- **DO NOT delay on-scene for vascular access or fluid replacement; wherever possible obtain vascular access and administer fluid EN-ROUTE TO HOSPITAL stopping if practicable to insert the cannula.**

6 Drugs SECTION

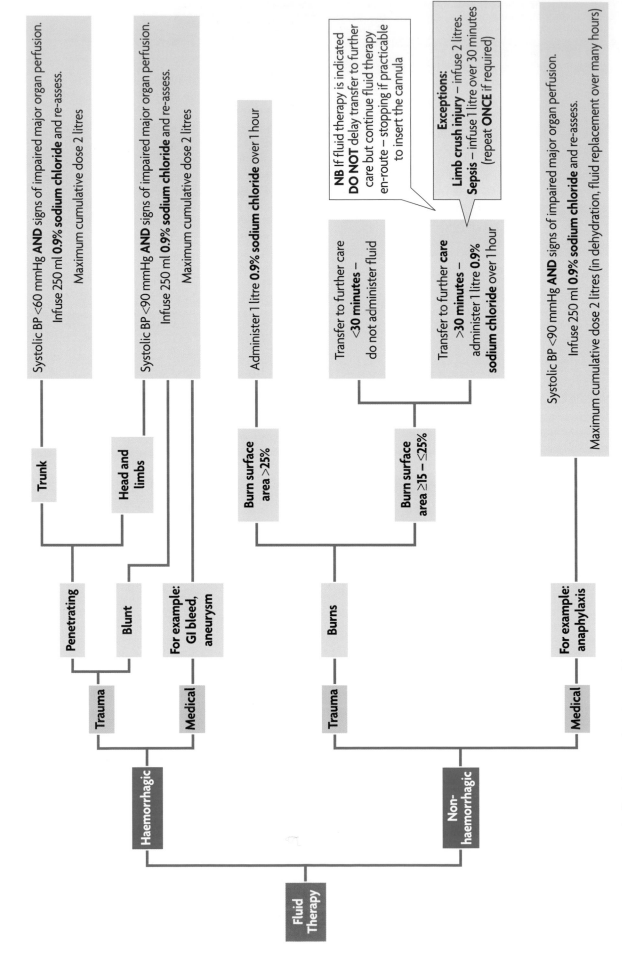

Figure 6.2 – Intravascular fluid therapy algorithm – adults

SECTION **6** Drugs

Intravascular Fluid Therapy (Children)

1. Introduction
- There has been no significant research in paediatric fluid administration in the literature and thus advice is dependent on that of adult studies and expert consensus.

2. Pathophysiology
- Although the basic pathophysiology is similar to adults, children have one very important difference. Their relatively healthy hearts and vasculature make the compensatory mechanisms very efficient. This means that only subtle signs of circulatory failure (shock) may be evident even in children with severe intravascular fluid depletion. When compensatory mechanisms start to fail, the child is in extremis and will deteriorate very quickly.

3. Assessment
- It is crucial that children with shock are treated before decompensation occurs whenever possible. There is no one sign that reliably dictates the state of shock a child may be in and a combination of all the markers of shock, along with an assessment of the mechanism of the shock (the history) must all be taken into account when deciding how shocked a child is.

- Blood pressure drops late in children for the reasons given above, and therefore is not a good indicator of the degree of volume depletion of the child. It is therefore of limited use in the prehospital setting, but if it is taken and found to be low (for the age of the child) this can be regarded as a pre-terminal sign.

- The following should be assessed:
  - pulse rate and volume
  - capillary refill measured on the forehead or sternum
  - respiratory rate
  - colour (pallor etc)
  - cold peripheries
  - conscious level (AVPU) including drowsiness.

These must be considered as a whole in the light of what is known about the mechanism (i.e. volume of blood or fluid lost).

Only when all these are taken together can a rough estimate of the degree of shock be made. Each one of these is not reliable when measured on its own.

NB There is no place for 'permissive hypotension' in children. To keep the blood pressure low deliberately is very dangerous. However, the reasons behind not fluid loading trauma victims are probably as applicable to children as adults so it is very important not to overload traumatised children. This is done by frequent re-assessment when giving fluid – see below.

4. Management
For the management of burns and scalds see below and refer to Figure 6.3.

4.1 Medical causes of shock
It is usually difficult to measure volumes of fluid lost in children with medical causes of shock.

- 20 ml/kg is used as standard medical fluid replacement (25% of the child's blood volume).
- This can be given intravenously or intra-osseously and is given as a bolus.
- The exact volume given must be documented.
- The child must be re-assessed after each bolus.
- It may be repeated once – total 40 ml/kg.

4.2 Exceptions
- Diabetic Ketoacidosis (DKA). Children with DKA are very prone to cerebral oedema if given IV fluids and can die because of it. Children with renal failure and heart failure should also be treated with extreme caution. IV fluids should not be given unless there is significant shock (as opposed to dehydration) and only 10 ml/kg given. If there is no improvement following this, it may be repeated once (total 20 ml/kg) except in DKA where the dose is 10 ml/kg over 15 minutes. NB If these patients deteriorate during fluid administration, stop administering fluid immediately. If it is felt that further fluid will not wait until hospital, senior medical advice should be sought.

4.3 Traumatic causes of shock
- Fluid overload should be avoided. For ease and because all trauma patients should not be overloaded, it is not necessary to distinguish between compressible and non compressible haemorrhage.
- 5 ml/kg aliquots of fluid should be given.
- Re-assessment should be undertaken after each 5 ml/kg dose, using the signs described above.
- The 5 ml/kg dose can be repeated until the child is **significantly** improved. The vital signs (eg pulse) need not be normalised, but the child must be obviously more stable. There is no absolute upper dose.
- The child must be constantly re-assessed during transport.
- Fluids can be recommenced at 5 ml/kg if there is deterioration, until improvement again occurs.

4.4 Burns
- Children lose fluids rapidly from severe burns and scalds and should have intravenous sodium chloride 0.9% started early.
- If the child has a >10% but <20% burn and the hospital time is more than 30 mins, fluids should be started, and if greater than 20% burn fluid should be given regardless of the time to hospital.

Where burn surface area is:
- <10% do not administer fluid.
- ≥10 – <20% and time to hospital is greater than 30 minutes then administer **sodium chloride 0.9%** 10ml/kg over an hour.
- ≥20% administer **sodium chloride 0.9%** 10 ml/kg over an hour.
- The total dose must be calculated and given as regular, tiny portions of this to aim to have infused the correct amount over the hour.

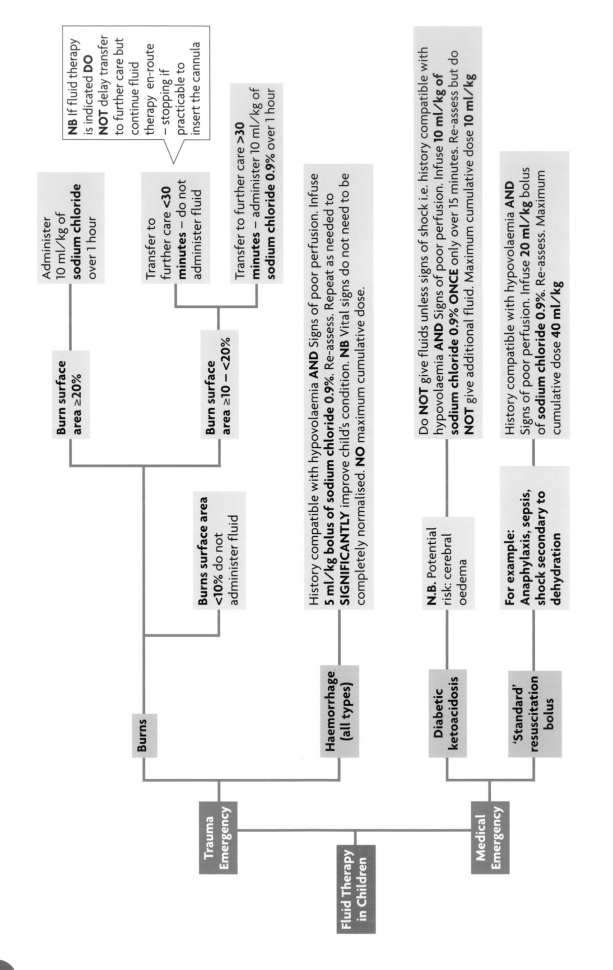

Figure 6.3 – Assessment and management of intravascular fluid therapy in children.

- If fluid therapy is indicated **DO NOT** delay transfer to further care but continue fluid therapy en-route – stopping if practicable to insert the cannula.
- Vascular access also means analgesia can be administered.

NB There is **NO** evidence that the absence of the radial pulse correlates with the blood pressure or degree of shock in a consistent manner in children. Do not monitor the need for fluids against the presence of the radial pulse.

Methodology

For details of the methodology used in the development of this guideline refer to the guideline webpage.

KEY POINTS

Intravascular Fluid Therapy in Children

- **Children compensate well for shock.**
- **Once decompensated, they deteriorate very rapidly.**
- **All physiological signs must be taken in combination to diagnose shock.**
- **20 ml/kg is the standard bolus for medically caused shock.**
- **5 ml/kg is the standard bolus for traumatic shock.**
- **10 ml/kg over one hour should be given to children with burns ≥20% and also to children with burns of ≥10 and <20% whose journey time will be more than 30 minutes. This procedure must not delay the time to hospital admission.**
- **Re-assessment after each bolus is vital to avoid fluid overload.**
- **Fluids should be used with extreme caution in DKA, renal failure and cardiac failure.**

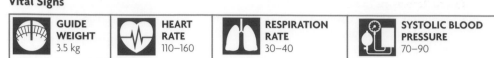

Page for Age

Vital Signs

	GUIDE WEIGHT 3.5 kg		HEART RATE 110–160		RESPIRATION RATE 30–40		SYSTOLIC BLOOD PRESSURE 70–90

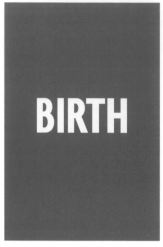

BIRTH

Airway Size by Type

OROPHARYNGEAL AIRWAY	LARYNGEAL MASK	I-GEL AIRWAY	ENDOTRACHEAL TUBE
000	1	1	Diameter: **3 mm**; Length: **10 cm**

Defibrillation – Cardiac Arrest

MANUAL	AUTOMATED EXTERNAL DEFIBRILLATOR
20 Joules	Where possible, use a manual defibrillator. If an AED is the only defibrillator available, it should be used (preferably using paediatric attenuation pads or else in paediatric mode).

Intravascular Fluid

FLUID	INITIAL DOSE	REPEAT DOSE	DOSE INTERVAL	CONCENTRATION	VOLUME	MAXIMUM DOSE	ROUTE
Sodium chloride (5 ml/kg)	20 ml	20 ml	PRN	0.9%	20 ml	140 ml	IV/IO
Sodium chloride (10 ml/kg)	35 ml	35 ml	PRN	0.9%	35 ml	140 ml	IV/IO
Sodium chloride (20 ml/kg)	70 ml	70 ml	PRN	0.9%	70 ml	140 ml	IV/IO

Cardiac Arrest

DRUG	INITIAL DOSE	REPEAT DOSE	DOSE INTERVAL	CONCENTRATION	VOLUME	MAXIMUM DOSE	ROUTE
ADRENALINE	35 micrograms	35 micrograms	3–5 minutes	1 milligram in 10 ml (1:10,000)	0.35 ml	No limit	IV/IO
AMIODARONE	18 milligrams (After 3rd shock)	18 milligrams	After 5th shock	300 milligrams in 10 ml	0.6 ml	36 milligrams	IV/IO
ATROPINE[a]	100 micrograms	NONE	N/A	100 micrograms in 1 ml	1 ml	100 micrograms	IV/IO
ATROPINE[a]	100 micrograms	NONE	N/A	200 micrograms in 1 ml	0.5 ml	100 micrograms	IV/IO
ATROPINE[a]	100 micrograms	NONE	N/A	300 micrograms in 1 ml	0.3 ml	100 micrograms	IV/IO
ATROPINE[a]	100 micrograms	NONE	N/A	600 micrograms in 1 ml	0.17 ml	100 micrograms	IV/IO

[a] **BRADYCARDIA** in children is most commonly caused by **HYPOXIA**, requiring immediate **ABC** care, **NOT** drug therapy; therefore **ONLY** administer atropine in cases of bradycardia caused by vagal stimulation (e.g. suction).

Reversal of respiratory and central nervous system depression in a neonate following maternal opioid use during labour – single dose only

DRUG	INITIAL DOSE	REPEAT DOSE	DOSE INTERVAL	CONCENTRATION	VOLUME	MAXIMUM DOSE	ROUTE
Naloxone* NB cautions	200 micrograms	NONE	N/A	400 micrograms in 1 ml	0.5 ml	200 micrograms	IM

*Reversal of respiratory arrest/extreme respiratory depression.

Quick Reference Table

DRUG	INITIAL DOSE	REPEAT DOSE	DOSE INTERVAL	CONCENTRATION	VOLUME	MAXIMUM DOSE	ROUTE
ADRENALINE anaphylaxis/asthma	150 micrograms	150 micrograms	5 minutes	1 milligram in 1 ml (1:1,000)	0.15 ml	No limit	IM
BENZYLPENICILLIN (IV/IO)	300 milligrams	NONE	N/A	600 milligrams in 9.6 ml	5 ml	300 milligrams	IV/IO
BENZYLPENICILLIN (IM)	300 milligrams	NONE	N/A	600 milligrams in 1.6 ml	1 ml	300 milligrams	IM
CHLORPHENAMINE (Oral)	N/A	N/A	N/A	N/A	N/A	N/A	Oral
CHLORPHENAMINE (IV/IO)	N/A	N/A	N/A	N/A	N/A	N/A	IV/IO
DEXAMETHASONE-croup	N/A	N/A	N/A	N/A	N/A	N/A	Oral
DIAZEPAM (IV/IO)	1 milligram	NONE	N/A	10 milligrams in 2 ml	0.2 ml	1 milligram	IV/IO
DIAZEPAM (PR)	1.25 or 2.5 milligrams	NONE	N/A	2.5 milligrams in 1.25 ml	½ × 2.5 milligram tube or 1 × 2.5 milligram tube	1.25 or 2.5 milligrams	PR
GLUCAGON	100 micrograms	NONE	N/A	1 milligram per vial	0.1 vial	100 micrograms	IM
GLUCOSE 10%	900 milligrams	900 milligrams	5 minutes	50 grams in 500 ml	9 ml	2.7 grams	IV/IO
HYDROCORTISONE	10 milligrams	NONE	N/A	100 milligrams in 1 ml	0.1 ml	10 milligrams	IV/IO/IM
HYDROCORTISONE	10 milligrams	NONE	N/A	100 milligrams in 2 ml	0.2 ml	10 milligrams	IV/IO/IM
IBUPROFEN	N/A	N/A	N/A	N/A	N/A	N/A	Oral
IPRATROPIUM	N/A	N/A	N/A	N/A	N/A	N/A	Neb
PATIENT'S OWN MIDAZOLAM[b]	1 milligram	NONE	N/A	10 milligrams in 1 ml	0.1 ml	1 milligram	Buccal
MORPHINE (IV/IO)	N/A	N/A	N/A	N/A	N/A	N/A	IV/IO
MORPHINE (Oral)	N/A	N/A	N/A	N/A	N/A	N/A	Oral
NALOXONE**[†] NB cautions (IV/IO)	40 micrograms	40 micrograms	3 minutes	400 micrograms in 1 ml	0.1 ml	440 micrograms	IV/IO
NALOXONE[†]-INITIAL DOSE (IM)	40 micrograms	See below	3 minutes	400 micrograms in 1 ml	0.1 ml	See below	IM
NALOXONE[†]-REPEAT DOSE (IM)	–	400 micrograms	–	400 micrograms in 1 ml	1 ml	440 micrograms	IM
ONDANSETRON	N/A	N/A	N/A	N/A	N/A	N/A	Oral
PARACETAMOL (Oral)	N/A	N/A	N/A	N/A	N/A	N/A	Oral
PARACETAMOL (IV/IO)	N/A	N/A	N/A	N/A	N/A	N/A	IV/IO
SALBUTAMOL	N/A	N/A	N/A	N/A	N/A	N/A	Neb
TRANEXAMIC ACID	50 mg	NONE	N/A	100 mg/ml	0.5 ml	50 mg	IV

[b] Give the dose as prescribed in the child's individualised treatment plan (the dosages described above reflect the recommended dosages for a child of this age).

**Reversal of respiratory and central nervous system depression in a neonate following maternal opioid use during labour – single dose only.

[†]Intramuscular naloxone is used to reverse respiratory and central nervous system depression in a neonate following maternal opioid use during labour. For this specific indication, the dose is described in a separate box on page 374.

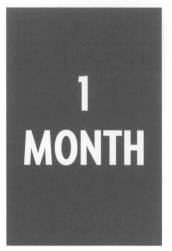

1 MONTH

Vital Signs

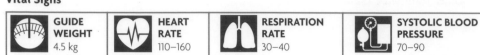

	GUIDE WEIGHT 4.5 kg		HEART RATE 110–160		RESPIRATION RATE 30–40		SYSTOLIC BLOOD PRESSURE 70–90

Airway Size by Type

OROPHARYNGEAL AIRWAY	LARYNGEAL MASK	I-GEL AIRWAY	ENDOTRACHEAL TUBE
00	1	1	Diameter: **3 mm**; Length: **10 cm**

Defibrillation – Cardiac Arrest

MANUAL	AUTOMATED EXTERNAL DEFIBRILLATOR
20 Joules	Where possible, use a manual defibrillator. If an AED is the only defibrillator available, it should be used (preferably using paediatric attenuation pads or else in paediatric mode).

Intravascular Fluid

FLUID	INITIAL DOSE	REPEAT DOSE	DOSE INTERVAL	CONCENTRATION	VOLUME	MAXIMUM DOSE	ROUTE
Sodium chloride (5 ml/kg)	20 ml	20 ml	PRN	0.9%	20 ml	180 ml	IV/IO
Sodium chloride (10 ml/kg)	45 ml	45 ml	PRN	0.9%	45 ml	180 ml	IV/IO
Sodium chloride (20 ml/kg)	90 ml	90 ml	PRN	0.9%	90 ml	180 ml	IV/IO

Cardiac Arrest

DRUG	INITIAL DOSE	REPEAT DOSE	DOSE INTERVAL	CONCENTRATION	VOLUME	MAXIMUM DOSE	ROUTE
ADRENALINE	50 micrograms	50 micrograms	3–5 minutes	1 milligram in 10 ml (1:10,000)	0.5 ml	No limit	IV/IO
AMIODARONE	25 milligrams (After 3rd shock)	25 milligrams	After 5th shock	300 milligrams in 10 ml	0.8 ml	50 milligrams	IV/IO
ATROPINE[a]	100 micrograms	NONE	N/A	100 micrograms in 1 ml	1 ml	100 micrograms	IV/IO
ATROPINE[a]	100 micrograms	NONE	N/A	200 micrograms in 1 ml	0.5 ml	100 micrograms	IV/IO
ATROPINE[a]	100 micrograms	NONE	N/A	300 micrograms in 1 ml	0.3 ml	100 micrograms	IV/IO
ATROPINE[a]	100 micrograms	NONE	N/A	600 micrograms in 1 ml	0.17 ml	100 micrograms	IV/IO

[a] **BRADYCARDIA** in children is most commonly caused by **HYPOXIA**, requiring immediate **ABC** care, **NOT** drug therapy; therefore **ONLY** administer atropine in cases of bradycardia caused by vagal stimulation (e.g. suction).

Quick Reference Table

DRUG	INITIAL DOSE	REPEAT DOSE	DOSE INTERVAL	CONCENTRATION	VOLUME	MAXIMUM DOSE	ROUTE
ADRENALINE anaphylaxis/asthma	150 micrograms	150 micrograms	5 minutes	1 milligram in 1 ml (1:1,000)	0.15 ml	No limit	IM
BENZYLPENICILLIN (IV/IO)	300 milligrams	NONE	N/A	600 milligrams in 9.6 ml	5 ml	300 milligrams	IV/IO
BENZYLPENICILLIN (IM)	300 milligrams	NONE	N/A	600 milligrams in 1.6 ml	1 ml	300 milligrams	IM
CHLORPHENAMINE (Oral)	N/A	N/A	N/A	N/A	N/A	N/A	Oral
CHLORPHENAMINE (IV/IO)	N/A	N/A	N/A	N/A	N/A	N/A	IV/IO
DEXAMETHASONE-croup	2 milligrams	NONE	N/A	4 milligrams per ml (use intravenous preparation orally)	0.5 ml	2 milligrams	Oral
DIAZEPAM (IV/IO)	1.5 milligrams	NONE	N/A	10 milligrams in 2 ml	0.3 ml	1.5 milligrams	IV/IO
DIAZEPAM (PR)	5 milligrams	NONE	N/A	5 milligrams in 2.5 ml	1 × 5 milligram tube	5 milligrams	PR
GLUCAGON	500 micrograms	NONE	N/A	1 milligram per vial	0.5 vial	500 micrograms	IM
GLUCOSE 10%	1 gram	1 gram	5 minutes	50 grams in 500 ml	10 ml	3 grams	IV/IO
HYDROCORTISONE	25 milligrams	NONE	N/A	100 milligrams in 1 ml	0.25 ml	25 milligrams	IV/IO/IM
HYDROCORTISONE	25 milligrams	NONE	N/A	100 milligrams in 2 ml	0.5 ml	25 milligrams	IV/IO/IM
IBUPROFEN	N/A	N/A	N/A	N/A	N/A	N/A	Oral
IPRATROPIUM	125 – 250 micrograms	NONE	N/A	250 micrograms in 1 ml	0.5 ml – 1 ml	125 – 250 micrograms	Neb
IPRATROPIUM	125 – 250 micrograms	NONE	N/A	500 micrograms in 2 ml	0.5 ml – 1 ml	125 – 250 micrograms	Neb
PATIENT'S OWN MIDAZOLAM[b]	1.5 milligrams	NONE	N/A	10 milligrams in 1 ml	0.15 ml	1.5 milligrams	Buccal
MORPHINE (IV/IO)	N/A	N/A	N/A	N/A	N/A	N/A	IV/IO
MORPHINE (Oral)	N/A	N/A	N/A	N/A	N/A	N/A	Oral
NALOXONE NB cautions (IV/IO)	40 micrograms	40 micrograms	3 minutes	400 micrograms in 1 ml	0.1 ml	440 micrograms	IV/IO
NALOXONE-INITIAL DOSE (IM)	40 micrograms	See below	3 minutes	400 micrograms in 1 ml	0.1 ml	See below	IM
NALOXONE-REPEAT DOSE (IM)	–	400 micrograms	–	400 micrograms in 1 ml	1 ml	440 micrograms	
ONDANSETRON	0.5 milligrams	NONE	N/A	2 milligrams in 1 ml	0.25 ml	0.5 milligrams	IV/IO/IM
PARACETAMOL (Oral)	N/A	N/A	N/A	N/A	N/A	N/A	Oral
PARACETAMOL (IV/IO)	N/A	N/A	N/A	N/A	N/A	N/A	IV/IO
SALBUTAMOL	2.5 milligrams	2.5 micrograms	5 minutes	2.5 milligrams in 2.5 ml	2.5 ml	N/A	Neb
SALBUTAMOL	2.5 milligrams	2.5 micrograms	5 minutes	5 milligrams in 2.5 ml	1.25 ml	N/A	Neb
TRANEXAMIC ACID	50 mg	NONE	N/A	100 mg/ml	0.5 ml	50 mg	IV

[a] **BRADYCARDIA** in children is most commonly caused by **HYPOXIA**, requiring immediate **ABC** care, **NOT** drug therapy; therefore **ONLY** administer atropine in cases of bradycardia caused by vagal stimulation (e.g. suction).

[b] Give the dose as prescribed in the child's individualised treatment plan (the dosages described above reflect the recommended dosages for a child of this age).

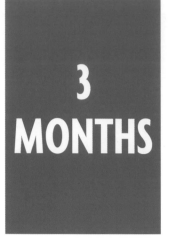

3 MONTHS

Vital Signs

	GUIDE WEIGHT 6 kg		HEART RATE 110–160		RESPIRATION RATE 30–40		SYSTOLIC BLOOD PRESSURE 70–90

Airway Size by Type

OROPHARYNGEAL AIRWAY	LARYNGEAL MASK	I-GEL AIRWAY	ENDOTRACHEAL TUBE
00	1.5	1.5	Diameter: **3.5 mm**; Length: **11 cm**

Defibrillation – Cardiac Arrest

MANUAL	AUTOMATED EXTERNAL DEFIBRILLATOR
25 Joules	Where possible, use a manual defibrillator. If an AED is the only defibrillator available, it should be used (preferably using paediatric attenuation pads or else in paediatric mode).

Intravascular Fluid

FLUID	INITIAL DOSE	REPEAT DOSE	DOSE INTERVAL	CONCENTRATION	VOLUME	MAXIMUM DOSE	ROUTE
Sodium chloride (5 ml/kg)	30 ml	30 ml	PRN	0.9%	30 ml	240 ml	IV/IO
Sodium chloride (10 ml/kg)	60 ml	60 ml	PRN	0.9%	60 ml	240 ml	IV/IO
Sodium chloride (20 ml/kg)	120 ml	120 ml	PRN	0.9%	120 ml	240 ml	IV/IO

Cardiac Arrest

DRUG	INITIAL DOSE	REPEAT DOSE	DOSE INTERVAL	CONCENTRATION	VOLUME	MAXIMUM DOSE	ROUTE
ADRENALINE	60 micrograms	60 micrograms	3–5 minutes	1 milligram in 10 ml (1:10,000)	0.6 ml	No limit	IV/IO
AMIODARONE	30 milligrams (after 3rd shock)	30 milligrams	After 5th shock	300 milligrams in 10 ml	1 ml	60 milligrams	IV/IO
ATROPINE[a]	120 micrograms	NONE	N/A	100 micrograms in 1 ml	1.2 ml	120 micrograms	IV/IO
ATROPINE[a]	120 micrograms	NONE	N/A	200 micrograms in 1 ml	0.6 ml	120 micrograms	IV/IO
ATROPINE[a]	120 micrograms	NONE	N/A	300 micrograms in 1 ml	0.4 ml	120 micrograms	IV/IO
ATROPINE[a]	120 micrograms	NONE	N/A	600 micrograms in 1 ml	0.2 ml	120 micrograms	IV/IO

[a] **BRADYCARDIA** in children is most commonly caused by **HYPOXIA**, requiring immediate **ABC** care, **NOT** drug therapy; therefore **ONLY** administer atropine in cases of bradycardia caused by vagal stimulation (e.g. suction).

Quick Reference Table

DRUG	INITIAL DOSE	REPEAT DOSE	DOSE INTERVAL	CONCENTRATION	VOLUME	MAXIMUM DOSE	ROUTE
ADRENALINE anaphylaxis/asthma	150 micrograms	150 micrograms	5 minutes	1 milligram in 1 ml (1:1,000)	0.15 ml	No limit	IM
BENZYLPENICILLIN (IV/IO)	300 milligrams	NONE	N/A	600 milligrams in 9.6 ml	5 ml	300 milligrams	IV/IO
BENZYLPENICILLIN (IM)	300 milligrams	NONE	N/A	600 milligrams in 1.6 ml	1 ml	300 milligrams	IM
CHLORPHENAMINE (Oral)	N/A	N/A	N/A	N/A	N/A	N/A	Oral
CHLORPHENAMINE (IV/IO)	N/A	N/A	N/A	N/A	N/A	N/A	IV/IO
DEXAMETHASONE-croup	2 milligrams	NONE	N/A	4 milligrams per ml (use intravenous preparation orally)	0.5 ml	2 milligrams	Oral
DIAZEAM (IV/IO)	2 milligrams	NONE	N/A	10 milligrams in 2 ml	0.4 ml	2 milligrams	IV/IO
DIAZEPAM (PR)	5 milligrams	NONE	N/A	5 milligrams in 2.5 ml	1 × 5 milligram tube	5 milligrams	PR
GLUCAGON	500 micrograms	NONE	N/A	1 milligram per vial	0.5 vial	500 micrograms	IM
GLUCOSE 10%	1 gram	1 gram	5 minutes	50 grams in 500 ml	10 ml	3 grams	IV/IO
HYDROCORTISONE	25 milligrams	NONE	N/A	100 milligrams in 1 ml	0.25 ml	25 milligrams	IV/IO/IM
HYDROCORTISONE	25 milligrams	NONE	N/A	100 milligrams in 2 ml	0.5 ml	25 milligrams	IV/IO/IM
IBUPROFEN	50 milligrams	50 milligrams	8 hours	100 milligrams in 5 ml	2.5 ml	150 milligrams	Oral
IPRATROPIUM	125–250 micrograms	NONE	N/A	250 micrograms in 1 ml	0.5 ml – 1 ml	125–250 micrograms	Neb
IPRATROPIUM	125–250 micrograms	NONE	N/A	500 micrograms in 2 ml	0.5 ml – 1 ml	125–250 micrograms	Neb
PATIENT'S OWN MIDAZOLAM[b]	2 milligrams	NONE	N/A	10 milligrams in 1 ml	0.2 ml	2 milligrams	Buccal
MORPHINE (IV/IO)	N/A	N/A	N/A	N/A	N/A	N/A	IV/IO
MORPHINE (Oral)	N/A	N/A	N/A	N/A	N/A	N/A	Oral
NALOXONE NB cautions (IV/IO)	60 micrograms	60 micrograms	3 minutes	400 micrograms in 1 ml	0.15 ml	660 micrograms	IV/IO
NALOXONE-INITIAL DOSE (IM)	60 micrograms	See below	3 minutes	400 micrograms in 1 ml	0.15 ml	See below	IM
NALOXONE-REPEAT DOSE (IM)	–	400 micrograms	–	400 micrograms in 1 ml	1 ml	460 micrograms	
ONDANSETRON	0.5 milligrams	NONE	N/A	2 milligrams in 1 ml	0.25 ml	0.5 milligrams	IV/IO/IM
PARACETAMOL (Oral)	60 milligrams	60 milligrams	4–6 hours	120 milligrams in 5 ml – infant paracetamol suspension	2.5 ml	240 milligrams in 24 hours	Oral
PARACETAMOL (IV/IO)	N/A	N/A	N/A	N/A	N/A	N/A	IV/IO
SALBUTAMOL	2.5 milligrams	2.5 milligrams	5 minutes	2.5 milligrams in 2.5 ml	2.5 ml	N/A	Neb
SALBUTAMOL	2.5 milligrams	2.5 milligrams	5 minutes	5 milligrams in 2.5 ml	1.25 ml	N/A	Neb
TRANEXAMIC ACID	100 mg	NONE	N/A	100 mg/ml	1 ml	100 mg	IV

[b] Give the dose as prescribed in the child's individualised treatment plan (the dosages described above reflect the recommended dosages for a child of this age).

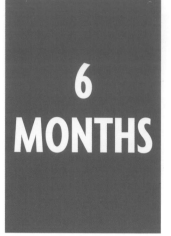

6 MONTHS

Vital Signs

GUIDE WEIGHT	HEART RATE	RESPIRATION RATE	SYSTOLIC BLOOD PRESSURE
8 kg	110–160	30–40	70–90

Airway Size by Type

OROPHARYNGEAL AIRWAY	LARYNGEAL MASK	I-GEL AIRWAY	ENDOTRACHEAL TUBE
00	1.5	1.5	Diameter: **4 mm**; Length: **12 cm**

Defibrillation – Cardiac Arrest

MANUAL	AUTOMATED EXTERNAL DEFIBRILLATOR
40 Joules	Where possible, use a manual defibrillator. If an AED is the only defibrillator available, it should be used (preferably using paediatric attenuation pads or else in paediatric mode).

Intravascular Fluid

FLUID	INITIAL DOSE	REPEAT DOSE	DOSE INTERVAL	CONCENTRATION	VOLUME	MAXIMUM DOSE	ROUTE
Sodium chloride (5 ml/kg)	40 ml	40 ml	PRN	0.9%	40 ml	320 ml	IV/IO
Sodium chloride (10 ml/kg)	80 ml	80 ml	PRN	0.9%	80 ml	320 ml	IV/IO
Sodium chloride (20 ml/kg)	160 ml	160 ml	PRN	0.9%	160 ml	320 ml	IV/IO

Cardiac Arrest

DRUG	INITIAL DOSE	REPEAT DOSE	DOSE INTERVAL	CONCENTRATION	VOLUME	MAXIMUM DOSE	ROUTE
ADRENALINE	80 micrograms	80 micrograms	3–5 minutes	1 milligram in 10 ml (1:10,000)	0.8 ml	No limit	IV/IO
AMIODARONE	40 milligrams (after 3rd shock)	40 milligrms	After 5th shock	300 milligrams in 10 ml	1.3 ml	80 milligrams	IV/IO
ATROPINE[a]	120 micrograms	NONE	N/A	100 micrograms in 1 ml	1.2 ml	120 micrograms	IV/IO
ATROPINE[a]	120 micrograms	NONE	N/A	200 micrograms in 1 ml	0.6 ml	120 micrograms	IV/IO
ATROPINE[a]	120 micrograms	NONE	N/A	300 micrograms in 1 ml	0.4 ml	120 micrograms	IV/IO
ATROPINE[a]	120 micrograms	NONE	N/A	600 micrograms in 1 ml	0.2 ml	120 micrograms	IV/IO

[a] **BRADYCARDIA** in children is most commonly caused by **HYPOXIA**, requiring immediate **ABC** care, **NOT** drug therapy; therefore **ONLY** administer atropine in cases of bradycardia caused by vagal stimulation (e.g. suction).

Quick Reference Table

DRUG	INITIAL DOSE	REPEAT DOSE	DOSE INTERVAL	CONCENTRATION	VOLUME	MAXIMUM DOSE	ROUTE
ADRENALINE anaphylaxis/asthma	150 micrograms	150 micrograms	5 minutes	1 milligram in 1 ml (1:1,000)	0.15 ml	No limit	IM
BENZYLPENICILLIN (IV/IO)	300 milligrams	NONE	N/A	600 milligrams in 9.6 ml	5 ml	300 milligrams	IV/IO
BENZYLPENICILLIN (IM)	300 milligrams	NONE	N/A	600 milligrams in 1.6 ml	1 ml	300 milligrams	IM
CHLORPHENAMINE (Oral)	N/A	N/A	N/A	N/A	N/A	N/A	Oral
CHLORPHENAMINE (IV/IO)	N/A	N/A	N/A	N/A	N/A	N/A	IV/IO
DEXAMETHASONE-croup	2 milligrams	NONE	N/A	4 milligrams per ml (use intravenous preparation orally)	0.5 ml	2 milligrams	Oral
DIAZEPAM (IV/IO)	2.5 milligrams	NONE	N/A	10 milligrams in 2 ml	0.5 ml	2.5 milligrams	IV/IO
DIAZEPAM (PR)	5 milligrams	NONE	N/A	5 milligrams in 2.5 ml	1 × 5 milligram tube	5 milligrams	PR
GLUCAGON	500 micrograms	NONE	N/A	1 milligram per vial	0.5 vial	500 micrograms	IM
GLUCOSE 10%	1.5 grams	1.5 grams	5 minutes	50 grams in 500 ml	16 ml	4.5 grams	IV/IO
HYDROCORTISONE	50 milligrams	NONE	N/A	100 milligrams in 1 ml	0.5 ml	50 milligrams	IV/IO/IM
HYDROCORTISONE	50 milligrams	NONE	N/A	100 milligrams in 2 ml	1 ml	50 milligrams	IV/IO/IM
IBUPROFEN	50 milligrams	50 milligrams	8 hours	100 milligrams in 5 ml	2.5 ml	150 milligrams	Oral
IPRATROPIUM	125–250 micrograms	NONE	N/A	250 micrograms in 1 ml	0.5ml – 1 ml	125–250 micrograms	Neb
IPRATROPIUM	125–250 micrograms	NONE	N/A	500 micrograms in 2 ml	0.5ml – 1 ml	125–250 micrograms	Neb
PATIENT'S OWN MIDAZOLAM[b]	2.5 milligrams	NONE	N/A	10 milligrams in 1 ml	0.25 ml	2.5 milligrams	Buccal
MORPHINE (IV/IO)	N/A	N/A	N/A	N/A	N/A	N/A	IV/IO
MORPHINE (Oral)	N/A	N/A	N/A	N/A	N/A	N/A	Oral
NALOXONE NB cautions (IV/IO)	80 micrograms	80 micrograms	3 minutes	400 micrograms in 1 ml	0.2 ml	880 micrograms	IV/IO
NALOXONE – INITIAL DOSE (IM)	80 micrograms	See below	3 minutes	400 micrograms in 1 ml	0.2 ml	See below	IM
NALOXONE-REPEAT DOSE (IM)	–	400 micrograms	–	400 micrograms in 1 ml	1 ml	480 micrograms	IM
ONDANSETRON	1 milligram	NONE	N/A	2 milligrams in 1 ml	0.5 ml	1 milligram	IV/IO/IM
PARACETAMOL (Oral)	120 milligrams	120 milligrams	4–6 hours	120 milligrams in 5 ml (infant suspension)	5 ml	480 milligrams in 24 hours	Oral
PARACETAMOL (IV/IO)	50 milligrams	50 milligrams	4–6 hours	10 milligrams in 1 ml	5 ml	200 milligrams in 24 hours	IV/IO
SALBUTAMOL	2.5 milligrams	2.5 milligrams	5 minutes	2.5 milligrams in 2.5 ml	2.5 ml	No limit	Neb
SALBUTAMOL	2.5 milligrams	2.5 milligrams	5 minutes	5 milligrams in 2.5 ml	1.25 ml	No limit	Neb
TRANEXAMIC ACID	100 mg	NONE	N/A	100 mg/ml	1 ml	100 mg	IV

[b] Give the dose as prescribed in the child's individualised treatment plan (the dosages described above reflect the recommended dosages for a child of this age).

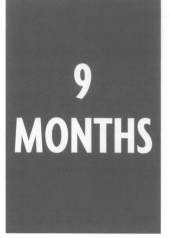

9 MONTHS

Vital Signs

| | GUIDE WEIGHT 9 kg | | HEART RATE 110–160 | | RESPIRATION RATE 30–40 | | SYSTOLIC BLOOD PRESSURE 70–90 |

Airway Size by Type

OROPHARYNGEAL AIRWAY	LARYNGEAL MASK	I-GEL AIRWAY	ENDOTRACHEAL TUBE
00	1.5	1.5	Diameter: **4 mm**; Length: **12 cm**

Defibrillation – Cardiac Arrest

MANUAL	AUTOMATED EXTERNAL DEFIBRILLATOR
40 Joules	Where possible, use a manual defibrillator. If an AED is the only defibrillator available, it should be used (preferably using paediatric attenuation pads or else in paediatric mode).

Intravascular Fluid

FLUID	INITIAL DOSE	REPEAT DOSE	DOSE INTERVAL	CONCENTRATION	VOLUME	MAXIMUM DOSE	ROUTE
Sodium chloride (5 ml/kg)	45 ml	45 ml	PRN	0.9%	45 ml	360 ml	IV/IO
Sodium chloride (10 ml/kg)	90 ml	90 ml	PRN	0.9%	90 ml	360 ml	IV/IO
Sodium chloride (20 ml/kg)	180 ml	180 ml	PRN	0.9%	180 ml	360 ml	IV/IO

Cardiac Arrest

DRUG	INITIAL DOSE	REPEAT DOSE	DOSE INTERVAL	CONCENTRATION	VOLUME	MAXIMUM DOSE	ROUTE
ADRENALINE	90 micrograms	90 micrograms	3–5 minutes	1 milligram in 10 ml (1:10,000)	0.9 ml	No limit	IV/IO
AMIODARONE	45 milligrams (after 3rd shock)	45 milligrams	After 5th shock	300 milligrams in 10 ml	1.5 ml	90 milligrams	IV/IO
ATROPINE[a]	120 micrograms	NONE	N/A	100 micrograms in 1 ml	1.2 ml	120 micrograms	IV/IO
ATROPINE[a]	120 micrograms	NONE	N/A	200 micrograms in 1 ml	0.6 ml	120 micrograms	IV/IO
ATROPINE[a]	120 micrograms	NONE	N/A	300 micrograms in 1 ml	0.4 ml	120 micrograms	IV/IO
ATROPINE[a]	120 micrograms	NONE	N/A	600 micrograms in 1 ml	0.2 ml	120 micrograms	IV/IO

[a] **BRADYCARDIA** in children is most commonly caused by **HYPOXIA**, requiring immediate **ABC** care, **NOT** drug therapy; therefore **ONLY** administer atropine in cases of bradycardia caused by vagal stimulation (e.g. suction).

Quick Reference Table

DRUG	INITIAL DOSE	REPEAT DOSE	DOSE INTERVAL	CONCENTRATION	VOLUME	MAXIMUM DOSE	ROUTE
ADRENALINE anaphylaxis/asthma	150 micrograms	150 micrograms	5 minutes	1 milligram in 1 ml (1:1,000)	0.15 ml	No limit	IM
BENZYLPENICILLIN (IV/IO)	300 milligrams	NONE	N/A	600 milligrams in 9.6 ml	5 ml	300 milligrams	IV/IO
BENZYLPENICILLIN (IM)	300 milligrams	NONE	N/A	600 milligrams in 1.6 ml	1 ml	300 milligrams	IM
CHLORPHENAMINE (Oral)	N/A	N/A	N/A	N/A	N/A	N/A	Oral
CHLORPHENAMINE (IV/IO)	N/A	N/A	N/A	N/A	N/A	N/A	IV/IO
DEXAMETHASONE-croup	2 milligrams	NONE	N/A	4 milligrams per ml (use intravenous preparation orally)	0.5 ml	2 milligrams	Oral
DIAZEPAM (IV/IO)	2.5 milligrams	NONE	N/A	10 milligrams in 2 ml	0.5 ml	2.5 milligrams	IV/IO
DIAZEPAM (PR)	5 milligrams	NONE	N/A	5 milligrams in 2.5 ml	1 × 5 milligram tube	5 milligrams	PR
GLUCAGON	500 micrograms	NONE	N/A	1 milligram per vial	0.5 vial	500 micrograms	IM
GLUCOSE 10%	2 grams	2 grams	5 minutes	50 grams in 500 ml	20 ml	6 grams	IV/IO
HYDROCORTISONE	50 milligrams	NONE	N/A	100 milligrams in 1 ml	0.5 ml	50 milligrams	IV/IO/IM
HYDROCORTISONE	50 milligrams	NONE	N/A	100 milligrams in 2 ml	1 ml	50 milligrams	IV/IO/IM
IBUPROFEN	50 milligrams	50 milligrams	8 hours	100 milligrams in 5 ml	2.5 ml	150 milligrams	Oral
IPRATROPIUM	125–250 micrograms	NONE	N/A	250 micrograms in 1 ml	0.5 ml – 1 ml	125–250 micrograms	Neb
IPRATROPIUM	125–250 micrograms	NONE	N/A	500 micrograms in 2 ml	0.5 ml – 1 ml	125–250 micrograms	Neb
PATIENT'S OWN MIDAZOLAM[b]	2.5 milligrams	NONE	N/A	10 milligrams in 1 ml	0.25 ml	2.5 milligrams	Buccal
MORPHINE (IV/IO)	N/A	N/A	N/A	N/A	N/A	N/A	IV/IO
MORPHINE (Oral)	N/A	N/A	N/A	N/A	N/A	N/A	Oral
NALOXONE NB cautions (IV/IO)	80 micrograms	80 micrograms	3 minutes	400 micrograms in 1 ml	0.2 ml	No limit	IV/IO
NALOXONE-INITIAL DOSE (IM)	80 micrograms	See below	3 minutes	400 micrograms in 1 ml	0.2 ml	See below	IM
NALOXONE-REPEAT DOSE (IM)	–	400 micrograms	–	400 micrograms in 1 ml	1 ml	480 micrograms	IM
ONDANSETRON	1 milligram	NONE	N/A	2 milligrams/ml	0.5 ml	1 milligram	IV/IO/IM
PARACETAMOL (Oral)	120 milligrams	120 milligrams	4–6 hours	120 milligrams in 5 ml (infant suspension)	5 ml	480 milligrams in 24 hours	Oral
PARACETAMOL (IV/IO)	50 milligrams	50 milligrams	4–6 hours	10 milligrams in 1 ml	5 ml	200 milligrams in 24 hours	IV/IO
SALBUTAMOL	2.5 milligrams	2.5 milligrams	5 minutes	2.5 milligrams in 2.5 ml	2.5 ml	No limit	Neb
SALBUTAMOL	2.5 milligrams	2.5 milligrams	5 minutes	5 milligrams in 2.5 ml	1.25 ml	No limit	Neb
TRANEXAMIC ACID	150 mg	NONE	N/A	100 mg/ml	1.5 mls	150 mg	IV

[b] Give the dose as prescribed in the child's individualised treatment plan (the dosages described above reflect the recommended dosages for a child of this age).

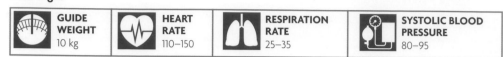
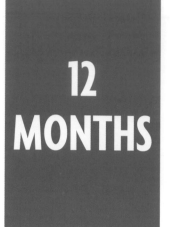

12 MONTHS

Vital Signs

	GUIDE WEIGHT 10 kg		HEART RATE 110–150		RESPIRATION RATE 25–35		SYSTOLIC BLOOD PRESSURE 80–95

Airway Size by Type

OROPHARYNGEAL AIRWAY	LARYNGEAL MASK	I-GEL AIRWAY	ENDOTRACHEAL TUBE
00 OR 0	1.5	1.5 OR 2	Diameter: **4.5 mm**; Length: **13 cm**

Defibrillation – Cardiac Arrest

MANUAL	AUTOMATED EXTERNAL DEFIBRILLATOR
40 Joules	A standard AED (either with paediatric attenuation pads or else in paediatric mode) can be used. If paediatric pads are not available, standard adult pads can used (but must not overlap).

Intravascular Fluid

FLUID	INITIAL DOSE	REPEAT DOSE	DOSE INTERVAL	CONCENTRATION	VOLUME	MAXIMUM DOSE	ROUTE
Sodium chloride (5 ml/kg)	50 ml	50 ml	PRN	0.9%	50 ml	400 ml	IV/IO
Sodium chloride (10 ml/kg)	100 ml	100 ml	PRN	0.9%	100 ml	400 ml	IV/IO
Sodium chloride (20 ml/kg)	200 ml	200 ml	PRN	0.9%	200 ml	400 ml	IV/IO

Cardiac Arrest

DRUG	INITIAL DOSE	REPEAT DOSE	DOSE INTERVAL	CONCENTRATION	VOLUME	MAXIMUM DOSE	ROUTE
ADRENALINE	100 micrograms	100 micrograms	3–5 minutes	1 milligram in 10 ml (1:10,000)	1 ml	No limit	IV/IO
AMIODARONE	50 milligrams (after 3rd shock)	50 milligrams	After 5th shock	300 milligrams in 10 ml	1.7 ml	100 milligrams	IV/IO
ATROPINE[a]	200 micrograms	NONE	N/A	100 micrograms in 1 ml	2 ml	200 micrograms	IV/IO
ATROPINE[a]	200 micrograms	NONE	N/A	200 micrograms in 1 ml	1 ml	200 micrograms	IV/IO
ATROPINE[a]	200 micrograms	NONE	N/A	300 micrograms in 1 ml	0.7 ml	200 micrograms	IV/IO
ATROPINE[a]	200 micrograms	NONE	N/A	600 micrograms in 1 ml	0.3 ml	200 micrograms	IV/IO

[a] **BRADYCARDIA** in children is most commonly caused by **HYPOXIA**, requiring immediate **ABC** care, **NOT** drug therapy; therefore **ONLY** administer atropine in cases of bradycardia caused by vagal stimulation (e.g. suction).

Quick Reference Table

DRUG	INITIAL DOSE	REPEAT DOSE	DOSE INTERVAL	CONCENTRATION	VOLUME	MAXIMUM DOSE	ROUTE
ADRENALINE anaphylaxis/asthma	150 micrograms	150 micrograms	5 minutes	1 milligram in 1 ml (1:1,000)	0.15 ml	No limit	IM
BENZYLPENICILLIN (IV/IO)	600 milligrams	NONE	N/A	600 milligrams in 9.6 ml	10 ml	600 milligrams	IV/IO
BENZYLPENICILLIN (IM)	600 milligrams	NONE	N/A	600 milligrams in 1.6 ml	2 ml	600 milligrams	IM
CHLORPHENAMINE (Oral)	1 milligram	NONE	N/A	Various	N/A	N/A	Oral
CHLORPHENAMINE (IV/IO)	2.5 milligrams	NONE	N/A	10 milligrams in 1 ml	0.25 ml	2.5 milligrams	IV/IO
DEXAMETHASONE-croup	2 milligrams	NONE	N/A	4 milligrams per ml (use intravenous preparation orally)	0.5 ml	2 milligrams	Oral
DIAZEPAM (IV/IO)	3 milligrams	NONE	N/A	10 milligrams in 2 ml	0.6 ml	3 milligrams	IV/IO
DIAZEPAM (PR)	5 milligrams	NONE	N/A	5 milligrams in 2.5 ml	1 × 5 milligram tube	5 milligrams	PR
GLUCAGON	500 micrograms	NONE	N/A	1 milligram per vial	0.5 vial	500 micrograms	IM
GLUCOSE 10%	2 grams	2 grams	5 minutes	50 grams in 500 ml	20 ml	6 grams	IV/IO
HYDROCORTISONE	50 milligrams	NONE	N/A	100 milligrams in 1 ml	0.5 ml	50 milligrams	IV/IO/IM
HYDROCORTISONE	50 milligrams	NONE	N/A	100 milligrams in 2 ml	1 ml	50 milligrams	IV/IO/IM
IBUPROFEN	100 milligrams	100 milligrams	8 hours	100 milligrams in 5 ml	5 ml	300 milligrams	Oral
IPRATROPIUM	125–250 micrograms	NONE	N/A	250 micrograms in 1 ml	0.5 ml – 1 ml	125–250 micrograms	Neb
IPRATROPIUM	125–250 micrograms	NONE	N/A	500 micrograms in 2 ml	0.5ml – 1 ml	125–250 micrograms	Neb
PATIENT'S OWN MIDAZOLAM[b]	5 milligrams	NONE	N/A	10 milligrams in 1 ml	0.5 ml	5 milligrams	Buccal
MORPHINE (IV/IO)	1 milligram	1 milligram	5 minutes	10 milligrams in 10 ml	1 ml	2 milligrams	IV/IO
MORPHINE (Oral)	2 milligrams	NONE	N/A	10 milligrams in 5 ml	1 ml	2 milligrams	Oral
NALOXONE NB cautions (IV/IO)	100 micrograms	100 micrograms	3 minutes	400 micrograms in 1 ml	0.25 ml	No limit	IV/IO
NALOXONE-INITIAL DOSE (IM)	100 micrograms	See below	3 minutes	400 micrograms in 1 ml	0.25 ml	See below	IM
NALOXONE-REPEAT DOSE (IM)	–	400 micrograms	–	400 micrograms in 1 ml	1 ml	500 micrograms	
ONDANSETRON	1 milligram	NONE	N/A	2 milligrams in 1 ml	0.5 ml	1 milligram	IV/IO/IM
PARACETAMOL (Oral)	120 milligrams	120 milligrams	4–6 hours	120 milligrams in 5 ml (infant suspension)	5 ml	480 milligrams in 24 hours	Oral
PARACETAMOL (IV/IO)	125 milligrams	125 milligrams	4–6 hours	10 milligrams in 1 ml	12.5 ml	500 milligrams in 24 hours	IV/IO
SALBUTAMOL	2.5 milligrams	2.5 milligrams	5 minutes	2.5 milligrams in 2.5 ml	2.5 ml	No limit	Neb
SALBUTAMOL	2.5 milligrams	2.5 milligrams	5 minutes	5 milligrams in 2.5 ml	1.25 ml	No limit	Neb
TRANEXAMIC ACID	150 mg	NONE	N/A	100 mg/ml	1.5 mls	150 mg	IV

[b] Give the dose as prescribed in the child's individualised treatment plan (the dosages described above reflect the recommended dosages for a child of this age).

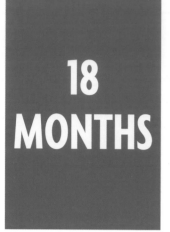

18 MONTHS

Vital Signs

	GUIDE WEIGHT 11 kg		HEART RATE 110–150		RESPIRATION RATE 25–35		SYSTOLIC BLOOD PRESSURE 80–95

Airway Size by Type

OROPHARYNGEAL AIRWAY	LARYNGEAL MASK	I-GEL AIRWAY	ENDOTRACHEAL TUBE
00 OR 0	2	1.5 OR 2	Diameter: **4.5 mm**; Length: **13 cm**

Defibrillation – Cardiac Arrest

MANUAL	AUTOMATED EXTERNAL DEFIBRILLATOR
50 Joules	A standard AED (either with paediatric attenuation pads or else in paediatric mode) can be used. If paediatric pads are not available, standard adult pads can used (but must not overlap).

Intravascular Fluid

FLUID	INITIAL DOSE	REPEAT DOSE	DOSE INTERVAL	CONCENTRATION	VOLUME	MAXIMUM DOSE	ROUTE
Sodium chloride (5 ml/kg)	55 ml	55 ml	PRN	0.9%	55 ml	440 ml	IV/IO
Sodium chloride (10 ml/kg)	110 ml	110 ml	PRN	0.9%	100 ml	440 ml	IV/IO
Sodium chloride (20 ml/kg)	220 ml	220 ml	PRN	0.9%	220 ml	440 ml	IV/IO

Cardiac Arrest

DRUG	INITIAL DOSE	REPEAT DOSE	DOSE INTERVAL	CONCENTRATION	VOLUME	MAXIMUM DOSE	ROUTE
ADRENALINE	110 micrograms	110 micrograms	3–5 minutes	1 milligram in 10 ml (1:10,000)	1.1 ml	No limit	IV/IO
AMIODARONE	55 milligrams (after 3rd shock)	55 milligrams	After 5th shock	300 milligrams in 10 ml	1.8 ml	110 milligrams	IV/IO
ATROPINE[a]	200 micrograms	NONE	N/A	100 micrograms in 1 ml	2 ml	200 micrograms	IV/IO
ATROPINE[a]	200 micrograms	NONE	N/A	200 micrograms in 1 ml	1 ml	200 micrograms	IV/IO
ATROPINE[a]	200 micrograms	NONE	N/A	300 micrograms in 1 ml	0.7 ml	200 micrograms	IV/IO
ATROPINE[a]	200 micrograms	NONE	N/A	600 micrograms in 1 ml	0.3 ml	200 micrograms	IV/IO

[a] **BRADYCARDIA** in children is most commonly caused by **HYPOXIA**, requiring immediate **ABC** care, **NOT** drug therapy; therefore **ONLY** administer atropine in cases of bradycardia caused by vagal stimulation (e.g. suction).

Quick Reference Table

DRUG	INITIAL DOSE	REPEAT DOSE	DOSE INTERVAL	CONCENTRATION	VOLUME	MAXIMUM DOSE	ROUTE
ADRENALINE anaphylaxis/asthma	150 micrograms	150 micrograms	5 minutes	1 milligram in 1 ml (1:1,000)	0.15 ml	No limit	IM
BENZYLPENICILLIN (IV/IO)	600 milligrams	NONE	N/A	600 milligrams in 9.6 ml	10 ml	600 milligrams	IV/IO
BENZYLPENICILLIN (IM)	600 milligrams	NONE	N/A	600 milligrams in 1.6 ml	2 ml	600 milligrams	IM
CHLORPHENAMINE (Oral)	1 milligram	NONE	N/A	Various	N/A	1 milligram	Oral
CHLORPHENAMINE (IV/IO)	2.5 milligrams	NONE	N/A	10 milligrams in 1 ml	0.25 ml	2.5 milligrams	IV/IO
DEXAMETHASONE-croup	4 milligrams	NONE	N/A	4 milligrams per ml (use intravenous preparation orally)	1 ml	4 milligrams	Oral
DIAZEPAM (IV/IO)	3.5 milligrams	NONE	N/A	10 milligrams in 2 ml	0.7 ml	3.5 milligrams	IV/IO
DIAZEPAM (PR)	5 milligrams	NONE	N/A	5 milligrams in 2.5 ml	1 × 5 milligram tube	5 milligrams	PR
GLUCAGON	500 micrograms	NONE	N/A	1 milligram per vial	0.5 vial	500 micrograms	IM
GLUCOSE 10%	2 grams	2 grams	5 minutes	50 grams in 500 ml	20 ml	6 grams	IV/IO
HYDROCORTISONE	50 milligrams	NONE	N/A	100 milligrams in 1 ml	0.5 ml	50 milligrams	IV/IO/IM
HYDROCORTISONE	50 milligrams	NONE	N/A	100 milligrams in 2 ml	1 ml	50 milligrams	IV/IO/IM
IBUPROFEN	100 milligrams	100 milligrams	8 hours	100 milligrams in 5 ml	5 ml	300 milligrams	Oral
IPRATROPIUM	125–250 micrograms	NONE	N/A	250 micrograms in 1 ml	0.5 ml – 1 ml	125–250 micrograms	Neb
IPRATROPIUM	125–250 micrograms	NONE	N/A	500 micrograms in 2 ml	0.5 ml – 1 ml	125–250 micrograms	Neb
PATIENT'S OWN MIDAZOLAM[b]	5 milligrams	NONE	N/A	10 milligrams in 1 ml	0.5 ml	5 milligrams	Buccal
MORPHINE (IV/IO)	1 milligram	1 milligram	5 minutes	10 milligrams in 10 ml	1 ml	2 milligrams	IV/IO
MORPHINE (Oral)	2 milligrams	NONE	N/A	10 milligrams in 5 ml	1 ml	2 milligrams	Oral
NALOXONE NB cautions (IV/IO)	120 micrograms	120 micrograms	3 minutes	400 micrograms in 1 ml	0.3 ml	1320 micrograms	IV/IO
NALOXONE–INITIAL DOSE (IM)	120 micrograms	See below	3 minutes	400 micrograms in 1 ml	0.3 ml	See below	IM
NALOXONE-REPEAT DOSE (IM)	–	400 micrograms	–	400 micrograms in 1 ml	1 ml	520 micrograms	IM
ONDANSETRON	1 milligram	NONE	N/A	2 milligrams in 1 ml	0.5 ml	1 milligram	IV/IO/IM
PARACETAMOL (Oral)	120 milligrams	120 milligrams	4–6 hours	120 milligrams in 5 ml (infant suspension)	5 ml	480 milligrams in 24 hours	Oral
PARACETAMOL (IV/IO)	125 milligrams	125 milligrams	4–6 hours	10 milligrams in 1 ml	12.5 ml	500 milligrams in 24 hours	IV/IO
SALBUTAMOL	2.5 milligrams	2.5 milligrams	5 minutes	2.5 milligrams in 2.5 ml	2.5 ml	No limit	Neb
SALBUTAMOL	2.5 milligrams	2.5 milligrams	5 minutes	5 milligrams in 2.5 ml	1.25 ml	No limit	Neb
TRANEXAMIC ACID	150 mg	NONE	N/A	100 mg/ml	1.5 mls	150 mg	IV

[b] Give the dose as prescribed in the child's individualised treatment plan (the dosages described above reflect the recommended dosages for a child of this age).

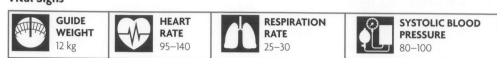

Page for Age

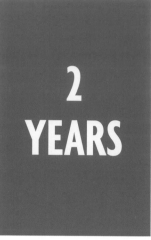

2 YEARS

Vital Signs

	GUIDE WEIGHT 12 kg		HEART RATE 95–140		RESPIRATION RATE 25–30		SYSTOLIC BLOOD PRESSURE 80–100

Airway Size by Type

OROPHARYNGEAL AIRWAY	LARYNGEAL MASK	I-GEL AIRWAY	ENDOTRACHEAL TUBE
0 OR 1	2	1.5 OR 2	Diameter: **5 mm**; Length: **14 cm**

Defibrillation – Cardiac Arrest

MANUAL	AUTOMATED EXTERNAL DEFIBRILLATOR
50 Joules	A standard AED (either with paediatric attenuation pads or else in paediatric mode) can be used. If paediatric pads are not available, standard adult pads can be used (but must not overlap).

Intravascular Fluid

FLUID	INITIAL DOSE	REPEAT DOSE	DOSE INTERVAL	CONCENTRATION	VOLUME	MAXIMUM DOSE	ROUTE
Sodium chloride (5 ml/kg)	60 ml	60 ml	PRN	0.9%	60 ml	480 ml	IV/IO
Sodium chloride (10 ml/kg)	120 ml	120 ml	PRN	0.9%	120 ml	480 ml	IV/IO
Sodium chloride (20 ml/kg)	240 ml	240 ml	PRN	0.9%	240 ml	480 ml	IV/IO

Cardiac Arrest

DRUG	INITIAL DOSE	REPEAT DOSE	DOSE INTERVAL	CONCENTRATION	VOLUME	MAXIMUM DOSE	ROUTE
ADRENALINE	120 micrograms	120 micrograms	3–5 minutes	1 milligram in 10 ml (1:10,000)	1.2 ml	No limit	IV/IO
AMIODARONE	60 milligrams (after 3rd shock)	60 milligrams	After 5th shock	300 milligrams in 10 ml	2 ml	120 milligrams	IV/IO
ATROPINE[a]	240 micrograms	NONE	N/A	100 micrograms in 1 ml	2.4 ml	240 micrograms	IV/IO
ATROPINE[a]	240 micrograms	NONE	N/A	200 micrograms in 1 ml	1.2 ml	240 micrograms	IV/IO
ATROPINE[a]	240 micrograms	NONE	N/A	300 micrograms in 1 ml	0.8 ml	240 micrograms	IV/IO
ATROPINE[a]	240 micrograms	NONE	N/A	600 micrograms in 1 ml	0.4 ml	240 micrograms	IV/IO

[a] **BRADYCARDIA** in children is most commonly caused by **HYPOXIA**, requiring immediate **ABC** care, **NOT** drug therapy; therefore **ONLY** administer atropine in cases of bradycardia caused by vagal stimulation (e.g. suction).

Quick Reference Table

DRUG	INITIAL DOSE	REPEAT DOSE	DOSE INTERVAL	CONCENTRATION	VOLUME	MAXIMUM DOSE	ROUTE
ADRENALINE anaphylaxis/asthma	150 micrograms	150 micrograms	5 minutes	1 milligram in 1ml (1:1,000)	0.15 ml	No limit	IM
BENZYLPENICILLIN (IV/IO)	600 milligrams	NONE	N/A	600 milligrams in 9.6 ml	10 ml	600 milligrams	IV/IO
BENZYLPENICILLIN (IM)	600 milligrams	NONE	N/A	600 milligrams in 1.6 ml	2 ml	600 milligrams	IM
CHLORPHENAMINE (Oral)	1 milligram	NONE	N/A	Various	N/A	1 milligram	Oral
CHLORPHENAMINE (IV/IO)	2.5 milligrams	NONE	N/A	10 milligrams in 1 ml	0.25 ml	2.5 milligrams	IV/IO
DEXAMETHASONE-croup	4 milligrams	NONE	N/A	4 milligrams per ml (use intravenous preparation orally)	1 ml	4 milligrams	Oral
DIAZEPAM (IV/IO)	3.5 milligrams	NONE	N/A	10 milligrams in 2 ml	0.7 ml	3.5 milligrams	IV/IO
DIAZEPAM (PR)	5 or 10 milligrams	NONE	N/A	5 milligrams in 2.5 ml or 10 milligrams in 2.5 ml	1 × 5 milligram tube or 1 × 10 milligram tube	5 or 10 milligrams	PR
GLUCAGON	500 micrograms	NONE	N/A	1 milligram per vial	0.5 vial	500 micrograms	IM
GLUCOSE 10%	2.5 grams	2.5 grams	5 minutes	50 grams in 500 ml	25 ml	7.5 grams	IV/IO
HYDROCORTISONE	50 milligrams	NONE	N/A	100 milligrams in 1 ml	0.5 ml	50 milligrams	IV/IO/IM
HYDROCORTISONE	50 milligrams	NONE	N/A	100 milligrams in 2 ml	1 ml	50 milligrams	IV/IO/IM
IBUPROFEN	100 milligrams	100 milligrams	8 hours	100 milligrams in 5 ml	5 ml	300 milligrams	Oral
IPRATROPIUM	250 micrograms	NONE	N/A	250 micrograms in 1 ml	1 ml	250 micrograms	Neb
IPRATROPIUM	250 micrograms	NONE	N/A	500 micrograms in 2 ml	1 ml	250 micrograms	Neb
PATIENT'S OWN MIDAZOLAM[b]	5 milligrams	NONE	N/A	10 milligrams in 1 ml	0.5 ml	5 milligrams	Buccal
MORPHINE (IV/IO)	1 milligram	1 milligram	5 minutes	10 milligrams in 10 ml	1 ml	2 milligrams	IV/IO
MORPHINE (Oral)	2 milligrams	NONE	N/A	10 milligrams in 5 ml	1 ml	2 milligrams	Oral
NALOXONE NB cautions (IV/IO)	120 micrograms	120 micrograms	3 minutes	400 micrograms in 1 ml	0.3 ml	1320 micrograms	IV/IO
NALOXONE– INITIAL DOSE (IM)	120 micrograms	See below	3 minutes	400 micrograms in 1 ml	0.3 ml	See below	IM
NALOXONE– REPEAT DOSE (IM)	–	400 micrograms	–	400 micrograms in 1 ml	1 ml	520 micrograms	
ONDANSETRON	1 milligram	NONE	N/A	2 milligrams in 1 ml	0.5 ml	1 milligram	IV/IO/IM
PARACETAMOL (Oral)	180 milligrams	180 milligrams	4–6 hours	120 milligrams in 5 ml (infant suspension)	7.5 ml	720 milligrams in 24 hours	Oral
PARACETAMOL (IV/IO)	125 milligrams	125 milligrams	4–6 hours	10 milligrams in 1 ml	12.5 ml	500 milligrams in 24 hours	IV/IO
SALBUTAMOL	2.5 milligrams	2.5 milligrams	5 minutes	2.5 milligrams in 2.5 ml	2.5 ml	No limit	Neb
SALBUTAMOL	2.5 milligrams	2.5 milligrams	5 minutes	5 milligrams in 2.5 ml	1.25 ml	No limit	Neb
TRANEXAMIC ACID	200 mg	NONE	N/A	100 mg/ml	2 mls	200 mg	IV

[b] Give the dose as prescribed in the child's individualised treatment plan (the dosages described above reflect the recommended dosages for a child of this age).

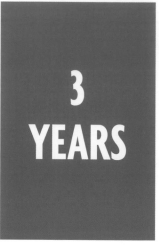

3 YEARS

Vital Signs

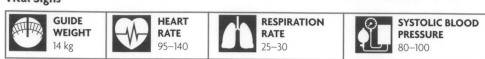

| | GUIDE WEIGHT 14 kg | | HEART RATE 95–140 | | RESPIRATION RATE 25–30 | | SYSTOLIC BLOOD PRESSURE 80–100 |

Airway Size by Type

OROPHARYNGEAL AIRWAY	LARYNGEAL MASK	I-GEL AIRWAY	ENDOTRACHEAL TUBE
1	2	2	Diameter: **5 mm**; Length: **14 cm**

Defibrillation – Cardiac Arrest

MANUAL	AUTOMATED EXTERNAL DEFIBRILLATOR
60 Joules	A standard AED (either with paediatric attenuation pads or else in paediatric mode) can be used. If paediatric pads are not available, standard adult pads can be used (but must not overlap).

Intravascular Fluid

FLUID	INITIAL DOSE	REPEAT DOSE	DOSE INTERVAL	CONCENTRATION	VOLUME	MAXIMUM DOSE	ROUTE
Sodium chloride (5 ml/kg)	70 ml	70 ml	PRN	0.9%	70 ml	560 ml	IV/IO
Sodium chloride (10 ml/kg)	140 ml	140 ml	PRN	0.9%	140 ml	560 ml	IV/IO
Sodium chloride (20 ml/kg)	280 ml	280 ml	PRN	0.9%	280 ml	560 ml	IV/IO

Cardiac Arrest

DRUG	INITIAL DOSE	REPEAT DOSE	DOSE INTERVAL	CONCENTRATION	VOLUME	MAXIMUM DOSE	ROUTE
ADRENALINE	140 micrograms	140 micrograms	3–5 minutes	1 milligram in 10 ml (1:10,000)	1.4 ml	No limit	IV/IO
AMIODARONE	70 milligrams (after 3rd shock)	70 milligrams	After 5th shock	300 milligrams in 10 ml	2.3 ml	140 milligrams	IV/IO
ATROPINE[a]	240 micrograms	NONE	N/A	100 micrograms in 1 ml	2.4 ml	240 micrograms	IV/IO
ATROPINE[a]	240 micrograms	NONE	N/A	200 micrograms in 1 ml	1.2 ml	240 micrograms	IV/IO
ATROPINE[a]	240 micrograms	NONE	N/A	300 micrograms in 1 ml	0.8 ml	240 micrograms	IV/IO
ATROPINE[a]	240 micrograms	NONE	N/A	600 micrograms in 1 ml	0.4 ml	240 micrograms	IV/IO

[a] **BRADYCARDIA** in children is most commonly caused by **HYPOXIA**, requiring immediate **ABC** care, **NOT** drug therapy; therefore **ONLY** administer atropine in cases of bradycardia caused by vagal stimulation (e.g. suction).

Quick Reference Table

DRUG	INITIAL DOSE	REPEAT DOSE	DOSE INTERVAL	CONCENTRATION	VOLUME	MAXIMUM DOSE	ROUTE
ADRENALINE anaphylaxis/asthma	150 micrograms	150 micrograms	5 minutes	1 milligram in 1 ml (1:1,000)	0.15 ml	No limit	IM
BENZYLPENICILLIN (IV/IO)	600 milligrams	NONE	N/A	600 milligrams in 9.6 ml	10 ml	600 milligrams	IV/IO
BENZYLPENICILLIN (IM)	600 milligrams	NONE	N/A	600 milligrams in 1.6 ml	2 ml	600 milligrams	IM
CHLORPHENAMINE (Oral)	1 milligram	NONE	N/A	Various	N/A	1 milligram	Oral
CHLORPHENAMINE (IV/IO)	2.5 milligrams	NONE	N/A	10 milligrams in 1 ml	0.25 ml	2.5 milligrams	IV/IO
DEXAMETHASONE-croup	4 milligrams	NONE	N/A	4 milligrams per ml (use intravenous preparation orally)	1 ml	4 milligrams	Oral
DIAZEPAM (IV/IO)	4.5 milligrams	NONE	N/A	10 milligrams in 2 ml	0.9 ml	4.5 milligrams	IV/IO
DIAZEPAM (PR)	5 or 10 milligrams	NONE	N/A	5 milligrams in 2.5 ml or 10 milligrams in 2.5 ml	1 × 5 milligram tube or 1 × 10 milligram tube	5 or 10 milligrams	PR
GLUCAGON	500 micrograms	NONE	N/A	1 milligram per vial	0.5 vial	500 micrograms	IM
GLUCOSE 10%	3 grams	3 grams	5 minutes	50 grams in 500 ml	30 ml	9 grams	IV/IO
HYDROCORTISONE	50 milligrams	NONE	N/A	100 milligrams in 1 ml	0.5 ml	50 milligrams	IV/IO/IM
HYDROCORTISONE	50 milligrams	NONE	N/A	100 milligrams in 2 ml	1 ml	50 milligrams	IV/IO/IM
IBUPROFEN	100 milligrams	100 milligrams	8 hours	100 milligrams in 5 ml	5 ml	300 milligrams	Oral
IPRATROPIUM	250 micrograms	NONE	N/A	250 micrograms in 1 ml	1 ml	250 micrograms	Neb
IPRATROPIUM	250 micrograms	NONE	N/A	500 micrograms in 2 ml	1 ml	250 micrograms	Neb
PATIENT'S OWN MIDAZOLAM[b]	5 milligrams	NONE	N/A	10 milligrams in 1 ml	0.5 ml	5 milligrams	Buccal
MORPHINE (IV/IO)	1.5 milligrams	1.5 milligrams	5 minutes	10 milligrams in 10 ml	1.5 ml	3 milligrams	IV/IO
MORPHINE (Oral)	3 milligrams	NONE	N/A	10 milligrams in 5 ml	1.5 ml	3 milligrams	Oral
NALOXONE NB cautions (IV/IO)	160 micrograms	160 micrograms	3 minutes	400 micrograms in 1 ml	0.4 ml	1760 micrograms	IV/IO
NALOXONE– INITIAL DOSE (IM)	160 micrograms	See below	3 minutes	400 micrograms in 1 ml	0.4 ml	See below	IM
NALOXONE– REPEAT DOSE (IM)	–	400 micrograms	–	400 micrograms in 1 ml	1 ml	560 micrograms	
ONDANSETRON	1.5 milligrams	NONE	N/A	2 milligrams in 1 ml	0.75 ml	1.5 milligrams	IV/IO/IM
PARACETAMOL (Oral)	180 milligrams	180 milligrams	4–6 hours	120 milligrams in 5 ml (infant suspension)	7.5 ml	720 milligrams in 24 hours	Oral
PARACETAMOL (IV/IO)	250 milligrams	250 milligrams	4–6 hours	10 milligrams in 1 ml	25 ml	1 gram in 24 hours	IV/IO
SALBUTAMOL	2.5 milligrams	2.5 milligrams	5 minutes	2.5 milligrams in 2.5 ml	2.5 ml	No limit	Neb
SALBUTAMOL	2.5 milligrams	2.5 milligrams	5 minutes	5 milligrams in 2.5 ml	1.25 ml	No limit	Neb
TRANEXAMIC ACID	200 mg	NONE	N/A	100 mg/ml	2 mls	200 mg	IV

[b]Give the dose as prescribed in the child's individualised treatment plan (the dosages described above reflect the recommended dosages for a child of this age).

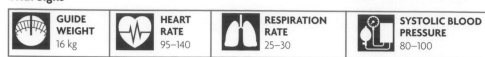

Page for Age

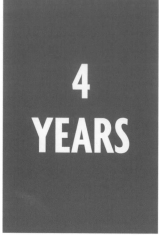

4 YEARS

Vital Signs

	GUIDE WEIGHT		HEART RATE		RESPIRATION RATE		SYSTOLIC BLOOD PRESSURE
	16 kg		95–140		25–30		80–100

Airway Size by Type

OROPHARYNGEAL AIRWAY	LARYNGEAL MASK	I-GEL AIRWAY	ENDOTRACHEAL TUBE
1	2	2	Diameter: **5 mm**; Length: **15 cm**

Defibrillation – Cardiac Arrest

MANUAL	AUTOMATED EXTERNAL DEFIBRILLATOR
70 Joules	A standard AED (either with paediatric attenuation pads or else in paediatric mode) can be used. If paediatric pads are not available, standard adult pads can be used (but must not overlap).

Intravascular Fluid

FLUID	INITIAL DOSE	REPEAT DOSE	DOSE INTERVAL	CONCENTRATION	VOLUME	MAXIMUM DOSE	ROUTE
Sodium chloride (5 ml/kg)	80 ml	80 ml	PRN	0.9%	80 ml	640 ml	IV/IO
Sodium chloride (10 ml/kg)	160 ml	160 ml	PRN	0.9%	160 ml	640 ml	IV/IO
Sodium chloride (20 ml/kg)	320 ml	320 ml	PRN	0.9%	320 ml	640 ml	IV/IO

Cardiac Arrest

DRUG	INITIAL DOSE	REPEAT DOSE	DOSE INTERVAL	CONCENTRATION	VOLUME	MAXIMUM DOSE	ROUTE
ADRENALINE	160 micrograms	160 micrograms	3–5 minutes	1 milligram in 10 ml (1:10,000)	1.6 ml	No limit	IV/IO
AMIODARONE	80 milligrams (after 3rd shock)	80 milligrams	After 5th shock	300 milligrams in 10 ml	2.7 ml	160 milligrams	IV/IO
ATROPINE[a]	300 micrograms	NONE	N/A	100 micrograms in 1 ml	3 ml	300 micrograms	IV/IO
ATROPINE[a]	300 micrograms	NONE	N/A	200 micrograms in 1 ml	1.5 ml	300 micrograms	IV/IO
ATROPINE[a]	300 micrograms	NONE	N/A	300 micrograms in 1 ml	1 ml	300 micrograms	IV/IO
ATROPINE[a]	300 micrograms	NONE	N/A	600 micrograms in 1 ml	0.5 ml	300 micrograms	IV/IO

[a] **BRADYCARDIA** in children is most commonly caused by **HYPOXIA**, requiring immediate **ABC** care, **NOT** drug therapy; therefore **ONLY** administer atropine in cases of bradycardia caused by vagal stimulation (e.g. suction).

Quick Reference Table

DRUG	INITIAL DOSE	REPEAT DOSE	DOSE INTERVAL	CONCENTRATION	VOLUME	MAXIMUM DOSE	ROUTE
ADRENALINE anaphylaxis/asthma	150 micrograms	150 micrograms	5 minutes	1 milligram in 1 ml (1:1,000)	0.15 ml	No limit	IM
BENZYLPENICILLIN (IV/IO)	600 milligrams	NONE	N/A	600 milligrams in 9.6 ml	10 ml	600 milligrams	IV/IO
BENZYLPENICILLIN (IM)	600 milligrams	NONE	N/A	600 milligrams in 1.6 ml	2 ml	600 milligrams	IM
CHLORPHENAMINE (Oral)	1 milligram	NONE	N/A	Various	N/A	1 milligram	Oral
CHLORPHENAMINE (IV/IO)	2.5 milligrams	NONE	N/A	10 milligrams in 1 ml	0.25 ml	2.5 milligrams	IV/IO
DEXAMETHASONE-croup	4 milligrams	NONE	N/A	4 milligrams per ml (use intravenous preparation orally)	1 ml	4 milligrams	Oral
DIAZEPAM (IV/IO)	5 milligrams	NONE	N/A	10 milligrams in 2 ml	1 ml	5 milligrams	IV/IO
DIAZEPAM (PR)	5 or 10 milligrams	NONE	N/A	5 milligrams in 2.5 ml or 10 milligrams in 2.5 ml	1 × 5 milligram tube or 1 × 10 milligram tube	5 or 10 milligrams	PR
GLUCAGON	500 micrograms	NONE	N/A	1 milligram per vial	0.5 vial	500 micrograms	IM
GLUCOSE 10%	3 grams	3 grams	5 minutes	50 grams in 500 ml	30 ml	9 grams	IV/IO
HYDROCORTISONE	50 milligrams	NONE	N/A	100 milligrams in 1 ml	0.5 ml	50 milligrams	IV/IO/IM
HYDROCORTISONE	50 milligrams	NONE	N/A	100 milligrams in 2 ml	1 ml	50 milligrams	IV/IO/IM
IBUPROFEN	150 milligrams	150 milligrams	8 hours	100 milligrams in 5 ml	7.5 ml	450 milligrams	Oral
IPRATROPIUM	250 micrograms	NONE	N/A	250 micrograms in 1 ml	1 ml	250 micrograms	Neb
IPRATROPIUM	250 micrograms	NONE	N/A	500 micrograms in 2 ml	1 ml	250 micrograms	Neb
PATIENT'S OWN MIDAZOLAM[b]	5 milligrams	NONE	N/A	10 milligrams in 1 ml	0.5 ml	5 milligrams	Buccal
MORPHINE (IV/IO)	1.5 milligrams	1.5 milligrams	5 minutes	10 milligrams in 10 ml	1.5 ml	3 milligrams	IV/IO
MORPHINE (Oral)	3 milligrams	NONE	N/A	10 milligrams in 5 ml	1.5 ml	3 milligrams	Oral
NALOXONE NB cautions (IV/IO)	160 micrograms	160 micrograms	3 minutes	400 micrograms in 1 ml	0.4 ml	1760 micrograms	IV/IO
NALOXONE–INITIAL DOSE (IM)	160 micrograms	See below	3 minutes	400 micrograms in 1 ml	0.4 ml	See below	IM
NALOXONE–REPEAT DOSE (IM)	–	400 micrograms	–	400 micrograms in 1 ml	1 ml	560 micrograms	
ONDANSETRON	1.5 milligrams	NONE	N/A	2 micrograms in 1 ml	0.75 ml	1.5 milligrams	IV/IO/IM
PARACETAMOL (Oral)	240 milligrams	240 milligrams	4–6 hours	120 milligrams in 5 ml (infant suspension)	10 ml	960 milligrams in 24 hours	Oral
PARACETAMOL (IV/IO)	250 milligrams	250 milligrams	4–6 hours	10 milligrams in 1 ml	25 ml	1 gram in 24 hours	IV/IO
SALBUTAMOL	2.5 milligrams	2.5 milligrams	5 minutes	2.5 milligrams in 2.5 ml	2.5 ml	No limit	Neb
SALBUTAMOL	2.5 milligrams	2.5 milligrams	5 minutes	5 milligrams in 2.5 ml	1.25 ml	No limit	Neb
TRANEXAMIC ACID	250 mg	NONE	N/A	100 mg/ml	2.5 mls	250 mg	IV

[b]Give the dose as prescribed in the child's individualised treatment plan (the dosages described above reflect the recommended dosages for a child of this age).

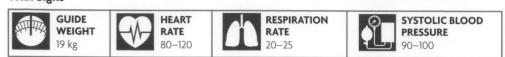

Page for Age

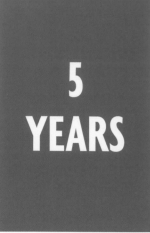

5 YEARS

Vital Signs

	GUIDE WEIGHT 19 kg		HEART RATE 80–120		RESPIRATION RATE 20–25		SYSTOLIC BLOOD PRESSURE 90–100

Airway Size by Type

OROPHARYNGEAL AIRWAY	LARYNGEAL MASK	I-GEL AIRWAY	ENDOTRACHEAL TUBE
1	2	2	Diameter: **5.5 mm**; Length: **15 cm**

Defibrillation – Cardiac Arrest

MANUAL	AUTOMATED EXTERNAL DEFIBRILLATOR
80 Joules	A standard AED (either with paediatric attenuation pads or else in paediatric mode) can be used. If paediatric pads are not available, standard adult pads can be used (but must not overlap).

Intravascular Fluid

FLUID	INITIAL DOSE	REPEAT DOSE	DOSE INTERVAL	CONCENTRATION	VOLUME	MAXIMUM DOSE	ROUTE
Sodium chloride (5 ml/kg)	95 ml	95 ml	PRN	0.9%	95 ml	760 ml	IV/IO
Sodium chloride (10 ml/kg)	190 ml	190 ml	PRN	0.9%	190 ml	760 ml	IV/IO
Sodium chloride (20 ml/kg)	380 ml	380 ml	PRN	0.9%	380 ml	760 ml	IV/IO

Cardiac Arrest

DRUG	INITIAL DOSE	REPEAT DOSE	DOSE INTERVAL	CONCENTRATION	VOLUME	MAXIMUM DOSE	ROUTE
ADRENALINE	190 micrograms	190 micrograms	3–5 minutes	1 milligram in 10 ml (1:10,000)	1.9 ml	No limit	IV/IO
AMIODARONE	100 milligrams (after 3rd shock)	100 milligrams	After 5th shock	300 milligrams in 10 ml	3.3 ml	200 milligrams	IV/IO
ATROPINE[a]	300 micrograms	NONE	N/A	100 micrograms in 1 ml	3 ml	300 micrograms	IV/IO
ATROPINE[a]	300 micrograms	NONE	N/A	200 micrograms in 1 ml	1.5 ml	300 micrograms	IV/IO
ATROPINE[a]	300 micrograms	NONE	N/A	300 micrograms in 1 ml	1 ml	300 micrograms	IV/IO
ATROPINE[a]	300 micrograms	NONE	N/A	600 micrograms in 1 ml	0.5 ml	300 micrograms	IV/IO

[a] **BRADYCARDIA** in children is most commonly caused by **HYPOXIA**, requiring immediate **ABC** care, **NOT** drug therapy; therefore **ONLY** administer atropine in cases of bradycardia caused by vagal stimulation (e.g. suction).

Quick Reference Table

DRUG	INITIAL DOSE	REPEAT DOSE	DOSE INTERVAL	CONCENTRATION	VOLUME	MAXIMUM DOSE	ROUTE
ADRENALINE anaphylaxis/asthma	150 micrograms	150 micrograms	5 minutes	1 milligram in 1 ml (1:1,000)	0.15 ml	No limit	IM
BENZYLPENICILLIN (IV/IO)	600 milligrams	NONE	N/A	600 milligrams in 9.6 ml	10 ml	600 milligrams	IV/IO
BENZYLPENICILLIN (IM)	600 milligrams	NONE	N/A	600 milligrams in 1.6 ml	2 ml	600 milligrams	IM
CHLORPHENAMINE (Oral)	1 milligram	NONE	N/A	Various	N/A	1 milligram	Oral
CHLORPHENAMINE (IV/IO)	2.5 milligrams	NONE	N/A	10 milligrams in 1 ml	0.25 ml	2.5 milligrams	IV/IO
DEXAMETHASONE-croup	4 milligrams	NONE	N/A	4 milligrams per ml (use intravenous preparation orally)	1 ml	4 milligrams	Oral
DIAZEPAM (IV/IO)	6 milligrams	NONE	N/A	10 milligrams in 2 ml	1.2 ml	6 milligrams	IV/IO
DIAZEPAM (PR)	5 or 10 milligrams	NONE	N/A	5 milligrams in 2.5 ml or 10 milligrams in 2.5 ml	1 × 5 milligram tube or 1 × 10 milligram tube	5 or 10 milligrams	PR
GLUCAGON	500 micrograms	NONE	N/A	1 milligram per vial	0.5 vial	500 micrograms	IM
GLUCOSE 10%	4 grams	4 grams	5 minutes	50 grams in 500 ml	40 ml	12 grams	IV/IO
HYDROCORTISONE	50 milligrams	NONE	N/A	100 milligrams in 1 ml	0.5 ml	50 milligrams	IV/IO/IM
HYDROCORTISONE	50 milligrams	NONE	N/A	100 milligrams in 2 ml	1 ml	50 milligrams	IV/IO/IM
IBUPROFEN	150 milligrams	150 milligrams	8 hours	100 milligrams in 5 ml	7.5 ml	450 milligrams	Oral
IPRATROPIUM	250 micrograms	NONE	N/A	250 micrograms in 1 ml	1 ml	250 micrograms	Neb
IPRATROPIUM	250 micrograms	NONE	N/A	500 micrograms in 2 ml	1 ml	250 micrograms	Neb
PATIENT'S OWN MIDAZOLAM[b]	7.5 milligrams	NONE	N/A	10 milligrams in 1 ml	0.75 ml	7.5 milligrams	Buccal
MORPHINE (IV/IO)	2 milligrams	2 milligrams	5 minutes	10 milligrams in 10 ml	2 ml	4 milligrams	IV/IO
MORPHINE (Oral)	4 milligrams	NONE	N/A	10 milligrams in 5 ml	2 ml	4 milligrams	Oral
NALOXONE NB cautions (IV/IO)	200 micrograms	200 micrograms	3 minutes	400 micrograms in 1 ml	0.5 ml	2200 micrograms	IV/IO
NALOXONE–INITIAL DOSE (IM)	200 micrograms	See below	3 minutes	400 micrograms in 1 ml	0.5 ml	See below	IM
NALOXONE–REPEAT DOSE (IM)	–	400 micrograms	–	400 micrograms in 1 ml	1 ml	600 micrograms	
ONDANSETRON	2 milligrams	NONE	N/A	2 milligrams in 1 ml	1 ml	2 milligrams	IV/IO/IM
PARACETAMOL (Oral)	240 milligrams	240 milligrams	4–6 hours	120 milligrams in 5 ml (infant suspension)	10 ml	960 milligrams in 24 hours	Oral
PARACETAMOL (IV/IO)	250 milligrams	250 milligrams	4–6 hours	10 milligrams in 1 ml	25 ml	1 gram in 24 hours	IV/IO
SALBUTAMOL	2.5 milligrams	2.5 milligrams	5 minutes	2.5 milligrams in 2.5 ml	2.5 ml	No limit	Neb
SALBUTAMOL	2.5 milligrams	2.5 milligrams	5 minutes	5 milligrams in 2.5 ml	1.25 ml	No limit	Neb
TRANEXAMIC ACID	300 mg	NONE	N/A	100 mg/ml	3 mls	300 mg	IV

[b] Give the dose as prescribed in the child's individualised treatment plan (the dosages described above reflect the recommended dosages for a child of this age).

Page for Age

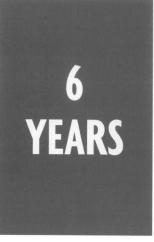

6 YEARS

Vital Signs

GUIDE WEIGHT 21 kg	HEART RATE 80–120	RESPIRATION RATE 20–25	SYSTOLIC BLOOD PRESSURE 80–110

Airway Size by Type

OROPHARYNGEAL AIRWAY	LARYNGEAL MASK	I-GEL AIRWAY	ENDOTRACHEAL TUBE
1	2.5	2	Diameter: **6 mm**; Length: **16 cm**

Defibrillation – Cardiac Arrest

MANUAL	AUTOMATED EXTERNAL DEFIBRILLATOR
80 Joules	A standard AED (either with paediatric attenuation pads or else in paediatric mode) can be used. If paediatric pads are not available, standard adult pads can be used (but must not overlap).

Intravascular Fluid

FLUID	INITIAL DOSE	REPEAT DOSE	DOSE INTERVAL	CONCENTRATION	VOLUME	MAXIMUM DOSE	ROUTE
Sodium chloride (5 ml/kg)	105 ml	105 ml	PRN	0.9%	105 ml	840 ml	IV/IO
Sodium chloride (10 ml/kg)	210 ml	210 ml	PRN	0.9%	210 ml	840 ml	IV/IO
Sodium chloride (20 ml/kg)	420 ml	420 ml	PRN	0.9%	420 ml	840 ml	IV/IO

Cardiac Arrest

DRUG	INITIAL DOSE	REPEAT DOSE	DOSE INTERVAL	CONCENTRATION	VOLUME	MAXIMUM DOSE	ROUTE
ADRENALINE	210 micrograms	210 micrograms	3–5 minutes	1 milligram in 10 ml (1:10,000)	2.1 ml	No limit	IV/IO
AMIODARONE	100 milligrams (after 3rd shock)	100 milligrams	After 5th shock	300 milligrams in 10 ml	3.3 ml	200 milligrams	IV/IO
ATROPINE[a]	400 micrograms	NONE	N/A	100 micrograms in 1 ml	4 ml	400 micrograms	IV/IO
ATROPINE[a]	400 micrograms	NONE	N/A	200 micrograms in 1 ml	2 ml	400 micrograms	IV/IO
ATROPINE[a]	400 micrograms	NONE	N/A	300 micrograms in 1 ml	1.3 ml	400 micrograms	IV/IO
ATROPINE[a]	400 micrograms	NONE	N/A	600 micrograms in 1 ml	0.7 ml	400 micrograms	IV/IO

[a] **BRADYCARDIA** in children is most commonly caused by **HYPOXIA**, requiring immediate **ABC** care, **NOT** drug therapy; therefore **ONLY** administer atropine in cases of bradycardia caused by vagal stimulation (e.g. suction).

Quick Reference Table

DRUG	INITIAL DOSE	REPEAT DOSE	DOSE INTERVAL	CONCENTRATION	VOLUME	MAXIMUM DOSE	ROUTE
ADRENALINE anaphylaxis/asthma	300 micrograms	300 micrograms	5 minutes	1 milligram in 1 ml (1:1,000)	0.3 ml	No limit	IM
BENZYLPENICILLIN (IV/IO)	600 milligrams	NONE	N/A	600 milligrams in 9.6 ml	10 ml	600 milligrams	IV/IO
BENZYLPENICILLIN (IM)	600 milligrams	NONE	N/A	600 milligrams in 1.6 ml	2 ml	600 milligrams	IM
CHLORPHENAMINE (Oral)	2 milligrams	NONE	N/A	Various	N/A	2 milligram	Oral
CHLORPHENAMINE (IV/IO)	5–10 milligrams	NONE	N/A	10 milligrams in 1 ml	0.5–1 ml	5–10 milligrams	IV/IO
DEXAMETHASONE – croup	4 milligrams	NONE	N/A	4 milligrams per ml (use intravenous preparation orally)	1 ml	4 milligrams	Oral
DIAZEPAM (IV/IO)	6.5 milligrams	NONE	N/A	10 milligrams in 2 ml	1.3 ml	6.5 milligrams	IV/IO
DIAZEPAM (PR)	5 or 10 milligrams	NONE	N/A	5 milligrams in 2.5 ml or 10 milligrams in 2.5 ml	1 × 5 milligram tube or 1 × 10 milligram tube	5 or 10 milligrams	PR
GLUCAGON	500 micrograms	NONE	N/A	1 milligram per vial	0.5 vial	500 micrograms	IM
GLUCOSE 10%	4 grams	4 grams	5 minutes	50 grams in 500 ml	40 ml	12 grams	IV/IO
HYDROCORTISONE	100 milligrams	NONE	N/A	100 milligrams in 1 ml	1 ml	100 milligrams	IV/IO/IM
HYDROCORTISONE	100 milligrams	NONE	N/A	100 milligrams in 2 ml	2 ml	100 milligrams	IV/IO/IM
IBUPROFEN	150 milligrams	150 milligrams	8 hours	100 milligrams in 5 ml	7.5 ml	450 milligrams	Oral
IPRATROPIUM	250 micrograms	NONE	N/A	250 micrograms in 1 ml	1 ml	250 micrograms	Neb
IPRATROPIUM	250 micrograms	NONE	N/A	500 micrograms in 2 ml	1 ml	250 micrograms	Neb
PATIENT'S OWN MIDAZOLAM[b]	7.5 milligrams	NONE	N/A	10 milligrams in 1 ml	0.75 ml	7.5 milligrams	Buccal
MORPHINE (IV/IO)	2 milligrams	2 milligrams	5 minutes	10 milligrams in 10 ml	2 ml	4 milligrams	IV/IO
MORPHINE (Oral)	4 milligrams	NONE	N/A	10 milligrams in 5 ml	2 ml	4 milligrams	Oral
NALOXONE NB cautions (IV/IO)	200 micrograms	200 micrograms	3 minutes	400 micrograms in 1 ml	0.5 ml	2200 micrograms	IV/IO
NALOXONE– INITIAL DOSE (IM)	200 micrograms	See below	3 minutes	400 micrograms in 1 ml	0.5 ml	See below	IM
NALOXONE– REPEAT DOSE (IM)	–	400 micrograms	–	400 micrograms in 1 ml	1 ml	600 micrograms	
ONDANSETRON	2 milligrams	NONE	N/A	2 milligrams in 1 ml	1 ml	2 milligrams	IV/IO/IM
PARACETAMOL (Oral)	250 milligrams	250 milligrams	4–6 hours	250 milligrams in 5 ml (six plus suspension)	5 ml	1 grams in 24 hours	Oral
PARACETAMOL (IV/IO)	300 milligrams	300 milligrams	4–6 hours	10 milligrams in 1 ml	30 ml	1.2 gram in 24 hours	IV/IO
SALBUTAMOL	5 milligrams	5 milligrams	5 minutes	2.5 milligrams in 2.5 ml	5 ml	No limit	Neb
SALBUTAMOL	5 milligrams	5 milligrams	5 minutes	5 milligrams in 2.5 ml	2.5 ml	No limit	Neb
TRANEXAMIC ACID	300 mg	NONE	N/A	100 mg/ml	3 mls	300 mg	IV

[b] Give the dose as prescribed in the child's individualised treatment plan (the dosages described above reflect the recommended dosages for a child of this age).

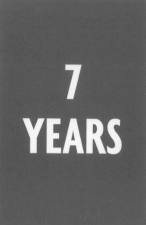

7 YEARS

Vital Signs

	GUIDE WEIGHT 23 kg		HEART RATE 80–120		RESPIRATION RATE 20–25		SYSTOLIC BLOOD PRESSURE 90–110

Airway Size by Type

OROPHARYNGEAL AIRWAY	LARYNGEAL MASK	I-GEL AIRWAY	ENDOTRACHEAL TUBE
1 OR 2	2.5	2	Diameter: **6 mm**; Length: **16 cm**

Defibrillation – Cardiac Arrest

MANUAL	AUTOMATED EXTERNAL DEFIBRILLATOR
100 Joules	A standard AED (either with paediatric attenuation pads or else in paediatric mode) can be used. If paediatric pads are not available, standard adult pads can be used (but must not overlap).

Intravascular Fluid

FLUID	INITIAL DOSE	REPEAT DOSE	DOSE INTERVAL	CONCENTRATION	VOLUME	MAXIMUM DOSE	ROUTE
Sodium chloride (5 ml/kg)	115 ml	115 ml	PRN	0.9%	115 ml	920 ml	IV/IO
Sodium chloride (10 ml/kg)	230 ml	230 ml	PRN	0.9%	230 ml	920 ml	IV/IO
Sodium chloride (20 ml/kg)	460 ml	460 ml	PRN	0.9%	460 ml	920 ml	IV/IO

Cardiac Arrest

DRUG	INITIAL DOSE	REPEAT DOSE	DOSE INTERVAL	CONCENTRATION	VOLUME	MAXIMUM DOSE	ROUTE
ADRENALINE	230 micrograms	230 micrograms	3–5 minutes	1 milligram in 10 ml (1:10,000)	2.3 ml	No limit	IV/IO
AMIODARONE	120 milligrams (after 3rd shock)	120 milligrams	After 5th shock	300 milligrams in 10 ml	4 ml	240 milligrams	IV/IO
ATROPINE[a]	400 micrograms	NONE	N/A	100 micrograms in 1 ml	4 ml	400 micrograms	IV/IO
ATROPINE[a]	400 micrograms	NONE	N/A	200 micrograms in 1 ml	2 ml	400 micrograms	IV/IO
ATROPINE[a]	400 micrograms	NONE	N/A	300 micrograms in 1 ml	1.3 ml	400 micrograms	IV/IO
ATROPINE[a]	400 micrograms	NONE	N/A	600 micrograms in 1 ml	0.7 ml	400 micrograms	IV/IO

[a] **BRADYCARDIA** in children is most commonly caused by **HYPOXIA**, requiring immediate **ABC** care, **NOT** drug therapy; therefore **ONLY** administer atropine in cases of bradycardia caused by vagal stimulation (e.g. suction).

Quick Reference Table

DRUG	INITIAL DOSE	REPEAT DOSE	DOSE INTERVAL	CONCENTRATION	VOLUME	MAXIMUM DOSE	ROUTE
ADRENALINE anaphylaxis/asthma	300 micrograms	300 micrograms	5 minutes	1 milligram in 1 ml (1:1,000)	0.3 ml	No limit	IM
BENZYLPENICILLIN (IV/IO)	600 milligrams	NONE	N/A	600 milligrams in 9.6 ml	10 ml	600 milligrams	IV/IO
BENZYLPENICILLIN (IM)	600 milligrams	NONE	N/A	600 milligrams in 1.6 ml	2 ml	600 milligrams	IM
CHLORPHENAMINE (Oral)	2 milligrams	NONE	N/A	Various	N/A	2 milligram	Oral
CHLORPHENAMINE (IV/IO)	5–10 milligrams	NONE	N/A	10 milligrams in 1 ml	0.5–1 ml	5–10 milligrams	IV/IO
DEXAMETHASONE – croup	N/A	NONE	N/A	N/A	N/A	N/A	Oral
DIAZEPAM (IV/IO)	7 milligrams	NONE	N/A	10 milligrams in 2 ml	1.4 ml	7 milligrams	IV/IO
DIAZEPAM (PR)	5 or 10 milligrams	NONE	N/A	5 milligrams in 2.5 ml or 10 milligrams in 2.5 ml	1 × 5 milligram tube or 1 × 10 milligram tube	5 or 10 milligrams	PR
GLUCAGON	500 micrograms	NONE	N/A	1 milligram per vial	0.5 vial	500 micrograms	IM
GLUCOSE 10%	5 grams	5 grams	5 minutes	50 grams in 500 ml	50 ml	15 grams	IV/IO
HYDROCORTISONE	100 milligrams	NONE	N/A	100 milligrams in 1 ml	1 ml	100 milligrams	IV/IO/IM
HYDROCORTISONE	100 milligrams	NONE	N/A	100 milligrams in 2 ml	2 ml	100 milligrams	IV/IO/IM
IBUPROFEN	200 milligrams	200 milligrams	8 hours	100 milligrams in 5 ml	10 ml	600 milligrams	Oral
IPRATROPIUM	250 micrograms	NONE	N/A	250 micrograms in 1 ml	1 ml	250 micrograms	Neb
IPRATROPIUM	250 micrograms	NONE	N/A	500 micrograms in 2 ml	1 ml	250 micrograms	Neb
PATIENT'S OWN MIDAZOLAM[b]	7.5 milligrams	NONE	N/A	10 milligrams in 1 ml	0.75 ml	7.5 milligrams	Buccal
MORPHINE (IV/IO)	2.5 milligrams	2.5 milligrams	5 minutes	10 milligrams in 10 ml	2.5 ml	5 milligrams	IV/IO
MORPHINE (Oral)	5 milligrams	NONE	N/A	10 milligrams in 5 ml	2.5 ml	5 milligrams	Oral
NALOXONE NB cautions (IV/IO)	240 micrograms	240 micrograms	3 minutes	400 micrograms in 1 ml	0.6 ml	2640 micrograms	IV/IO
NALOXONE– INITIAL DOSE (IM)	240 micrograms	See below	3 minutes	400 micrograms in 1 ml	0.6 ml	See below	IM
NALOXONE– REPEAT DOSE (IM)	–	400 micrograms	–	400 micrograms in 1 ml	1 ml	640 micrograms	
ONDANSETRON	2.5 milligrams	NONE	N/A	2 milligrams in 1 ml	1.3 ml	2.5 milligrams	IV/IO/IM
PARACETAMOL (Oral)	250 milligrams	250 milligrams	4–6 hours	250 milligrams in 5 ml (six plus suspension)	5 ml	1 grams in 24 hours	Oral
PARACETAMOL (IV/IO)	300 milligrams	300 milligrams	4–6 hours	10 milligrams in 1 ml	30 ml	1.2 gram in 24 hours	IV/IO
SALBUTAMOL	5 milligrams	5 milligrams	5 minutes	2.5 milligrams in 2.5 ml	5 ml	No limit	Neb
SALBUTAMOL	5 milligrams	5 milligrams	5 minutes	5 milligrams in 2.5 ml	2.5 ml	No limit	Neb
TRANEXAMIC ACID	350 mg	NONE	N/A	100 mg/ml	3.5 mls	350 mg	IV

[b] Give the dose as prescribed in the child's individualised treatment plan (the dosages described above reflect the recommended dosages for a child of this age).

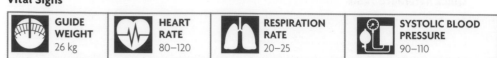

Page for Age

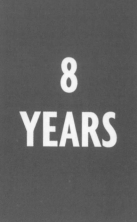

8 YEARS

Vital Signs

	GUIDE WEIGHT 26 kg		HEART RATE 80–120		RESPIRATION RATE 20–25		SYSTOLIC BLOOD PRESSURE 90–110

Airway Size by Type

OROPHARYNGEAL AIRWAY	LARYNGEAL MASK	I-GEL AIRWAY	ENDOTRACHEAL TUBE
1 OR 2	2.5	2.5	Diameter: **6.5 mm**; Length: **17 cm**

Defibrillation – Cardiac Arrest

MANUAL	AUTOMATED EXTERNAL DEFIBRILLATOR
100 Joules	A standard AED (either with paediatric attenuation pads or else in paediatric mode) can be used. If paediatric pads are not available, standard adult pads can be used (but must not overlap).

Intravascular Fluid

FLUID	INITIAL DOSE	REPEAT DOSE	DOSE INTERVAL	CONCENTRATION	VOLUME	MAXIMUM DOSE	ROUTE
Sodium chloride (5 ml/kg)	130 ml	130 ml	PRN	0.9%	130 ml	1000 ml	IV/IO
Sodium chloride (10 ml/kg)	250 ml	250 ml	PRN	0.9%	250 ml	1000 ml	IV/IO
Sodium chloride (20 ml/kg)	500 ml	500 ml	PRN	0.9%	500 ml	1000 ml	IV/IO

Cardiac Arrest

DRUG	INITIAL DOSE	REPEAT DOSE	DOSE INTERVAL	CONCENTRATION	VOLUME	MAXIMUM DOSE	ROUTE
ADRENALINE	260 micrograms	260 micrograms	3–5 minutes	1 milligram in 10 ml (1:10,000)	2.6 ml	No limit	IV/IO
AMIODARONE	130 milligrams (after 3rd shock)	130 milligrams	After 5th shock	300 milligrams in 10 ml	4.3 ml	260 milligrams	IV/IO
ATROPINE[a]	500 micrograms	NONE	N/A	100 micrograms in 1 ml	5 ml	500 micrograms	IV/IO
ATROPINE[a]	500 micrograms	NONE	N/A	200 micrograms in 1 ml	2.5 ml	500 micrograms	IV/IO
ATROPINE[a]	500 micrograms	NONE	N/A	300 micrograms in 1 ml	1.7 ml	500 micrograms	IV/IO
ATROPINE[a]	500 micrograms	NONE	N/A	600 micrograms in 1 ml	0.8 ml	500 micrograms	IV/IO

[a] **BRADYCARDIA** in children is most commonly caused by **HYPOXIA**, requiring immediate **ABC** care, **NOT** drug therapy; therefore **ONLY** administer atropine in cases of bradycardia caused by vagal stimulation (e.g. suction).

Quick Reference Table

DRUG	INITIAL DOSE	REPEAT DOSE	DOSE INTERVAL	CONCENTRATION	VOLUME	MAXIMUM DOSE	ROUTE
ADRENALINE anaphylaxis/asthma	300 micrograms	300 micrograms	5 minutes	1 milligram in 1 ml (1:1,000)	0.3 ml	No limit	IM
BENZYLPENICILLIN (IV/IO)	600 milligrams	NONE	N/A	600 milligrams in 9.6 ml	10 ml	600 milligrams	IV/IO
BENZYLPENICILLIN (IM)	600 milligrams	NONE	N/A	600 milligrams in 1.6 ml	2 ml	600 milligrams	IM
CHLORPHENAMINE (Oral)	2 milligrams	NONE	N/A	Various	N/A	2 milligram	Oral
CHLORPHENAMINE (IV/IO)	5–10 milligrams	NONE	N/A	10 milligrams in 1 ml	0.5–1 ml	5–10 milligrams	IV/IO
DEXAMETHASONE – croup	N/A	N/A	N/A	N/A	N/A	N/A	Oral
DIAZEPAM (IV/IO)	8 milligrams	NONE	N/A	10 milligrams in 2 ml	1.6 ml	8 milligrams	IV/IO
DIAZEPAM (PR)	5 or 10 milligrams	NONE	N/A	5 milligrams in 2.5 ml or 10 milligrams in 2.5 ml	1 × 5 milligram tube or 1 × 10 milligram tube	5 or 10 milligrams	PR
GLUCAGON	1 milligram	NONE	N/A	1 milligram per vial	1 vial	1 milligram	IM
GLUCOSE 10%	5 grams	5 grams	5 minutes	50 grams in 500 ml	50 ml	15 grams	IV/IO
HYDROCORTISONE	100 milligrams	NONE	N/A	100 milligrams in 1 ml	1 ml	100 milligrams	IV/IO/IM
HYDROCORTISONE	100 milligrams	NONE	N/A	100 milligrams in 2 ml	2 ml	100 milligrams	IV/IO/IM
IBUPROFEN	200 milligrams	200 milligrams	8 hours	100 milligrams in 5 ml	10 ml	600 milligrams	Oral
IPRATROPIUM	250 micrograms	NONE	N/A	250 micrograms in 1 ml	1 ml	250 micrograms	Neb
IPRATROPIUM	250 micrograms	NONE	N/A	500 micrograms in 2 ml	1 ml	250 micrograms	Neb
PATIENT'S OWN MIDAZOLAM[b]	7.5 milligrams	NONE	N/A	10 milligrams in 1 ml	0.75 ml	7.5 milligrams	Buccal
MORPHINE (IV/IO)	2.5 milligrams	2.5 milligrams	5 minutes	10 milligrams in 10 ml	2.5 ml	5 milligrams	IV/IO
MORPHINE (Oral)	5 milligrams	NONE	N/A	10 milligrams in 5 ml	2.5 ml	5 milligrams	Oral
NALOXONE NB cautions (IV/IO)	280 micrograms	280 micrograms	3 minutes	400 micrograms in 1 ml	0.7 ml	3080 micrograms	IV/IO
NALOXONE– INITIAL DOSE (IM)	280 micrograms	See below	3 minutes	400 micrograms in 1 ml	0.7 ml	See below	IM
NALOXONE– REPEAT DOSE (IM)	–	400 micrograms	–	400 micrograms in 1 ml	1 ml	680 micrograms	
ONDANSETRON	2.5 milligrams	NONE	N/A	2 milligrams in 1 ml	1.3 ml	2.5 milligrams	IV/IO/IM
PARACETAMOL (Oral)	375 milligrams	375 milligrams	4–6 hours	250 milligrams in 5 ml (six plus suspension)	7.5 ml	1.5 grams in 24 hours	Oral
PARACETAMOL (IV/IO)	300 milligrams	300 milligrams	4–6 hours	10 milligrams in 1 ml	30 ml	1.2 gram in 24 hours	IV/IO
SALBUTAMOL	5 milligrams	5 milligrams	5 minutes	2.5 milligrams in 2.5 ml	5 ml	No limit	Neb
SALBUTAMOL	5 milligrams	5 milligrams	5 minutes	5 milligrams in 2.5 ml	2.5 ml	No limit	Neb
TRANEXAMIC ACID	400 mg	NONE	N/A	100 mg/ml	4 mls	400 mg	IV

[b] Give the dose as prescribed in the child's individualised treatment plan (the dosages described above reflect the recommended dosages for a child of this age).

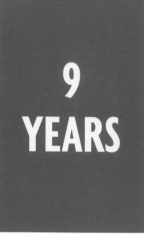

9 YEARS

Vital Signs

	GUIDE WEIGHT		HEART RATE		RESPIRATION RATE		SYSTOLIC BLOOD PRESSURE
	29 kg		80–120		20–25		90–110

Airway Size by Type

OROPHARYNGEAL AIRWAY	LARYNGEAL MASK	I-GEL AIRWAY	ENDOTRACHEAL TUBE
1 OR 2	2.5	2.5	Diameter: **6.5 mm**; Length: **17 cm**

Defibrillation – Cardiac Arrest

MANUAL	AUTOMATED EXTERNAL DEFIBRILLATOR
120 Joules	A standard AED can be used (without the need for paediatric attenuation pads).

Intravascular Fluid

FLUID	INITIAL DOSE	REPEAT DOSE	DOSE INTERVAL	CONCENTRATION	VOLUME	MAXIMUM DOSE	ROUTE
Sodium chloride (5 ml/kg)	145 ml	145 ml	PRN	0.9%	145 ml	1000 ml	IV/IO
Sodium chloride (10 ml/kg)	290 ml	290 ml	PRN	0.9%	290 ml	1000 ml	IV/IO
Sodium chloride (20 ml/kg)	500 ml	500 ml	PRN	0.9%	500 ml	1000 ml	IV/IO

Cardiac Arrest

DRUG	INITIAL DOSE	REPEAT DOSE	DOSE INTERVAL	CONCENTRATION	VOLUME	MAXIMUM DOSE	ROUTE
ADRENALINE	300 micrograms	300 micrograms	3–5 minutes	1 milligram in 10 ml (1:10,000)	3 ml	No limit	IV/IO
AMIODARONE	150 milligrams (after 3rd shock)	150 milligrams	After 5th shock	300 milligrams in 10 ml	5 ml	300 milligrams	IV/IO
ATROPINE[a]	500 micrograms	NONE	N/A	100 micrograms in 1 ml	5 ml	500 micrograms	IV/IO
ATROPINE[a]	500 micrograms	NONE	N/A	200 micrograms in 1 ml	2.5 ml	500 micrograms	IV/IO
ATROPINE[a]	500 micrograms	NONE	N/A	300 micrograms in 1 ml	1.7 ml	500 micrograms	IV/IO
ATROPINE[a]	500 micrograms	NONE	N/A	600 micrograms in 1 ml	0.8 ml	500 micrograms	IV/IO

[a] **BRADYCARDIA** in children is most commonly caused by **HYPOXIA**, requiring immediate **ABC** care, **NOT** drug therapy; therefore **ONLY** administer atropine in cases of bradycardia caused by vagal stimulation (e.g. suction).

Quick Reference Table

DRUG	INITIAL DOSE	REPEAT DOSE	DOSE INTERVAL	CONCENTRATION	VOLUME	MAXIMUM DOSE	ROUTE
ADRENALINE anaphylaxis/asthma	300 micrograms	300 micrograms	5 minutes	1 milligram in 1 ml (1:1,000)	0.3 ml	No limit	IM
BENZYLPENICILLIN (IV/IO)	600 milligrams	NONE	N/A	600 milligrams in 9.6 ml	10 ml	600 milligrams	IV/IO
BENZYLPENICILLIN (IM)	600 milligrams	NONE	N/A	600 milligrams in 1.6 ml	2 ml	600 milligrams	IM
CHLORPHENAMINE (Oral)	2 milligrams	NONE	N/A	Various	N/A	2 milligram	Oral
CHLORPHENAMINE (IV/IO)	5–10 milligrams	NONE	N/A	10 milligrams in 1 ml	0.5–1 ml	5–10 milligrams	IV/IO
DEXAMETHASONE – croup	N/A	N/A	N/A	N/A	N/A	N/A	Oral
DIAZEPAM (IV/IO)	9 milligrams	NONE	N/A	10 milligrams in 2 ml	1.8 ml	9 milligrams	IV/IO
DIAZEPAM (PR)	5 or 10 milligrams	NONE	N/A	5 milligrams in 2.5 ml or 10 milligrams in 2.5 ml	1 × 5 milligram tube or 1 × 10 milligram tube	5 or 10 milligrams	PR
GLUCAGON	1 milligrams	NONE	N/A	1 milligram per vial	1 vial	1 milligram	IM
GLUCOSE 10%	6 grams	6 grams	5 minutes	50 grams in 500 ml	60 ml	18 grams	IV/IO
HYDROCORTISONE	100 milligrams	NONE	N/A	100 milligrams in 1 ml	1 ml	100 milligrams	IV/IO/IM
HYDROCORTISONE	100 milligrams	NONE	N/A	100 milligrams in 2 ml	2 ml	100 milligrams	IV/IO/IM
IBUPROFEN	200 milligrams	200 milligrams	8 hours	100 milligrams in 5 ml	10 ml	600 milligrams	Oral
IPRATROPIUM	250 micrograms	NONE	N/A	250 micrograms in 1 ml	1 ml	250 micrograms	Neb
IPRATROPIUM	250 micrograms	NONE	N/A	500 micrograms in 2 ml	1 ml	250 micrograms	Neb
PATIENT'S OWN MIDAZOLAM[b]	7.5 milligrams	NONE	N/A	10 milligrams in 1 ml	0.75 ml	7.5 milligrams	Buccal
MORPHINE (IV/IO)	3 milligrams	3 milligrams	5 minutes	10 milligrams in 10 ml	3 ml	6 milligrams	IV/IO
MORPHINE (Oral)	6 milligrams	NONE	N/A	10 milligrams in 5 ml	3 ml	6 milligrams	Oral
NALOXONE NB cautions (IV/IO)	280 micrograms	280 micrograms	3 minutes	400 micrograms in 1 ml	0.7 ml	3080 micrograms	IV/IO
NALOXONE– INITIAL DOSE (IM)	280 micrograms	See below	3 minutes	400 micrograms in 1 ml	0.7 ml	See below	IM
NALOXONE– REPEAT DOSE (IM)	–	400 micrograms	–	400 micrograms in 1 ml	1 ml	680 micrograms	
ONDANSETRON	3 milligrams	NONE	N/A	2 milligrams in 1 ml	1.5 ml	3 milligrams	IV/IO/IM
PARACETAMOL (Oral)	375 milligrams	375 milligrams	4–6 hours	250 milligrams in 5 ml (six plus suspension)	7.5 ml	1.5 grams in 24 hours	Oral
PARACETAMOL (IV/IO)	500 milligrams	500 milligrams	4–6 hours	10 milligrams in 1 ml	50 ml	2 grams in 24 hours	IV/IO
SALBUTAMOL	5 milligrams	5 milligrams	5 minutes	2.5 milligrams in 2.5 ml	5 ml	No limit	Neb
SALBUTAMOL	5 milligrams	5 milligrams	5 minutes	5 milligrams in 2.5 ml	2.5 ml	No limit	Neb
TRANEXAMIC ACID	450 mg	NONE	N/A	100 mg/ml	4.5 mls	450 mg	IV

[b] Give the dose as prescribed in the child's individualised treatment plan (the dosages described above reflect the recommended dosages for a child of this age).

Page for Age

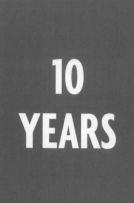

10 YEARS

Vital Signs

	GUIDE WEIGHT 32 kg		HEART RATE 80–120		RESPIRATION RATE 20–25		SYSTOLIC BLOOD PRESSURE 90–110

Airway Size by Type

OROPHARYNGEAL AIRWAY	LARYNGEAL MASK	I-GEL AIRWAY	ENDOTRACHEAL TUBE
2 OR 3	3	2.5 OR 3	Diameter: **7 mm**; Length: **18 cm**

Defibrillation – Cardiac Arrest

MANUAL	AUTOMATED EXTERNAL DEFIBRILLATOR
130 Joules	A standard AED can be used (without the need for paediatric attenuation pads).

Intravascular Fluid

FLUID	INITIAL DOSE	REPEAT DOSE	DOSE INTERVAL	CONCENTRATION	VOLUME	MAXIMUM DOSE	ROUTE
Sodium chloride (5 ml/kg)	160 ml	160 ml	PRN	0.9%	160 ml	1000 ml	IV/IO
Sodium chloride (10 ml/kg)	320 ml	320 ml	PRN	0.9%	320 ml	1000 ml	IV/IO
Sodium chloride (20 ml/kg)	500 ml	500 ml	PRN	0.9%	500 ml	1000 ml	IV/IO

Cardiac Arrest

DRUG	INITIAL DOSE	REPEAT DOSE	DOSE INTERVAL	CONCENTRATION	VOLUME	MAXIMUM DOSE	ROUTE
ADRENALINE	320 micrograms	320 micrograms	3–5 minutes	1 milligram in 10 ml (1:10,000)	3.2 ml	No limit	IV/IO
AMIODARONE	160 milligrams (after 3rd shock)	160 milligrams	After 5th shock	300 milligrams in 10 ml	5.3 ml	320 milligrams	IV/IO
ATROPINE[a]	500 micrograms	NONE	N/A	100 micrograms in 1 ml	5 ml	500 micrograms	IV/IO
ATROPINE[a]	500 micrograms	NONE	N/A	200 micrograms in 1 ml	2.5 ml	500 micrograms	IV/IO
ATROPINE[a]	500 micrograms	NONE	N/A	300 micrograms in 1 ml	1.7 ml	500 micrograms	IV/IO
ATROPINE[a]	500 micrograms	NONE	N/A	600 micrograms in 1 ml	0.8 ml	500 micrograms	IV/IO

[a] **BRADYCARDIA** in children is most commonly caused by **HYPOXIA**, requiring immediate **ABC** care, **NOT** drug therapy; therefore **ONLY** administer atropine in cases of bradycardia caused by vagal stimulation (e.g. suction).

Quick Reference Table

DRUG	INITIAL DOSE	REPEAT DOSE	DOSE INTERVAL	CONCENTRATION	VOLUME	MAXIMUM DOSE	ROUTE
ADRENALINE anaphylaxis/asthma	300 micrograms	300 micrograms	5 minutes	1 milligram in 1 ml (1:1,000)	0.3 ml	No limit	IM
BENZYLPENICILLIN (IV/IO)	1.2 grams	NONE	N/A	600 milligrams in 9.6 ml	20 ml	1.2 grams	IV/IO
BENZYLPENICILLIN (IM)	1.2 grams	NONE	N/A	600 milligrams in 1.6 ml	4 ml	1.2 grams	IM
CHLORPHENAMINE (Oral)	2 milligrams	NONE	N/A	Various	N/A	2 milligrams	Oral
CHLORPHENAMINE (IV/IO)	5–10 milligrams	NONE	N/A	10 milligrams in 1 ml	0.5–1 ml	5–10 milligrams	IV/IO
DEXAMETHASONE – croup	N/A	N/A	N/A	N/A	N/A	N/A	Oral
DIAZEPAM (IV/IO)	10 milligrams	NONE	N/A	10 milligrams in 2 ml	2 ml	10 milligrams	IV/IO
DIAZEPAM (PR)	5 or 10 milligrams	NONE	N/A	5 milligrams in 2.5 ml or 10 milligrams in 2.5 ml	1 × 5 milligram tube or 1 × 10 milligram tube	5 or 10 milligrams	PR
GLUCAGON	1 milligram	NONE	N/A	1 milligram per vial	1 vial	1 milligram	IM
GLUCOSE 10%	6.5 grams	6.5 grams	5 minutes	50 grams in 500 ml	65 ml	19.5 grams	IV/IO
HYDROCORTISONE	100 milligrams	NONE	N/A	100 milligrams in 1 ml	1 ml	100 milligrams	IV/IO/IM
HYDROCORTISONE	100 milligrams	NONE	N/A	100 milligrams in 2 ml	2 ml	100 milligrams	IV/IO/IM
IBUPROFEN	300 milligrams	300 milligrams	8 hours	100 milligrams in 5 ml	15 ml	900 milligrams	Oral
IPRATROPIUM	250 micrograms	NONE	N/A	250 micrograms in 1 ml	1 ml	250 micrograms	Neb
IPRATROPIUM	250 micrograms	NONE	N/A	500 micrograms in 2 ml	1 ml	250 micrograms	Neb
PATIENT'S OWN MIDAZOLAM[b]	10 milligrams	NONE	N/A	10 milligrams in 1 ml	1 ml	10 milligrams	Buccal
MORPHINE (IV/IO)	3 milligrams	3 milligrams	5 minutes	10 milligrams in 10 ml	3 ml	6 milligrams	IV/IO
MORPHINE (Oral)	6 milligrams	NONE	N/A	10 milligrams in 5 ml	3 ml	6 milligrams	Oral
NALOXONE NB cautions (IV/IO)	320 micrograms	320 micrograms	3 minutes	400 micrograms in 1 ml	0.8 ml	3520 micrograms	IV/IO
NALOXONE– INITIAL DOSE (IM)	320 micrograms	See below	3 minutes	400 micrograms in 1 ml	0.8 ml	See below	IM
NALOXONE– REPEAT DOSE (IM)	–	400 micrograms	–	400 micrograms in 1 ml	1 ml	720 micrograms	
ONDANSETRON	3 milligrams	NONE	N/A	2 milligrams in 1 ml	1.5 ml	3 milligrams	IV/IO/IM
PARACETAMOL (Oral)	500 milligrams	500 milligrams	4–6 hours	250 milligrams in 5 ml (six plus suspension)	10 ml	2 grams in 24 hours	Oral
PARACETAMOL (IV/IO)	500 milligrams	500 milligrams	4–6 hours	10 milligrams in 1 ml	50 ml	2 grams in 24 hours	IV/IO
SALBUTAMOL	5 milligrams	5 milligrams	5 minutes	2.5 milligrams in 2.5 ml	5 ml	No limit	Neb
SALBUTAMOL	5 milligrams	5 milligrams	5 minutes	5 milligrams in 2.5 ml	2.5 ml	No limit	Neb
TRANEXAMIC ACID	500 mg	NONE	N/A	100 mg/ml	5 mls	500 mg	IV

[b] Give the dose as prescribed in the child's individualised treatment plan (the dosages described above reflect the recommended dosages for a child of this age).

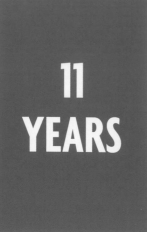

11 YEARS

Vital Signs

	GUIDE WEIGHT 35 kg		HEART RATE 80–120		RESPIRATION RATE 20–25		SYSTOLIC BLOOD PRESSURE 90–110

Airway Size by Type

OROPHARYNGEAL AIRWAY	LARYNGEAL MASK	I-GEL AIRWAY	ENDOTRACHEAL TUBE
2 OR 3	3	2.5 OR 3	Diameter: **7 mm**; Length: **18 cm**

Defibrillation – Cardiac Arrest

MANUAL	AUTOMATED EXTERNAL DEFIBRILLATOR
140 Joules	A standard AED can be used (without the need for paediatric attenuation pads).

Intravascular Fluid

FLUID	INITIAL DOSE	REPEAT DOSE	DOSE INTERVAL	CONCENTRATION	VOLUME	MAXIMUM DOSE	ROUTE
Sodium chloride (5 ml/kg)	175 ml	175 ml	PRN	0.9%	175 ml	1000 ml	IV/IO
Sodium chloride (10 ml/kg)	350 ml	350 ml	PRN	0.9%	350 ml	1000 ml	IV/IO
Sodium chloride (20 ml/kg)	500 ml	500 ml	PRN	0.9%	500 ml	1000 ml	IV/IO

Cardiac Arrest

DRUG	INITIAL DOSE	REPEAT DOSE	DOSE INTERVAL	CONCENTRATION	VOLUME	MAXIMUM DOSE	ROUTE
ADRENALINE	350 micrograms	350 micrograms	3–5 minutes	1 milligram in 10 ml (1:10,000)	3.5 ml	No limit	IV/IO
AMIODARONE	180 milligrams (after 3rd shock)	180 milligrams	After 5th shock	300 milligrams in 10 ml	6 ml	360 milligrams	IV/IO
ATROPINE[a]	500 micrograms	NONE	N/A	100 micrograms in 1 ml	5 ml	500 micrograms	IV/IO
ATROPINE[a]	500 micrograms	NONE	N/A	200 micrograms in 1 ml	2.5 ml	500 micrograms	IV/IO
ATROPINE[a]	500 micrograms	NONE	N/A	300 micrograms in 1 ml	1.7 ml	500 micrograms	IV/IO
ATROPINE[a]	500 micrograms	NONE	N/A	600 micrograms in 1 ml	0.8 ml	500 micrograms	IV/IO

[a] **BRADYCARDIA** in children is most commonly caused by **HYPOXIA**, requiring immediate **ABC** care, **NOT** drug therapy; therefore **ONLY** administer atropine in cases of bradycardia caused by vagal stimulation (e.g. suction).

Quick Reference Table

DRUG	INITIAL DOSE	REPEAT DOSE	DOSE INTERVAL	CONCENTRATION	VOLUME	MAXIMUM DOSE	ROUTE
ADRENALINE anaphylaxis/asthma	300 micrograms	300 micrograms	5 minutes	1 milligram in 1 ml (1:1,000)	0.3 ml	No limit	IM
BENZYLPENICILLIN (IV/IO)	1.2 grams	NONE	N/A	600 milligrams in 9.6 ml	20 ml	1.2 grams	IV/IO
BENZYLPENICILLIN (IM)	1.2 grams	NONE	N/A	600 milligrams in 1.6 ml	4 ml	1.2 grams	IM
CHLORPHENAMINE (Oral)	2 milligrams	NONE	N/A	Various	N/A	2 milligrams	Oral
CHLORPHENAMINE (IV/IO)	5–10 milligrams	NONE	N/A	10 milligrams in 1 ml	0.5–1 ml	5–10 milligrams	IV/IO
DEXAMETHASONE – croup	N/A	N/A	N/A	N/A	N/A	N/A	Oral
DIAZEPAM (IV/IO)	10 milligrams	NONE	N/A	10 milligrams in 2 ml	2 ml	10 milligrams	IV/IO
DIAZEPAM (PR)	5 or 10 milligrams	NONE	N/A	5 milligrams in 2.5 ml or 10 milligrams in 2.5 ml	1 × 5 milligram tube or 1 × 10 milligram tube	5 or 10 milligrams	PR
GLUCAGON	1 milligram	NONE	N/A	1 milligram per vial	1 vial	1 milligram	IM
GLUCOSE 10%	7 grams	7 grams	5 minutes	50 grams in 500 ml	70 ml	21 grams	IV/IO
HYDROCORTISONE	100 milligrams	NONE	N/A	100 milligrams in 1 ml	1 ml	100 milligrams	IV/IO/IM
HYDROCORTISONE	100 milligrams	NONE	N/A	100 milligrams in 2 ml	2 ml	100 milligrams	IV/IO/IM
IBUPROFEN	300 milligrams	300 milligrams	8 hours	100 milligrams in 5 ml	15 ml	900 milligrams	Oral
IPRATROPIUM	250 micrograms	NONE	N/A	250 micrograms in 1 ml	1 ml	250 micrograms	Neb
IPRATROPIUM	250 micrograms	NONE	N/A	500 micrograms in 2 ml	1 ml	250 micrograms	Neb
PATIENT'S OWN MIDAZOLAM[b]	10 milligrams	NONE	N/A	10 milligrams in 1 ml	1 ml	10 milligrams	Buccal
MORPHINE (IV/IO)	3.5 milligrams	3.5 milligrams	5 minutes	10 milligrams in 10 ml	3.5 ml	7 milligrams	IV/IO
MORPHINE (Oral)	7 milligrams	NONE	N/A	10 milligrams in 5 ml	3.5 ml	7 milligrams	Oral
NALOXONE NB cautions (IV/IO)	350 micrograms	350 micrograms	3 minutes	400 micrograms in 1 ml	0.9 ml	3850 micrograms	IV/IO
NALOXONE– INITIAL DOSE (IM)	350 micrograms	See below	3 minutes	400 micrograms in 1 ml	0.9 ml	See below	IM
NALOXONE– REPEAT DOSE (IM)	–	400 micrograms	–	400 micrograms in 1 ml	1 ml	750 micrograms	
ONDANSETRON	3 milligrams	NONE	N/A	2 milligrams in 1 ml	1.5 ml	3 milligrams	IV/IO/IM
PARACETAMOL (Oral)	500 milligrams	500 milligrams	4–6 hours	250 milligrams in 5 ml (six plus suspension)	10 ml	2 grams in 24 hours	Oral
PARACETAMOL (IV/IO)	500 milligrams	500 milligrams	4–6 hours	10 milligrams in 1 ml	50 ml	2 grams in 24 hours	IV/IO
SALBUTAMOL	5 milligrams	5 milligrams	5 minutes	2.5 milligrams in 2.5 ml	5 ml	No limit	Neb
SALBUTAMOL	5 milligrams	5 milligrams	5 minutes	5 milligrams in 2.5 ml	2.5 ml	No limit	Neb
TRANEXAMIC ACID	500 mg	NONE	N/A	100 mg/ml	5 mls	500 mg	IV

[b] Give the dose as prescribed in the child's individualised treatment plan (the dosages described above reflect the recommended dosages for a child of this age).

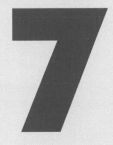

Special Situations

Special Situations

Major Incident Management

Safety First

Carry out a dynamic risk assessment and undertake measures to preserve your own safety, and where possible, that of the patient, bystanders, and other rescuers. Safety is a dynamic process and needs to be continually re-assessed throughout the incident.

- Be alert to the incident surroundings in addition to the incident.
- Appropriate Personal Protective Equipment must be worn – this may include:
  - helmets
  - eye protection
  - high visibility apparel
  - overalls
  - waterproofs
  - gloves
  - boots
  - identity cards.
- Consider the resources required to manage the major incident.
- Consider the possibility of major chemical, biological, radiological, nuclear or explosive (CBRNE) incident (**refer to CBRNE guideline**).
- Provide an early situation report using the '**METHANE**' report format (Table 7.1).
- Check the scene for other patients who are not immediately or easily visible, for example, patients ejected from vehicles during an RTC.

Table 7.1 – METHANE REPORT FORMAT

M	Major incident standby or declared
E	Exact location of incident
T	Type of incident
H	Hazards (present and potential)
A	Access and egress routes
N	Number, severity and type of casualties
E	Emergency services present on scene and further resources required

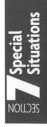

1. Introduction

- Chemical, biological, radiological and nuclear (CBRN) incidents present unique difficulties for ambulance services.

- CBRN incidents may also be associated with explosions and therefore the terminology has changed to CBRN**E** in recognition of this.

- Explosions can be accidental or terrorist related, taking place in industrial or community settings.

- The cause of the explosion will determine the explosive force; this together with the environment and distance from the source will determine the nature of the injuries sustained (Table 7.2).

- Confined space explosions usually cause more severe injury due to confinement of the blast and resultant barotrauma. This has nothing to do with structural collapse, which mitigates some of the blast injury effects by absorbing energy. Reflection of the blast wave from the walls and ceiling may also exaggerate the effects of barotrauma.

The materials involved in CBRNE incidents are all very different; they present four main types of hazard, depending on the physical properties and characteristics of the agent released:

I.   contact hazard

II. inhalation hazard

III. injection hazard

IV. ingestion hazard.

I.   **Contact hazards** – are created by chemical, biological or radioactive agents that can be absorbed into the skin. These agents can be in solid, liquid or vapour form. Most biological agents do not pose contact hazards, unless the skin is cut or abraded.

II. **Inhalation hazards** – are created by vapour, aerosols or contaminated dust that can be inhaled into the lungs.

III. **Injection hazards** – result from chemical, biological or radiological agents being absorbed into open wounds (injected) – either by the agent moving from the injection scene into the blood stream or being injected directly into a vein or artery.

Table 7.2 – MECHANISMS OF INJURY AND RELATED INJURIES

Phase	Cause	Area affected/Injuries
Primary	**Injuries caused by the interaction of the blast (shock) wave with the patient's body.**	**Area affected:** • gas-containing organs – barotrauma. **Injuries:** • pulmonary bleeding, pneumothorax • air emboli • perforation of the GI tract • burns. NB Death may occur in absence of any outward signs.
Secondary	**Injuries caused by flying fragments/debris blown against the patient.**	**Area affected:** • body surface • skeletal system. **Injuries:** • lacerations • fractures • burns.[a] NB Some fragments may be human tissue i.e. suicide bombers.
Tertiary	**Injuries caused by the patient being blown against an object due to the blast wind (dynamic overpressure).**	**Area affected:** • area of impact or referred energy. **Injuries:** • lacerations • fractures.
Quaternary	**All explosion-related injuries, illnesses, or diseases not due to primary, secondary, or tertiary mechanisms.**	**Area affected:** • body surface • skeletal system. **Injuries:** • burns[a] • crush • toxic chemical injury.

[a] Burns following an explosion may be superficial flash burns confined to exposed skin, typically the face and hands. Full thickness burns may also be seen in patients close to the point of explosion.

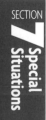

SECTION **7** Special Situations

IV. **Ingestion hazards** – result from chemical, biological or radiological agents being ingested.

In addition, radioactive agents present a significant additional hazard because of the radiation they emit from radioactive material, vapours or liquids. Exposure may result from explosion, fire damage, or direct radiation effects.

Suspect Package(s)/Material(s)

● If you are called to, or identify, a suspect package/material alert ambulance control to call the police.

● Isolate the package/material and do not open, move or handle.

Personal protective equipment (PPE)

● PPE is designed to protect you, the patient, and other patients and colleagues from contamination and from other hazards, but only if selected, worn and discarded correctly.

● Specially trained staff will wear appropriate PPE; advice will be provided at the time to ambulance clinicians by Public Health experts, Ambulance Trust Medical Director, and Hazardous Area Response Teams (HART) Medical Advisors.

● Appropriate PPE may include:
  – simple face masks
  – gloves and aprons
  – gas tight chemical suits with breathing apparatus
  – CR1 police style overalls with respirator
  – PRPS (powered respirator protective suits).

Decontamination – will be managed by HART, Special Operations Response Team (SORT) and Fire Service colleagues (Figure 7.1).

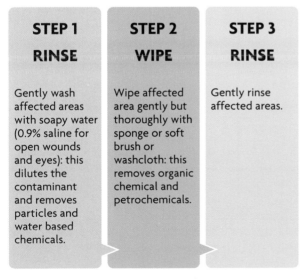

STEP 1 RINSE	STEP 2 WIPE	STEP 3 RINSE
Gently wash affected areas with soapy water (0.9% saline for open wounds and eyes): this dilutes the contaminant and removes particles and water based chemicals.	Wipe affected area gently but thoroughly with sponge or soft brush or washcloth: this removes organic chemical and petrochemicals.	Gently rinse affected areas.

Figure 7.1 – Decontamination technique.

The equipment necessary for decontamination will be provided by the HART/SORT/Fire Service.

Incident Identification – Consider whether this is or potentially is a CBRNE incident – refer to Figure 7.2, Table 7.3, Table 7.4 and Appendix 1.

STEP 1	STEP 2	STEP 3
One collapsed casualty: • approach using normal procedures • CBRN contamination unlikely.	Two collapsed casualties at one location: • CBRN contamination possible • approach with caution • if CBRN possible or suspected follow the advice for STEP 3.	Three or more collapsed casualties at one location: • CBRN contamination possible • DO NOT approach the scene – CBRN contamination likely.

Figure 7.2 – Identification of CBRNE incident and approach.

● On identification or if you have a high suspicion of a CBRNE incident advise Ambulance Control using the METHANE report protocol (Table 7.3).

Table 7.3 – METHANE REPORT PROTOCOL

M **My call sign**, or name and appointment. Major incident, **STANDBY** or **DECLARED**.

E **Exact location** – where possible, map reference.

T **Type of incident** – e.g. chemical, explosion, road traffic collision (RTC).

H **Hazards** – present and potential.

A **Access** – best routes for access and egress to scene and rendezvous point(s) (RVP).

N **Number of casualties** – approximate numbers and types of casualties (**T**[a]**1, T2, T3, DEAD** and whether contaminated).

E **Emergency services report** – on emergency services already on scene and if further services required.

[a] In this guideline the letter 'T' stands for triage, but in some documents 'P' may be used, which stands for priority; these terms are interchangeable.

2. Assessment and Management

For the assessment and management of unspecified CBRNE incidents refer to Figure 7.3.

3. Additional Information

CBRNE Detection

● There are a wide range of products available to aid with the detection of chemical and radiological incidents. Detection of the agent will be undertaken by the Fire Service, HART or Emergency Department staff as appropriate.

● Emergency Departments (ED) have been supplied with Toxi-Boxes (toxicological analytical sampling kits). These are to be used for toxicological sampling.

● When provided, electronic personal dosimeters (EPD) or other personal monitors should be worn to give advance notice of other hazards that may not have been identified.

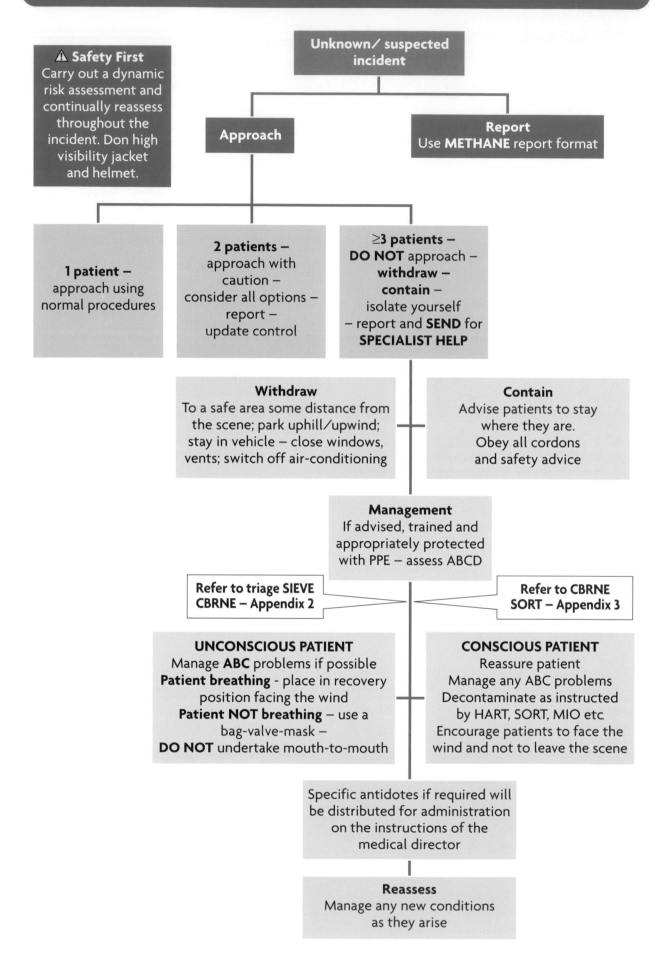

Safety First
Carry out a dynamic risk assessment and continually reassess throughout the incident. Don high visibility jacket and helmet.

Unknown/ suspected incident

Approach

Report
Use **METHANE** report format

1 patient – approach using normal procedures

2 patients – approach with caution – consider all options – report – update control

≥3 patients – DO NOT approach – **withdraw – contain –** isolate yourself – report and **SEND** for **SPECIALIST HELP**

Withdraw
To a safe area some distance from the scene; park uphill/upwind; stay in vehicle – close windows, vents; switch off air-conditioning

Contain
Advise patients to stay where they are. Obey all cordons and safety advice

Management
If advised, trained and appropriately protected with PPE – assess ABCD

Refer to triage SIEVE CBRNE – Appendix 2

Refer to CBRNE SORT – Appendix 3

UNCONSCIOUS PATIENT
Manage **ABC** problems if possible
Patient breathing - place in recovery position facing the wind
Patient NOT breathing – use a bag-valve-mask –
DO NOT undertake mouth-to-mouth

CONSCIOUS PATIENT
Reassure patient
Manage any ABC problems
Decontaminate as instructed by HART, SORT, MIO etc.
Encourage patients to face the wind and not to leave the scene

Specific antidotes if required will be distributed for administration on the instructions of the medical director

Reassess
Manage any new conditions as they arise

Figure 7.3 – General management for an unspecified CBRNE incident.

Chemical, Biological, Radiological, Nuclear and Explosive Incidents

Table 7.4 – Incident descriptions[a]

Incident	Characteristics	Casualties	Decontamination
Chemical – Refer to Appendix 1	<ul><li>Rapid action producing mass casualties.</li><li>Persistent liquid contact and downwind vapour hazards.</li><li>Casualties can contaminate first responders.</li><li>Decontamination will probably be necessary and needs to start quickly.</li><li>Most effective in confined spaces where there are lots of people.</li></ul>	<ul><li>Mass casualties at scene.</li><li>Rapid onset of symptoms/signs.</li><li>Rapid treatment is essential.</li></ul>	<ul><li>Wear PPE as appropriate.</li><li>Most contamination will be on clothing **which should be removed as soon as possible**.</li><li>Skin must be decontaminated rapidly – **wet decontamination is advised**. Where possible get contaminated patients out of doors to prevent ongoing further exposure from off gassing. (Chemical evaporation from clothing, etc., producing further chemical exposure.)</li></ul>
Biological	<ul><li>Slow action producing mass casualties over time.</li><li>Could go undetected until people become ill and attend their GP or Emergency Departments.</li><li>Potential for epidemic with some diseases.</li><li>The need for decontamination will depend on agent used.</li><li>Deliberate releases are most effective in confined spaces where there are lots of people.</li></ul>	<ul><li>Unlikely to be any casualties at the scene.</li><li>Window for treatment in first 12–24 hours.</li><li>Cannot tell who has been exposed.</li><li>First casualties will start to appear 2–3 days later.</li><li>It may be very difficult to be sure the incident is over.</li><li>Recommended prophylaxis for potential biological agents will be available as advised by incident officers.</li></ul>	<ul><li>Wear PPE as appropriate.</li><li>Washing skin and clothing should be effective.</li></ul>
Radiological	<ul><li>Few immediate casualties.</li><li>**Some may have blast injuries.**</li><li>Need to monitor those present for contamination.</li><li>Persistent radiation hazard.</li><li>Persistent contact and downwind hazards.</li><li>Casualties can contaminate first responders.</li></ul>	<ul><li>Few casualties at scene.</li><li>Damage is dosage related and cumulative.</li><li>Casualties will become ill over a period of days to weeks.</li><li>Casualties will need reassurance.</li><li>Most contamination on clothing.</li><li>Skin must be decontaminated rapidly.</li></ul>	<ul><li>Wear PPE as appropriate.</li><li>Decontamination will be necessary **and needs to start quickly with removal of clothing and wet decontamination**.</li></ul>
Nuclear	There are two types of deliberate release involving radiological substances: 1. 'Dirty Bomb' – explosive device delivering radioactive material. 2. Exposure to radioactive material deliberately left in a public place.	There are three classic symptoms of radiation sickness: 1. Vomiting 2. Diarrhoea 3. Skin burns.	<ul><li>Wear PPE as appropriate.</li></ul>

[a] Specific advice will be available to the ambulance service on specific measure(s) required.

- Most EDs have access to RAM GENE-1 (combined dose-rate/contamination monitors) monitoring equipment to screen patients for radioactive contaminants.

Specific treatments for CBRNE

- In extreme circumstances you may be asked to administer specific antidotes and drugs for CBRNE. This will be on the instructions of your Ambulance Service Medical Director who will take advice from the Public Health Service – **refer to specific CBRNE drug guidelines as instructed**.

- You may be asked to assist in taking samples for toxicological or biological analysis. You will receive directions from your Ambulance Service Medical Director.

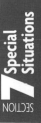

Table 7.5 – Conditions associated with agents

Disease /agent	Chlorine/ irritant gases	Mustard/ vesicants	Riot control agents	Ricin/abrin – toxalbumins	Phosgene	Nerve agents/ organo- phosphate	Hydrogen cyanide/ cyanogens
Exposure – skin							
Vesicant		●					
Irritant	●	●	●		●		
Corrosive	●				●		
Erythema or Redness	●	●	●				
Blisters		●	●				
Sweating						●	
Fasiculations							
Muscle paralysis						●	
Itching		●					
Burns or Frosbite	●				●		
Exposure – eyes							
Lacrimation	●	●	●		●	●	
Stinging/burning	●		●			●	
Blepharospasm	●	●	●		●		
Periorbital oedema		●					●
Blurred vision			●			●	
Blindness		●					
Corneal ulceration/clouding		●	●				
Burns or frostbite	●				●		
Airway							
Salivation			●			●	
Runny nose			●			●	
Bronchospasm	●	●	●		●	●	
Breathing							
Throat pain			●				
Cough	●	●		●	●	●	●
Choking	●						●
Chest pain	●				●		
Chest tightness	●		●	●	●		●
Laryngospasm					●		
Wheezing	●				●	●	
Dyspnoea	●	●		●	●	●	●
Increased respiration	●						
Hoarseness/loss of voice		●	●				
Respiratory arrest				●		●	●
Pseudomembrane		●					
Pneumonitis/pneumonia	●	●			●		
Pulmonary oedema	●	●	●	●	●	●	●

Chemical, Biological, Radiological, Nuclear and Explosive Incidents

Table 7.5 – Conditions associated with agents – *continued*

Disease /Agent	Chlorine/ irritant gases	Mustard/ vesicants	Riot control agents	Ricin/abrin – toxalbumins	Phosgene	Nerve agents/ organo- phosphate	Hydrogen cyanide/ cyanogens
Circulation/cardiac							
Arrhythmias		●			●	●	
Cardiac arrest	●					●	●
Hypotension				●	●		●
Hypoxia	●				●		
Headache				●		●	●
Cyanosis							●
Dehydration				●			
Hypovolaemic shock				●			
Disability							
Pinpoint pupils						●	●
Fixed dilated pupils							●
Confusion/agitation						●	●
Dizziness						●	●
Miosis						●	
Convulsions				●		●	●
Arthralgia				●			
Myalgia				●			
CNS depression		●				●	
Unconscious						●	●
Other							
Fever		●		●			
Nausea	●	●			●		●
Vomiting	●	●		●	●	●	●
Diarrhoea		●		●		●	●
GI bleeding				●			
Abdominal pain				●			
Faecal/urinary incontinence						●	

Methodology

For details of the methodology used in the development of this guideline refer to the guideline webpage

KEY POINTS

Chemical, Biological, Radiological, Nuclear and Explosive Incidents

- CBRN incidents may also be associated with explosions – the new terminology is CBRNE.
- Make an early METHANE call once a chemical incident is identified.
- Do not enter the scene unless protected in appropriate PPE and trained to do so.
- Encourage walking casualties to disrobe and self-decontaminate where possible.
- If ambulance clinicians become contaminated they are considered to be patients.

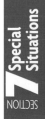

SECTION 7 Special Situations

NaCTSO
National Counter Terrorism Security Office

CPNI
Centre for the Protection of National Infrastructure

DO NOT TOUCH!

Overleaf is a list of chemicals which are precursors for home made explosives (HMEs). Many of these chemicals are also used in the manufacture of illicit drugs and are additionally marked with a smiley face symbol. ☺ A small number of the drugs precursors are controlled under various pieces of drugs legislation and these also feature a key symbol. 🔑

DO NOT assume that any packaging or labelling is correct or corresponds to the contents of the container. Treat any unidentified substances with caution.

REMEMBER: Chemicals may present a multitude of hazards, some of which may not be immediately apparent.

All of these chemicals have a legitimate use, HOWEVER, if you encounter;

- any of the listed chemicals
- any combinations of the listed chemicals
- any potential laboratory equipment such as glassware, scales, funnels, filter papers etc, either dedicated or improvised,

in unusual or suspicious circumstances you should;

For suspected explosives related activity, inform your CT section and your CTSA, or your relevant agency contact immediately on; (insert number)..

For suspected illicit drugs manufacture contact;
Serious Organised Crime Agency (SOCA)
Chemical Control Team (CCT) on 020 7238 2426 or
Hazardous Environment Search Team (HEST) (24hr) on 0870 496 0093 and
ask for the 'HEST Operations Manager'.

Produced jointly by the NaCTSO and CPNI.

OCTOBER 2011

DO NOT TOUCH!
INCLUDING ANYTHING WHICH MAY BE ON THE FLOOR!

	Chemical	Formula
☺	Acetic Acid	CH_3COOH
☺ 🔑	Acetone	C_3H_6O / CH_3COCH_3
☺	Alcohol (Ethanol, Methanol)	C_2H_5OH / CH_3CH_2OH or CH_3OH
☺	Ammonium Nitrate	NH_4NO_3
☺	Anything Chlorate / Perchlorate	$NaClO_3$ / $KClO_3$ or $NAClO_4$ / $KClO_4$ / NH_4ClO_4
☺	Anything Nitrate	KNO_3 / $NaNO_3$
	Calcium Hypochlorite	$Ca(OCl)_2$
☺	Citric Acid	$C_6H_8O_7$
	Ethylene Glycol	$C_2H_6O_2$ / $HOCH_2CH_2OH$
	Glycerine	$C_3H_8O_3$
☺	Hexamine	$C_6H_{12}N_4$
☺ 🔑	Hydrochloric Acid	HCl
☺	Hydrogen Peroxide	H_2O_2
	Lead Nitrate	$Pb(NO_3)_2$
☺	Mercury	Hg
☺ 🔑	Methyl Ethyl Ketone	C_4H_8O / $CH_3COCH_2CH_3$
☺	Nitric Acid	HNO_3
☺	Nitrobenzene	$C_6H_5NO_2$
☺	Nitromethane	CH_3NO_2
	Pentaerythritol	$C_5H_{12}O_4$ / $C(CH_2OH)_4$
☺ 🔑	Potassium Permanganate	$KMnO_4$
☺	Powdered Metals (Aluminium (Al) Magnesium (Mg) Magnalium (Al/Mg) Zinc (Zn))	
	Sodium Azide	NaN_3
☺	Sulphur	S
☺ 🔑	Sulphuric Acid	H_2SO_4
☺	Urea	CH_4N_2O / $CO(NH_2)_2$

Appendix 1 – Chemical Incident[a]

In the case of a chemical incident – **DO NOT TOUCH** any of the chemicals, including anything which may be on the floor.

Do not assume that any packaging or labelling is correct and treat any unidentified substance with caution.

Do not assume the only hazard is explosive. There may be other health and safety hazards present from a variety of sources.

All of these chemicals have a legitimate use. **HOWEVER**, if you come across:

- Any of the listed chemicals
- Any combinations of the listed chemicals
- Any potential laboratory equipment such as flasks, scales, funnels, filter papers etc.

in unusual or suspicious circumstances you should inform Ambulance Control **IMMEDIATELY**.

[a] Produced by the National Counter Terrorism Security Office/ACPOS.

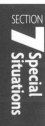

SECTION 7 Special Situations

Appendix 2

CBRNE (SPECIAL AGENT) TRIAGE SIEVE: For use before and during decontamination.

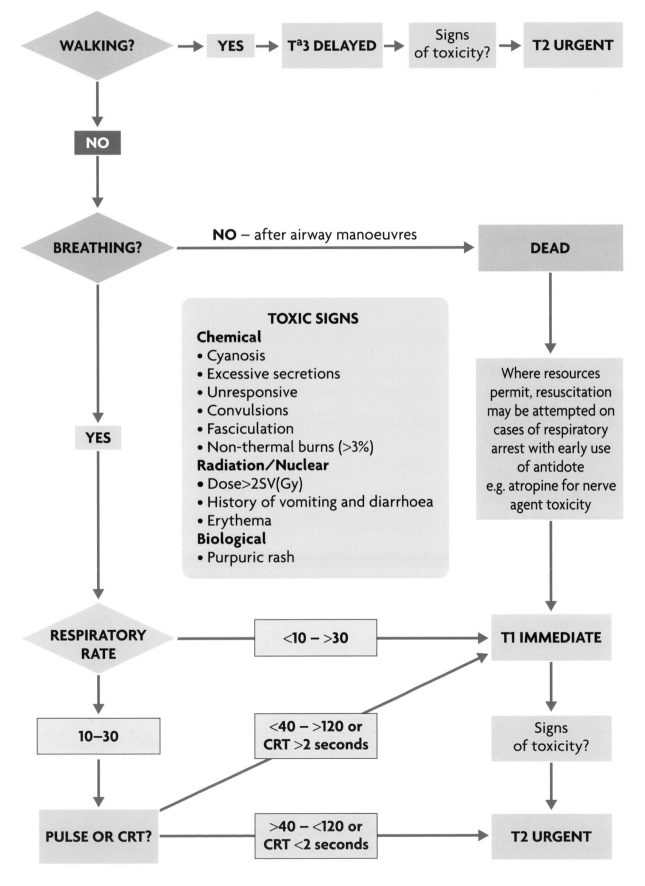

TOXIC SIGNS

Chemical
- Cyanosis
- Excessive secretions
- Unresponsive
- Convulsions
- Fasciculation
- Non-thermal burns (>3%)

Radiation/Nuclear
- Dose>2SV(Gy)
- History of vomiting and diarrhoea
- Erythema

Biological
- Purpuric rash

[a] In this guideline the letter 'T' stands for triage, but in some documents 'P' may be used, which stands for priority; these terms are interchangeable.

Section 7 Special Situations

Chemical, Biological, Radiological, Nuclear and Explosive Incidents

Appendix 3

CBRNE SORT (for use after decontamination).

RESPIRATION		
	10–29 per minute	+4
	>30 per minute	+2
	>30 per minute + cyanosis	+0
	≤9 per minute	+0
	RESPIRATORY ARREST	**Immediate or expectant**

HEART RATE		
	60–100 per minute	+4
	40–59 OR 101–120 per minute	+2
	<40 per minute + cyanosis	+0
	>120 per minute	+0
	CARDIAC ARREST	**DEAD**

SYSTOLIC BLOOD PRESSURE		
	≥90 mmHg	+4
	70–89 mmHg	+3
	50–69 mmHg	+2
	1–49 mmHg	+1
	CARDIAC ARREST	**DEAD**

GLASGOW COMA SCALE		
	13–15	+4
	9–12	+3
	6–8	+2
	4–5	+1
	3 OR CONVULSIONS	**+0**

FASCICULATION		
	None	+4
	Local/intermittent	+2
	General/continuous	+0
	Flaccidity	+0

BIOLOGICAL RADIOLOGICAL		
	If purpuric rash	−2
	If vomiting, diarrhoea, erythema or dose >2Sv	−2

TOTAL SCORE OUT OF 20 [ ]

EVACUATION SCORE		EVACUATION PRIORITY
20	**DELAYED**	T3
18–19	**URGENT**	T2
0–17	**IMMEDIATE**	T1

SECTION 7 Special Situations

Atropine (CBRNE)
ATR

Presentation

- Pre-filled syringe containing 1 milligram atropine in 5ml.
- Pre-filled syringe containing 1 milligram atropine in 10ml.
- Pre-filled syringe containing 3 milligrams atropine in 10 ml.
- An ampoule containing 600 micrograms in 1 ml.
- Nerve Agent Antidote Kit (NAAK) containing 2 milligrams of atropine sulphate.

Indications

Organophosphate (OP) poisoning.

Adults and children with a clinical diagnosis of poisoning by OP nerve agents, as an adjunct to maintenance of oxygenation.

Atropine should be administered for confirmed OP poisoning, or where features of OP poisoning develop. Clinical diagnosis of nerve agent poisoning (see below) is suggested by the characteristic features of nerve agent poisoning, associated with a history of possible exposure. Clinical features must include one or more of the following: bronchorrhoea, bronchospasm, severe bradycardia (<40 bpm).

Actions

Reduction or elimination of bronchorrhoea and bronchospasm in nerve agent poisoning.

Contra-indications

Hypersensitivity to Atropine Sulphate or excipients in nerve agent poisoning.

Cautions

There are no other absolute criteria for the exclusion from administration of atropine in the treatment of OP poisoning, as the consequences of not instituting prompt treatment in poisoned patients will usually outweigh the risks associated with treatment. However, caution needs to be administered in the following:

- Patients with ulcerative colitis.
- Patients with risk of urinary retention.
- Patients with glaucoma.
- Patients with conditions characterised by tachycardia e.g. thyrotoxicosis, heart failure.
- Patients with myasthenia gravis.

Side Effects

Reactions are mostly dose related and usually reversible and include:

- Loss of visual accommodation
- Photophobia
- Arrhythmias, transient bradycardia followed by tachycardia
- Palpitations
- Difficulty in micturition.

Additional Information

Toxic doses may cause CNS stimulation manifesting as restlessness, confusion, ataxia, lack of coordination, hallucinations and delirium. In severe intoxication CNS stimulation may give way to CNS depression, coma, circulatory and respiratory failure and death.

Characteristic features of nerve agent poisoning:

- Miosis, excess secretions (e.g. lacrimation and bronchorrhoea).
- Respiratory difficulty (e.g. bronchospasm or respiratory depression)
- Altered consciousness, convulsions, together with a history of possible exposure.

Dosage and Administration

Nerve Agent Poisoning

- Atropine must only be administered after the patient is adequately oxygenated.

- In organophosphate poisoning there is no maximum dose and large doses e.g. 20 milligrams may be required to achieve atropinisation.[a]

- **When administering atropine via the intramuscular route:** administering large volumes intramuscularly could lead to poor absorption and/or tissue damage, therefore administer the smallest volume possible and divide where necessary and practicable. Vary the site of injection for repeated doses; appropriate sites include: buttock (gluteus maximus), thigh (vastus lateralis), lateral hip (gluteus medius) and upper arm (deltoid).

Route: Intramuscular.

AGE	INITIAL DOSE	REPEAT DOSE	DOSE INTERVAL	CONCENTRATION	VOLUME	MAXIMUM DOSE
≥12 years – adult	2 milligrams	2 milligrams	5 minutes	2 milligrams per auto-injector	0.7 ml automatically delivered	No limit
11 years	2 milligrams	2 milligrams	5 minutes	2 milligrams per auto-injector	0.7 ml automatically delivered	No limit
10 years	2 milligrams	2 milligrams	5 minutes	2 milligrams per auto-injector	0.7 ml automatically delivered	No limit
9 years	2 milligrams	2 milligrams	5 minutes	2 milligrams per auto-injector	0.7 ml automatically delivered	No limit
8 years	2 milligrams	2 milligrams	5 minutes	2 milligrams per auto-injector	0.7 ml automatically delivered	No limit

NB See charts on following pages for doses for children <8 years.

[a] **Signs of atropinisation include:** dry skin and mouth and an absence of bradycardia (e.g. heart rate adult ≥80; heart rate child HR ≥100 bpm). NB DO NOT rely on reversal of pinpoint pupils as a guide to atropinisation.

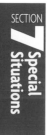

Atropine (CBRNE)

Route: Intravenous/intraosseous/intramuscular (as appropriate).

AGE	INITIAL DOSE	REPEAT DOSE	DOSE INTERVAL	CONCENTRATION	VOLUME	MAXIMUM DOSE
≥12 years – adult	2 milligrams	2 milligrams	5 minutes	1 milligram in 5 ml	10 ml	No limit
11 years	2 milligrams	2 milligrams	5 minutes	1 milligram in 5 ml	10 ml	No limit
10 years	2 milligrams	2 milligrams	5 minutes	1 milligram in 5 ml	10 ml	No limit
9 years	2 milligrams	2 milligrams	5 minutes	1 milligram in 5 ml	10 ml	No limit
8 years	2 milligrams	2 milligrams	5 minutes	1 milligram in 5 ml	10 ml	No limit
7 years	600 micrograms	600 micrograms	5 minutes	1 milligram in 5 ml	3 ml	No limit
6 years	600 micrograms	600 micrograms	5 minutes	1 milligram in 5 ml	3 ml	No limit
5 years	600 micrograms	600 micrograms	5 minutes	1 milligram in 5 ml	3 ml	No limit
4 years	600 micrograms	600 micrograms	5 minutes	1 milligram in 5 ml	3 ml	No limit
3 years	600 micrograms	600 micrograms	5 minutes	1 milligram in 5 ml	3 ml	No limit
2 years	600 micrograms	600 micrograms	5 minutes	1 milligram in 5 ml	3 ml	No limit
18 months	600 micrograms	600 micrograms	5 minutes	1 milligram in 5 ml	3 ml	No limit
12 months	600 micrograms	600 micrograms	5 minutes	1 milligram in 5 ml	3 ml	No limit
9 months	200 micrograms	200 micrograms	5 minutes	1 milligram in 5 ml	1 ml	No limit
6 months	200 micrograms	200 micrograms	5 minutes	1 milligram in 5 ml	1 ml	No limit
3 months	200 micrograms	200 micrograms	5 minutes	1 milligram in 5 ml	1 ml	No limit
1 month	200 micrograms	200 micrograms	5 minutes	1 milligram in 5 ml	1 ml	No limit
Birth	200 micrograms	200 micrograms	5 minutes	1 milligram in 5 ml	1 ml	No limit

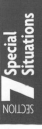

SECTION 7 Special Situations

Atropine (CBRNE)

Route: Intravenous/intraosseous/intramuscular (administer the smallest volume possible and divide where necessary and practicable).

AGE	INITIAL DOSE	REPEAT DOSE	DOSE INTERVAL	CONCENTRATION	VOLUME	MAXIMUM DOSE
≥12 years – adult	2 milligrams	2 milligrams	5 minutes	1 milligram in 10 ml	20 ml	No limit
11 years	2 milligrams	2 milligrams	5 minutes	1 milligram in 10 ml	20 ml	No limit
10 years	2 milligrams	2 milligrams	5 minutes	1 milligram in 10 ml	20 ml	No limit
9 years	2 milligrams	2 milligrams	5 minutes	1 milligram in 10 ml	20 ml	No limit
8 years	2 milligrams	2 milligrams	5 minutes	1 milligram in 10 ml	20 ml	No limit
7 years	600 micrograms	600 micrograms	5 minutes	1 milligram in 10 ml	6 ml	No limit
6 years	600 micrograms	600 micrograms	5 minutes	1 milligram in 10 ml	6 ml	No limit
5 years	600 micrograms	600 micrograms	5 minutes	1 milligram in 10 ml	6 ml	No limit
4 years	600 micrograms	600 micrograms	5 minutes	1 milligram in 10 ml	6 ml	No limit
3 years	600 micrograms	600 micrograms	5 minutes	1 milligram in 10 ml	6 ml	No limit
2 years	600 micrograms	600 micrograms	5 minutes	1 milligram in 10 ml	6 ml	No limit
18 months	600 micrograms	600 micrograms	5 minutes	1 milligram in 10 ml	6 ml	No limit
12 months	600 micrograms	600 micrograms	5 minutes	1 milligram in 10 ml	6 ml	No limit
9 months	200 micrograms	200 micrograms	5 minutes	1 milligram in 10 ml	2 ml	No limit
6 months	200 micrograms	200 micrograms	5 minutes	1 milligram in 10 ml	2 ml	No limit
3 months	200 micrograms	200 micrograms	5 minutes	1 milligram in 10 ml	2 ml	No limit
1 month	200 micrograms	200 micrograms	5 minutes	1 milligram in 10 ml	2 ml	No limit
Birth	200 micrograms	200 micrograms	5 minutes	1 milligram in 10 ml	2 ml	No limit

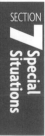

Atropine (CBRNE)

Route: Intravenous/intraosseous/intramuscular (as appropriate).

AGE	INITIAL DOSE	REPEAT DOSE	DOSE INTERVAL	CONCENTRATION	VOLUME	MAXIMUM DOSE
≥12 years – adult	2 milligrams	2 milligrams	5 minutes	3 milligrams in 10 ml	6.7 ml	No limit
11 years	2 milligrams	2 milligrams	5 minutes	3 milligrams in 10 ml	6.7 ml	No limit
10 years	2 milligrams	2 milligrams	5 minutes	3 milligrams in 10 ml	6.7 ml	No limit
9 years	2 milligrams	2 milligrams	5 minutes	3 milligrams in 10 ml	6.7 ml	No limit
8 years	2 milligrams	2 milligrams	5 minutes	3 milligrams in 10 ml	6.7 ml	No limit
7 years	600 micrograms	600 micrograms	5 minutes	3 milligrams in 10 ml	2 ml	No limit
6 years	600 micrograms	600 micrograms	5 minutes	3 milligrams in 10 ml	2 ml	No limit
5 years	600 micrograms	600 micrograms	5 minutes	3 milligrams in 10 ml	2 ml	No limit
4 years	600 micrograms	600 micrograms	5 minutes	3 milligrams in 10 ml	2 ml	No limit
3 years	600 micrograms	600 micrograms	5 minutes	3 milligrams in 10 ml	2 ml	No limit
2 years	600 micrograms	600 micrograms	5 minutes	3 milligrams in 10 ml	2 ml	No limit
18 months	600 micrograms	600 micrograms	5 minutes	3 milligrams in 10 ml	2 ml	No limit
12 months	600 micrograms	600 micrograms	5 minutes	3 milligrams in 10 ml	2 ml	No limit
9 months	200 micrograms	200 micrograms	5 minutes	3 milligrams in 10 ml	0.6 ml	No limit
6 months	200 micrograms	200 micrograms	5 minutes	3 milligrams in 10 ml	0.6 ml	No limit
3 months	200 micrograms	200 micrograms	5 minutes	3 milligrams in 10 ml	0.6 ml	No limit
1 month	200 micrograms	200 micrograms	5 minutes	3 milligrams in 10 ml	0.6 ml	No limit
Birth	200 micrograms	200 micrograms	5 minutes	3 milligrams in 10 ml	0.6 ml	No limit

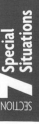

SECTION 7 Special Situations

Atropine (CBRNE)

Route: Intravenous/intraosseous/intramuscular.

AGE	INITIAL DOSE	REPEAT DOSE	DOSE INTERVAL	CONCENTRATION	VOLUME	MAXIMUM DOSE
≥12 years – adult	2 milligrams	2 milligrams	5 minutes	600 micrograms in 1 ml	3.3 ml	No limit
11 years	2 milligrams	2 milligrams	5 minutes	600 micrograms in 1 ml	3.3 ml	No limit
10 years	2 milligrams	2 milligrams	5 minutes	600 micrograms in 1 ml	3.3 ml	No limit
9 years	2 milligrams	2 milligrams	5 minutes	600 micrograms in 1 ml	3.3 ml	No limit
8 years	2 milligrams	2 milligrams	5 minutes	600 micrograms in 1 ml	3.3 ml	No limit
7 years	600 micrograms	600 micrograms	5 minutes	600 micrograms in 1 ml	1 ml	No limit
6 years	600 micrograms	600 micrograms	5 minutes	600 micrograms in 1 ml	1 ml	No limit
5 years	600 micrograms	600 micrograms	5 minutes	600 micrograms in 1 ml	1 ml	No limit
4 years	600 micrograms	600 micrograms	5 minutes	600 micrograms in 1 ml	1 ml	No limit
3 years	600 micrograms	600 micrograms	5 minutes	600 micrograms in 1 ml	1 ml	No limit
2 years	600 micrograms	600 micrograms	5 minutes	600 micrograms in 1 ml	1 ml	No limit
18 months	600 micrograms	600 micrograms	5 minutes	600 micrograms in 1 ml	1 ml	No limit
12 months	600 micrograms	600 micrograms	5 minutes	600 micrograms in 1 ml	1 ml	No limit
9 months	200 micrograms	200 micrograms	5 minutes	600 micrograms in 1 ml	0.3 ml	No limit
6 months	200 micrograms	200 micrograms	5 minutes	600 micrograms in 1 ml	0.3 ml	No limit
3 months	200 micrograms	200 micrograms	5 minutes	600 micrograms in 1 ml	0.3 ml	No limit
1 month	200 micrograms	200 micrograms	5 minutes	600 micrograms in 1 ml	0.3 ml	No limit
Birth	200 micrograms	200 micrograms	5 minutes	600 micrograms in 1 ml	0.3 ml	No limit

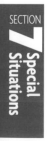

Ciprofloxacin (CBRNE) [994, 995]

Presentation

500 milligrams ciprofloxacin (as hydrochloride) in tablet form.

Indications

Patients who have been exposed to a known or suspected biological agent:

- Anthrax – (licensed indication).
- Plague.
- Tularaemia.
- Other biological agent.

Dispensed on the instruction of the public health advice or Medical Director.

Actions

Antibiotic active against Gram-positive and Gram-negative bacteria.

Prophylaxis against these potentially life-threatening conditions.

Contra-indications

Known hypersensitivity to ciprofloxacin or other quinolones (seek further guidance if contra-indicated).

Cautions

In the following cases the benefits of using ciprofloxacin to prevent the onset of disease outweigh the potential risks of the drug:

- Growing adolescents.
- Pregnancy and nursing mothers. **NOTE** nursing mothers should not breastfeed during treatment with ciprofloxacin.
- Older patients.

Seek medical advice for patients with:

- Epilepsy or a history of central nervous system disorders.
- A family history of or actual defects in glucose-6-phosphate dehydrogenase (G6PD).
- Severe renal impairment.
- Patients taking any of the following medication:
  - corticosteroid therapy
  - phenytoin
  - theophylline
  - anticoagulants including warfarin.
- NSAIDS.
- Ciclosporin.
- Glibenclamide.
- Probenecid.

Side Effects

Nausea, vomiting, dyspepsia, abdominal pain, diarrhoea (rarely antibiotic associated colitis), headache, restlessness, rash, renal disturbances, blurred vision, dizziness and pruritis.

Increases in liver enzymes, arthralgia, myalgia, leucopenia, thrombocytopenia also reported.

Tendon inflammation[a] and rupture may occur with ciprofloxacin. Such reactions have been observed particularly in older patients and in those treated concurrently with corticosteroids.

[a] At the first sign of pain or inflammation, patients taking quinolones should discontinue the treatment and rest the affected limb until tendon symptoms have resolved.

Dosage and Administration

NOTE: The initial treatment for adults is one tablet to be taken twice daily for 3 days until laboratory results are known. The dose and course of treatment may be amended and the medical director will advise.

AGE	INITIAL DOSE	REPEAT DOSE	DOSE INTERVAL	CONCENTRATION	TABLET	MAXIMUM DOSE
Adult	500 milligrams	Given in secondary care	N/A	500 milligrams per tablet	1 tablet	500 milligrams
< 12 years	10/30 milligrams/kilogram	Given in secondary care	N/A	500 milligrams per tablet	–	1 dose

Presentation

Each 20 ml ampoule contains 300 mg (15 mg/ml) dicobalt edetate.

Indications

Adults and children with a clinical diagnosis of severe poisoning with hydrogen cyanide, or cyanide salts; in the presence of respiratory depression, and impaired consciousness e.g. Glasgow Coma Score <8.

NB Dicobalt edetate can be toxic in the absence of cyanide ions – **IT MUST ONLY BE GIVEN WHEN POISONING IS SEVERE**.

Cyanide is rapidly detoxified in the body. Any casualty who is fully conscious and breathing normally more than five minutes after removal from exposure of hydrogen cyanide will recover spontaneously and does **NOT** require treatment with an antidote.

Dispensed on the instruction of the Health Protection Agency or Medical Director.

Actions

Chelating agent to diminish the effects of cyanide poisoning.

Contra-indications

Hypersensitivity to dicobalt edetate.

There are no other absolute criteria for the exclusion from administration of dicobalt edetate as the consequences of not instituting prompt treatment in severely poisoned patients will usually outweigh the risks associated with treatment.

Cautions

ONLY BE ADMINISTERED WHEN POISONING IS SEVERE (i.e. coma, respiratory depression <9 and apparent cyanosis).

Side Effects

The initial effects of dicobalt edetate are vomiting, a fall in blood pressure and compensatory tachycardia.

Signs and symptoms may be due to cobalt toxicity or to an anaphylactic type reaction (**refer to anaphylaxis guidelines**), which may be severe.

Facial, laryngeal and pulmonary oedema, vomiting, chest pain, sweating, hypotension, cardiac irregularities and rashes may occur.

Anaphylaxis should be treated in the usual way.

Dosage and Administration

NOTE:

- Administer oxygen.
- Follow administration by an intravenous infusion of 250 ml 10% glucose (**refer to glucose 10% guideline**) in adults.
- Children receive 12.5 ml of 10% glucose for each 1 ml (15 mg) of dicobalt edetate.

Route: Intravenous injection at a regular rate over one minute.

AGE	INITIAL DOSE	REPEAT DOSE	DOSE INTERVAL	CONCENTRATION	VOLUME	MAXIMUM DOSE
Adult	300 milligrams	300 milligrams	30 minutes if no improvement	15 milligrams per ml	20 ml	600 milligrams
Children	7.5 milligrams/kilogram	7.5 mg/kg	30 minutes if no improvement	15 milligrams per ml	0.5 ml/kg	15 mg/kg

Adults

The dose required is related to the quantity of cyanide absorbed into the body, if the patient shows an inadequate response, a second 300 mg dose of dicobalt edetate may be administered followed by a further 250 ml intravenous infusion of 10% (500g/l) glucose (**refer to glucose 10% guideline**).

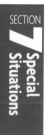

Presentation

100 milligram of doxycycline in capsules.

Indications

Patients who have been exposed to a known or suspected biological agent:

- Anthrax (licensed indication).
- Plague.
- Tularaemia.
- Other biological agent.

Actions

Prophylaxis against potentially life-threatening biological agents.

Contra-indications

Known hypersensitivity to doxycycline or other tetracyclines.

Children under 12 years **UNLESS** specifically recommended by a medical advisor.

Cautions

Doxycycline is not usually recommended for use in pregnant women. In this case the benefits of using doxycycline to prevent the onset of disease outweigh the potential risks of the drug. Adverse effects on developing teeth and bones are dose related. Therefore, doxycycline may be used for a short course of therapy (7-14 days) prior to the 6th month of pregnancy. Nursing mothers should not breastfeed during treatment with doxycycline.

Obtain medical advice for patients with the following conditions/medications:

- Women more than six months pregnant.
- Patient with any exclusion criteria.
- Systemic lupus erythematosus.
- Patient declines treatment.
- Hepatic impairment.
- Porphyria.

- Myasthenia gravis.
- Achorhydria.
- Ciclosporin.
- Retinoids (isotretinoin, acitretin, tretinoin).
- Anticoagulants (e.g. warfarin).
- Antiepileptics (e.g. carbamazepine, phenytoin).
- Oral contraceptives.
- Antacids.
- Sucralfate.
- Barbiturates.
- Penicillins.

Advise the patient to sit upright, swallow the capsule whole with plenty of water.

Side Effects

Nausea, vomiting, diarrhoea, dysphagia, oesophageal irritation, hypersensitivity reactions (including rash, exfoliative dermatitis, urticaria, angioedema, anaphylaxis, pericarditis), headache and vision disturbances may indicate benign intracranial hypertension, hepatotoxicity, pancreatitis and antibiotic-associated colitis.

Rarely photosensitivity, blood dyscrasias.

Dosage and Administration

NOTE: The initial treatment for adults is one tablet to be taken twice daily for 3 days until laboratory results are known.

Route: Oral.

AGE	INITIAL DOSE	REPEAT DOSE	DOSE INTERVAL	CONCENTRATION	VOLUME	MAXIMUM DOSE
All ages	100 milligrams	100 milligrams	12 hours	100 milligrams per capsule	1 capsule	200 milligrams per 24 hours

Page **1** of **1**

2013

Special Situations

7 Special Situations

SECTION

429

Obidoxime Chloride (CBRNE)

Presentation

Obidoxime chloride (Toxogonin), 250 mg ampoules, 250 mg per ml, for intravenous injection.

Indications

An adjunct to atropine in the treatment of organophosphorus (OP) poisoning by nerve agents.

Adults and children with a clinical diagnosis of poisoning by organophosphorus (OP) nerve agents, as an adjunct to maintenance of oxygenation and atropine administration.

Characteristic features of nerve agent poisoning include miosis, excess secretions (e.g. lacrimation and bronchorrhoea), respiratory difficulty (e.g. bronchospasm or respiratory depression), altered consciousness, and convulsions, together with a history of possible exposure.

Dispensed on the instruction of the Health Protection Agency or Medical Director.

Actions

Binds to organophosphate thus restoring enzyme function.

Contra-indications

Hypersensitivity to obidoxime or excipients.

NOTE: There are no other absolute criteria for the exclusion from administration of obidoxime chloride, as the consequences of not instituting prompt treatment in poisoned patients will often outweigh the risks associated with treatment.

Cautions

Patients with impaired renal function.

Patients with myasthenia gravis.

Side Effects

Sensation of heat or flushing of the face 5–10 minutes after injection lasting several hours, pain at the injection site, numbness of the face, dry mouth, mild to moderate hypertension and tachycardia.

Patients with organophosphorus poisoning treated with obidoxime have developed abnormal liver function tests and renal impairment.

Dosage and Administration

NOTE: Only administer after oxygenation (**refer to oxygen guideline**) and atropinisation (**refer to atropine guideline**) of the patient.

Route: Intravenous injection. If necessary obidoxime chloride may be diluted with 0.9% saline for IV injection.

AGE	INITIAL DOSE	REPEAT DOSE	DOSE INTERVAL	CONCENTRATION	VOLUME	MAXIMUM DOSE
Adult	250 milligrams	250 milligrams	2 hourly	250 milligrams in 1 ml	1 ml	5 mg
Children	2 mg/kg	2 mg/kg	2 hourly	250 milligrams in 1 ml	–	4 mg/kg

Severe poisoning in children

In cases of severe poisoning 2 milligrams/per kilogram body weight may be administered slowly every 2 hours, until clinical recovery is achieved and maintained.

NOTE: Undertake a medical review after second and third dose.

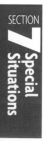

Presentation

Potassium iodate 85 milligram tablets (50 mg equivalent mass of iodine).

Indications

Known, expected or suspected exposure to radioactive iodine, at or above a level judged appropriate by a Director of Public Health (or delegate).

On the direction of a Director of Public Health (or delegate) or Ambulance Service Medical Director.

Actions

One treatment will provide protection for 24 hours.

Contra-indications

Iodine sensitivity.

Hypocomplementaemic vasculitis.

Dermatitis herpetiformis.

Cautions

Pregnancy.

Hypothyroidism.

Side Effects

Allergic reactions, usually mild nausea, vomiting and skin rash.

Relapse of thyrotoxicosis.

Iodine-induced hyperthyroidism.

Additional Information

Priority should be given to young children (under the age of 10 years).

Pregnant and nursing mothers should receive the normal adult treatment.

It is not necessary to exclude those with previously treated or active thyroid disease.

Dosage and Administration

On the instructions of the Director of Public Health (or delegate) administer a single treatment of potassium iodate.
NOTE: Dose should be taken immediately.

Route: Oral – may be broken up and stirred into a drink or mixed with a small quantity of food to ease swallowing.

AGE	INITIAL DOSE Equivalent Mass of Iodine (mg)	REPEAT DOSE	DOSE INTERVAL	CONCENTRATION	TABLET	MAXIMUM DOSE
Birth – <1 month	12.5 milligrams	NONE	N/A	50 equivalent mass of Iodine	¼ tablet	¼ tablet
1 month – <3 years	25 milligrams	NONE	N/A	50 equivalent mass of Iodine	½ tablet	½ tablet
3–12 years	50 milligrams	NONE	N/A	50 equivalent mass of Iodine	1 tablet	1 tablet
>12 years	100 milligrams	NONE	N/A	50 equivalent mass of Iodine	2 tablets	2 tablets

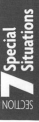

SECTION 7 Special Situations

Pralidoxime (CBRNE)

Presentation

A 5 ml ampoule containing 1 gram of pralidoxime.

Indications

Adults and children with a clinical diagnosis of poisoning by organophosphorus (OP) nerve agents, as an adjunct to maintenance of oxygenation and atropine administration.

Characteristic features of nerve agent poisoning include miosis, excess secretions (e.g. lacrimation and bronchorrhoea), respiratory difficulty (e.g. bronchospasm or respiratory depression), altered consciousness, convulsions, together with a history of possible exposure.

Actions

An antidote for poisoning with organophosphates.

Contra-indications

Hypersensitivity to pralidoxime or excipients.

There are no other absolute criteria for the exclusion from administration of pralidoxime mesylate, as the consequences of not instituting prompt treatment in poisoned patients will usually outweigh the risks associated with treatment.

Cautions

Patients with impaired renal function.

Patients with myasthenia gravis.

Side Effects

Drowsiness, dizziness, visual disturbances, nausea, tachycardia, headache, hyperventilation and muscular weakness.

Large doses may cause transient neuromuscular blockade.

Dosage and Administration

NOTE: Pralidoxime must only be administered after oxygenation and atropinisation of the patient.

Route: Intravenous – slowly over 5–10 minutes.

AGE	INITIAL DOSE	REPEAT DOSE	DOSE INTERVAL	CONCENTRATION	TABLETS	MAXIMUM DOSE
Adult	2 grams	30 mg/kg	4 hourly	200 milligrams in 1 ml	20 ml	12 grams per 24 hours

Route: Intravenous – slowly over 5–10 minutes.

AGE	INITIAL DOSE	REPEAT DOSE	DOSE INTERVAL	CONCENTRATION	TABLETS	MAXIMUM DOSE
Children	30 milligrams/kg	30 mg/kg	4 hourly	200 milligrams in 1 ml	20 ml	12 grams per 24 hours

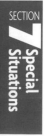

1. Introduction

- The deployment of incapacitating agents on individuals and/or groups can lead to conditions requiring prehospital care.
- The aim of this guideline is to support clinical decision making for the management of patients following the deployment of:
  - i. Conducted Electrical Weapon (CEW) for example TASER®, and stun guns.
  - ii. Incapacitant sprays.
  - iii. Projectiles.
  - iv. Batons.
- Not all patients exposed to incapacitating agents will require hospital assessment; however, all patients should undergo a primary assessment.
- ⚠ **Safety first** – carry out a dynamic risk assessment; continually re-assess throughout the incident.

i. Conducted Electrical Weapon (CEW)

- Conducted Electrical Weapons (CWE) are battery operated hand-held devices which deliver up to 50,000 volts of electricity, in rapid pulses, via two barbed electrodes (Figure 7.4).

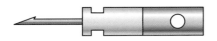

Figure 7.4 – CEW barb. Reproduction of CEW barb image by kind permission of TASER International.

- The barbs are designed to stick into skin or clothes, and connect to the device by fine long copper wires, or via two probes directly applied to the skin or clothes.
- Firing the weapon results in pain and a loss of voluntary control of muscles. These devices are currently in use by all police forces in the United Kingdom.
- ⚠ Before touching the patient ensure the wires are disconnected from the device; the wires break easily by cutting with scissors.
- ⚠ There is an increased risk of combustion if a CWE is deployed after the deployment of incapacitant sprays or following contact with flammable liquids such as petrol.

2. Assessment and Management

- Most people incapacitated with an CEW do not require hospital assessment; however, patients should undergo a primary survey specially assessing for the presence of:
  - neck and back injuries
  - secondary injuries
  - cardiac symptoms
  - excited delirium
  - attached electrodes.
- For the assessment and management of symptoms, conditions and injuries following deployment of CEW refer to Table 7.6.

Table 7.6 – ASSESSMENT and MANAGEMENT following

The Deployment of a Conducted Electrical Weapon (CEW)

PRIMARY EFFECTS

EFFECT	ASSESSMENT/MANAGEMENT
PAIN	For specific guidance **refer to the guidelines for**: • **Management of pain in adults.** • **Management of pain in children.**
Electrode attachment: • The electrodes vary in length and have a 'fish hook' type end which is designed to stick to clothes and into the skin. NB Although the lengths of the barbs may vary, the management principles remain the same.	**Electrode removal:** 1. Slightly stretch the skin around the electrode and pull sharply on the electrode. 2. Dispose of the electrode as contaminated waste. 3. Clean the area with an alcohol/antiseptic wipe. 4. Cover the site with a dressing e.g. a plaster. 5. Advise tetanus booster within 72 hours if not covered for tetanus. NB If the electrode cannot be removed at the first attempt or breaks during attempted removal, leave in situ and transfer to further care. DO NOT attempt to remove the electrode if it is: • Attached to skin where blood vessels are close to the skin surface e.g. neck and groin. • Attached to one or both eye/s.

SECTION 7 Special Situations

Table 7.6 – ASSESSMENT and MANAGEMENT following

The Deployment of a Conducted Electrical Weapon (CEW) *continued*

PRIMARY EFFECTS *continued*

EFFECT	ASSESSMENT/MANAGEMENT
Electrode attachment: *continued*	<ul><li>Attached to the face.</li><li>Attached to the genitalia.</li><li>Attached to the mouth, throat or if the electrode has been swallowed.</li><li>Firmly embedded in the scalp.</li><li>Embedded in a joint e.g. finger.</li><li>Broken.</li></ul>**In these circumstances** – cut the wire close to the electrode leaving approximately 4 cm attached to the electrode and transfer to further care.
Burns:<ul><li>Superficial burns are likely around the area where the electrode attached to the skin and electricity was delivered.</li><li>Burns may also occur if a CWE is deployed after the deployment of incapacitant sprays or following contact with flammable liquids such as petrol.</li></ul>	**For specific guidance refer to the guidelines for:**<ul><li>**Management of pain in adults.**</li><li>**Management of pain in children.**</li></ul>
Cardiac conditions/symptoms:<ul><li>Cardiac conditions have been reported following the deployment of a CEW including, increases in heart rate, cardiac rhythm disturbance, and cardiac arrest.</li></ul>	ECGs are not routinely necessary; however, always undertake a 12-lead ECG, and monitor blood pressure and oxygen saturation for patents:<ul><li>Complaining of chest pain.</li><li>With cardiac symptoms e.g. tachycardia, bradycardia.</li><li>With significant cardiac history e.g. angina, arrhythmias or a myocardial infarction.</li><li>Fitted with pacemakers or cardioverter defibrillator.</li><li>**Cardiac arrhythmia: Refer to the cardiac rhythm disturbance guidelines** for specific guidance.</li><li>**Cardiac arrest: Refer to the appropriate resuscitation guidelines.**</li></ul>
Convulsions:<ul><li>The deployment of a CEW may trigger a convulsion or epileptic fit.</li></ul>	For specific guidance **refer to the guidelines for:**<ul><li>**Convulsions in adults.**</li><li>**Convulsions in children.**</li></ul>
Obstetric and gynaecological conditions: Spontaneous abortion has been reported following the deployment of CWE.	<ul><li>**Refer to the appropriate obstetric and gynaecological guidelines.**</li></ul>
Soft tissue injury/injuries:<ul><li>Contusions</li><li>Tendons damage</li><li>Abrasions</li><li>Lacerations</li><li>Puncture wounds</li></ul>	**Abrasions, lacerations and puncture wounds:** 1. Clean the area with an alcohol/antiseptic wipe. 2. Cover the site with a dressing e.g. a plaster. 3. Advise tetanus booster within 72 hours if not covered for tetanus. **Contusions, damage to ligament and tendons:** These injuries should be managed accordingly.
Head injury:<ul><li>Head injuries and loss of consciousness may also result from intracranial penetration of an electrode.</li></ul>	**For specific guidance refer to the guidelines for:**<ul><li>**Head trauma.**</li><li>**Altered level of consciousness.**</li></ul>

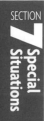

Incapacitating Agents

Table 7.6 – ASSESSMENT and MANAGEMENT following

The Deployment of a Conducted Electrical Weapon (CEW) *continued*

SECONDARY EFFECTS

EFFECT	ASSESSMENT/MANAGEMENT
Head, neck, and back injuries, contusions, abrasions, and lacerations: ● The powerful muscular contractions caused by the deployment of a CEW may result in thoraco-lumbar fractures. ● The loss of voluntary control of the muscles caused by the deployment of a CEW may result in falls, leading to injuries of the head, neck, and back, contusions, abrasions, lacerations, ligament and tendon injury, etc.	For specific guidance refer to the guidelines for: ● **Head trauma**. ● **Altered level of consciousness**. ● **Neck and back trauma**. **Contusions, abrasions, lacerations, ligament and tendon injury:** Manage as per soft tissue injuries above.

COINCIDENTAL EFFECTS

Injuries and conditions unrelated to CEW deployment: ● Injuries and or conditions may be sustained or develop that are unrelated to the deployment of a CEW, for example, as the result of a physical struggle, the consumption of drugs and of physical exhaustion.	Assess and manage coincidental injuries as per condition, cognisant of the effects of drugs, dehydration or exhaustion.
NB Excited delirium:	A CEW may be deployed on people in an aroused state which is sometimes described as 'excited delirium'. People in this state may be at a greater risk of collapse, arrhythmias, and sudden death following deployment of a CEW – undertake a **TIME CRITICAL** transfer and provide an alert/information call. The signs of excited delirium include: bizarre behaviour, physical aggression against people and objects, ripping off clothing, being under the influence of drugs or alcohol, abnormal physical strength, and reduced perception of pain. NB A doctor may be required to administer rapid tranquilisation; assistance from the police may also be required.

ii. Incapacitant sprays

● Incapacitant sprays/peripheral chemosensory irritants (PCSIs) such as pepper spray (oleoresin, capsicum, pelargonic acid, vanillylamide) and CS spray 2-chlorobenzalmalononitrile (O-chlorobenzylidene malononitrile) are prepared with methyl isobutyl ketone (MIBK).

● The sprays cause irritation (burning sensation) when in contact with exposed skin and mucus membranes including eye, nose, and mouth and respiratory tract causing lacrimation, rhinorrhoea, sialorrhoea, disorientation, dizziness, breathing difficulties, coughing, vomiting.

⚠ Try not to enter a contaminated or closed environment.

3. Assessment and Management

● Most people exposed to incapacitant sprays do not require hospital assessment.

● For the assessment and management of symptoms, and conditions following deployment of incapacitant sprays refer to Table 7.7.

iii. Projectiles

● Projectiles such as plastic or rubber bullets or bean bags can cause sudden death (after strikes to the head, chest and abdomen), dislocations, fractures,

SECTION 7 Special Situations

joint damage, ligaments and tendons, haemorrhage and haematoma, compartment syndrome, splenic rupture, subcapsular liver/haematoma, pneumothorax/haemothorax, pentrating injuries to thorax, abdomen, eye, arm, leg, blood vessels.

4. Assessment and Management

For the assessment and management of symptoms refer to Table 7.8.

iv. Batons

- Baton strikes can cause dislocations, fractures, joint damage, ligaments and tendons, haemorrhage and haematoma, compartment syndrome and death.

- Baton strikes to limbs will typically cause 'tramline bruising'; this is of no significant concern unless there is evidence of underlying fracture or neuromuscular condition.

5. Assessment and Management

- For the assessment and management of symptoms refer to Table 7.9.

Methodology

For details of the methodology used in the development of this guideline refer to the guideline webpage.

KEY POINTS

Incapacitating Agents

- Ensure the wires are disconnected from the CWE before touching the patient.
- DO NOT remove electrodes from any of the instances listed in Table 7.6.
- Patients may also sustain secondary injuries e.g. head injuries and fractures following a fall.
- Transfer to further care any patient with one or more of the following: cardiac symptoms, neck and back injuries, excited delirium.
- The symptoms of patients exposed to incapacitant sprays should settle after exposure to air. If symptoms do not settle after 15 minutes transfer to further care.

Table 7.7 – ASSESSMENT and MANAGEMENT following

The Deployment of Incapacitant Sprays

PRIMARY EFFECTS

EFFECT	ASSESSMENT/MANAGEMENT
Lacrimation, rhinorrhoea, sialorrhoea, dizziness, coughing and vomiting	• Move the patient away from the source of the contamination. • Expose to fresh air. • For patients with heavy contamination of the skin and eyes irrigate with tap water. • If symptoms persist for longer than 15 minutes transfer to further care.
Breathing difficulties	For specific guidance **refer to the guideline for**: • **Dyspnoea.**

Table 7.8 – ASSESSMENT and MANAGEMENT following

The Deployment of Projectiles

PRIMARY EFFECTS

EFFECT	ASSESSMENT/MANAGEMENT
Head injuries and loss of consciousness	For specific guidance refer to the guidelines for: • **Head trauma.** • **Altered level of consciousness.**
Chest injuries	For specific guidance **refer to the guideline for**: • **Thoracic trauma.**
Abdominal injuries	For specific guidance **refer to the guideline for**: • **Abdominal trauma.**

Table 7.9 – ASSESSMENT and MANAGEMENT following

The Deployment of Batons

PRIMARY EFFECTS

EFFECT	ASSESSMENT/MANAGEMENT
Dislocations, fractures, damage, ligaments and tendons	For specific guidance refer to the guidelines for: ● **Trauma emergencies in adults – overview**. ● **Trauma emergencies in children – overview**.
Haemorrhage and haematoma, compartment syndrome	For specific guidance refer to the guidelines for: ● **Trauma emergencies in adults – overview**. ● **Trauma emergencies in children – overview**.

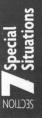

References

1. Health and Care Professions Council. *Standards of Conduct, Performance and Ethics: Your duties as a registrant*. London: Health Professions Council, 2003.

2. Gold M, Philip J, McIver S, Komesaroff PA. Between a rock and a hard place: exploring the conflict between respecting the privacy of patients and informing their carers. *Internal Medicine Journal* 2009, 39(9): 582–87.

3. Department of Health. *Confidentiality: NHS Code of Practice*. London: Stationery Office, 2003.

4. NHS Scotland. *NHS Code of Practice on Protecting Patient Confidentiality*. Available from: http://www.ehealth.scot.nhs.uk/wp-content/documents/nhs-code-of-practice-on-protecting-patient-confidentiality.pdf, 2003/2009.

5. Department of Health. *Confidentiality: NHS Code of Practice – supplementary guidance: public interest disclosures*. Available from: www.dh.gov.uk/publications, 2010.

6. General Medical Council. *Confidentiality: Protecting and providing information*. London: General Medical Council, 2004.

7. Thomas MG. Team learning: the issue of patient confidentiality. *Work Based Learning in Primary Care* 2004, 2(4): 377–80.

8. Department of Health. *The Caldicott Committee Report on the Review of Patient-identifiable Information*. London: Stationery Office, 1997.

9. Woodward B. The computer-based patient record and confidentiality. *The New England Journal of Medicine* 1995, 333(21): 1419–22.

10. Gostin LO. Health information privacy. *Cornell Law Review* 1995, 80(3): 451–528.

11. Brooks J. Caldicott Guardians: driving the confidentiality agenda. *British Journal of Healthcare Computing and Information Management* 2004, 21(3): 20–1.

12. White C, Hardy J. What do palliative care patients and their relatives think about research in palliative care? A systematic review. *Support Care Cancer* 2010, 18(8): 905–11.

13. Data Protection Act 1998. London: Stationery Office, 1998.

14. Department of Health. *The Caldicott Committee Report on the Review of Patient-identifiable Information*. London: Stationery Office, 1997.

15. General Medical Council. *Confidentiality*. Available from: http://www.gmc-uk.org/static/documents/content/Confidentiality_0910.pdf, 2009.

16. Griffith R, Tengnah C. Access to health records: the rights of the patient. *British Journal of Community Nursing* 2010, 15(7): 344–7.

17. Wougare J. Patient rights to privacy and dignity in the NHS. *Nursing Standard* 2005, 19(18): 33–7.

18. Ministry of Justice. *The Mental Capacity Act 2005 Code of Practice*. London: The Stationery Office, 2005.

19. British Medical Association. *The Mental Capacity Act 2005: Guidance for health professionals*. Available from: http://www.bma.org.uk/irnages/mentalcapacityactguidanceaug2009_tcm4l-190120.pdf, 2009.

20. Malviya S, Voepel-Lewis T, Burke C, Merkel 5, Tait AR. The revised FLACC observational pain tool: improved reliability and validity for pain assessment in children with cognitive impairment. *Pediatric Anesthesia* 2006, 16(3): 258–65.

21. Royal College of Paediatrics and Child Health. Available from: http://www.rcpch.ac.uk, 2012.

22. National Society for the Prevention of Cruelty to Children. Available from: http://www.nspcc.org.uk, 2012.

23. Department of Health. *National Service Framework for Children, Young People and Maternity Services*. London: The Stationery Office, 2004.

24. Department of Health Social Care Group. *No Secrets: Guidance on developing and implementing multi-agency policies and procedures to protect vulnerable adults from abuse*. London: The Stationery Office, 2000.

25. HM Government. *Children Act 2004*. Available from: http://www.legislation.gov.uk/ukpga/2004/31/pdfs/ukpga_20040031_en.pdf, 2004.

26. Lord Laming. *The Victoria Climbié Inquiry*. London: The Stationery Office, 2003. Available from: http://www.dh.gov.uk/prod_consum_dh/groups/dh_digitalassets/documents/digitalasset/dh_110711.pdf.

27. Lord Laming. *The Protection of Children in England: Progress report*. London: The Stationery Office, 2009.

28. Department for Children, Schools and Families. *Working Together to Safeguard Children: A guide to inter-agency working to safeguard and promote the welfare of children*. London: The Stationery Office, 2010. Available from: https: //www.education.gov.uk/publications/eOrderingDownload/00305-2010DOM-EN.pdf.

29. National Institute for Health and Clinical Excellence. *When to Suspect Child Maltreatment: NICE guideline (CG 89)*. London: NICE, 2009. Available from: http://www.nice.org.uk/nicemedia/live/12183/44914/44914.pdf.

30. Avegno J, Mills TJ, Mills LD. Sexual assault victims in the emergency department: analysis by demographic and event characteristics. *Journal of Emergency Medicine* 2009, 37(3). 328–34.

31. Dalton M. *Forensic Gynaecology: Towards better care of the female victim of sexual assault*. London: Royal College of Obstetricians and Gynaecologists Press, 2004.

32. Department of Health. *Improving Services for Women and Child Victims of Violence: the Department of Health Action Plan*. Available from: http://www.dh.gov.uk/prod_consum_dh/groups/dh_digitalassets/@dh/@ en/@ps/documents/digitalasset/dh_122094.pdf, 2010.

33. Du Mont J, White D, McGregor MJ. Investigating the medical forensic examination from the perspectives of sexually assaulted women. *Social Science & Medicine* 2009, 68(4): 774–80.

34. Martin EK, Taft CT, Resick PA. A review of marital rape. *Aggression and Violent Behavior* 2007, 12(3): 329–47.

35. Moin JK, Palmer CM, Shand MC, Templeton DJ, Parekh V, Mobbs M, et al. Management of acute adult sexual assault. *Medical Journal of Australia* 2003, 178(5): 226–30.

36. Metropolitan Specialist Crime Directorate. *Rape and Serious Sexual Assault*. Available from: http://www.met.police.uk/sapphire, 2011.

37. Pesola GR, Westfal RE, Kuffner CA. Emergency department characteristics of male sexual assault. *Academic Emergency Medicine* 1999, 6(8): 792–98.

38. Regan L, Lovett J, Kelly L. *Forensic Nursing: An option for improving responses to reported rape and sexual assault*. London: Home Office, 2004.

39. Taskforce on the Health Aspects of Violence Against Women and Children. *Responding to Violence Against Women and Children: The role of the NHS*. Available from: http://www.dh.gov.uk/prod_consum_dh/groups/dh_digitalassets/@dh/@ en/@ps/documents/digitalasset/dh_113824.pdf, 2010.

40. Office of the Public Guardian. *Office of the Public Guardian and Local Authorities: A protocol for working together to safeguard vulnerable adults*. Available from: http://www.justice.gov.uk/downloads/protecting-the-vulnerable/mca/sva-policyl-12081.pdf, 2008.

41. Office of the Public Guardian. *Safeguarding Vulnerable Adults Policy.* Available from: http://www.justice.gov.uk/downloads/protecting-the-vulnerable/mca/sva-policyl-12081.pdf, 2008.

42. Lord Chancellor's Department. *Who Decides? Making decisions on behalf of mentally incapacitated adults.* London: The Stationery Office, 1997.

43. Department of Health, Home Office. *Clinical Governance and Adult Safeguarding: An integrated process.* Available from: http://www.dh.gov.uk/prod_consum_dh/groups/dh_digitalassets/@dh/@en@ps/documents/digitalasset/dh_112341.pdf, 2010.

44. Department of Health, Home Office. *Safeguarding Adults: Report on the consultation on the review of No Secrets.* Available from: http://www.dh.gov.uk/prod_consum_dh/groups/dh_digitalassets/documents/digitalasset/dh_102981.pdf, 2009.

45. Department of Health, Home Office. *No Secrets: Guidance on developing and implementing multi-agency policies and procedures to protect vulnerable adults from abuse.* Available from: http://www.dh.gov.uk/prod_consum_dh/groups/dh_digitalassets/@dh/@en/documents/digitalasset/dh_4074540.pdf, 2000.

46. Department of Health. *Safeguarding Adults: The role of health services.* Available from: http://www.dh.gov.uk/en/Publicationsandstatistics/Publications/PublicationsPolicyAndGuidance/DH_124882, 2011.

47. Biarent D, Bingham R, Eich C, López-Herce J, Maconochie I, Rodriguez-Nunez A, et al. European Resuscitation Council Guidelines for Resuscitation 2010 Section 6: Paediatric life support. *Resuscitation* 2010, 81(10): 1364–88.

48. Richmond S, Wyllie J. European Resuscitation Council Guidelines for Resuscitation 2010: Section 7: Resuscitation of babies at birth. *Resuscitation* 2010, 81(10): 1389–99.

49. Porter A, Snooks H, Youren A, Gaze S, Whitfield R, Rapport F, et al. 'Covering our backs': ambulance crews' attitudes towards clinical documentation when emergency (999) patients are not conveyed to hospital. *Emergency Medicine Journal* 2008, 25(5): 292–95.

50. The Childhood Bereavement Network. Available from: http://www.childhoodbereavementnetwork.org.uk/index.htm, 2012.

51. Department of Health. *Reduce the Risk of Cot Death.* Available from: http://www.dh.gov.uk/en/Publicationsandstatistics/Publications/PublicationsPolicyAndGuidance/DH_4123625, 2009.

52. Loughrey CM, Preece MA, Green A. Sudden unexpected death in infancy (SUDI). *Journal of Clinical Pathology* 2005, 58(1): 20–1.

53. National End of Life Care Programme and National Nurse Consultant Group. *Guidance for Staff Responsible for Care after Death.* Available from: http://www.endoflifecareforadults.nhs.uk/publications/guidance-for-staff-responsible-for-care-after-death, 2005.

54. The University of Nottingham. *Bereavement Care Services: A synthesis of the literature.* Available from: http://www.endoflifecareforadults.nhs.uk/publications/bereavement-care-services-a-synthesis-of-the-literature, 2010.

55. The Royal College of Pathologists, The Royal College of Paediatrics and Child Health. *Sudden Unexpected Death in Infancy: A multi-agency protocol for care and investigation.* Available from: http://www.rcpath.org/Resources/RCPath/Migrated%20Resources/Documents/S/SUDI%20report%20for%20web.pdf, 2004.

56. The Royal College of Pathologists, The Royal College of Paediatrics and Child Health. *Sudden Unexpected Death in Infancy: A multi-agency protocol for care and investigation.* Available from: http://www.rcpath.org/Resources/RCPath/Migrated%20Resources/Documents/S/SUDI%20report%20for%20web.pdf, 2004.

57. Royal College of Paediatrics and Child Health. *Review of Child Deaths.* Available from: http://www.rcpch.ac.uk/child-health-review-uk/chr-uk-programme/child-health-reviews-uk, 2012.

58. Deakin CD, Nolan JP, Soar J, Sunde K, Koster RW, Smith GB, et al. European Resuscitation Council Guidelines for Resuscitation 2010 Section 4: Adult advanced life support. *Resuscitation* 2010, 81(10): 1305–52.

59. Koster RW, Baubin MA, Bossaert LL, Caballero A, Cassan P, Castren M, et al. European Resuscitation Council Guidelines for Resuscitation 2010 Section 2: Adult basic life support and use of automated external defibrillators. *Resuscitation* 2010, 81(10): 1277–92.

60. Soar J, Perkins GD, Abbas G, Alfonzo A, Barelli A, Bierens JJLM, et al. European Resuscitation Council Guidelines for Resuscitation 2010 Section 8: Cardiac arrest in special circumstances: electrolyte abnormalities, poisoning, drowning, accidental hypothermia, hyperthermia, asthma, anaphylaxis, cardiac surgery, trauma, pregnancy, electrocution. *Resuscitation* 2010, 81(10): 1400–33.

61. de Caen AR, Kleinman ME, Chameides L, Atkins DL, Berg RA, Berg MD, et al. Part 10: Paediatric basic and advanced life support: 2010 International Consensus on Cardiopulmonary Resuscitation and Emergency Cardiovascular Care Science with Treatment Recommendations. *Resuscitation* 2010, 81(1): e213–59.

62. Deakin CD, Clarke T, Nolan J, Zideman DA, Gwinnutt C, Moore F, et al. A critical reassessment of ambulance service airway management in prehospital care: Joint Royal Colleges Ambulance Liaison Committee Airway Working Group, June 2008. *Emergency Medicine Journal* 2010, 27(3): 226–33.

63. Deakin CD, Morrison LJ, Morley PT, Callaway CW, Kerber RE, Kronick SL, et al. Part 8: Advanced life support: 2010 International Consensus on Cardiopulmonary Resuscitation and Emergency Cardiovascular Care Science with Treatment Recommendations. *Resuscitation* 2010, 81(1): e93–174.

64. Koster RW, Sayre MR, Botha M, Cave DM, Cudnik MT, Handley AJ, et al. Part 5: Adult basic life support: 2010 International Consensus on Cardiopulmonary Resuscitation and Emergency Cardiovascular Care Science with Treatment Recommendations. *Resuscitation* 2010, 81(1): e48–70.

65. Wyllie J, Perlman JM, Kattwinkel J, Atkins DL, Chameides L, Goldsmith JP, et al. Part 11: Neonatal resuscitation: 2010 International Consensus on Cardiopulmonary Resuscitation and Emergency Cardiovascular Care Science with Treatment Recommendations. *Resuscitation* 2010, 81(1): e260–87.

66. Lim SH, Shuster M, Deakin CD, Kleinman ME, Koster RW, Morrison LJ, et al. Part 7: CPR techniques and devices: 2010 International Consensus on Cardiopulmonary Resuscitation and Emergency Cardiovascular Care Science with Treatment Recommendations. *Resuscitation* 2010, 81(1): e86–92.

67. Lockey D, Crewdson K, Davies G. Traumatic cardiac arrest: who are the survivors? *Annals of Emergency Medicine* 2006, 48(3): 240–4.

68. Lippert FK, Raffay V, Georgiou M, Steen PA, Bossaert L. European Resuscitation Council Guidelines for Resuscitation 2010 Section 10: The ethics of resuscitation and end-of-life decisions. *Resuscitation* 2010, 81(10): 1445–51.

References

69. Nolan JP, Soar J, Zideman DA, Biarent D, Bossaert LL, Deakin C, et al. European Resuscitation Council Guidelines for Resuscitation 2010 Section 1: Executive summary. *Resuscitation* 2010, 81(10): 1219–76.

70. British Medical Association, Resuscitation Council (UK), Royal College of Nursing. *Decisions Relating to Cardio-pulmonary Resuscitation: A joint statement.* London: RCN, 2007. Available from: http://www.rcn.org.uk/data/assets/pdf_file/0004/108337/003206.pdf.

71. Department of Health. *Mental Capacity Act 2005: Information about the transitional provisions for existing advance decisions to refuse life-sustaining treatment.* Available from: http://www.dh.gov.uk/en/Publicationsandstatistics/Publications/PublicationsPolicyAndGuidance/DH_078814, 2007.

72. Nolan JP, Soar J, Zideman DA, Biarent D, Bossaert LL, Deakin C, et al. European Resuscitation Council Guidelines for Resuscitation 2010 Section 1: Executive summary. *Resuscitation* 2010, 81(10): 1219–76.

73. Soar J, Mancini ME, Bhanji F, Billi JE, Dennett J, Finn J, et al. Part 12: Education, implementation, and teams: 2010 International Consensus on Cardiopulmonary Resuscitation and Emergency Cardiovascular Care Science with Treatment Recommendations. *Resuscitation* 2010, 81(1): e288–332.

74. Deakin CD, Nolan JP, Sunde K, Koster RW. European Resuscitation Council Guidelines for Resuscitation 2010 Section 3: Electrical therapies: automated external defibrillators, defibrillation, cardioversion and pacing. *Resuscitation* 2010, 81(10): 1293–304.

75. Sunde K, Jacobs I, Deakin CD, Hazinski MF, Kerber RE, Koster RW, et al. Part 6: Defibrillation: 2010 International Consensus on Cardiopulmonary Resuscitation and Emergency Cardiovascular Care Science with Treatment Recommendations. *Resuscitation* 2010, 81(1): e71–85.

76. Royal College of Obstetricians and Gynaecologists. *Maternal Collapse in Pregnancy and the Puerperium (Green-top Guideline 56).* London: RCOG, 2009.

77. Kavanagh S. The acute abdomen: assessment, diagnosis and pitfalls. *UK MPS Casebook* 2004, 12(1): 11–18.

78. Manterola C, Vial M, Moraga J, Astudillo P. Analgesia in patients with acute abdominal pain. *Cochrane Database of Systematic Reviews* 2011, 1. Available from: http://www.mrw.interscience.wiley.com/cochrane/clsysrev/articles/CD005660/frame.html: doi 10.1002/14651858.CD005660.pub3.

79. Agarwal T, Butt MA. Small bowel obstruction. *Emergency Medicine Journal* 2007, 24(5): 368.

80. Amoli HA, Golozar A, Keshavarzi S, Tavakoli H, Yaghoobi A. Morphine analgesia in patients with acute appendicitis: a randomised double-blind clinical trial. *Emergency Medicine Journal* 2008, 25(9): 586–89.

81. Beck J, Jang TB. Short answer question case series: controversies in the diagnosis and management of diverticulitis. *Emergency Medicine Journal* 2012, 29(6): 517–18.

82. Beck J, Jang TB. Short answer question case series: diagnosis of acute cholecystitis. *Emergency Medicine Journal* 2012, 29(5): 430–1.

83. Beckingham IJ, Bornman PC. Acute pancreatitis. *British Medical Journal* 2001, 322(7286): 595–8.

84. Car J. Urinary tract infections in women: diagnosis and management in primary care. *British Medical Journal* 2006, 332(7533): 94–7.

85. Cartwright SL, Knudson MP. Evaluation of acute abdominal pain in adults. *American Family Physician* 2008, 77(7): 971–8.

86. Chan SSW, Ng KC, Lyon DJ, Cheung WL, Cheng AFB, Rainer TH. Acute bacterial gastroenteritis: a study of adult patients with positive stool cultures treated in the emergency department. *Emergency Medicine Journal* 2003, 20(4): 335–8.

87. Chong CF, Wang TL, Chen CC, Ma HP, Chang H. Preconsultation use of analgesics on adults presenting to the emergency department with acute appendicitis. *Emergency Medicine Journal* 2004, 21(1): 41–3.

88. Gray J, Wardrope J, Fothergill DJ. The ABC of community emergency care: 7 Abdominal pain: abdominal pain in women, complications of pregnancy and labour. *Emergency Medicine Journal* 2004, 21(5): 606–13.

89. Hall J, Driscoll P. The ABC of community emergency care: 10 Nausea, vomiting and fever. *Emergency Medicine Journal* 2005, 22(3): 200–4.

90. Humes DJ, Simpson J. Acute appendicitis. *British Medical Journal* 2006, 333(7567): 530–4.

91. Kingsnorth A, O'Reilly D. Acute pancreatitis. *British Medical Journal* 2006, 332(7549): 1072–6.

92. Lehnert T, Sorge I, Till H, Rolle U. Intussusception in children: clinical presentation, diagnosis and management. *International Journal of Colorectal Disease* 2009, 24(10): 1187–92.

93. Lewis SRR, Mahony PJ, Simpson J. Appendicitis. *British Medical Journal* 2011, 343: d5976.

94. Little P, Merriman R, Turner S, Rumsby K, Warner G, Lowes JA, et al. Presentation, pattern, and natural course of severe symptoms, and role of antibiotics and antibiotic resistance among patients presenting with suspected uncomplicated urinary tract infection in primary care: observational study. *British Medical Journal* 2010, 340: b5633.

95. Lynch RM. Accuracy of abdominal examination in the diagnosis of non-ruptured abdominal aortic aneurysm. *Accident and Emergency Nursing* 2004, 12(2): 99–107.

96. Metcalfe D, Holt PIE, Thompson MM. The management of abdominal aortic aneurysms. *British Medical Journal* 2011, 342: d1384.

97. Ranji SR, Goldman L, Simel DL, Shojania KG. Do opiates affect the clinical evaluation of patients with acute abdominal pain? *Journal of the American Medical Association* 2006, 296(14): 764–74.

98. Royal College of Obstetricians and Gynaecologists. *Management of Acute Pelvic Inflammatory Disease (Green top Guideline 32).* London: RCOG, 2008. Available from: http://www.rcog.org.uk/files/rcog-corp/uploaded-files/T32PelvicInflammatoryDisease2008MinorRevision.pdf.

99. Sakalihasan N, Limet R, Defawe OD. Abdominal aortic aneurysm. *The Lancet* 2005, 365(9470): 1577–89.

100. Touzios JG, Dozois EJ. Diverticulosis and acute diverticulitis. *Gastroenterology Clinics of North America* 2009, 38(3): 513–25.

101. Trowbridge RL, Rutkowski NK, Shojania KG. Does this patient have acute cholecystitis? *Journal of the American Medical Association* 2003, 289(1): 80–6.

102. National Collaborating Centre for Women's and Children's Health. *Urinary Tract Infection in Children: Diagnosis, treatment and long-term management* (CG54). London: Royal College of Obstetricians and Gynaecologists, 2007. Available from: http://www.nice.org.uk/nicemedia/pdf/CG54fullguideline.pdf.

103. National Collaborating Centre for Women's and Children's Health. *Diarrhoea and Vomiting in Children: Diarrhoea and vomiting caused by gastroenteritis: diagnosis, assessment and management in children younger than 5 years* (CG84). London: National Institute for Health and Clinical Excellence, 2009. Available from: http://www.nice.org.uk/nicemedia/live/11846/47350/47350.pdf.

References

104. Scottish Intercollegiate Guidelines Network. *Management of Acute Upper and Lower Gastrointestinal Bleeding* (Guideline 105). Edinburgh: SIGN, 2008.

105. Arntz H-R, Bossaert LL, Danchin N, Nikolaou NI. European Resuscitation Council Guidelines for Resuscitation 2010 Section 5: Initial management of acute coronary syndromes. *Resuscitation* 2010, 81(10): 1353–63.

106. Bossaert L, O'Connor RE, Arntz H-R, Brooks SC, Diercks D, Feitosa-Filho G, et al. Part 9: Acute coronary syndromes: 2010 International Consensus on Cardiopulmonary Resuscitation and Emergency Cardiovascular Care Science with Treatment Recommendations. *Resuscitation* 2010, 81(1): e175–212.

107. National Collaborating Centre for Acute Care. *Head Injury: Triage, assessment, investigation and early management of head injury in infants, children and adults* (CG56). London: National Collaborating Centre for Acute Care at The Royal College of Surgeons of England, 2007. Available from: http://www.nice.orguk/nicemedia/pdf/CG56guidance.pdf.

108. National Institute for Health and Clinical Excellence. *Stroke: The diagnosis and initial management of acute stroke and transient ischaemic attack* (CG68). London: NICE, 2008.

109. National Institute for Health and Clinical Excellence. *The Epilepsies: The diagnosis and management of the epilepsies in adults and children in primary and secondary care* (CG137). London: NICE, 2012. Available from: http://guidance.nice.org.uk/CG137/NICEGuidance/pdf/English.

110. National Institute for Health and Clinical Excellence. *Transient Loss of Consciousness in Adults and Young People* (CG109). London: NICE, 2012. Available from: http://www.nice.org.uk/nicemedia/live/13111/50432/50432.pdf.

111. Task Force for the Diagnosis and Management of Syncope, European Society of Cardiology, European Heart Rhythm Association, Heart Failure Association, Heart Rhythm Society, Moya A, Sutton R, Ammirati F, Blanc JJ, Brignole M, Dahm JB, et al. Guidelines for the diagnosis and management of syncope (version 2009). *European Heart Journal* 2009, 30(21): 2631–71.

112. Lansing RW, Gracely RH, Banzett RB. The multiple dimensions of dyspnea: review and hypotheses. *Respiratory Physiology and Neurobiology* 2009, 167(1): 53–60.

113. Nardi AE, Freire RC, Zin WA. Panic disorder and control of breathing. *Respiratory Physiology and Neurobiology* 2009, 167(1): 133–43.

114. Peiffer C. Dyspnea relief: more than just the perception of a decrease in dyspnea. *Respiratory Physiology and Neurobiology* 2009, 167(1): 61–71.

115. Parshall MB, Schwartzstein RM, Adams L, Banzett RB, Manning HL, Bourbeau J, et al. An official American Thoracic Society statement: update on the mechanisms, assessment, and management of dyspnea. *American Journal of Respiratory and Critical Care Medicine* 2012, 185(4): 435–52.

116. Michelson E, Hollrah S. Evaluation of the patient with shortness of breath: an evidence based approach. *Emergency Medicine Clinics of North America* 1999, 17(1): 221–37.

117. Karras DJ, Sammon ME, Terregino CA, Lopez BL, Griswold SK, Arnold GK. Clinically meaningful changes in quantitative measures of asthma severity. *Academic Emergency Medicine* 2000, 7(4): 327–34.

118. National Institute for Health and Clinical Excellence. *Chest Pain of Recent Onset: Assessment and diagnosis of recent onset chest pain or discomfort of suspected cardiac origin* (CG95). London: NICE, 2010. Available from: http://www.nice.org.uk/nicemedia/live/12947/47938/47938.pdf.

119. NHS Evidence. *Dyspnoea*. Available from: http://www.evidence.nhs.uk/search?q=Dyspnoea, 2010.

120. NHS Evidence. *Headache Assessment/Management: How should I assess someone presenting with a headache?* Clinical Knowledge Summaries. London: NHS Evidence, 2010.

121. Scottish Intercollegiate Guidelines Network. *Diagnosis and Management of Headache in Adults* (Guideline 107). Edinburgh: SIGN, 2008. Available from: http://www.sign.ac.uk/pdf/signl07.pdf.

122. The Headache Classification Subcommittee of the International Headache Society. *The International Classification of Headache Disorders, 2nd Edition (ICHD-II)*, 1st revision. The International Headache Society, 2005.

123. World Health Organization. *Headache Disorders* (Fact sheet 277). Available from: http://www.who.int/mediacentre/factsheets/fs277/en, 2004.

124. Budassi Sheehy S, editor. *Emergency Nursing: Principles and practice*, third edition. London: Elsevier Health Sciences, 1992.

125. National Collaborating Centre for Mental Health. *Common Mental Health Disorders: Identification and pathways to care* (CG123). London: NCCMH, 2011. Available from: http://publications.nice.org.uk/common-mental-health-disorders-cg123.

126. Department of Health. *Improving the Management of Patients with Mental Ill Health in Emergency Care Settings*. Available from: http://its-services.org.ulc/silo/files/improving-the-management-of-patients-with-mental-ill-health-in-emergency-care-settings-pdf, 2004.

127. Anderson D, Aveyard B, Baldwin B, Barker A, Forsyth D, Holmes J, et al. *Who Cares Wins*. Leeds: The Royal College of Psychiatrists, 2005. Available from: http://www.rcpsych.ac.uk/PDF/WhoCaresWins.pdf.

128. National Institute for Health and Clinical Excellence. *Self-harm: The short-term physical and psychological management and secondary prevention of self-harm in primary and secondary care* (CG16). London: NICE, 2004. Available from: http://www.nice.org.uk/CG16.

129. Nicholson TRJ, Cutter W, Hotopf M. Assessing mental capacity: the Mental Capacity Act. *British Medical Journal* 2008, 336(7639): 322–5.

130. Zigmond T. *A Clinician's Brief Guide to the Mental Health Act*. London: Royal College of Psychiatrists, 2011.

131. Advanced Life Support Group. *Pre-hospital Paediatric Life Support. A practical approach to the out-of-hospital emergency care of children*, second edition. Oxford: Blackwell, 2005.

132. Maconochie I. Capillary refill time in the field: it's enough to make you blush. *Prehospital Immediate Care* 1998, 2: 95–6.

133. Revell M, Porter K, Greaves I. Fluid resuscitation in prehospital trauma care: a consensus view. *Emergency Medicine Journal* 2002,19(6): 494–8.

134. Samuels M, Wieteska S. *Advanced Paediatric Life Support: The practical approach*, fifth edition. Oxford: Blackwell, 2012.

135. Walls RM. *Manual of Emergency Airway Management*. Philadelphia, PA: Lippincott Williams and Wilkins, 2000.

136. Jewkes F, Woollard M. Assessment and management of paediatric primary survey negative patients. *Emergency Medicine Journal* 2004, 21(5): 595–605.

References

137. Hanna CM, Greenes DS. How much tachycardia in infants can be attributed to fever? *Annals of Emergency Medicine* 2004, 43(6): 699–705.

138. Hay AD, Costelloe C, Redmond NM, Montgomery AA, Fletcher M, Hollinghurst S, et al. Paracetamol plus ibuprofen for the treatment of fever in children (PITCH): randomised controlled trial. *British Medical Journal* 2008, 337: a1302.

139. National Collaborating Centre for Women's and Children's Health. *Feverish Illness in Children: Assessment and initial management in children younger than 5 years* (CG47). London: National Institute for Health and Clinical Excellence, 2007.

140. National Collaborating Centre for Women's and Children's Health. *Patient's Information Sheet.* London: National Institute for Health and Clinical Excellence, 2007.

141. National Collaborating Centre for Women's and Children's Health. *Bacterial Meningitis and Meningococcal Septicaemia: Management of bacterial meningitis and meningococcal septicaemia in children and young people younger than 16 years in primary and secondary care* (CG102). London: National Institute for Health and Clinical Excellence, 2010. Available from: http://publications.nice.org.ukjbacterial-meningitis-and-meningococcalsepticaemia-cg102.

142. Woollard M, Pitt K. Antipyretic prehospital therapy for febrile convulsions: does the treatment fit? A literature review. *Health Education* 2003, 62(1): 23–8.

143. Godden CW, Campbell MJ, Hussey M, Cogswell JJ. Double blind placebo controlled trial of nebulised budesonide for croup. *Archives of Disease in Childhood* 1997, 76(2): 155–8.

144. Russell KF, Liang Y, O'Gorman K, Johnson DW, Klassen TP. Glucocorticoids for croup. *Cochrane Database of Systematic Reviews* 2011(1): CD001955.

145. Scottish Intercollegiate Guidelines Network. *Management of Sore Throat and Indications for Tonsillectomy* (Guideline 117). Edinburgh: SIGN, 2010. Available from: http://www.sign.ac.uk/pdf/sign117.pdf.

146. Sparrow A, Geelhoed G. Prednisolone versus dexamethasone in croup: a randomised equivalence trial. *Archives of Disease in Childhood* 2006, 91(7): 580–3.

147. Scottish Intercollegiate Guidelines Network. *Bronchiolitis in Children* (Guideline 91). Edinburgh: SIGN, 2006. Available from: http://www.sign.ac.uk/pdf/sign9l.pdf.

148. Baumer JH. Glucocorticoid treatment in croup. *Archives of Disease in Childhood Education and Practice Edition* 2006, 91(2): ep58–60.

149. Sandell JM, Charman SC. Can age-based estimates of weight be safely used when resuscitating children? *Emergency Medicine Journal* 2009, 26(1): 43–7.

150. Taussig LM, Castro O, Beaudry PH, Fox WW, Bureau M. Treatment of laryngotracheobronchitis (croup): use of intermittent positive-pressure breathing and racemic epinephrine. *American Journal of Diseases of Children* 1975, 129(7): 790–3.

151. Centre for Clinical Practice at the National Institute for Health and Clinical Excellence. *Acutely Ill Patients in Hospital: Recognition of and response to acute illness in adults in hospital* (CG50). London: NICE, 2007. Available from: http://www.nice.org.uk/nicemedia/live/11810/58247/58247.pdf.

152. National Institute for Health and Clinical Excellence. *Respiratory Tract Infections – Antibiotic Prescribing: Prescribing of antibiotics for self-limiting respiratory tract infections in adults and children in primary care* (CG 69). London: NICE, 2008. Available from: http://www.nice.org.uk/nicemedia/live/12015/41323/41323.pdf.

153. The British National Formulary for Children. *Croup.* Available from: http://www.evidence.nhs.uk/formulary/bnfc/current/medical-emergencies-in-the-community/croup, 2011.

154. Soar J, Deakin CD, Nolan JP, Abbas G, Alfonzo A, Handley AJ, et al. European Resuscitation Council Guidelines for Resuscitation 2005 Section 7: Cardiac arrest in special circumstances. *Resuscitation* 2005, 67(suppl. 1): S135–570.

155. Bouchama A, Dehbi M, Mohamed G, Matthies F, Shoukri M, Menne B. Prognostic factors in heat wave related deaths: a meta-analysis. *Archives of Internal Medicine* 2007, 167(20): 2170–6.

156. Pease S, Bouadma L, Kermarrec N, Schortgen F, Regnier B, Wolff M. Early organ dysfunction course, cooling time and outcome in classic heatstroke. *Intensive Care Medicine* 2009, 35(8): 1454–8.

157. Allen A, Segal-Gidan F. Heat-related illness in the elderly. *Clinical Geriatrics* 2007, 15(7): 37–45.

158. Belmin J, Auffray J-C, Berbezier C, Boirin P, Mercier S, de Reviers B, et al. Level of dependency: a simple marker associated with mortality during the 2003 heatwave among French dependent elderly people living in the community or in institutions. *Age and Ageing* 2007, 36(3): 298–303.

159. Brody GM. Hyperthermia and hypothermia in the elderly. *Clinics in Geriatric Medicine* 1994, 10(1): 213–29.

160. Daniel V, Paladugu N, Fuentes G. Heat stroke and cocaine in an inner city New York hospital. *Internet Journal of Emergency and Intensive Care Medicine* 2008, 11(1): doi 10.5580/157e.

161. de Galan BE, Hoekstra JBL. Extremely elevated body temperature: case report and review of classical heat stroke. *Netherlands Journal of Medicine* 1995, 47(6): 281–7.

162. Hausfater P, Megarbane B, Dautheville S, Patzak A, Andronikof M, Santin A, et al. Prognostic factors in non-exertional heatstroke. *Intensive Care Medicine* 2010, 36(2): 272–80.

163. Stafoggia M, Forastiere F, Agostini D, Biggeri A, Bisanti L, Cadum E, et al. Vulnerability to heat-related mortality: a multicity, population-based, case-crossover analysis. *Epidemiology* 2006, 17(3): 315–23.

164. Vicario SJ, Okabajue R, Haltom T. Rapid cooling in classic heatstroke: effect on mortality rates. *American Journal of Emergency Medicine* 1986, 4(5): 394–8.

165. Bernardo LM, Crane PA, Veenema TG. Treatment and prevention of pediatric heat-related illnesses at mass gatherings and special events. *Dimensions of Critical Care Nursing* 2006, 25(4): 165–71.

166. Guard A, Gallagher SS. Heat related deaths to young children in parked cars: an analysis of 171 fatalities in the United States, 1995–2002. *Injury Prevention* 2005, 11(1): 33–7.

167. Gutierrez G. Solar injury and heat illness: treatment and prevention in children. *Physician and Sportsmedicine* 1995, 23(7): 43–8.

168. Krous HF, Nadeau JM, Fukumoto RI, Blackbourne BD, Byard RW. Environmental hyperthermic infant and early childhood death: circumstances, pathologic changes, and manner of death. *American Journal of Forensic Medicine and Pathology* 2001, 22(4): 374–82.

169. Ohshima T, Maeda H, Takayasu T, Fujioka Y, Nakaya T. An autopsy case of infant death due to heat stroke. *American Journal of Forensic Medicine and Pathology* 1992, 13(3): 217–21.

170. Rossi R. Emergency treatment of an infant with heat-stroke. *Notfallmedizin* 1993, 19(3): 109–11.

171. Wagner C, Boyd K. Pediatric heatstroke. *Air Medical Journal* 2008, 27(3): 118–22.

172. Martinez M, Devenport L, Saussy J, Martinez J. Drug-associated heat stroke. *Southern Medical Journal* 2002, 95(8): 799–802.

173. Aarseth HP, Eide I, Skeie B, Thaulow E. Heat stroke in endurance exercise. *Acta Medica Scandinavica* 1986, 220(3): 279–83.

174. Armstrong LE, Crago AE, Adams R, Roberts WO, Maresh CM. Whole-body cooling of hyperthermic runners: comparison of two field therapies. *American Journal of Emergency Medicine* 1996, 14(4): 355–8.

175. Binkley HM, Beckett J, Casa DJ, Kleiner DM, Plummer PE. National Athletic Trainers' Association position statement: exertional heat illnesses. *Journal of Athletic Training* 2002, 37(3): 329–43.

176. Clapp AJ, Bishop PA, Muir I, Walker IL. Rapid cooling techniques in joggers experiencing heat strain. *Journal of Science and Medicine in Sport* 2001, 4(2): 160–7.

177. Hansen RD, Olds TS, Richards DA, Richards CR, Leelarthaepin B. Infrared thermometry in the diagnosis and treatment of heat exhaustion. *International Journal of Sports Medicine* 1996, 17(1): 66–70.

178. Hee-Nee P, Rupeng M, Lee VJ, Chua W-C, Seet B. Treatment of exertional heat injuries with portable body cooling unit in a mass endurance event. *American Journal of Emergency Medicine* 2010, 28(2): 246–8.

179. McDermott BP, Casa DJ, O'Connor FG, Adams WB, Armstrong LE, Brennan AH, et al. Cold-water dousing with ice massage to treat exertional heat stroke: a case series. *Aviation Space and Environmental Medicine* 2009, 80(8): 720–2.

180. Centers for Disease Control and Prevention. Heat-related deaths among crop workers: United States, 1992–2006. *Morbidity and Mortality Weekly Report* 2008, 57(24): 649–53.

181. Maeda T, Kaneko S-Y, Ohta M, Tanaka K, Sasaki A, Fukushima T. Risk factors for heatstroke among Japanese forestry workers. *Journal of Occupational Health* 2006, 48(4): 223–9.

182. Tranter M. An assessment of heat stress among laundry workers in a Far North Queensland hotel. *Journal of Occupational Health and Safety Australia and New Zealand* 1998, 14(1): 61–3.

183. Yoshino K, Takano K, Nagasaka A, Shigeta S. An experimental study on the prediction of heat stress of workers in a hot environment. With special reference to the relation between wearing suits, work load and environmental temperature. *Japanese Journal of Industrial Health* 1987, 29(6): 466–79.

184. Angerer P, Kadlez-Gebhardt S, Delius M, Raluca P, Nowak D. Comparison of cardiocirculatory and thermal strain of male firefighters during fire suppression to exercise stress test and aerobic exercise testing. *American Journal of Cardiology* 2008, 102(11): 1551–6.

185. Barr D, Gregson W, Reilly T. The thermal ergonomics of firefighting reviewed. *Applied Ergonomics* 2010, 41(1): 161–72.

186. Barr D, Gregson W, Sutton L, Reilly T. A practical cooling strategy for reducing the physiological strain associated with firefighting activity in the heat. *Ergonomics* 2009, 52(4): 413–20.

187. Giesbrecht GG, Jamieson C, Cahill F. Cooling hyperthermic firefighters by immersing forearms and hands in 10 degrees C and 20 degrees C water. *Aviation Space and Environmental Medicine* 2007, 78(6): 561–7.

188. Patel HC, Rao NM, Saha A. Heat exposure effects among firefighters. *Indian Journal of Occupational and Environmental Medicine* 2006, 10(3): 121–3.

189. Bedno SA, Li Y, Han W, Cowan DN, Scott CT, Cavicchia MA, et al. Exertional heat illness among overweight U.S. Army recruits in basic training. *Aviation Space and Environmental Medicine* 2010, 81(2): 107–11.

190. Bruce ASW, Tunstall C, Boulter MJ, Coneybeare A. A treatment algorithm for mass heat casualties. *Journal of the Royal Army Medical Corps* 2008, 154(1): 19–20.

191. Carter R III, Cheuvront SN, Sawka MN. A case report of idiosyncratic hyperthermia and review of U.S. Army heat stroke hospitalizations. *Journal of Sport Rehabilitation* 2007, 16(3): 238–43.

192. Gardner JW, Kark JA. Fatal rhabdomyolysis presenting as mild heat illness in military training. *Military Medicine* 1994, 159(2): 160–3.

193. Keatinge WR, Donaldson GC, Cordioli E, Martinelli M, Kunst AE, Mackenbach W, et al. Heat related mortality in warm and cold regions of Europe: observational study. *British Medical Journal* 2000, 321(7262): 670–3.

194. Epstein Y, Albukrek D, Kalmovitc B, Moran DS, Shapiro Y. Heat intolerance induced by antidepressants. *Annals of the New York Academy of Sciences* 1997, 813: 553–8.

195. Fijnheer R, Van De Ven PJG, Erkelens DW. Psychiatric medication as a risk factor for fatal heat stroke. *Nederlands Tijdschrift voor Geneeskunde* 1995, 139(27): 1391–3.

196. Kao RL, Kelly LM. Fatal exertional heat stroke in a patient receiving zuclopenthixol, quetiapine and benztropine. *Canadian Journal of Clinical Pharmacology* 2007, 14(3): e322–5.

197. Kwok JSS, Chan TYK. Recurrent heat-related illnesses during antipsychotic treatment. *Annals of Pharmacotherapy* 2005, 39(11): 1940–2.

198. Feldman KW, Mazor S. Ecstasy ingestion causing heatstroke-like, multiorgan injury in a toddler. *Pediatric Emergency Care* 2007, 23(10): 725–6.

199. Jenkins RD, Woodhouse KW. Drug-induced fever. *Adverse Drug Reaction Bulletin* 1999, 197: 751–4.

200. Kilbourne EM. Cocaine use and death during heat waves. *Journal of the American Medical Association* 1828, 279(22): 1828–9.

201. Lan K-C, Lin Y-F, Yu F-C, Lin C-S, Chu P. Clinical manifestations and prognostic features of acute methamphetamine intoxication. *Journal of the Formosan Medical Association* 1998, 97(8): 528–33.

202. Dahmash NS, Al Harthi SS, Akhtar J. Invasive evaluation of patients with heat stroke. *Chest* 1993, 103(4): 1210–14.

203. Graham BS, Lichtenstein MJ, Hinson JM, Theis GB. Nonexertional heatstroke. Physiologic management and cooling in 14 patients. *Archives of Internal Medicine* 1986, 146(1): 87–90.

204. LoVecchio F, Pizon AF, Berrett C, Balls A. Outcomes after environmental hyperthermia. *American Journal of Emergency Medicine* 2007, 25(4): 442–4.

205. Misset B, De Jonghe B, Bastuji-Garin S, Gattolliat O, Boughrara E, Annane D, et al. Mortality of patients with heatstroke admitted to intensive care units during the 2003 heat wave in France: a national multiple-center risk-factor study. *Critical Care Medicine* 2006, 34(4): 1087–92.

206. Ramsey CB, Watson WA, Robinson WA. Effect of cooling time on survival in classical heatstroke. *Journal of Wilderness Medicine* 1993, 4(1): 27–31.

207. Varghese GM, John G, Thomas K, Abraham OC, Mathai D. Predictors of multi-organ dysfunction in heatstroke. *Emergency Medicine Journal* 2005, 22(3): 185–7.

208. Albukrek D, Bakon M, Moran DS, Faibel M, Epstein Y. Heat-stroke-induced cerebellar atrophy: clinical course, CT and MRI findings. *Neuroradiology* 1997, 39(3): 195–7.

209. Biary N, Madkour MM, Sharif H. Post-heatstroke parkinsonism and cerebellar dysfunction. *Clinical Neurology and Neurosurgery* 1995, 97(1): 55–7.

210. Deleu D, El Siddig A, Kamran S, Kamha AA, Al Omary IYM, Zalabany HA. Downbeat nystagmus following classical heat stroke. *Clinical Neurology and Neurosurgery* 2005, 108(1): 102–4.

211. Fink E, Brandom BW, Torp KD. Heatstroke in the super-sized athlete. *Pediatric Emergency Care* 2006, 22(7): 510–13.

212. Rav-Acha M, Shuvy M, Hagag S, Gomori M, Biran I. Unique persistent neurological sequelae of heat stroke. *Military Medicine* 2007, 172(6): 603–6.

213. Sudhir U, Anil Kumar T, Srinivasan G, Punith K. Post-heat stroke cerebellar atrophy. *Journal, Indian Academy of Clinical Medicine* 2009, 10(1–2): 60–2.

214. Bazille C, Megarbane B, Bensimhon D, Lavergne-Slove A, Baglin AC, Loirat P, et al. Brain damage after heat stroke. *Journal of Neuropathology and Experimental Neurology* 2005, 64(11): 70–5.

215. Cleary M, Ruiz D, Eberman L, Mitchell I, Binkley H. Dehydration, cramping, and exertional rhabdomyolysis: a case report with suggestions for recovery. *Journal of Sport Rehabilitation* 2007, 16(3): 244–59.

216. Shafie H, Abd Wahab M, Masilamany M, Abu Hassan AA. Exertional heat stroke: a lucky bunch of overly motivated policemen! *Hong Kong Journal of Emergency Medicine* 2007, 14(1): 37–44.

217. Sharma HS, Hoopes PJ. Hyperthermia induced pathophysiology of the central nervous system. *International Journal of Hyperthermia* 2003, 19(3): 325–54.

218. Wang AYM, Li PKT, Lui SF, Lai KN. Renal failure and heatstroke. *Renal Failure* 1995, 17(2): 171–9.

219. Wexler RK. Evaluation and treatment of heat-related illnesses. *American Family Physician* 2002, 65(11): 2307–15.

220. Yan Y-E, Zhao Y-Q, Wang H, Fan M. Pathophysiological factors underlying heatstroke. *Medical Hypotheses* 2006, 67(3): 609–17.

221. Bourdon L, Canini F, Saissy J-M, D'Aleo P, Koulmann N, Aubert M, et al. Exertional heatstroke: II – Pathophysiology. *Science and Sports* 2003, 18(5): 241–52.

222. Bouchama A, Hammami MM, Haq A, Jackson J, Al-Sedairy S. Evidence for endothelial cell activation/injury in heatstroke. *Critical Care Medicine* 1996, 24(7): 1173–8.

223. Lee SJ, Yang ES, Kim SY, Kim SY, Shin SW, Park J-W. Regulation of heat shockinduced apoptosis by sensitive to apoptosis gene protein. *Free Radical Biology and Medicine* 2008, 45(2): 167–76.

224. Wang Z, Shi Q, Li S, Du J, Liu J, Dai K. Hyperthermia induces platelet apoptosis and glycoprotein 1b ectodomain shedding. *Platelets* 2010, 21(3): 229–37.

225. Al-Aska AK, Abu-Aisha H, Yaqub B. Simplified cooling bed for heatstroke. *The Lancet* 1987, 329(8529): 381.

226. Mundel T, Bunn SJ, Hooper PL, Jones DA. The effects of face cooling during hyperthermic exercise in man: evidence for an integrated thermal, neuroendocrine and behavioural response. *Experimental Physiology* 2007, 92(1): 187–95.

227. Sinclair WH, Rudzki SJ, Leicht AS, Fogarty AL, Winter SK, Patterson MJ. Efficacy of field treatments to reduce body core temperature in hyperthermic subjects. *Medicine and Science in Sports and Exercise* 2009, 41(11): 1984–90.

228. Buono MJ, Jechort A, Marques R, Smith C, Welch J. Comparison of infrared versus contact thermometry for measuring skin temperature during exercise in the heat. *Physiological Measurement* 2007, 28(8): 855–9.

229. Gagnon D, Lemire BB, Jay O, Kenny GP. Aural canal, esophageal, and rectal temperatures during exertional heat stress and the subsequent recovery period. *Journal of Athletic Training* 2010, 45(2): 157–63.

230. Budd GM. Wet-bulb globe temperature (WBGT): its history and its limitations. *Journal of Science and Medicine in Sport* 2008, 11(1): 20–32.

231. Moran DS, Pandolf KB. Wet bulb globe temperature (WBGT): to what extent is GT essential? *Aviation Space and Environmental Medicine* 1999, 70(5): 480–4.

232. Smith JE. Cooling methods used in the treatment of exertional heat illness. *British Journal of Sports Medicine* 2005, 39(8): 503–7.

233. McDermott BP, Casa DJ, Ganlo MS, Lopez RM, Yeargin SW, Armstrong LE, et al. Acute whole-body cooling for exercise-induced hyperthermia: a systematic review. *Journal of Athletic Training* 2009, 44(1): 84–93.

234. Casa DJ, McDermott BP, Lee EC, Yeargin SW, Armstrong LE, Maresh CM. Cold water immersion: the gold standard for exertional heatstroke treatment. *Exercise and Sport Sciences Reviews* 2007, 35(3): 141–9.

235. Empana J-P, Sauval P, Ducimetiere P, Tafflet M, Carli P, Jouven X. Increase in out-of-hospital cardiac arrest attended by the medical mobile intensive care units, but not myocardial infarction, during the 2003 heat wave in Paris, France.[Erratum appears in *Critical Care Medicine* 2010, 38(2): 741.] *Critical Care Medicine* 2009, 37(12): 3079–84.

236. Lacunza J, San Roman I, Moreno S, Garcia-Molina E, Gimeno J, Valdes M. Heat stroke, an unusual trigger of Brugada electrocardiogram. *American Journal of Emergency Medicine* 2009, 27(5): 634.e1–3.

237. Wakino S, Hori S, Mimura T, Miyatake S, Fujishima S, Aikawa N. A case of severe heat stroke with abnormal cardiac findings. *International Heart Journal*. 2005, 46(3): 543–50.

238. Malmberg LP, Tamminen K, Sovijärvi ARA. Orthostatic increase of respiratory gas exchange in hyperventilation syndrome. *Thorax* 2000, 55(4): 295–301.

239. Maguire CA, Robson AG, Pentland J, McAllister D, Innes JA. Smoking status predicts benefit from breathing retraining for hyperventilation. *Thorax* 2010, 65(suppl. 4): A157.

240. Gardner W. Orthostatic increase of respiratory gas exchange in hyperventilation syndrome. *Thorax* 2000, 55(4): 257–9.

241. Bazin KA, Moosavi S, Murphy K, Perkins A, Hickson M, Howard LS. Carbon dioxide sensitivity in patients with hyperventilation syndrome. *Thorax* 2010, 65(suppl. 4): A134.

242. van den Hout MA, Boek C, van der Molen GM, Jansen A, Griez E. Rebreathing to cope with hyperventilation: experimental tests of the paper bag method. *Journal of Behavioral Medicine* 1988, 11(3): 303–10.

243. Tavel ME. Hyperventilation syndrome: hiding behind pseudonyms? *Chest* 1990, 97(6): 1285–8.

244. Saisch SGN, Wessely S, Gardner WN. Patients with acute hyperventilation presenting to an inner-city emergency department. *Chest* 1996, 110(4): 952–7.

245. Hornsveld HK, Garssen B, Fiedeldij Dop MJC, van Spiegel PI, de Haes J. Double-blind placebo-controlled study of the hyperventilation provocation test and the validity of the hyperventilation syndrome. *The Lancet* 1996, 348(9021): 154–8.

246. Gardner WN. The pathophysiology of hyperventilation disorders. *Chest* 1996, 109(2): 516–34.

247. Folgering H. The pathophysiology of hyperventilation syndrome. *Monaldi Archives for Chest Disease* 1999, 54(4): 365–72.

248. Callaham M. Hypoxic hazards of traditional paper bag rebreathing in hyperventilating patients. *Annals of Emergency Medicine* 1989, 18(6): 622–8.

249. The British Thoracic Society, Scottish Intercollegiate Guidelines Network. *British Guideline on the Management of Asthma* (Guideline 101). London/Edinburgh: BTS and SIGN, 2008 (revised May 2012). Available from: http://www.sign.ac.uk/pdf/qrgl0l.pdf.

250. Alfonzo A, Lomas A, Drummond I, McGugan E. Survival after 5-h resuscitation attempt for hypothermic cardiac arrest using CVVH for extracorporeal rewarming. *Nephrology Dialysis Transplantation* 2009, 24(3): 1054–6.

251. Brugger H, Etter HJ, Boyd J, Falk M. Causes of death from avalanche. *Wilderness and Environmental Medicine* 2009, 20(1): 93–6.

252. Brugger H, Paal P, Boyd J. Prehospital resuscitation of the buried avalanche victim. *High Altitude Medicine & Biology* 2011, 12(3): 199–205.

253. Caroselli C, Gabrieli A, Pisani A, Bruno G. Hypothermia: an under-estimated risk. *Internal and Emergency Medicine* 2009, 4(3): 227–30.

254. Cutter J. Recording patient temperature: are we getting it right? *Professional Nurse* 1994, 9(9): 608–10.

255. Danzl DF, Hedges JR, Pozos RS. Hypothermia outcome score: development and implications. *Critical Care Medicine* 1989, 17(3): 227–31.

256. Durrer B, Brugger H, Syme D. The medical on-site treatment of hypothermia: ICAR-MEDCOM recommendation. *High Altitude Medicine & Biology* 2003, 4(1): 99–103.

257. Hamilton RS, Paton BC. The diagnosis and treatment of hypothermia by mountain rescue teams: a survey. *Wilderness and Environmental Medicine* 1996, 7(1): 28–37.

258. Hasper D, Nee J, Schefold JC, Krueger A, Storm C. Tympanic temperature during therapeutic hypothermia. *Emergency Medicine Journal* 2011, 28(6): 483–5.

259. Helm M, Lampl L, Hauke J, Bock KH. Accidental hypothermia in trauma patients: is it relevant to prehospital emergency treatment? [In German]. *Anaesthesist* 1995, 44(2): 101–7.

260. Husby P, Andersen KS, Owen-Falkenberg A, Steien E, Solheim J. Accidental hypothermia with cardiac arrest: complete recovery after prolonged resuscitation and rewarming by extracorporeal circulation. *Intensive Care Medicine* 1990, 16(1): 69–72.

261. Incagnoli P, Bourgeois B, Teboul A, Laborie JM. Resuscitation from accidental hypothermia of 22 degrees C with circulatory arrest: importance of prehospital management. *Annales Françaises d'Anesthesie et de Reanimation* 2006, 25(5): 535–8.

262. Lee CH, Van Gelder C, Burns K, Cone DC. Advanced cardiac life support and defibrillation in severe hypothermic cardiac arrest. *Prehospital Emergency Care* 2009, 13(1): 85–9.

263. Long WB III, Edlich RF, Winters KL, Britt LD. Cold injuries. *Journal of Long Term Effects of Medical Implants* 2005, 15(1): 67–78.

264. Mallet ML. Pathophysiology of accidental hypothermia. *QJM: An International Journal of Medicine* 2002, 95(12): 775–85.

265. Oberhammer R, Beikircher W, Hormann C, Lorenz I, Pycha R, Adler-Kastner L, et al. Full recovery of an avalanche victim with profound hypothermia and prolonged cardiac arrest treated by extracorporeal re-warming. *Resuscitation* 2008, 76(3): 474–80.

266. Office for National Statistics. *Deaths from Hypothermia in England and Wales*. Available from: http://www.ons.gov.uk, 1999/2000.

267. Petersen MH, Hauke HN. Can training improve the results with infrared tympanic thermometers? *Acta Anaesthesiologica Scandinavica* 1997, 41(8): 1066–70.

268. Pugh Davies S. A comparison of mercury and digital clinical thermometers. *Journal of Advanced Nursing* 1986, 11(5): 535–43.

269. Southwick FS, Dalglish PHJ. Recovery after prolonged asystolic cardiac arrest in profound hypothermia: a case report and literature review. *Journal of the American Medical Association* 1980, 243(12): 1250–3.

270. van der Ploeg G-J, Goslings JC, Walpoth BH, Bierens JJLM. Accidental hypothermia: rewarming treatments, complications and outcomes from one university medical centre. *Resuscitation* 2010, 81(11): 1550–5.

271. Vayrynen T, Kuisma M, Maatta T, Boyd J. Medical futility in asystolic out-of-hospital cardiac arrest. *Acta Anaesthesiologica Scandinavica* 2008, 52(1): 81–7.

272. Young DM. Risk factors for hypothermia in psychiatric patients. *Annals of Clinical Psychiatry* 1996, 8(2): 93–7.

273. Azzopardi DV, Strohm B, Edwards AD, Dyet L, Halliday HL, Juszczak E, et al. Moderate hypothermia to treat perinatal asphyxial encephalopathy. *The New England Journal of Medicine* 2009, 361(14): 1349–58.

274. Edwards AD, Brocklehurst P, Gunn AJ, Halliday H, Juszczak E, Levene M, et al. Neurological outcomes at 18 months of age after moderate hypothermia for perinatal hypoxic ischaemic encephalopathy: synthesis and meta-analysis of trial data. *British Medical Journal* 2010, 340: c363.

275. Gluckman PD, Wyatt JS, Azzopardi D, Ballard R, Edwards AD, Ferriero DM, et al. Selective head cooling with mild systemic hypothermia after neonatal encephalopathy: multicentre randomised trial. *The Lancet* 2005, 365(9460): 663–70.

276. Johnson AG. *Report of a Working Party of the Standing Medical Advisory Committee on Sickle Cell, Thalassaemia and other Haemoglobinopathies: Policy in confidence*. London: HMSO, 1993.

277. Maxwell K, Streetly A, Bevan D. Experiences of hospital care and treatment-seeking behavior for pain from sickle cell disease: qualitative study. *Western Journal of Medicine* 1999, 171(5–6): 306–13.

278. Vichinsky EP, Neumayr LD, Earles AN, Williams R, Lennette ET, Dean D, et al. Causes and outcomes of the acute chest syndrome in sickle cell disease. National Acute Chest Syndrome Study Group. *The New England Journal of Medicine* 2000, 342(25): 1855–65.

279. Yale SH, Nagib N, Guthrie T. Acute chest syndrome in sickle cell disease: crucial considerations in adolescents and adults. *Postgraduate Medicine* 2000, 107(1): 215–22.

280. Thompson MJ, Ninis N, Perera R, Mayon-White R, Phillips C, Bailey L, et al. Clinical recognition of meningococcal disease in children and adolescents. *The Lancet* 2006, 367(9508): 397–403.

281. Strang JR, Pugh EJ. Meningococcal infections: reducing the case fatality rate by giving penicillin before admission to hospital. *British Medical Journal* 1992, 305(6846): 141–3.

282. Riordan FA, Thomson AP, Sills JA, Hart CA. Who spots the spots? Diagnosis and treatment of early meningococcal disease in children. *British Medical Journal* 1996, 313(7067): 1255–6.

283. Scottish Intercollegiate Guidelines Network. *Management of Invasive Meningococcal Disease in Children and Young People* (Guideline 102). Edinburgh: SIGN, 2008.

284. Chief Medical Officer. Meningococcal infection (letter, PL/CMO/99/1). London: Department of Health, 1999.

285. Hart CA, Thomson AP. Meningococcal disease and its management in children. *British Medical Journal* 2006, 333(7570): 685–90.

286. Hahne SJ, Charlett A, Purcell B, Samuelsson S, Camaroni I, Ehrhard I, et al. Effectiveness of antibiotics given before admission in reducing mortality from meningococcal disease: systematic review. *British Medical Journal* 2006, 332(7553): 1299–303.

287. Meningitis Research Foundation. *Meningococcal Septicaemia: Identification & management for ambulance personnel*, second edition. Bristol/Edinburgh/Belfast: Meningitis Research Foundation, 2008.

288. Cartwright K, Reilly S, White D, Stuart J. Early treatment with parenteral penicillin in meningococcal disease. *British Medical Journal* 1992, 305(6846): 143–7.

289. Booy R, Habibi P, Nadel S, de Munter C, Britto J, Morrison A, et al. Reduction in case fatality rate from meningococcal disease associated with improved healthcare delivery. *Archives of Disease in Childhood* 2001, 85(5): 386–90.

290. Pollard AJ, Cloke A, Glennie L, Faust SN, Haines C, Heath PT, et al. *Management of Meningococcal Disease in Children and Young People*, seventh edition. Bristol/Edinburgh/Belfast: Meningitis Research Foundation, 2010. Incorporates NICE *Bacterial Meningitis and Meningococcal Septicaemia* (CG102). Distributed in partnership with NICE.

291. Health Protection Agency. *Meningococcal Reference Unit isolates of Neisseria menengitidis: England and Wales, by region, age group & epidemiological year, 2000–2001 to 2009–2010*. London: HPA, 2010.

292. Surtees SJ, Stockton MG, Gietzen TW. Allergy to penicillin: fable or fact? *British Medical Journal* 1991, 302(6784): 1051–2.

293. Carcillo JA, Davis AL, Zaritsky A. Role of early fluid resuscitation in pediatric septic shock. *Journal of the American Medical Association* 1991, 266(9): 1242–5.

294. Burls A, Cabello JB, Emparanza JI, Bayliss S, Quinn T. Oxygen therapy for acute myocardial infarction: a systematic review and meta-analysis. *Emergency Medicine Journal* 2011, 28(11): 917–23.

295. Hamm CW, Bassand J-P, Agewall S, Bax J, Boersma E, Bueno H, et al. ESC Guidelines for the management of acute coronary syndromes in patients presenting without persistent ST-segment elevation. *European Heart Journal* 2011, 32(23): 2999–3054.

296. National Institute for Clinical Outcomes Research, British Cardiac Society. *Myocardial Ischaemia National Audit Project (MINAP)*. London: The Healthcare Quality Improvement Partnership, 2012. Available from: http://www.hqip.org.uk/myocardial-ischaemia-national-audit-project-minap.

297. National Institute for Health and Clinical Excellence. *Unstable Angina and NSTEMI: The early management of unstable angina and non-ST-segmentelevation myocardial infarction* (CG94). London: NICE, 2010. Available from: http://www.nice.org.uk/nicemedia/live/12949/47921/47921.pdf.

298. NHS Evidence. *Unstable Angina*. Available from: http://www.evidence.nhs.uk/search?q=unstable+angina, 2011.

299. Wijns W, Kolh P, Danchin N, Di Mario C, Falk V, Folliguet T, et al. Guidelines on myocardial revascularization. *European Heart Journal* 2010, 31(20): 2501–55.

300. NHS Evidence. *Pulmonary Embolism*. Available from: http://www.evidence.nhs.uk/topic/pulmonary-embolism, 2011.

301. National Institute for Health and Clinical Excellence. *Anaphylaxis: Assessment to confirm an anaphylactic episode and the decision to refer after emergency treatment for a suspected anaphylactic episode* (CG134). London: NICE, 2011. Available from: http://www.nice.org.uk/nicemedia/live/13626/57537/57537.pdf.

302. Brown SGA. Clinical features and severity grading of anaphylaxis. *Journal of Allergy and Clinical Immunology* 2004, 114(2): 371–6.

303. Kane KE, Cone DC. Anaphylaxis in the prehospital setting. *Journal of Emergency Medicine* 2004, 27(4): 371–7.

304. McLean-Tooke APC, Bethune CA, Fay AC, Spickett GP. Adrenaline in the treatment of anaphylaxis: what is the evidence? *British Medical Journal* 2003, 327(7427): 1332–5.

305. Langran M, Laird C. Management of allergy, rashes, and itching. *Emergency Medicine Journal* 2004, 21(6): 728–41.

306. Lieberman P, Nicklas RA, Oppenheimer J, Kemp SF, Lang DM, Bernstein DI, et al. The diagnosis and management of anaphylaxis practice parameter: 2010 update. *Journal of Allergy and Clinical Immunology* 2010, 126(3): 477–80.e1–42.

307. Pumphrey RSH. Lessons for management of anaphylaxis from a study of fatal reactions. *Clinical & Experimental Allergy* 2000, 30(8): 1144–50.

308. Sampson HA, Muñoz-Furlong A, Campbell RL, Adkinson NF Jr, Allan Bock S, Branum A, et al. Second symposium on the definition and management of anaphylaxis: summary report – second National Institute of Allergy and Infectious Disease/Food Allergy and Anaphylaxis Network symposium. *Annals of Emergency Medicine* 2006, 47(4): 373–80.

309. Brown AFT, McKinnon D, Chu K. Emergency department anaphylaxis: a review of 142 patients in a single year. *Journal of Allergy and Clinical Immunology* 2001, 108(5): 861–6.

310. Sheikh A, Shehata YA, Brown SGA, Simons FER. Adrenaline for the treatment of anaphylaxis: Cochrane Systematic Review. *Allergy* 2009, 64(2): 204–12.

311. Pumphrey RSH, Gowland MH. Further fatal allergic reactions to food in the United Kingdom, 1999–2006. *Journal of Allergy and Clinical Immunology* 2007, 119(4): 1018–19.

312. Visscher PK, Vetter RS, Camazine S. Removing bee stings. *The Lancet* 1996, 348(9023): 301–2.

313. Brown SGA, Blackman KE, Stenlake V, Heddle RJ. Insect sting anaphylaxis: prospective evaluation of treatment with intravenous adrenaline and volume resuscitation. *Emergency Medicine Journal* 2004, 21(2): 149–54.

314. Rubin BK, Dhand R, Ruppel GL, Branson RD, Hess DR. Respiratory care year in review 2010. Part 1: Asthma, COPD, pulmonary function testing, ventilator-associated pneumonia. *Respiratory Care* 2011, 56(4): 488–502.

315. Nunn AJ, Gregg I. New regression equations for predicting peak expiratory flow in adults. *British Medical Journal* 1989, 298(6680): 1068–70.

316. Austin MA, Wills KE, Blizzard L, Walters EH, Wood-Baker R. Effect of high flow oxygen on mortality in chronic obstructive pulmonary disease patients in prehospital setting: randomised controlled trial. *British Medical Journal* 2010, 341: c5462.

317. Austin MA, Wood-Baker R. Oxygen therapy in the pre-hospital setting for acute exacerbations of chronic obstructive pulmonary disease. *Cochrane Database of Systematic Reviews* 2006, 3: doi 10.1002/14651858.CD005534.pub2. Available from: http://www.mrw.interscience.wiley.com/cochrane/clsysrev/articles/CD005534/frame.html.

318. National Institute for Health and Clinical Excellence. *Chronic Obstructive Pulmonary Disease: Management of chronic obstructive pulmonary disease in adults in primary and secondary care (partial update)* (CG101). London: NICE, 2010. Available from: http://www.nice.org.uk/nicemedia/live/13029/49397/49397.pdf.

319. NHS Evidence. *COPD*. Available from: http://www.evidence.nhs.uk/topic/chronic-obstructive-pulmonarydisease?q=copd, 2012.

320. Ram FSF, Picot J, Lightowler J, Wedzicha JA. Non-invasive positive pressure ventilation for treatment of respiratory failure due to exacerbations of chronic obstructive pulmonary disease. *Cochrane Database of Systematic Reviews* 2004, 3: doi 10.1002/14651858.CD004104.pub3.

321. Schmidbauer W, Ahlers O, Spies C, Dreyer A, Mager G, Kerner T. Early prehospital use of non-invasive ventilation improves acute respiratory failure in acute exacerbation of chronic obstructive pulmonary disease. *Emergency Medicine Journal* 2011, 28(7): 626–7.

322. The Global Initiative for Chronic Obstructive Lung Disease. *Global Strategy for Diagnosis, Management, and Prevention of COPD*. Available from: http://www.goldcopd.org/uploads/users/files/GOLD _Report_2011_Feb2l.pdf, 2011.

323. Uronis H, McCrory DC, Samsa G, Currow D, Abernethy A. Symptomatic oxygen for non-hypoxaemic chronic obstructive pulmonary disease. *Cochrane Database of Systematic Reviews* 2011, 6: doi 10.1002/14651858.CD006429.pub2. Available from: http://www.mrw.interscience.wiley.com/cochrane/cls ysrev/articles/CD006429/frame.html.

324. O'Driscoll BR, Howard LS, Davison AG, on behalf of the British Thoracic Society. BTS guideline for emergency oxygen use in adult patients. *Thorax* 2008, 63(suppl. 6): vi1–vi68.

325. Healthcare Commission. *Clearing the Air: A national study of chronic obstructive pulmonary disease*. London: Healthcare Commission, 2006.

326. Michael GE, O'Connor RE. The diagnosis and management of seizures and status epilepticus in the prehospital setting. *Emergency Medicine Clinics of North America* 2011, 29(1): 29–39.

327. Chen JWY, Wasterlain CG. Status epilepticus: pathophysiology and management in adults. *The Lancet Neurology* 2006, 5(3): 246–56.

328. Larkin M. Seizures may be safely treated en route to hospital. *The Lancet* 2001, 358(9283): 733.

329. Woollard M, Hinshaw K, Simpson H, Wieteska S. Emergencies in late pregnancy. In *Pre-Hospital Obstetric Emergency Training*. India: Wiley-Blackwell, 2009: 62–110.

330. Cappell MS, Friedel D. Initial management of acute upper gastrointestinal bleeding: from initial evaluation up to gastrointestinal endoscopy. *Medical Clinics of North America* 2008, 92: 491–509.

331. Edwards AJ, Maskell GF. Acute lower gastrointestinal haemorrhage. *British Medical Journal* 2009, 339: b4156.

332. Michels SL, Collins J, Reynolds MW, Abramsky S, Paredes-Diaz A, McCarberg B. Over-the-counter ibuprofen and risk of gastrointestinal bleeding complications: a systematic literature review. *Current Medical Research and Opinion* 2012, 28(1): 89–99.

333. Palmer K. Acute upper gastrointestinal haemorrhage. *British Medical Bulletin* 2007, 83(1): 307–24.

334. Szajerka T, Jablecki J. Upper gastrointestinal bleeding in a young female with AIDS: a case report. *International Journal of STD & AIDS* 2012, 23(3): e33–4.

335. van Leerdam ME. Epidemiology of acute upper gastrointestinal bleeding. *Best Practice & Research in Clinical Gastroenterology* 2008, 22(2): 209–24.

336. Alkhatib AA, Elkhatib FA, Maldonado A, Abubakr SM, Adler DG. Acute upper gastrointestinal bleeding in elderly people: presentations, endoscopic findings, and outcomes. *Journal of the American Geriatrics Society* 2010, 58(1): 182–5.

337. Kent AJ, O'Beirne J, Negus R. The patient with haematemesis and melaena. *Acute Medicine* 2011, 10(1): 45–9.

338. Sampson HA. Anaphylaxis and emergency treatment. *Pediatrics* 2003, 111(suppl. 3): 1601–8.

339. Shah E, Pongracic J. Food-induced anaphylaxis: who, what, why, and where? *Pediatric Annals* 2008, 37(8): 536–41.

340. Boushey HA, Warnock DG, Smith LH. Hypoglycemia: a pitfall of insulin therapy. *Western Journal of Medicine* 1983, 139(5): 688–95.

341. Anderson S, Hogskilde PD, Wetterslev J, Bredgaard M, Moller JT, et al. Appropriateness of leaving emergency medical service treated hypoglycemic patients at home: a retrospective study. *Acta Anaesthesiologica/Scandinavica* 2002, 46(4): 464–8.

342. Asplund K, Wiholm BE, Lithner F. Glibenclamide-associated hypoglycaemia: a report on 57 cases. *Diabetologia* 1983, 24(6): 412–17.

343. Carter AJE, Keane PS, Dreyer JF. Transport refusal by hypoglycemic patients after on-scene intravenous dextrose. *Academic Emergency Medicine* 2002, 9(8): 855–7.

344. Fitzpatrick D, Duncan EAS. Improving post-hypoglycaemic patient safety in the prehospital environment: a systematic review. *Emergency Medicine Journal* 2009, 26(7): 472–8.

345. Mattila EM, Kuisma MJ, Sund KP, Voipio-Pulkki L-M. Out-of-hospital hypoglycaemia is safely and cost-effectively treated by paramedics. *European Journal of Emergency Medicine* 2004, 11(2): 70–4.

346. Roberts K, Smith A. Outcome of diabetic patients treated in the prehospital arena after a hypoglycaemic episode, and an exploration of treat and release protocols: a review of the literature. *Emergency Medicine Journal* 2003, 20(3): 274–6.

347. Fadini GP, Rigato M, Tiengo A, Avogaro A. Characteristics and mortality of Type 2 diabetic patients hospitalized for severe iatrogenic hypoglycemia. *Diabetes Research and Clinical Practice* 2009, 84(3): 267–72.

348. Chiasson J-L, Aris-Jilwan N, Belanger R, Bertrand S, Beauregard H, Ekoe J-M, et al. Diagnosis and treatment of diabetic ketoacidosis and the hyperglycemic hyperosmolar state. *Canadian Medical Association Journal* 2003, 168(7): 859–66.

349. Holstein A, Plaschke A, Vogel MY, Egberts EH. Prehospital management of diabetic emergencies: a population-based intervention study. *Acta Anaesthesiologica Scandinavica* 2003, 47(5): 610–15.

350. Ferner RE, Neil HAW. Sulphonylureas and hypoglycaemia. *British Medical Journal* 1988, 296(6627): 949–50.

351. Gangji AS, Cukierman T, Gerstein HC, Goldsmith CH, Clase CM. A systematic review and meta-analysis of hypoglycemia and cardiovascular events. *Diabetes Care* 2007, 30(2): 389–94.

352. Jennings AM, Wilson RM, Ward JD. Symptomatic hypoglycemia in NIDDM patients treated with oral hypoglycemic agents. *Diabetes Care* 1989, 12(3): 203–8.

353. Kelly A-M. The case for venous rather than arterial blood gases in diabetic ketoacidosis. *Emergency Medicine Australasia* 2006, 18(1): 64–7.

354. o WY, Chan JCN, Yeung VTF, Chow CC, Ko GTC, Li JKY, et al. Sulphonylurea-induced hypoglycaemia in institutionalized elderly in Hong Kong. *Diabetic Medicine* 2002, 19(11): 966–8.

355. Veitch PC, Clifton-Bligh RJ. Long-acting sulfonylureas: long-acting hypoglycaemia. *Medical Journal of Australia* 2004, 180(2): 84–5.

356. Wild D, von Maltzahn R, Brohan E, Christensen T, Clauson P, Gonder-Frederick L. A critical review of the literature on fear of hypoglycemia in diabetes: implications for diabetes management and patient education. *Patient Education and Counseling* 2007, 68(1): 10–15.

357. Brackenridge A, Wallbank H, Lawrenson RA, Russell-Jones D. Emergency management of diabetes and hypoglycaemia. *Emergency Medicine Journal* 2006, 23(3): 183–5.

358. Stanisstreet D, Walden E, Jones C, Graveling A. *The Hospital Management of Hypoglycaemia in Adults with Diabetes Mellitus.* London: NHS Diabetes, 2010. Available from: http://www.diabetes.nhs.uk/our_publications.

359. Steinmetz J, Nielsen SL, Rasmussen LS. Hypoglycaemia in patients with diabetes: do they prefer prehospital treatment or admission to hospital? *European Journal of Emergency Medicine* 2006, 13(5): 319–20.

360. Walker A, James C, Bannister M, Jobes E. Evaluation of a diabetes referral pathway for the management of hypoglycaemia following emergency contact with the ambulance service to a diabetes specialist nurse team. *Emergency Medicine Journal* 2006, 23(6): 449–51.

361. Akram K, Pedersen-Bjergaard U, Carstensen B, Borch-Johnsen K, Thorsteinsson B. Frequency and risk factors of severe hypoglycaemia in insulin-treated Type 2 diabetes: a cross-sectional survey. *Diabetic Medicine* 2006, 23(7): 750–6.

362. Ben-Ami H, Nagachandran P, Mendelson A, Edoute Y. Drug-induced hypoglycemic coma in 102 diabetic patients. *Archives of Internal Medicine* 1999, 159(3): 281–4.

363. Cain E, Ackroyd-Stolarz S, Alexiadis P, Murray D. Prehospital hypoglycemia: the safety of not transporting treated patients. *Prehospital Emergency Care* 2003, 7(4): 458–65.

364. Draeger KE, Wernicke-Panten K, Lomp HJ, Schuler E, Rosskamp R. Long-term treatment of Type 2 diabetic patients with the new oral antidiabetic agent glimepiride (Amaryl®): a double-blind comparison with glibenclamide. *Hormone and Metabolic Research* 1996, 28(09): 419–25.

365. Lerner EB, Billittier AJ, Lance OR, Janicke DM, Teuscher JA. Can paramedics safely treat and discharge hypoglycemic patients in the field? *American Journal of Emergency Medicine* 2003, 21(2): 115–20.

366. Amiel SA, Dixon T, Mann R, Jameson K. Hypoglycaemia in Type 2 diabetes. *Diabetic Medicine* 2008, 25(3): 245–54.

367. Ben Salem C, Fathallah N, Hmouda H, Bouraoui K. Drug-induced hypoglycaemia: an update. *Drug Safety* 2011, 34(1): 21–45.

368. Chansky ME, Corbett JG, Cohen E. Hyperglycemic emergencies in athletes. *Clinics in Sports Medicine* 2009, 28(3): 469–78.

369. National Institute for Health and Clinical Excellence. *Type 1 Diabetes in Adults (CG15).* London: NICE, 2004. Available from: http://www.nice.org.uk.

370. Joint British Diabetes Societies Inpatient Care Group, Savage MW, Sinclair-Hammersley M, Rayman G, Courtney H, Dhatariya K, Dyer P, et al. *The Management of Diabetic Ketoacidosis in Adults.* London: NHS Diabetes, 2010. Available from: http://www.diabetes.nhs.uk.

371. Department of Health. *Six Years On: Delivering the Diabetes National Service Framework.* Available from: http://www.dh.gov.uk/en/Publicationsandstatistics/Publications/PublicationsPolicyAndGuidance/DH_1125 09, 2010.

372. Dar O, Cowie MR. Acute heart failure in the intensive care unit: epidemiology. *Critical Care Medicine* 2008, 36: 53–8.

373. Murray-Thomas T, Cowie MR. Epidemiology and clinical aspects of congestive heart failure. *Journal of the Renin-Angiotensin-Aldosterone System* 2003, 4: 131–6.

374. Cowie MR, Mosterd A, Wood DA, Deckers JW, Poole-Wilson PA, Sutton GC, et al. The epidemiology of heart failure. *European Heart Journal* 1997, 18(2): 208–25.

375. Gibbs C, Davies M, Lip G, editors. *ABC of Heart Failure,* second edition. London: BMJ Books, 2002.

376. Fonarow GC. Acute decompensated heart failure: challenges and opportunities. *Reviews in Cardiovascular Medicine* 2007, 8(suppl. 5): S3–12.

377. Fonarow GC. Epidemiology and risk stratification in acute heart failure. *American Heart Journal* 2008, 155: 200–7.

378. Gibbs JSR, McCoy ASM, Gibbs LME, Rogers AE, Addington-Hall JM. Living with and dying from heart failure: the role of palliative care. *Heart* 2002, 88(suppl. 2): ii36–9.

379. Abraham WT, Adams KF, Fonarow GC, Costanzo MR, Berkowitz RL, Lejemtel TH, et al. In-hospital mortality in patients with acute decompensated heart failure requiring intravenous vasoactive medications: an analysis from the Acute Decompensated Heart Failure National Registry (ADHERE). *Journal of the American College of Cardiology* 2005, 46: 57–64.

380. Adams KF Jr, Fonarow GC, Emerman CL, Lejemtel TH, Costanzo MR, Abraham WT, et al. Characteristics and outcomes of patients hospitalized for heart failure in the United States: rationale, design, and preliminary observations from the first 100,000 cases in the Acute Decompensated Heart Failure National Registry (ADHERE). *American Heart Journal* 2005, 149: 209–16.

381. Barker WH, Mullooly JP, Getchell W. Changing incidence and survival for heart failure in a well-defined older population, 1970–1974 and 1990–1994. *Circulation* 2006, 113: 799–805.

382. Cleland JG, Swedberg K, Follath F, Komajda M, Cohen-Solal A, Aguilar JC, et al. The EuroHeart Failure Survey programme: a survey on the quality of care among patients with heart failure in Europe. Part 1: Patient characteristics and diagnosis. *European Heart Journal* 2003, 24: 442–63.

383. Kearney MT, Marber M. Trends in incidence and prognosis of heart failure: you always pass failure on the way to success. *European Heart Journal* 2004, 25: 2834.

384. Komajda M, Follath F, Swedberg K, Cleland J, Aguilar JC, Cohen-Solal A, et al. The EuroHeart Failure Survey programme: a survey on the quality of care among patients with heart failure in Europe. Part 2: Treatment. *European Heart Journal* 2003, 24: 464–74.

385. Macintyre K, Capewell S, Stewart S, Chalmers JW, Boyd J, Finlayson A, et al. Evidence of improving prognosis in heart failure: trends in case fatality in 66,547 patients hospitalized between 1986 and 1995. *Circulation* 2000, 102: 1126–31.

386. Nieminen MS, Brutsaert D, Dickstein K, Drexler H, Follath F, Harjola VP, et al. EuroHeart Failure Survey II (EHFS II): a survey on hospitalized acute heart failure patients: description of population. *European Heart Journal* 2006, 27: 2725–36.

387. Nieminen MS, Harjola VP, Hochadel M, Drexler H, Komajda M, Brutsaert D, et al. Gender related differences in patients presenting with acute heart failure. Results from EuroHeart Failure Survey II. *European Journal of Heart Failure* 2008, 10: 140–8.

388. Schaufelberger M, Swedberg K, Koster M, Rosen M, Rosengren A. Decreasing one-year mortality and hospitalization rates for heart failure in Sweden: data from the Swedish Hospital Discharge Registry 1988 to 2000. *European Heart Journal* 2004, 25: 300–7.

389. Anonymous. ACE inhibitors in the treatment of chronic heart failure: effective and cost effective. *Bandolier* 1994, 1(8): 59–61.

390. Cleland JG, Gemmell I, Khand A, Boddy A. Is the prognosis of heart failure improving? *European Journal of Heart Failure* 1999, 1: 229–41.

391. Dickstein K, Cohen-Solal A, Filippatos G, McMurray JJ, Ponikowski P, PooleWilson PA, et al. ESC guidelines for the diagnosis and treatment of acute and chronic heart failure 2008: The Task Force for the Diagnosis and Treatment of Acute and Chronic Heart Failure 2008 of the European Society of Cardiology. Developed in collaboration with the Heart Failure Association of the ESC (HFA) and endorsed by the European Society of Intensive Care Medicine (ESCIM). *European Heart Journal* 2008, 29: 2388–442.

392. McMurray JJ, Petrie MC, Murdoch DR, Davie AP. Clinical epidemiology of heart failure: public and private health burden. *European Heart Journal* 1998, 19(suppl. P): P9–16.

393. Murdoch DR, McDonagh TA, Byrne J, Blue L, Farmer R, Morton JJ, et al. Titration of vasodilator therapy in chronic heart failure according to plasma brain natriuretic peptide concentration: randomized comparison of the hemodynamic and neuroendocrine effects of tailored versus empirical therapy. *American Heart Journal* 1999, 138: 1126–32.

394. Wilhelmsen L, Rosengren A, Eriksson H, Lappas G. Heart failure in the general population of men: morbidity, risk factors and prognosis. *Journal of Internal Medicine* 2001, 249: 253–61.

395. Shamsham F, Mitchell J. Essentials of the diagnosis of heart failure. *American Family Physician* 2000, 61(5): 1319–28.

396. Talley NJ, O'Conner S. *Clinical Examination: A systematic guide to physical diagnosis.* Philadelphia, PA: Churchill Livingston, 2006.

397. Davie AP, Francis CM, Caruana L, Sutherland GR, McMurray JJ. Assessing diagnosis in heart failure: which features are any use? *QJM: An International Journal of Medicine* 1997, 90: 335–9.

398. Douglas G, Nicol F, Robertson C, editors. *Macleod's Clinical Examination.* Philadelphia, PA: Churchill Livingston, 2005.

399. Gray AJ, Goodacre S, Newby DE, Masson MA, Sampson F, Dixon S, et al. A multicentre randomised controlled trial of the use of continuous positive airway pressure and non-invasive positive pressure ventilation in the early treatment of patients presenting to the emergency department with severe acute cardiogenic pulmonary oedema: the 3CPO trial. *Health Technology Assessment* 2009, 13.

400. Agarwal R, Aggarwal AN, Gupta D. Is noninvasive pressure support ventilation as effective and safe as continuous positive airway pressure in cardiogenic pulmonary oedema? *Singapore Medical Journal* 2009, 50: 595–603.

401. Cabrini L, Idone C, Colombo S, Monti G, Bergonzi PC, Landoni G, et al. Medical emergency team and non-invasive ventilation outside ICU for acute respiratory failure. *Intensive Care Medicine* 2009, 35: 339–43.

402. Carvalho L, Carneiro R, Freire E, Pinheiro P, Aragao I, Martins A. Non-invasive ventilation in cardiogenic pulmonary edema in the emergency department. *Revista Portuguesa de Cardiologia* 2008, 27: 191–8.

403. Collins SP, Mielniczuk LM, Whittingham HA, Boseley ME, Schramm DR, Storrow AB. The use of noninvasive ventilation in emergency department patients with acute cardiogenic pulmonary edema: a systematic review. *Annals of Emergency Medicine* 2006, 48: 260–9.

404. Ho KM, Wong K. A comparison of continuous and bi-level positive airway pressure non-invasive ventilation in patients with acute cardiogenic pulmonary oedema: a meta-analysis. *Critical Care* 2006, 10: R49.

405. Masip J, Roque M, Sanchez B, Fernandez R, Subirana M, Exposito JA. Noninvasive ventilation in acute cardiogenic pulmonary edema: systematic review and meta-analysis. *Journal of the American Medical Association* 2005, 294: 3124–30.

406. Mebazaa A, Gheorghiade M, Pina IL, Harjola VP, Hollenberg SM, Follath F, et al. Practical recommendations for prehospital and early in-hospital management of patients presenting with acute heart failure syndromes. *Critical Care Medicine* 2008, 36: 5129–39.

407. Moritz F, Brousse B, Gellee B, Chajara A, L'her E, Hellot M-F, et al. Continuous positive airway pressure versus bilevel noninvasive ventilation in acute cardiogenic pulmonary edema: a randomized multicenter trial. *Annals of Emergency Medicine* 2003, 50: 666–75.

408. Vital FMR, Saconato H, Ladeira MT, Sen A, Hawkes CA, Soares B, et al. Non-invasive positive pressure ventilation (CPAP or bilevel NPPV) for cardiogenic pulmonary edema. *Cochrane Database of Systematic Reviews* 2008: doi 10.1002/14651858.CD005351.pub2.

409. Nava S, Carbone G, Dibattista N, Bellone A, Baiardi P, Cosentini R, et al. Noninvasive ventilation in cardiogenic pulmonary edema: a multicenter randomized trial. *American Journal of Respiratory & Critical Care Medicine* 2003, 168: 1432–7.

410. Park M, Sangean MC, Volpe MDS, Feltrim MIZ, Nozawa E, Leite PF, et al. Randomized, prospective trial of oxygen, continuous positive airway pressure, and bilevel positive airway pressure by face mask in acute cardiogenic pulmonary edema. *Critical Care Medicine* 2004, 32: 2407–15.

411. Peter JV, Moran JL, Phillips-Hughes J, Graham P, Bersten AD. Effect of noninvasive positive pressure ventilation (NIPPV) on mortality in patients with acute cardiogenic pulmonary oedema: a meta-analysis. *The Lancet* 2006, 367: 1155–63.

412. Pladeck T, Hader C, Von Orde A, Rasche K, Wiechmann HW. Non-invasive ventilation: comparison of effectiveness, safety, and management in acute heart failure syndromes and acute exacerbations of chronic obstructive pulmonary disease. *Journal of Physiology and Pharmacology* 2007, 58(suppl. 5): 539–49.

413. Plaisance P, Pirracchio R, Berton C, Vicaut E, Payen D, Berton C, et al. A randomized study of out-of-hospital continuous positive airway pressure for acute cardiogenic pulmonary oedema: physiological and clinical effects. *European Heart Journal* 2007, 28: 2895–901.

414. Pollack CJ, Torres MT, Alexander L. Feasibility study of the use of bilevel positive airway pressure for respiratory support in the emergency department *Annals of Emergency Medicine* 1996, 27: 189–92.

415. Poponick JM, Renston JP, Bennett RP, Emerman CL. Use of a ventilatory support system (BiPAP) for acute respiratory failure in the emergency department. *Chest* 1999, 116: 166–71.

416. Potts M. Noninvasive positive pressure ventilation: effect on mortality in acute cardiogenic pulmonary edema: a pragmatic meta-analysis. *Polskie Archiwum Medycyny Wewnetrznej* 2009, 119: 349–53.

417. Sacchetti AD, Harris RH, Paston C, Hernandez Z. Bi-level positive airway pressure support system use in acute congestive heart failure: preliminary case series. *Academic Emergency Medicine* 1995, 2: 714–18.

418. Winck JC, Azevedo LF, Costa-Pereira A, Antonelli M, Wyatt JC. Efficacy and safety of non-invasive ventilation in the treatment of acute cardiogenic pulmonary edema: a systematic review and meta-analysis. *Critical Care* 2006, 10(2): R69.

419. Wood KA, Lewis L, Von Harz B, Kollef MH. The use of noninvasive positive pressure ventilation in the emergency department: results of a randomized clinical trial. *Chest* 1998, 113: 1339–46.

420. Bruge P, Jabre P, Dru M, Jbeili C, Lecarpentier E, Khalid M, et al. An observational study of noninvasive positive pressure ventilation in an out-of-hospital setting. *American Journal of Emergency Medicine* 2008, 26: 165–9.

421. Craven RA, Singletary N, Bosken L, Sewell E, Payne M, Lipsey R. Use of bilevel positive airway pressure in out-of-hospital patients. *Academic Emergency Medicine* 2000, 7: 1065–8.

422. Dieperink W, Weelink EEM, van der Horst ICC, de Vos R, Jaarsma T, Aarts LPHJ, et al. Treatment of presumed acute cardiogenic pulmonary oedema in an ambulance system by nurses using Boussignac continuous positive airway pressure. *Emergency Medicine Journal* 2009, 26(2): 141–4.

423. Fort P-A, Boussarie C, Hilbert G, Habachi M. Prehospital noninvasive ventilation: study of importance and feasibility (7 cases). *Presse Medicale* 2002, 31: 1886–9.

424. Gardtman M, Waagstein L, Karlsson T, Herlitz J. Has an intensified treatment in the ambulance of patients with acute severe left heart failure improved the outcome? *European Journal of Emergency Medicine* 2000, 7: 15–24.

425. Hubble MW, Richards ME, Jarvis R, Millikan T, Young D. Effectiveness of prehospital continuous positive airway pressure in the management of acute pulmonary edema. *Prehospital Emergency Care* 2006, 10: 430–9.

426. Kallio T, Kuisma M, Alaspaa A, Rosenberg PH. The use of prehospital continuous positive airway pressure treatment in presumed acute severe pulmonary edema. *Prehospital Emergency Care* 2003, 7: 209–13.

427. Kosowsky JM, Stephanides SL, Branson RD, Sayre MR. Prehospital use of continuous positive airway pressure (CPAP) for presumed pulmonary edema: a preliminary case series. *Prehospital Emergency Care* 2001, 5: 190–6.

428. Templier F, Dolveck F, Baer M, Chauvin M, Fletcher D. 'Boussignac' continuous positive airway pressure system: practical use in a prehospital medical care unit. *European Journal of Emergency Medicine* 2003, 10: 87–93.

429. Thompson J, Petrie DA, Ackroyd-Stolarz S, Bardua DJ. Out-of-hospital continuous positive airway pressure ventilation versus usual care in acute respiratory failure: a randomized controlled trial. *Annals of Emergency Medicine* 2008, 52: 232–41.

430. Weitz G, Struck J, Zonak A, Balnus S, Perras B, Dodt C. Prehospital noninvasive pressure support ventilation for acute cardiogenic pulmonary edema. *European Journal of Emergency Medicine* 2007, 14(5): 276–9.

431. Yosefy C, Hay E, Ben-Barak A, Derazon H, Magen E, Reisin L, et al. BiPAP ventilation as assistance for patients presenting with respiratory distress in the department of emergency medicine. *American Journal of Respiratory Medicine* 2003, 2: 343–47.

432. Costanzo MR, Johannes RS, Pine M, Gupta V, Saltzberg M, Hay J, et al. The safety of intravenous diuretics alone versus diuretics plus parenteral vasoactive therapies in hospitalized patients with acutely decompensated heart failure: a propensity score and instrumental variable analysis using the Acutely Decompensated Heart Failure National Registry (ADHERE) database. *American Heart Journal* 2007, 154: 267–77.

433. European Resuscitation Council. Part 6: Advanced cardiovascular life support. Section 6: Pharmacology II: agents to optimize cardiac output and blood pressure. *Resuscitation* 2000, 46: 155–62.

434. Francis GS, Siegel RM, Goldsmith SR, Olivari MT, Levine TB, Cohn JN. Acute vasoconstrictor response to intravenous furosemide in patients with chronic congestive heart failure: activation of the neurohumoral axis. *Annals of Internal Medicine* 1985, 103: 1–6.

435. Kraus PA, Lipman J, Becker PJ. Acute preload effects of furosemide. *Chest* 1990, 98(1): 124–8.

436. Jhund PS, Davie AP, McMurray JJ. Aspirin inhibits the acute venodilator response to furosemide in patients with chronic heart failure. *Journal of the American College of Cardiology* 2001, 37(5): 1234–8.

437. Cotter G, Metzkor E, Kaluski E, Faigenberg Z, Miller R, Simovitz A, et al. Randomised trial of high-dose isosorbide dinitrate plus low-dose furosemide versus high-dose furosemide plus low-dose isosorbide dinitrate in severe pulmonary oedema. *The Lancet* 1998, 351: 389–93.

438. Faris RF, Flather M, Purcell H, Poole-Wilson PA, Coats AJS. Diuretics for heart failure. *Cochrane Database of Systematic Reviews* 2006, 1: doi 10.1002/14651858.CD003838.pub2.

439. Hoffman JR, Reynolds S. Comparison of nitroglycerin, morphine and furosemide in treatment of presumed pre-hospital pulmonary edema. *Chest* 1987, 92: 586–93.

440. Jaronik J, Mikkelson P, Fales W, Overton DT. Evaluation of prehospital use of furosemide in patients with respiratory distress. *Prehospital Emergency Care* 2006, 10(2): 194–7.

441. Singer AJ, Emerman C, Char DM, Heywood JT, Kirk JD, Hollander JE, et al. Bronchodilator therapy in acute decompensated heart failure patients without a history of chronic obstructive pulmonary disease. *Annals of Emergency Medicine* 2008, 51: 25–34.

442. Sparer KA, Tabas JA, Tam RK, Sellers KL, Rosenson J, Barton CW, et al. Do medications affect vital signs in the prehospital treatment of acute decompensated heart failure? *Prehospital Emergency Care* 2006, 10: 41–5.

443. Mosesso VN Jr, Dunford J, Blackwell T, Criswell JK. Prehospital therapy for acute congestive heart failure: state of the art. *Prehospital Emergency Care* 2003, 7: 13–23.

444. Bruns BM, Dieckmann R, Shagoury C, Dingerson A, Swartzell C. Safety of pre-hospital therapy with morphine sulfate. *American Journal of Emergency Medicine* 1992, 10(1): 53–7.

445. Fiutowski M, Waszyrowski T, Krzeminska-Pakula M, Kasprzak JD. Clinical presentation and pharmacological therapy in patients with cardiogenic pulmonary oedema. *Kardiologia Polska* 2004, 61: 561–9.

446. Sacchetti A, Ramoska E, Moakes ME, McDermott P, Moyer V. Effect of ED management on ICU use in acute pulmonary edema. *American Journal of Emergency Medicine* 1999, 17: 571–4.

447. Peacock WF, Hollander JE, Diercks DB, Lopatin M, Fonarow C, Emerman CL. Morphine and outcomes in acute decompensated heart failure: an ADHERE analysis. *Emergency Medicine Journal* 2008, 25: 205–9.

448. Bertini G, Giglioli C, Biggeri A, Margheri M, Simonetti I, Sica ML, et al. Intravenous nitrates in the prehospital management of acute pulmonary edema. *Annals of Emergency Medicine* 1997, 30: 493–9.

449. Channer KS, McLean KA, Lawson-Matthew P, Richardson M. Combination diuretic treatment in severe heart failure: a randomised controlled trial, *British Heart Journal* 1994, 71: 146–50.

450. Cotter G. High-dose intravenous isosorbide-dinitrate is safer and better than BiPAP ventilation combined with conventional treatment for severe pulmonary edema. *Journal of the American College of Cardiology* 2000, 36: 832–7.

451. Levy P, Compton S, Welch R, Delgado G, Jennett A, Penugonda N, et al. Treatment of severe decompensated heart failure with high-dose intravenous nitroglycerin: a feasibility and outcome analysis. *Annals of Emergency Medicine* 2007, 50: 144–52.

452. Peacock WF, Costanzo MR, De Marco T, Lopatin M, Wynne J, Mills RM, et al. Impact of intravenous loop diuretics on outcomes of patients hospitalized with acute decompensated heart failure: insights from the ADHERE registry. *Cardiology* 2009, 113: 12–19.

453. Peacock WF, Emerman CL, Costanzo MR. Early initiation of intravenous vasoactive therapy improves heart failure outcomes: an analysis from the ADHERE registry database. In Aghababian R, Jackson EJ, Boyer EW, Braen RG, Manno MM, Moorhead JC, et al., editors. *Essentials of Emergency Medicine*. Sudbury, MA: Jones and Bartlett, 2003.

454. Sharon A, Shpirer I, Kaluski E, Moshkovitz Y, Milovanov O, Polak R, et al. High-dose intravenous isosorbide-dinitrate is safer and better than BiPAP ventilation combined with conventional treatment for severe pulmonary edema. *Journal of the American College of Cardiology* 2000, 36: 832–7.

455. Wuerz RC, Meador SA. Effects of prehospital medications on mortality and length of stay in congestive heart failure. *Annals of Emergency Medicine* 1992, 21: 669–74.

456. Johnson A, Mackway-Jones K. Frusemide or nitrates in acute left ventricular failure. *Emergency Medicine Journal* 2001, 18(1): 59–60.

457. Gunnell D, Bennewith O, Peters TJ, House A, Hawton K. The epidemiology and management of self-harm amongst adults in England. *Journal of Public Health* 2005, 27(1): 67–73.

458. Gwini SM, Shaw D, Iqbal M, Spaight A, Siriwardena AN. Exploratory study of factors associated with adverse clinical features in patients presenting with non-fatal drug overdose/self-poisoning to the ambulance service. *Emergency Medicine Journal* 2011, 28(10): 892–94.

459. Health Protection Agency, Centre for Radiation, Chemical and Environmental Hazards. *National Poisons Information Service Annual Report 2010/2011*. Available from: http://www.hpa.org.uk/webc/HPAwebFile/HPAweb_C/1317130944236, 2011.

460. Health Protection Agency, Centre for Radiation, Chemical and Environmental Hazards. *Current Awareness in Clinical Toxicology*. Available from: http://www.hpa.org.uk/web/HPAweb&Page&HPAweb AutoListName/Page/1217835684945, 2012.

461. Health Protection Agency, Centre for Radiation, Chemical and Environmental Hazards. *Chemicals & Poisons A–Z and Compendium*. Available from: http://www.hpa.org.uk/Topics/ChemicalsAndPoisons/ChemicalsPoisonsAZ, 2012.

462. Health Protection Agency, Centre for Radiation, Chemical and Environmental Hazards. *Chemicals and Poisons*. Available from: http://www.hpa.org.uk/Topics/ChemicalsAndPoisons, 2012.

463. National Poisons Information Service. *TOXBASE*. Available from: http://www.npis.org/toxbase.html, 2012.

464. National Poisons Information Service. Available from: http://www.npis.org/index.html, 2012.

465. The British National Formulary. Emergency treatment of poisoning. *BNF 63*. Available from: http://www.medicinescomplete.com/mc/bnf/current/203970.htm, 2012.

466. The British National Formulary. Medicines information services. *BNF 63*. Available from: http://www.medicinescomplete.com/mc/bnf/current/203953.htm, 2012.

467. NHS Evidence. *Overdose*. Available from: http://www.evidence.nhs.uk/search?q=overdose, 2011.

468. NHS Evidence. *Poisoning*. Available from: http://www.evidence.nhs.uk/search?q=poisoning, 2011.

469. National Institute for Health and Clinical Excellence. *Venous Thromboembolism: Reducing the risk. Reducing the risk of venous thromboembolism (deep vein thrombosis and pulmonary embolism) in patients admitted to hospital (CG 92)*. London: NICE, 2010. Available from: http://www.nice.org.uk/nicemedia/live/12695/47195/47195.pdf.

470. Torbicki A, Perrier A, Konstantinides S, Agnelli G, Galie N, Pruszczyk P, et al. Guidelines on the diagnosis and management of acute pulmonary embolism. *European Heart Journal* 2008, 29(18): 2276–315.

471. Wells PS, Anderson DR, Rodger M, Ginsberg JS, Kearon C, Gent M. Derivation of a simple clinical model to categorize patients' probability of pulmonary embolism: increasing the models utility with the SimpliRED D-dimer. *Thrombosis and Haemostasis* 2000, 83: 416–20.

472. Cohen AT, Agnelli G, Anderson FA, Arcelus JI, Bergqvist D, Brecht JG, et al. Venous thromboembolism (VTE) in Europe: the number of VTE events and associated morbidity and mortality. *Thrombosis and Haemostasis* 2007, 98(4): 756–64.

473. Farmer RDT, Lawrenson RA, Todd JC, Williams TJ, MacRae KD, Tyrer F, et al. A comparison of the risks of venous thromboembolic disease in association with different combined oral contraceptives. *British Journal of Clinical Pharmacology* 2000, 49 (6): 580–90.

474. Goldhaber SZ, Morrison RB. Pulmonary embolism and deep vein thrombosis. *Circulation* 2002, 106(12): 1436–8.

475. Meyer G, Roy P-M, Gilberg S, Perrier A. Pulmonary embolism. *British Medical Journal* 2010, 340: c1421.

476. White RH. The epidemiology of venous thromboembolism. *Circulation* 2003, 107: I-4–8.

477. Wolf SJ, McCubbin T, Feldhaus KM, Faragher JP, Adcock DM. Prospective validation of Wells Criteria in the evaluation of patients with suspected pulmonary embolism. *Annals of Emergency Medicine* 2004, 44(5): 503–10.

478. Department of Health. *National Stroke Strategy*. Available from: http://www.dh.gov.uk/en/Publicationsandstatistics/Publications/PublicationsPolicyAndGuidance/DH_081062, 2007.

479. Harbison J, Hossain O, Jenkinson D, Davis J, Louw SJ, Ford GA. Diagnostic accuracy of stroke referrals from primary care, emergency room physicians, and ambulance staff using the face arm speech test. *Stroke: A Journal of Cerebral Circulation* 2003, 34(1): 71–6.

480. NHS Evidence. *Stroke*. Available from: http://www.evidence.nhs.uk/topic/stroke, 2012.

References

481. NHS Improvement. *Stroke: Supporting the development of stroke care networks*. Available from: http://www.improvement.nhs.uk/stroke, 2008.

482. Nor AM, McAllister C, Louw SJ, Dyker AG, Davis M, Jenkinson D, et al. Agreement between ambulance paramedic- and physician-recorded neurological signs with Face Arm Speech Test (FAST) in acute stroke patients. *Stroke: A Journal of Cerebral Circulation* 2004, 35(6): 1355–9.

483. The Stroke Association. *About Stroke*. Available from: http://www.stroke.org.uk/about/about-stroke, 2012.

484. Soar J, Pumphrey R, Cant A, Clarke S, Corbett A, Dawson P, et al. *Emergency Treatment of Anaphylactic Reactions: Guidelines for healthcare providers*. London: Resuscitation Council (UK), 2008. Available from: http://www.resus.org.uk/pages/reaction.pdf.

485. Resuscitation Council (UK). What is the guidance for emergency oxygen use in children? Available from: http://www.resus.org.uk/pages/faqPLS.htm, 2011.

486. Yoong M, Chin RFM, Scott RC. Management of convulsive status epilepticus in children. *Archives of Disease in Childhood Education and Practice Edition* 2009, 94(1): 1–9.

487. The Status Epilepticus Working Party, Appleton R, Choonara I, Martland T, Phillips B, Scott R, et al. The treatment of convulsive status epilepticus in children. *Archives of Disease in Childhood* 2000, 83(5): 415–19.

488. Sadleir LG, Scheffer IE. Febrile seizures. *British Medical Journal* 2007, 334(7588): 307–11.

489. Baysun S, Aydin ÖF, Atmaca E, Gürer YKY. A comparison of buccal midazolam and rectal diazepam for the acute treatment of seizures. *Clinical Pediatrics* 2005, 44(9): 771–6.

490. Sadleir LG, Scheffer IE. Febrile seizures. *British Medical Journal* 2007, 334(7588): 307–11.

491. Armon K, Stephenson T, MacFaul R, Eccleston P, Werneke U. An evidence and consensus based guideline for acute diarrhoea management. *Archives of Disease in Childhood* 2001, 85(2): 132–42.

492. Health Protection Agency. *Avoiding Infection on Farm Visits: Advice for the public*. Available from: http://www.hpa.org.uk/webc/HPAwebFile/HPAweb_C/1270122184581, 2011.

493. Murphy MS. Guidelines for managing acute gastroenteritis based on a systematic review of published research. *Archives of Disease in Childhood* 1998, 79(3): 279–84.

494. Dunger DB, Sperling MA, Acerini CL, Bohn DJ, Daneman D, Danne TPA, et al. ESPE/LWPES consensus statement on diabetic ketoacidosis in children and adolescents. *Archives of Disease in Childhood* 2004, 89(2): 188–94.

495. Achoki R, Opiyo N, English M. Mini-review: management of hypoglycaemia in children aged 0–59 months. *Journal of Tropical Pediatrics* 2010, 56(4): 227–34.

496. National Collaborating Centre for Women's and Children's Health. *Type 1 Diabetes: Diagnosis and management of Type 1 diabetes in children and young people* (CG86). London: National Institute for Health and Clinical Excellence, 2009. Available from: http://www.nice.org.uk/nicemedia/live/10944/29394/29394.pdf.

497. The British National Formulary. *Treatment of Hypoglycaemia*. Available from: http://www.evidence.nhs.uk/formulary/bnf/current/6-endocrine-system/61-drugs-used-in-diabetes/614-treatment-of-hypoglycaemia, 2011.

498. The British National Formulary for Children. *Treatment of Hypoglycaemia*. Available from: http://www.evidence.nhs.uk/formulary/bnfc/current/6-endocrine-system/61-drugs-used-in-diabetes/614-treatment-of-hypoglycaemia, 2011.

499. Wolfsdorf J, Craig ME, Daneman D, Dunger D, Edge J, Lee WW, et al. Diabetic ketoacidosis. *Pediatric Diabetes* 2007, 8: 28–43.

500. Hawdon JM. Investigation, prevention and management of neonatal hypoglycaemia (impaired postnatal metabolic adaptation). *Paediatrics and Child Health* 2012, 22(4): 131–5.

501. Cornblath M, Hawdon JM, Williams AF, Aynsley-Green A, Ward-Platt MP, Schwartz R, et al. Controversies regarding definition of neonatal hypoglycemia: suggested operational thresholds. *Pediatrics* 2000, 105 (5): 1141–5.

502. The British National Formulary for Children. *Emergency Treatment of Poisoning*. Available from: http://www.evidence.nhs.uk/formulary/bnfc/current/emergency-treatment-of-poisoning, 2012–2013.

503. Jorgensen H, Jensen CH, Dirks J. Does prehospital ultrasound improve treatment of the trauma patient? A systematic review. *European Journal of Emergency Medicine* 2010, 17(5): 249–53.

504. Best Evidence Topics. Does the 'Seatbelt Sign' predict intra-abdominal injury after motor vehicle trauma in children? *Emergency Medicine Journal* 2012, 29(2): 163–4.

505. Demetriades D, Murray J, Brown C, Velmahos G, Salim A, Alo K, et al. High-level falls: type and severity of injuries and survival outcome according to age. *Journal of Trauma and Acute Care Surgery* 2005, 58(2): 342–5.

506. England RJ, Dalton R, Walker J. Penetrating handlebar injury causing bowel evisceration. *Injury Extra* 2004, 35(4): 40–1.

507. Feliciano DV, Burch JM, Spjut-Patrinely V, Mattox KL, Jordan GL Jr. Abdominal gunshot wounds: an urban trauma center's experience with 300 consecutive patients. *Annals of Surgery* 1988, 208(3): 362–70.

508. Hardcastle TC, Coetzee GJN, Wasserman L. Evisceration from blunt trauma in adults: an unusual injury pattern: 3 cases and a literature review. *Scandinavian Journal of Trauma, Resuscitation & Emergency Medicine* 2005, 13: 234–5.

509. Holmes IF, Sokolove PE, Brant WE, Palchak MJ, Vance CW, Owings JT, et al. Identification of children with intra-abdominal injuries after blunt trauma. *Annals of Emergency Medicine* 2002, 39(5): 500–9.

510. Mulholland SA, Cameron PA, Gabbe BJ, Williamson OD, Young K, Smith KL, et al. Prehospital prediction of the severity of blunt anatomic injury. *Journal of Trauma and Acute Care Surgery* 2008, 64(3): 754–60: doi 10.1097/01.ta.0000244384.85267.c5.

511. Newgard CD, Lewis RJ, Kraus JF. Steering wheel deformity and serious thoracic or abdominal injury among drivers and passengers involved in motor vehicle crashes. *Annals of Emergency Medicine* 2005, 45(1): 43–50.

512. Nishijima DK, Simel DL, Wisner DH, Holmes JF. Does this adult patient have a blunt intra-abdominal injury? *Journal of the American Medical Association* 2012, 307(14): 1517–27.

513. Owers C, Morgan JL, Garner JP. Abdominal trauma in primary blast injury. *British Journal of Surgery* 2011, 98(2): 168–79.

514. Plurad DS. Blast injury. *Military Medicine* 2011, 176(3): 276–82.

515. Smith J, Caldwell E, D'Amours S, Jalaludin B, Sugrue M. Abdominal trauma: a disease in evolution. *ANZ Journal of Surgery* 2005, 75(9): 790–4.

References

516. Sugrue M, Balogh Z, Lynch J, Bardsley J, Sisson G, Weigelt J. Guidelines for the management of haemodynamically stable patients with stab wounds to the anterior abdomen. *ANZ Journal of Surgery* 2007, 77(8): 614–20.

517. Demetriades D, Murray J, Martin M, Velmahos G, Salim A, Alo K, et al. Pedestrians injured by automobiles: relationship of age to injury type and severity. *Journal of the American College of Surgeons* 2004, 199(3): 382–7.

518. Scottish Intercollegiate Guidelines Network. *Early Management of Patients with a Head Injury* (Guideline 110). Edinburgh: SIGN, 2007.

519. Pandor A, Goodacre S, Harnan S, Holmes M, Pickering A, Fitzgerald P, et al. Diagnostic management strategies for adults and children with minor head injury: a systematic review and an economic evaluation. *Health Technology Assessment* 2011, 15(27).

520. Macpherson A, Spinks A. Bicycle helmet legislation for the uptake of helmet use and prevention of head injuries. *Cochrane Database of Systematic Reviews* 2009: doi 10.1002/14651858.CD005401.pub3.

521. Antoniou D, Kyriakidis A, Zaharopoulos A, Moskoklaidis S. Degloving injury. *European Journal of Trauma* 2005, 31(6): 593–6.

522. Arnez ZM, Khan U, Tyler MPH. Classification of soft-tissue degloving in limb trauma. *Journal of Plastic, Reconstructive & Aesthetic Surgery* 2010, 63(11): 1865–9.

523. Beekley AC, Sebesta JA, Blackbourne LH, Herbert GS, Kauvar DS, Baer DG, et al. Prehospital tourniquet use in Operation Iraqi Freedom: effect on hemorrhage control and outcomes. *Journal of Trauma* 2008, 64 (suppl. 2): S28–37; discussion S37.

524. Burns BJ, Sproule J, Smyth H. Acute compartment syndrome of the anterior thigh following quadriceps strain in a footballer. *British Journal of Sports Medicine* 2004, 38(2): 218–20.

525. Cooper C, Dennison FM, Leufkens HGM, Bishop N, van Staa TP. Epidemiology of childhood fractures in Britain: a study using the General Practice Research Database. *Journal of Bone and Mineral Research* 2004, 19(12): 976–81.

526. Daniels JM, Zook EG, Lynch JM. Hand and wrist injuries. Part II: Emergent evaluation. *American Family Physician* 2004, 69(8): 1949–56.

527. Dykes PC. Minding the five Ps of neurovascular assessment. *American Journal of Nursing* 1993, 93(6): 38–9.

528. Griffiths R, Alper J, Beckingsale A, Goldhill D, Heyburn G, Holloway J, et al. Management of proximal femoral fractures 2011. *Anaesthesia* 2012, 67(1): 85–98.

529. Hodgetts TJ, Mahoney PF, Russell MQ, Byers M. ABC to ‹C›ABC: redefining the military trauma paradigm. *Emergency Medical Journal* 2006, 23(10): 745–6.

530. Jagdeep N, Durai N, Umraz K, Christopher M, Stephen B, Frances S, et al. *Standards for the Management of Open Fractures of the Lower Limb.* London: British Association of Plastic Reconstructive and Aesthetic Surgeons, British Orthopaedic Association, 2009. Available from: http://www.bapras.org.uk/downloaddoc.asp?id=141.

531. Kaye JA, Jick H. Epidemiology of lower limb fractures in general practice in the United Kingdom. *Injury Prevention* 2004, 10(6): 368–74.

532. Klos K, Muckley T, Gras F, Hofmann GO, Schmidt R. Early posttraumatic rotationplasty after severe degloving and soft tissue avulsion injury: a case report. *Journal of Orthopaedic Trauma* 2010, 24(2): el–5.

533. Kragh JF Jr, Walters TJ, Baer DG, Fox CJ, Wade CE, Salinas J, et al. Practical use of emergency tourniquets to stop bleeding in major limb trauma. *Journal of Trauma* 2008, 64 (suppl. 2): S38–49; discussion S49–50.

534. Lee C, Porter KM. Prehospital management of lower limb fractures. *Emergency Medicine Journal* 2005, 22(9): 660–3.

535. Lee C, Porter KM, Hodgetts TJ. Tourniquet use in the civilian prehospital setting. *Emergency Medicine Journal* 2007, 24(8): 584–7.

536. Lisle DA, Shepherd GJ, Cowderoy GA, O'Connell PT. MR imaging of traumatic and overuse injuries of the wrist and hand in athletes. *Magnetic Resonance Imaging Clinics of North America* 2009, 17(4): 639–54.

537. National Library of Medicine. *Fractures.* Available from: http://www.nlm.nih.gov/medlineplus/fractures.html, 2011.

538. Pearse MF, Harry L, Nanchahal J. Acute compartment syndrome of the leg. *British Medical Journal* 2002, 325(7364): 557–8.

539. Power RA, Greengross P. Acute lower leg compartment syndrome. *British Journal of Sports Medicine* 1991, 25(4): 218–20.

540. Taxter AJ, Konstantakos EK, Ames DW. Lateral compartment syndrome of the lower extremity in a recreational athlete: a case report. *American Journal of Emergency Medicine* 2008, 26(8): 973.el–2.

541. van Staa TP, Dennison EM, Leufkens HGM, Cooper C. Epidemiology of fractures in England and Wales. *Bone* 2001, 29(6): 517–22.

542. Weinmann M. Compartment syndrome. *Emergency Medical Services* 2003, 32(9): 36.

543. Wood SP, Vrahas M, Wedel SK. Femur fracture immobilization with traction splints in multisystem trauma patients. *Prehospital Emergency Care* 2003, 7(2): 241–3.

544. British Orthopaedic Association, British Association of Plastic Reconstructive and Aesthetic Surgeons. *The Management of Severe Open Lower Limb Fractures.* Available from: http://www.boa.ac.uk, 2009.

545. Melamed E, Blumenfeld A, Kalmovich B, Kosashvili Y, Lin G, Israel Defense Forces Medical Corps Consensus Group on Prehospital Care of Orthopedic Injuries. Prehospital care of orthopedic injuries. *Prehospital Disaster Medicine* 2007, 22(1): 22–5.

546. Bragg S. Avulsion amputation of the hand. *Journal of Emergency Nursing* 2005, 31(3): 282.

547. Bragg S. The boxers' fracture. *Journal of Emergency Nursing* 2005, 31(5): 473.

548. Bragg S. Vertical deceleration: falls from height. *Journal of Emergency Nursing* 2007, 33(4): 377–8.

549. Lovell ME, Evans JR. A comparison of the spinal board and the vacuum stretcher, spinal stability and interface pressure. *Injury* 1994, 25(3): 179–80.

550. Stiell IG, Wells GA, Vandemheen KL, Clement CM, Lesiuk H, De Maio VJ, et al. The Canadian C-spine rule for radiography in alert and stable trauma patients. *Journal of the American Medical Association* 2001, 286(15): 1841–8.

551. Gardner B, Kluger PJ. (iv) The overall care of the spinal cord injured patient. *Current Orthopaedics* 2004, 18(1): 33–48.

552. Ersoy G, Karcioglu O, Enginbas Y, Eray O, Ayrik C. Are cervical spine X-rays mandatory in all blunt trauma patients? *European Journal of Emergency Medicine* 1995, 2(4): 191–5.

553. Sekhon LH, Fehlings MG. Epidemiology, demographics, and pathophysiology of acute spinal cord injury. *Spine* 2001, 26(suppl. 24): S2–12.

554. Kwon BK, Tetzlaff W, Grauer JN, Beiner J, Vaccaro AR. Pathophysiology and pharmacologic treatment of acute spinal cord injury. *The Spine Journal* 2004, 4(4): 451–64.

555. Kwan I, Brunn F, Roberts I. Spinal immobilisation for trauma patients (review). *Cochrane Database of Systematic Reviews* 2009 (reprint): doi 10.1002/14651858.CD002803(1).

556. Gertzbein SD, Khoury D, Bullington A, St John TA, Larson AI. Thoracic and lumbar fractures associated with skiing and snowboarding injuries according to the AO Comprehensive Classification. *American Journal of Sports Medicine* 2012, 40(8): 1750–4

557. Milby AH, Halpern CH, Guo W, Stein SC. Prevalence of cervical spinal injury in trauma. *Neurosurgical Focus* 2008, 25(5): E10.

558. Polk-Williams A, Carr BG, Blinman TA, Masiakos PT, Wiebe DJ, Nance ML. Cervical spine injury in young children: a National Trauma Data Bank review. *Journal of Pediatric Surgery* 2008, 43(9): 1718–21.

559. Qaiyum M, Tyrrell PN, McCall IW, Cassar-Pullicino VN. MRI detection of unsuspected vertebral injury in acute spinal trauma: incidence and significance. *Skeletal Radiology* 2001, 30(6): 299–304.

560. Sultan HY, Boyle A, Pereira M, Antoun N, Maimaris C. Application of the Canadian CT head rules in managing minor head injuries in a UK emergency department: implications for the implementation of the NICE guidelines. *Emergency Medicine Journal* 2004, 21(4): 420–5.

561. Hinds JD, Allen G, Morris CG. Trauma and motorcyclists: born to be wild, bound to be injured? *Injury* 2007, 38(10): 1131–8.

562. Barry B, George G, Oag H, Shafighian B. Fractures of the atlas: can we rely on the NICE guidelines for imaging the cervical spine after head injury? *Emergency Medicine Journal* 2006, 23(9): e52.

563. Brown RL, Brunn MA, Garcia VF. Cervical spine injuries in children: a review of 103 patients treated consecutively at a level I pediatric trauma center. *Journal of Pediatric Surgery* 2001, 36(8): 1107–14.

564. Cirak B, Ziegfeld S, Knight VM, Chang D, Avellino AM, Paidas CN. Spinal injuries in children. *Journal of Pediatric Surgery* 2004, 39(4): 607–12.

565. Claytor B, MacLennan PA, McGwin GJ, Rue LWI, Kirkpatrick JS. Cervical spine injury and restraint system use in motor vehicle collisions. *Spine* 2004, 29(4): 386–9.

566. Donaldson WFI, Hanks SE, Nassr A, Vogt MT, Lee JY. Cervical spine injuries associated with the incorrect use of airbags in motor vehicle collisions. *Spine* 2008, 33(6): 631–4: doi 10.1097/BRS.0b013e318166e06d.

567. Reed MA, Naftel RP, Carter S, MacLennan PA, McGwin G, Rue LW. Motor vehicle restraint system use and risk of spine injury. *Traffic Injury Prevention* 2006, 7(3): 256–63.

568. Smith JA, Siegel JH, Siddiqi SQ. Spine and spinal cord injury in motor vehicle crashes: a function of change in velocity and energy dissipation on impact with respect to the direction of crash. *Journal of Trauma and Acute Care Surgery* 2005, 59(1): 117–31.

569. Stein DM, Kufera JA, Ho SM, Ryb GE, Dischinger PC, O'Connor JV, et al. Occupant and crash characteristics for case occupants with cervical spine injuries sustained in motor vehicle collisions. *Journal of Trauma and Acute Care Surgery* 2011, 70(2): 299–309: doi 10.1097/TA.0b013e3181f8aa91.

570. Yanar H, Demetriades D, Hatzizacharia P, Nomoto S, Salim A, Inaba K, et al. Pedestrians injured by automobiles: risk factors for cervical spine injuries. *Journal of the American College of Surgeons* 2007, 205(6): 794–9.

571. Boden BP, Jarvis CG. Spinal injuries in sports. *Physical Medicine and Rehabilitation Clinics of North America* 2009, 20(1): 55–68.

572. King DA, Hume PA, Gianotti S, Clark T. Neck, back and spine injuries in amateur rugby league: a review of nine years of Accident Compensation Corporation injury entitlement claims and costs. *Journal of Science and Medicine in Sport/Sports Medicine Australia* 2011, 14(2): 126–9.

573. Kruse D, Lemmen B. Spine injuries in the sport of gymnastics. *Current Sports Medicine Reports* 2009, 8(1): 20–8: doi 10.1249/JSR.0b013e3181967ca6.

574. Siebenga J, Segers MJ, Elzinga MJ, Bakker FC, Haarman HJ, Patka P. Spine fractures caused by horse riding. *European Spine Journal* 2006, 15(4): 465–71.

575. Morisod J, Coutaz M. Falls in the elderly: think about cervical fracture! *Revue Médicale Suisse* 2009, 5(224): 2195–6, 2198–9.

576. Lomoschitz FM, Blackmore CC, Mirza SK, Mann FA. Cervical spine injuries in patients 65 years old and older. *American Journal of Roentgenology* 2002, 178(3): 573–7.

577. Kent A, Pearce A. Review of morbidity and mortality associated with falls from heights among patients presenting to a major trauma centre. *Emergency Medicine Australasia* 2006, 18(1): 23–30.

578. Kannus P, Palvanen M, Niemi S, Parkkari J. Alarming rise in the number and incidence of fall-induced cervical spine injuries among older adults. *Journals of Gerontology Series A: Biological Sciences and Medical Sciences* 2007, 62(2): 180–3.

579. Miller CP, Brubacher JW, Biswas D, Lawrence BD, Whang PG, Grauer JN. The incidence of noncontiguous spinal fractures and other traumatic injuries associated with cervical spine fractures: a 10-year experience at an academic medical center. *Spine* 2011, 36(19): 1532–40: doi 10.097/BRS.0b013e3181f550a6.

580. Keenen TL, Antony J, Benson DR. Non-contiguous spinal fractures. *Journal of Trauma* 1990, 30(4): 489–91.

581. Wittenberg RH, Hargus S, Steffen R, Muter G, Botel U. Noncontiguous unstable spine fractures. *Spine* 2002, 27(3): 254–7.

582. The College of Emergency Medicine. *Guideline on the Management of Alert, Adult Patients with Potential Cervical Spine Injury in the Emergency Department.* Available from: http://www.collemergencymed.ac.uk/Shop-Floor/Clinical Guidelines, 2011.

583. Podolsky S, Baraff LJ, Simon RR, Hoffman JR, Larmon B, Ablon W. Efficacy of cervical spine immobilization methods. *Journal of Trauma* 1983, 23(6): 461–5.

584. Huerta C, Griffith R, Joyce SM. Cervical spine stabilization in pediatric patients: Evaluation of current techniques. *Annals of Emergency Medicine* 1987, 16(10): 1121–6.

585. McCabe JB, Nolan DJ. Comparison of the effectiveness of different cervical immobilization collars. *Annals of Emergency Medicine* 1986, 15: 93–6.

586. Ahn H, Singh J, Nathens A, MacDonald RD, Travers A, Tallon J, et al. Prehospital care management of a potential spinal cord injured patient: a systematic review of the literature and evidence-based guidelines. *Journal of Neurotrauma* 2010, 28(8): 1341–61.

587. Chandler DR, Nemejc C, Adkins RH, Waters RL. Emergency cervical-spine immobilization. *Annals of Emergency Medicine* 1992, 21(10): 1185–8.

588. De Lorenzo RA. A review of spinal immobilization techniques. *Journal of Emergency Medicine* 1996, 14(5): 603–13.

589. Graziano AF, Scheidel EA, Cline JR, Baer LJ. A radiographic comparison of prehospital cervical immobilization methods. *Annals of Emergency Medicine* 1987, 16(10): 1127–31.

590. Howell JM, Burrow R, Dumontier C, Hillyard A. A practical radiographic comparison of short board technique and Kendrick extrication device. *Annals of Emergency Medicine* 1989, 18(9): 943–6.

591. Chan D, Goldberg R, Tascone A, Harmon S, Chan L. The effect of spinal immobilization on healthy volunteers. *Annals of Emergency Medicine* 1994, 23(1): 48–51.

592. Cordell WH, Hollingsworth JC, Olinger ML, Stroman SJ, Nelson DR. Pain and tissue-interface pressures during spine-board immobilization. *Annals of Emergency Medicine* 1995, 26(1): 31–6.

593. Hamilton RS, Pons PT. The efficacy and comfort of full-body vacuum splints for cervical-spine immobilization. *Journal of Emergency Medicine* 1996, 14(5): 553–9.

594. McGuire RA, Neville S, Green BA, Watts C. Spinal instability and the log-rolling maneuver. *Journal of Trauma* 1987, 27(5): 525–31.

595. Del Rossi G, Rechtine GR, Conrad BP, Horodyski M. Are scoop stretchers suitable for use on spine-injured patients? *American Journal of Emergency Medicine* 2010, 28(7): 751–6.

596. Kaups KL, Davis JW. Patients with gunshot wounds to the head do not require cervical spine immobilization and evaluation. *Journal of Trauma, Injury, Infection, & Critical Care* 1998, 44(5): 865–7.

597. Kennedy F, Gonzalez P, Dang C, Fleming A, Sterling-Scott R. The Glasgow Coma Scale and prognosis in gunshot wounds to the brain. *Journal of Trauma* 1993, 35(1): 75–7.

598. Medzon R, Rothenhaus T, Bono CM, Grindlinger G, Rathlev NK. Stability of cervical spine fractures after gunshot wounds to the head and neck. *Spine* 2005, 30(20): 2274–9: doi 10.1097/01.brs.0000182083.43553.fa.

599. Lanoix R, Gupta R, Leak L, Pierre, Jean. C-spine injury associated with gunshot wounds to the head: retrospective study and literature review. *Journal of Trauma and Acute Care Surgery* 2000, 49(5): 860–3.

600. Kaups KL, Davis JW. Patients with gunshot wounds to the head do not require cervical spine immobilization and evaluation. *Journal of Trauma and Acute Care Surgery* 1998, 44(5): 865–7.

601. DuBose J, Teixeira PGR, Hadjizacharia P, Harmon M, Inaba K, Green DG, et al. The role of routine spinal imaging and immobilisation in asymptomatic patients after gunshot wounds. *Injury* 2009, 40(8): 860–3.

602. Barkana Y, Stein M, Scope A, Maor R, Abramovich Y, Friedman Z. Prehospital stabilization of the cervical spine for penetrating injuries of the neck: is it necessary? *Injury* 2000, 31(5): 305–9.

603. Ramasamy A, Midwinter M, Mahoney P, Clasper J. Learning the lessons from conflict: pre-hospital cervical spine stabilisation following ballistic neck trauma. *Injury* 2009, 40(12): 1342–5.

604. Brywczynski JJ, Barrett TW, Lyon JA, Cotton BA. Management of penetrating neck injury in the emergency department: a structured literature review. *Emergency Medicine Journal* 2008, 25(11): 711–15.

605. Domeier RM, Swor RA, Evans RW, Hancock JB, Fales W, Krohmer J. Multicenter prospective validation of pre-hospital clinical spinal clearance criteria. *Journal of Trauma* 2002, 53(4): 744–50.

606. Stroh G, Braude D. Can an out-of-hospital cervical spine clearance protocol identify all patients with injuries? An argument for selective immobilization. *Annals of Emergency Medicine* 2001, 37(6): 609–15.

607. Sahni R, Menegazzi JJ, Mosesso VNJ. Paramedic evaluation of clinical indicators of cervical spinal injury. *Prehospital Emergency Care* 1997, 1(1): 16–18.

608. Domeier RM, Evans RW, Swor RA, Hancock JB, Fales W, Krohmer J. The reliability of prehospital clinical evaluation for potential spinal injury is not affected by the mechanism of injury. *Prehospital Emergency Care* 1999, 3(4): 332–7.

609. Muhr MD, Seabrook DL, Wittwer LK. Paramedic use of a spinal injury clearance algorithm reduces spinal immobilization in the out-of-hospital setting. *Prehospital Emergency Care* 1999, 3(1): 1–6.

610. Totten VY, Sugarman DB. Respiratory effects of spinal immobilization. *Prehospital Emergency Care* 1999, 3(4): 347–52.

611. Raphael JH, Chotai R. Effects of the cervical collar on cerebrospinal fluid pressure. *Anaesthesia* 1994, 49: 437–9.

612. Kolb JC, Summers RL, Galli RL. Cervical collar induced changes in intracranial pressure. *American Journal of Emergency Medicine* 1999, 17: 135–7.

613. Ferguson J, Mardel SN, Beattie TF, Wytch R. Cervical collars: a potential risk to the head-injured patient. *Injury* 1993, 24(7): 454–6.

614. Davies G, Deakin C, Wilson A. The effect of a rigid collar on intracranial pressure. *Injury* 1996, 27(9): 647–9.

615. Craig GR, Nielsen MS. Rigid cervical collars and intracranial pressure. *Intensive Care Medicine* 1991, 17: 504–5.

616. Hunt K, Hallworth S, Smith M. The effects of rigid collar placement on intracranial and cerebral perfusion pressures. *Anaesthesia* 2001, 56: 511–13.

617. Butman AM, Schelble DT, Vomacka RW. The relevance of the occult cervical spine controversy and mechanism of injury to pre-hospital protocols: a review of the issues and literature. *Prehospital Disaster Medicine* 1996, 11(3): 228–33.

618. Dodd FM, Simon E, McKeown D, Patrick MR. The effect of a cervical collar on the tidal volume of anaesthetised adult patients. *Anaesthesia* 1995, 50(11): 961–3.

619. Houghton DJ. Dysphagia caused by a hard cervical collar. *British Journal of Neurosurgery* 1996, 10(5): 501–2.

620. Black CA, Buderer NMF, Blaylock B, Hogan BJ. Comparative study of risk factors for skin breakdown with cervical orthotic devices. *Journal of Trauma Nursing* 1998, 5(3): 62–6.

621. Hewitt S. Skin necrosis caused by a semi-rigid cervical collar in a ventilated patient with multiple injuries. *Injury* 1994, 25(5): 323–4.

622. Liew SC, Hill DA. Complication of hard cervical collars in multi-trauma patients. *Archives of Pediatrics & Adolescent Medicine* 1994, 64(2): 139–40.

623. Chan D, Goldberg RM, Mason J, Chan L. Backboard versus mattress splint immobilization: a comparison of symptoms generated. *Journal of Emergency Medicine* 1996, 14(3): 293–8.

624. Browne GJ, Lam LT, Barker RA. The usefulness of a modified adult protocol for the clearance of paediatric cervical spine injury in the emergency department. *Emergency Medicine Australasia* 2003, 15(2): 133–42.

625. Slack SE, Clancy MJ. Clearing the cervical spine of paediatric trauma patients. *Emergency Medical Journal* 2004, 21(2): 189–93.

626. Curran C, Dietrich AM, Bowman MJ, Ginn-Pease ME, King DR, Kosnik E. Pediatric cervical-spine immobilization: achieving neutral position? *Journal of Trauma* 1995, 39(4): 729–32.

627. Bracken MB. Steroids for acute spinal cord injury. *Cochrane Database Systematic Reviews* 2012, 1: CD001046.

628. Sorensen P. High-dose methylprednisolone in acute spinal injury. *Ugeskrift for Laeger* 2008, 170(5): 315–17.

629. Sayer FT, Kronvall E, Nilsson OG. Methylprednisolone treatment in acute spinal cord injury: the myth challenged through a structured analysis of published literature. *The Spine Journal: Official Journal of the North American Spine Society* 2006, 6(3): 335–43.

630. Kronvall E, Sayer FT, Nilsson OG. Methylprednisolone in the treatment of acute spinal cord injury has become more and more questioned. *Lakartidningen* 2005, 102(24–25): 1887–8.

631. Hugenholtz H, Cass DE, Dvorak MF, Fewer DH, Fox RJ, Izukawa DM, et al. High-dose methylprednisolone for acute closed spinal cord injury: only a treatment option. *Canadian Journal of Neurological Sciences* 2002, 29(3): 227–35.

632. Manix T. The tying game: how effective are body-to-board strapping techniques? *Emergency Medical Services* 1995, 20(6): 44–50.

633. Jones L, Bagnall AM. Spinal injuries centres (SICs) for acute traumatic spinal cord injury. *Cochrane Database of Systematic Reviews* 2008 (reprint), 4: doi 10.1002/14651858.CD004442.pub2.

634. Stagg MJ, Lovell ME. A repeat audit of spinal board usage in the emergency department. *Injury* 2008, 39(3): 323–6.

635. Porter KM, Allison KP. The UK emergency department practice for spinal board unloading: is there conformity? *Resuscitation* 2003, 58(1): 117–20.

636. Cooke MW. Use of the spinal board within the accident and emergency department. *Journal of Accident & Emergency Medicine* 1998, 15(2): 108–9.

637. Walton R, DeSalvo JF, Ernst AA, Shahane A. Padded vs unpadded spine board for cervical spine immobilization. *Annals of Emergency Medicine* 1995, 2(8): 725–8.

638. Brown JK, Jing Y, Wang S, Ehrlich PF. Patterns of severe injury in pediatric car crash victims: Crash Injury Research Engineering Network database. *Journal of Pediatric Surgery* 2006, 41(2): 362–7.

639. O'Brien DP, Luchette FA, Pereira SJ, Lim E, Seeskin CS, James L, et al. Pelvic fracture in the elderly is associated with increased mortality. *Surgery* 2002, 132(4): 710–14.

640. Stein DM, O'Connor JV, Kufera JA, Ho SM, Dischinger PC, Copeland CE, et al. Risk factors associated with pelvic fractures sustained in motor vehicle collisions involving newer vehicles. *Journal of Trauma* 2006, 61(1): 21–30.

641. Dalai SA, Burgess AR, Siegel JH, Young JW, Brumback RJ, Poka A, et al. Pelvic fracture in multiple trauma: classification by mechanism is key to pattern of organ injury, resuscitative requirements, and outcome. *Journal of Trauma* 1989, 29(7): 981–1000; discussion 1000–2.

642. Demetriades D, Karaiskakis M, Toutouzas K, Alo K, Velmahos G, Chan L. Pelvic fractures: epidemiology and predictors of associated abdominal injuries and outcomes. *Journal of the American College of Surgeons* 2002, 195(1): 1–10.

643. Demetriades D, Murray J, Brown C, Velmahos G, Salim A, Alo K, et al. High-level falls: type and severity of injuries and survival outcome according to age. *Journal of Trauma* 2005, 58(2): 342–5.

644. Ferrera PC, Hill DA. Good outcomes of open pelvic fractures. *Injury* 1999, 30(3): 187–90.

645. Gustavo Parreira J, Coimbra R, Rasslan S, Oliveira A, Fregoneze M, Mercadante M. The role of associated injuries on outcome of blunt trauma patients sustaining pelvic fractures. *Injury* 2000, 31(9): 677–82.

646. Inaba K, Sharkey PW, Stephen DJG, Redelmeier DA, Brenneman FD. The increasing incidence of severe pelvic injury in motor vehicle collisions. *Injury* 2004, 35(8): 759–65.

647. Kimbrell BJ, Velmahos GC, Chan LS, Demetriades D. Angiographic embolization for pelvic fractures in older patients. *Archives of Surgery* 2004, 139(7): 728–32.

648. Tarman GJ, Kaplan GW, Lerman SL, McAleer IM, Losasso BE. Lower genitourinary injury and pelvic fractures in pediatric patients. *Urology* 2002, 59(1): 123–6.

649. Demetriades D, Murray J, Martin M, Velmahos G, Salim A, Alo K, et al. Pedestrians injured by automobiles: relationship of age to injury type and severity. *Journal of the American College of Surgeons* 2004, 199(3): 382–7.

650. Hill RMF, Robinson CM, Keating JF. Fractures of the pubic rami. *Journal of Bone & Joint Surgery, British Volume* 2001, 83-B(8): 1141–4.

651. Baxter NN, Habermann EB, Tepper JE, Durham SB, Virnig BA. Risk of pelvic fractures in older women following pelvic irradiation. *Journal of the American Medical Association* 2005, 294(20): 2587–93.

652. Boufous S, Finch C, Lord S, Close J. The increasing burden of pelvic fractures in older people, New South Wales, Australia. *Injury* 2005, 36(11): 1323–9.

653. Hauschild O, Strohm PC, Culemann U, Pohlemann T, Suedkamp NP, Koestler W, et al. Mortality in patients with pelvic fractures: results from the German pelvic injury register. *Journal of Trauma* 2008, 64(2): 449–55.

654. Gansslen A, Pohlemann T, Paul C, Lobenhoffer P, Tscherne H. Epidemiology of pelvic ring injuries. *Injury* 1996, 27(1001): S/A13–20, S/A51.

655. Moreno C, Moore EE, Rosenberger A, Cleveland HC. Hemorrhage associated with major pelvic fracture: a multispecialty challenge. *Journal of Trauma* 1986, 26(11): 987–94.

656. Mucha P Jr, Farnell MB. Analysis of pelvic fracture management. *Journal of Trauma* 1984, 24(5): 379–86.

657. Siegel JH, Mason-Gonzalez S, Dischinger P, Cushing B, Read K, Robinson R, et al. Safety belt restraints and compartment intrusions in frontal and lateral motor vehicle crashes: mechanisms of injuries, complications, and acute care costs. *Journal of Trauma* 1993, 34(5): 736–58.

658. Brenneman FD, Katyal D, Boulanger BR, Tile M, Redelmeier DA. Long-term outcomes in open pelvic fractures. *Journal of Trauma and Acute Care Surgery* 1997, 42(5): 773–7.

659. Poole GV, Ward EF, Muakkassa FF, Hsu HSH, Griswold JA, Rhodes RS. Pelvic fracture from major blunt trauma: outcome is determined by associated injuries. *Annals of Surgery* 1991, 213(6): 532–9.

660. Croce MA, Magnotti LJ, Savage SA, Wood IGW, Fabian TC. Emergent pelvic fixation in patients with exsanguinating pelvic fractures. *Journal of the American College of Surgeons* 2007, 204(5): 935–9.

661. Duane TM, Tan BB, Golay D, Cole FJ Jr, Weireter LJ Jr, Britt LD. Blunt trauma and the role of routine pelvic radiographs: a prospective analysis. *Journal of Trauma* 2002, 53(3): 463–8.

662. Gonzalez RP, Fried PQ, Bukhalo M. The utility of clinical examination in screening for pelvic fractures in blunt trauma. *Journal of the American College of Surgeons* 2002, 194(2): 121–5.

663. Ham SJ, Van Walsum ADP, Vierhout PAM. Predictive value of the hip flexion test for fractures of the pelvis. *Injury Prevention* 1996, 27(8): 543–4.

664. Heath FR, Blum F, Rockwell S. Physical examination as a screening test for pelvic fractures in blunt trauma patients. *West Virginia Medical Journal* 1997, 93(5): 267–9.

665. Kaneriya PP, Schweitzer ME, Spettell C, Cohen MJ, Karasick D. The costeffectiveness of routine pelvic radiography in the evaluation of blunt trauma patients. *Skeletal Radiology* 1999, 28(5): 271–3.

666. Khoury G, Sfeir R, Khalifeh M, Khoury SJ, Nabbout G. Penetrating trauma to the abdominal vessels. *Cardiovascular Surgery* 1996, 4(3): 405–7.

667. Salvino CK, Esposito TJ, Smith D, Dries D, Marshall W, Flisak M, et al. Routine pelvic x-ray studies in awake blunt trauma patients: a sensible policy? *Journal of Trauma* 1992, 33(3): 413–16.

668. Tien IY, Dufel SE. Does ethanol affect the reliability of pelvic bone examination in blunt trauma? *Annals of Emergency Medicine* 2000, 36(5): 451–5.

669. Yugueros P, Sarmiento JM, Garcia AF, Ferrada R. Unnecessary use of pelvic x-ray in blunt trauma. *Journal of Trauma* 1995, 39(4): 722–5.

670. Boulanger BR, Milzman D, Mitchell K, Rodriguez A. Body habitus as a predictor of injury pattern after blunt trauma. *Journal of Trauma* 1992, 33(2): 228–32.

671. Hanson PB, Milne JC, Chapman MW. Open fractures of the pelvis: review of 43 cases. *Journal of Bone & Joint Surgery, British Volume* 1991, 73(2): 325–9.

672. Malangoni MA, Miller FB, Cryer HM, Mullins RJ, Richardson JD. The management of penetrating pelvic trauma. *American Surgeon* 1990, 56(2): 61–5.

673. Perry IF Jr. Pelvic open fractures. *Clinical Orthopaedics* 1980(151): 41–5.

674. Chong KH, DeCoster T, Osler T, Robinson B. Pelvic fractures and mortality. *Iowa Orthopaedic Journal* 1997, 17: 110–14.

675. Cryer HM, Miller FB, Evers BM, Rouben LR, Seligson DL. Pelvic fracture classification: correlation with hemorrhage. *Journal of Trauma* 1988, 28(7): 973–80.

676. Evers BM, Cryer HM, Miller FB. Pelvic fracture hemorrhage: priorities in management. *Archives of Surgery* 1989, 124(4): 422–4.

677. Heetveld MJ, Harris I, Schlaphoff G, Balogh Z, D'Amours SK, Sugrue M. Hemodynamically unstable pelvic fractures: recent care and new guidelines. *Journal of Surgery* 2004, 28(9): 904–9.

678. Heetveld MJ, Harris I, Schlaphoff G, Sugrue M. Guidelines for the management of haemodynamically unstable pelvic fracture patients. *ANZ Journal of Surgery* 2004, 74(7): 520–9.

679. Poole GV, Ward EF. Causes of mortality in patients with pelvic fractures. *Orthopedics* 1994, 17(8): 691–6.

680. Burgess AR, Eastridge BJ, Young JW, Ellison TS, Ellison PSJ, Poka A, et al. Pelvic ring disruptions: effective classification system and treatment protocols. *Journal of Trauma* 1990, 30(7): 848–56.

681. Failinger MS, McGanity PLJ. Unstable fractures of the pelvic ring. *Journal of Bone & Joint Surgery, American Volume* 1992, 74(5): 781–91.

682. Henry SM, Tometta IP, Scalea TM. Damage control for devastating pelvic and extremity injuries. *Surgical Clinics of North America* 1997, 77(4): 879–95.

683. Richardson JD, Harty J, Amin M, Flint LM. Open pelvic fractures. *Journal of Trauma* 1982, 22(7): 533–8.

684. Rothenberger DA, Fischer RP, Perry JF Jr. Major vascular injuries secondary to pelvic fractures: an unsolved clinical problem. *American Journal of Surgery* 1978, 136(6): 660–2.

685. Grotz MRW, Gummerson NW, Gansslen A, Petrowsky H, Keel M, Allami MK, et al. Staged management and outcome of combined pelvic and liver trauma: an international experience of the deadly duo. *Injury* 2006, 37(7): 642–51.

686. Wubben RC. Mortality rate of pelvic fracture patients. *Wisconsin Medical Journal* 1996, 95(10): 702–4.

687. Starr AJ, Griffen, MA. Pelvic ring disruptions: mechanisms, fracture pattern, morbidity and mortality. An analysis of 325 patients. OTA Annual Meeting, Texas, USA, 2000.

688. Koury HI, Peschiera JL, Welling RE. Selective use of pelvic roentgenograms in blunt trauma patients. *Journal of Trauma, Injury, Infection, & Critical Care* 1993, 34(2): 236–7.

689. Sriussadaporn S. Abdominopelvic vascular injuries. *Journal of the Medical Association of Thailand* 2000, 83(1): 13–20.

690. Moss MC, Bircher MD. Volume changes within the true pelvis during disruption of the pelvic ring: where does the haemorrhage go? *Injury* 1996, 27(suppl. 1): S-A21–3.

691. Rowe SA, Sochor MS, Staples KS, Wahl WL, Wang SC. Pelvic ring fractures: implications of vehicle design, crash type, and occupant characteristics. *Surgery* 2004, 136(4): 842–7.

692. Ben-Menachem Y, Coldwell DM, Young JWR, Burgess AR. Hemorrhage associated with pelvic fractures: causes, diagnosis, and emergent management. *American Journal of Roentgenology* 1991, 157(5): 1005–14.

693. Dyer GSM, Vrahas MS. Review of the pathophysiology and acute management of haemorrhage in pelvic fracture. *Injury* 2006, 37(7): 602–13.

694. Fleming WH, Bowen JC III. Control of hemorrhage in pelvic crush injuries. *Journal of Trauma* 1973, 13(6): 567–70.

695. Davidson BS, Simmons GT, Williamson PR, Buerk CA. Pelvic fractures associated with open perineal wounds: a survivable injury. *Journal of Trauma* 1993, 35(1): 36–9.

696. Govender S, Sham A, Singh B. Open pelvic fractures. *Injury* 1990, 21(6): 373–6.

697. Sinnott R, Rhodes M, Brader A. Open pelvic fracture: an injury for trauma centers. *American Journal of Surgery* 1992, 163(3): 283–7.

698. Barach E, Martin G, Tomlanovich M. Blunt pelvic trauma with urethral injury in the female: a case report and review of the literature. *Journal of Emergency Medicine* 1984, 2(2): 101–5.

699. Bottlang M, Simpson T, Sigg J, Krieg JC, Madey SM, Long WB. Noninvasive reduction of open-book pelvic fractures by circumferential compression. *Journal of Orthopaedic Trauma* 2002, 16(6): 367–73.

700. Smith RJ. Avulsion of the nongravid uterus due to pelvic fracture. *Southern Medical Journal* 1989, 82(1): 70–3.

701. Sandler CM, Hall JT, Rodriguez MB, Corriere JN Jr. Bladder injury in blunt pelvic trauma. *Radiology* 1985, 158(3): 633–8.

702. Lunt HR. Entrapment of bowel within fractures of the pelvis. *Injury* 1970, 2(2): 121–6.

703. Reiff DA, McGwin G Jr, Metzger J, Windham ST, Doss M, Rue LW III. Identifying injuries and motor vehicle collision characteristics that together are suggestive of diaphragmatic rupture. *Journal of Trauma* 2002, 53(6): 1139–45.

704. Waydhas C, Nast-Kolb D, Ruchholtz S. Pelvic ring fractures: utility of clinical examination in patients with impaired consciousness or tracheal intubation. *European Journal of Trauma and Emergency Surgery* 2007, 33(2): 170–5.

705. Fox MA, Mangiante EC, Fabian TC, Voeller GR, Kudsk KA. Pelvic fractures: an analysis of factors affecting prehospital triage and patient outcome. *Southern Medical Journal* 1990, 83(7): 785–8.

706. MacLeod M, Powell JN. Evaluation of pelvic fractures: clinical and radiologic. *Orthopedic Clinics of North America* 1997, 28(3): 299–319.

707. Sauerland S, Bouillon B, Rixen D, Raum MR, Koy T, Neugebauer EAM. The reliability of clinical examination in detecting pelvic fractures in blunt trauma patients: a meta-analysis. *Archives of Orthopaedic and Trauma Surgery* 2004, 124(2): 123–8.

708. Lee C, Porter K. The prehospital management of pelvic fractures. *Emergency Medicine Journal* 2007, 24(2): 130-3.

709. Waikakul S, Harnroongroj T, Vanadurongwan V. Immediate stabilization of unstable pelvic fractures versus delayed stabilization. *Journal of the Medical Association of Thailand* 1999, 82(7): 637–42.

710. Grimm MR, Vrahas MS, Thomas KA. Pressure-volume characteristics of the intact and disrupted pelvic retroperitoneum. *Journal of Trauma* 1998, 44(3): 454–9.

711. Bottlang M, Krieg JC, Mohr M, Simpson TS, Madey SM. Emergent management of pelvic ring fractures with use of circumferential compression. *Journal of Orthopaedic Trauma* 2002, 16(6): 367–73.

712. Brunette DD, Fifield G, Ruiz E. Use of pneumatic antishock trousers in the management of pediatric pelvic hemorrhage. *Pediatric Emergency Care* 1987, 3(2): 86–90.

713. Connolly B, Gerlinger T, Pitcher JD. Complete masking of a severe open-book pelvic fracture by a pneumatic antishock garment. *Journal of Trauma* 1999, 46(2): 340–2.

714. Friese G, LaMay G. Emergency stabilization of unstable pelvic fractures. *Emergency Medical Services* 2005, 34(5): 65.

715. Jowett AJL, Bowyer GW. Pressure characteristics of pelvic binders. *Injury* 2007, 38(1): 118–21.

716. Katsoulis E, Drakoulakis E, Giannoudis PV. (iii) Management of open pelvic fractures. *Current Orthopaedics* 2005, 19(5): 345–53.

717. Krieg JC, Mohr M, Ellis TJ, Simpson TS, Madey SM, Bottlang M. Emergent stabilization of pelvic ring injuries by controlled circumferential compression: a clinical trial. *Journal of Trauma, Injury, Infection, & Critical Care* 2005, 59(3): 659–64.

718. Routt MLC Jr, Simonian PT, Swiontkowski MF. Stabilization of pelvic ring disruptions. *Orthopedic Clinics of North America* 1997, 28(3): 369–88.

719. Salomone JP, Ustin JS, McSwain NE Jr, Feliciano DV. Opinions of trauma practitioners regarding prehospital interventions for critically injured patients. *Journal of Trauma* 2005, 58(3): 509–15; discussion 515–17.

720. Scurr JH, Cutting P. Tight jeans as a compression garment after major trauma. *British Medical Journal (Clinical Research Edition)* 1984, 288(6420): 828.

721. Simpson T, Krieg JC, Heuer F, Bottlang M. Stabilization of pelvic ring disruptions with a circumferential sheet. *Journal of Trauma, Injury, Infection, & Critical Care* 2002, 52(1): 158–61.

722. Vermeulen B, Peter R, Hoffmeyer P, Unger PF. Prehospital stabilization of pelvic dislocations: a new strap belt to provide temporary hemodynamic stabilization. *Swiss Surgery* 1999, 5(2): 43–6.

723. Nunn T, Cosker TDA, Bose D, Pallister I. Immediate application of improvised pelvic binder as first step in extended resuscitation from life-threatening hypovolaemic shock in conscious patients with unstable pelvic injuries. *Injury* 2007, 38(1): 125–8.

724. Krieg JC, Mohr M, Mirza AJ, Bottlang M. Pelvic circumferential compression in the presence of soft-tissue injuries: a case report. *Journal of Trauma, Injury, Infection, & Critical Care* 2005, 59(2): 470–2.

725. Ismail N, Bellemare JF, Mollitt DL, DiScala C, Koeppel B, Tepas IJJ. Death from pelvic fracture: children are different. *Journal of Pediatric Surgery* 1996, 31(1): 82–5.

726. Junkins EPJ, Nelson DS, Carroll KL, Hansen K, Furnival RA. A prospective evaluation of the clinical presentation of pediatric pelvic fractures. *Journal of Trauma* 2001, 51(1): 64–8.

727. Silber JS, Flynn JM, Koffler KM, Dormans JP, Drummond DS. Analysis of the cause, classification, and associated injuries of 166 consecutive pediatric pelvic fractures. *Journal of Pediatric Orthopaedics* 2001, 21(4): 446–50.

728. Junkins EP, Furnival RA, Bake RG. The clinical presentation of pediatric pelvic fractures. *Pediatric Emergency Care* 2001, 17(1): 15–18.

729. Lee C, Revell M, Porter K, Steyn R. The prehospital management of chest injuries: a consensus statement Faculty of Pre-hospital Care, Royal College of Surgeons of Edinburgh. *Emergency Medicine Journal* 2007, 24(3): 220–4.

730. Warner KJ, Copass MK, Bulger EM. Paramedic use of needle thoracostomy in the prehospital environment. *Prehospital Emergency Care* 2008, 12(2): 162–8.

731. Waydhas C, Sauerland S. Pre-hospital pleural decompression and chest tube placement after blunt trauma: a systematic review. *Resuscitation* 2007, 72(1): 11–25.

732. Dretzke J, Sandercock J, Bayliss S, Burls A. Clinical effectiveness and costeffectiveness of prehospital intravenous fluids in trauma patients. *Health Technology Assessment* 2004, 8(23).

733. Turner J, Nicholl J, Webber L, Cox H, Dixon S, Yates D. A randomised controlled trial of prehospital intravenous fluid replacement therapy in serious trauma. *Health Technology Assessment* 2000, 4(31).

734. Bickell WH, Wall MJJ, Pepe PE, Martin RR, Ginger VF, Allen M K, et al Immediate versus delayed fluid resuscitation in patients with trauma. *New England Journal of Medicine* 1994, 331: 1105–9.

735. Stern SA. Low-volume fluid resuscitation for presumed hemorrhagic shock: helpful or harmful? *Current Opinion in Critical Care* 2001, 7(6): 422–30.

736. Pepe PE, Mosesso VNJ, Falk JL. Prehospital fluid resuscitation of the patient with major trauma. *Prehospital Emergency Care* 2002, 6(1): 81–91.

737. de Guzman E, Shankar MN, Mattox KL. Limited volume resuscitation in penetrating thoracoabdominal trauma. *AACN Advanced Critical Care* 1999, 10(1): 61–8.

738. Borman JB, Aharonson-Daniel L, Savitsky B, Peleg K. Unilateral flail chest is seldom a lethal injury. *Emergency Medicine Journal* 2006, 23(12): 903–5.

739. BMJ Evidence Centre. *Best Practice: Cardiac tamponade.* Available from: http://bestpractice.bmj.com/best-practice/monograph/459.html, 2012.

740. Fitzgerald M, Spencer J, Johnson F, Marasco S, Atkin C, Kossmann T. Definitive management of acute cardiac tamponade secondary to blunt trauma. *Emergency Medicine Australasia* 2005, 17(5–6): 494–9.

741. Friend KD. Prehospital recognition of tension pneumothorax. *Prehospital Emergency Care* 2000, 4(1): 75–7.

742. Massarutti D, Trillo G, Berlot G, Tomasini A, Bacer B, D'Orlando L, et al. Simple thoracostomy in prehospital trauma management is safe and effective: a 2-year experience by helicopter emergency medical crews. *European Journal of Emergency Medicine* 2006, 13(5): 276–80.

743. Wanek S, Mayberry JC. Blunt thoracic trauma: flail chest, pulmonary contusion, and blast injury. *Critical Care Clinics* 2004, 20(1): 71–81.

744. Blaivas M. Inadequate needle thoracostomy rate in the prehospital setting for presumed pneumothorax. *Journal of Ultrasound in Medicine* 2010, 29(9): 1285–9.

745. Ayers DE, Kay AR. Management of burns in the wilderness. *Travel Medicine and Infectious Disease* 2005, 3(4): 239–48.

746. Boots RJ, Dulhunty JM, Paratz J, Lipman J. Respiratory complications in burns: an evolving spectrum of injury. *Clinical Pulmonary Medicine* 2009, 16(3): 132–8.

747. Cancio LC. Airway management and smoke inhalation injury in the burn patient. *Clinics in Plastic Surgery* 2009, 36(4): 555–67.

748. National Institute for Health and Clinical Excellence. *Clinical Knowledge Summaries: Burns and scalds.* London: NICE, 2007. Available from: http://www.cks.nhs.uk/burns_and_scalds.

749. Enoch S, Roshan A, Shah M. Emergency and early management of burns and scalds. *British Medical Journal* 2009, 338(7700): 937–41.

750. Hassan Z, Wong JK, Bush J, Bayat A, Dunn KW. Assessing the severity of inhalation injuries in adults. *Burns: Journal of the International Society for Burn Injuries* 2010, 36(2): 212–16.

751. Hermans MHE. A general overview of burn care. *International Wound Journal* 2005, 2(3): 206–20, 222–3.

752. Karpelowsky JS, Rode H. Basic principles in the management of thermal injuries. *South African Family Practice* 2008, 50(3): 24–31.

753. KarpelowskyJS, Wallis L, Madaree A, Rode H. South African Burn Society burn stabilisation protocol. *South African Medical Journal* 2007, 97(8): 574–7.

754. Marek K, Piotr W, Stanislaw S, Stefan G, Justyna G, Mariusz N, et al. Fibreoptic bronchoscopy in routine clinical practice in confirming the diagnosis and treatment of inhalation burns. *Burns: Journal of the International Society for Burn Injuries* 2007, 33(5): 554–60.

755. Mlcak RP, Suman OE, Herndon DN. Respiratory management of inhalation injury. *Burns: Journal of the International Society for Burn Injuries* 2007, 33(1): 2–13.

756. Muehlberger T, Ottomann C, Toman N, Daigeler A, Lehnhardt M. Emergency pre-hospital care of burn patients. *The Surgeon: Journal of the Royal Colleges of Surgeons of Edinburgh & Ireland* 2010, 8(2): 101–4.

757. New Zealand Guidelines Group. *Management of Burns and Scalds in Primary Care.* Wellington: Accident Compensation Corporation, 2007. Available from: http://www.guideline.gov/content.aspx?id=11509.

758. Palmieri TL. Inhalation injury: research progress and needs. *Journal of Burn Care and Research* 2007, 28(4): 549–54.

759. Pham TN, Gibran NS. Thermal and electrical injuries. *Surgical Clinics of North America* 2007, 87(1): 185–206.

760. Singh S, Handy J. The respiratory insult in burns injury. *Current Anaesthesia and Critical Care* 2008, 19(5–6): 264–8.

761. Spanholtz TA, Theodorou P, Amini P, Spilker G. Severe burn injuries: acute and long-term treatment. *Deutsches Arzteblatt* 2009, 106(38): 607–13.

762. Suzuki M, Aikawa N, Kobayashi K, Higuchi R. Prognostic implications of inhalation injury in burn patients in Tokyo. *Burns: Journal of the International Society for Burn Injuries* 2005, 31(3): 331–6.

763. Walton JJ, Manara AR. Burns and smoke inhalation. *Anaesthesia & Intensive Care Medicine* 2005, 6(9): 317–21.

764. Wasiak J, Cleland H, Campbell F. Dressings for superficial and partial thickness burns. *Cochrane Database of Systematic Reviews* 2007, 3: CD002106.

765. Durrant CAT, Simpson AR, Williams G. Thermal injury: the first 24 h. *Current Anaesthesia and Critical Care* 2008, 19(5–6): 256–63.

766. Freiburg C, Igneri P, Sartorelli K, Rogers F. Effects of differences in percent total body surface area estimation on fluid resuscitation of transferred burn patients. *Journal of Burn Care and Research* 2007, 28(1): 42–8.

767. Hackenschmidt A. Burn trauma priorities for a patient with 80% total body surface area burns. *Journal of Emergency Nursing* 2007, 33(4): 405–8.

768. Hussain S, Ferguson C. Assessing the size of burns: which method works best? *Emergency Medicine Journal* 2009, 26(9): 664–6.

769. Singer AJ, Dagum AB. Current management of acute cutaneous wounds. *New England Journal of Medicine* 2008, 359(10): 1037–46.

770. Williams C. Successful assessment and management of burn injuries. *Nursing Standard* 2009, 23(32): 53–4.

771. Allison K, Porter K. Consensus on the prehospital approach to burns patient management. *Emergency Medicine Journal* 2004, 21(1): 112–14.

772. Williams G, Dziewulski P. Intravascular fluid therapy in burns injury. In Group. TJRCALGD, editor, 2011.

773. Blackhurst H. Estimation of burn surface area using the hand. *BestBets* 2007. Available from: http://www.bestbets.org/bets/bet.php?id=01516.

774. Jose RM, Roy DK, Vidyadharan R, Erdmann M. Burns area estimation: an error perpetuated. *Burns: Journal of the International Society for Burn Injuries* 2004, 30(5): 481–2.

775. Jose RM, Roy DK, Wright PK, Erdmann M. Hand surface area: do racial differences exist? *Burns: Journal of the International Society for Burn Injuries* 2006, 32(2): 216–17.

776. Lee J-Y, Choi J-W, Kim H. Determination of hand surface area by sex and body shape using alginate. *Journal of Physiological Anthropology* 2007, 26(4): 475–83.

777. Liao C-Y, Chen S-L, Chou T-D, Lee T-P, Dai N-T, Chen T-M. Use of twodimensional projection for estimating hand surface area of Chinese adults. *Burns: Journal of the International Society for Burn Injuries* 2008, 34(4): 556–9.

778. Yu C-Y, Hsu Y-W, Chen C-Y. Determination of hand surface area as a percentage of body surface area by 3D anthropometry. *Burns: Journal of the International Society for Burn Injuries* 2008, 34(8): 1183–9.

779. Hidvegi N, Nduka C, Myers S, Dziewulski P. Estimation of breast burn size. *Plastic and Reconstructive Surgery* 2004, 113(6): 1591–7.

780. Ichiki Y, Kato Y, Kitajima Y. Assessment of burn area: most objective method. *Burns: Journal of the International Society for Burn Injuries* 2008, 34(3): 425–6.

781. Singer AJ, Brebbia J, Soroff HH. Management of local burn wounds in the ED. *American Journal of Emergency Medicine* 2007, 25(6): 666–71.

782. Cuttle L, Kravchuk O, Wallis B, Kimble RM. An audit of first-aid treatment of pediatric burns patients and their clinical outcome. *Journal of Burn Care & Research: Official publication of the American Burn Association* 2009, 30(6): 1028–34.

783. Health Protection Agency. *HPA Compendium of Chemical Hazards: Benzene.* London: HPA, 2007. Available from: http://www.hpa.org.uk/Topics/ChemicalsAndPoisons/CompendiumOfChemicalHazards.

784. Health Protection Agency. *HPA Compendium of Chemical Hazards: Cadmium.* London: HPA, 2007. Available from: http://www.hpa.org.uk/Topics/ChemicalsAndPoisons/CompendiumOfChemicalHazards.

785. Health Protection Agency. *HPA Compendium of Chemical Hazards: Carbolic acid.* London: HPA, 2007. Available from: http://www.hpa.org.uk/Topics/ChemicalsAndPoisons/CompendiumOfChemicalHazards.

786. Health Protection Agency. *HPA Compendium of Chemical Hazards: Chlorine.* London: HPA, 2007. Available from: http://www.hpa.org.uk/Topics/ChemicalsAndPoisons/CompendiumOfChemicalHazards.

787. Health Protection Agency. *HPA Compendium of Chemical Hazards: Chloroform.* London: HPA, 2007. Available from: http://www.hpa.org.uk/Topics/ChemicalsAndPoisons/CompendiumOfChemicalHazards.

788. Health Protection Agency. *HPA Compendium of Chemical Hazards: Chromium.* London: HPA, 2007. Available from: http://www.hpa.org.uk/Topics/ChemicalsAndPoisons/CompendiumOfChemicalHazards.

789. Health Protection Agency. *HPA Compendium of Chemical Hazards: Diesel.* London: HPA, 2007. Available from: http://www.hpa.org.uk/Topics/ChemicalsAndPoisons/CompendiumOfChemicalHazards.

790. Health Protection Agency. *HPA Compendium of Chemical Hazards: Ethylene glycol.* London: HPA, 2007. Available from: http://www.hpa.org.uk/Topics/Chemicals AndPoisons/CompendiumOfChemical Hazards.

791. Health Protection Agency. *HPA Compendium of Chemical Hazards: Gasoline.* London: HPA, 2007. Available from: http://www.hpa.org.uk/Topics/ChemicalsAndPoisons/CompendiumOfChemicalHazards.

792. Health Protection Agency. *HPA Compendium of Chemical Hazards: Hydrochloric acid.* London: HPA, 2007. Available from: http://www.hpa.org.uk/Topics/ChemicalsAndPoisons/CompendiumOfChemicalHazards.

793. Health Protection Agency. *HPA Compendium of Chemical Hazards: Hydrogen cyanide.* London: HPA, 2007. Available from: http://www.hpa.org.uk/Topics/ChemicalsAndPoisons/CompendiumOfChemicalHazards.

794. Health Protection Agency. *HPA Compendium of Chemical Hazards: Hydrogen sulphide.* London: HPA, 2007. Available from: http://www.hpa.org.uk/Topics/ChemicalsAndPoisons/CompendiumOfChemicalHazards.

795. Health Protection Agency. *HPA Compendium of Chemical Hazards: Methanol.* London: HPA, 2007. Available from: http://www.hpa.org.uk/Topics/ChemicalsAndPoisons/CompendiumOfChemicalHazards.

796. Health Protection Agency. *HPA Compendium of Chemical Hazards: Naphthalene.* London: HPA, 2007. Available from: http://www.hpa.org.uk/Topics/ChemicalsAndPoisons/CompendiumOfChemicalHazards.

797. Health Protection Agency. *HPA Compendium of Chemical Hazards: Nitric acid.* London: HPA, 2007. Available from: http://www.hpa.org.uk/Topics/ChemicalsAndPoisons/CompendiumOfChemicalHazards.

798. Health Protection Agency. *HPA Compendium of Chemical Hazards: Phosgene.* London: HPA, 2007. Available from: http://www.hpa.org.uk/Topics/ChemicalsAndPoisons/CompendiumOfChemicalHazards.

799. Health Protection Agency. *HPA Compendium of Chemical Hazards: Phosphine.* London: HPA, 2007. Available from: http://www.hpa.org.uk/Topics/ChemicalsAndPoisons/CompendiumOfChemicalHazards.

800. Health Protection Agency. *HPA Compendium of Chemical Hazards: Phosphorus.* London: HPA, 2007. Available from: http://www.hpa.org.uk/Topics/ChemicalsAndPoisons/CompendiumOfChemicalHazards.

801. Health Protection Agency. *HPA Compendium of Chemical Hazards: Styrene.* London: HPA, 2007. Available from: http://www.hpa.org.uk/Topics/ChemicalsAndPoisons/CompendiumOfChemicalHazards.

802. Health Protection Agency. *HPA Compendium of Chemical Hazards: Sulphuric acid.* London: HPA, 2007. Available from: http://www.hpa.org.uk/Topics/ChemicalsAndPoisons/CompendiumOfChemicalHazards.

803. Health Protection Agency. *HPA Compendium of Chemical Hazards: Ammonia.* London: HPA, 2008. Available from: http://www.hpa.org.uk/Topics/ChemicalsAndPoisons/CompendiumOfChemicalHazards.

804. Health Protection Agency. *HPA Compendium of Chemical Hazards: Arsenic.* London: HPA, 2008. Available from: http://www.hpa.org.uk/Topics/ChemicalsAndPoisons/CompendiumOfChemicalHazards.

805. Health Protection Agency. *HPA Compendium of Chemical Hazards: Benzopyrine.* London: HPA, 2008. Available from: http://www.hpa.org.uk/Topics/ChemicalsAndPoisons/CompendiumOfChemicalHazards.

806. Health Protection Agency. *HPA Compendium of Chemical Hazards: Chloroethylene.* London: HPA, 2008. Available from: http://www.hpa.org.uk/Topics/ChemicalsAndPoisons/CompendiumOfChemicalHazards.

807. Health Protection Agency. *HPA Compendium of Chemical Hazards: Formaldehyde.* London: HPA, 2008. Available from: http://www.hpa.org.uk/Topics/ChemicalsAndPoisons/CompendiumOfChemicalHazards.

808. Health Protection Agency. *HPA Compendium of Chemical Hazards: Nitrobenzene.* London: HPA, 2008. Available from: http://www.hpa.org.uk/Topics/ChemicalsAndPoisons/CompendiumOfChemicalHazards.

809. Health Protection Agency. *HPA Compendium of Chemical Hazards: Sodium fluoride.* London: HPA, 2008. Available from: http://www.hpa.org.uk/Topics/ChemicalsAndPoisons/CompendiumOfChemicalHazards.

810. Health Protection Agency. *HPA Compendium of Chemical Hazards: Sodium hypochlorite.* London: HPA, 2008. Available from: http://www.hpa.org.uk/Topics/ChemicalsAndPoisons/CompendiumOfChemicalHazards.

811. Health Protection Agency. *HPA Compendium of Chemical Hazards: Tetrachloroethylene.* London: HPA, 2008. Available from: http://www.hpa.org.uk/Topics/ChemicalsAndPoisons/CompendiumOfChemicalHazards.

812. Health Protection Agency. *HPA Compendium of Chemical Hazards: Trichloroethylene.* London: HPA, 2008. Available from: http://www.hpa.org.uk/Topics/ChemicalsAndPoisons/CompendiumOfChemicalHazards.

813. Health Protection Agency. *HPA Compendium of Chemical Hazards: Acrylonitrile.* London: HPA, 2009. Available from: http://www.hpa.org.uk/Topics/ChemicalsAndPoisons/CompendiumOfChemicalHazards.

814. Health Protection Agency. *HPA Compendium of Chemical Hazards: Bromine.* London: HPA, 2009. Available from: http://www.hpa.org.uk/Topics/ChemicalsAndPoisons/CompendiumOfChemicalHazards.

815. Health Protection Agency. *HPA Compendium of Chemical Hazards: Carbon tetrachloride.* London: HPA, 2009. Available from: http://www.hpa.org.uk/Topics/ChemicalsAndPoisons/CompendiumOfChemicalHazards.

816. Health Protection Agency. *HPA Compendium of Chemical Hazards: Jet fuel.* London: HPA, 2009. Available from: http://www.hpa.org.uk/Topics/ChemicalsAndPoisons/CompendiumOfChemicalHazards.

817. Health Protection Agency. *HPA Compendium of Chemical Hazards: Mercury.* London: HPA, 2009. Available from: http://www.hpa.org.uk/Topics/ChemicalsAndPoisons/CompendiumOfChemicalHazards.

818. Health Protection Agency. *HPA Compendium of Chemical Hazards: Nickel.* London: HPA, 2009. Available from: http://www.hpa.org.uk/Topics/ChemicalsAndPoisons/CompendiumOfChemicalHazard

819. Health Protection Agency. *HPA Compendium of Chemical Hazards: Perfluorooctane sulfonate*. London: HPA, 2009. Available from: http://www.hpa.org.uk/Topics/ChemicalsAndPoisons/CompendiumOfChemicalHazards.

820. Health Protection Agency. *HPA Compendium of Chemical Hazards: Hydrogen peroxide*. London: HPA, 2009. Available from: http://www.hpa.org.uk/Topics/ChemicalsAndPoisons/CompendiumOfChemicalHazards.

821. Health Protection Agency. *HPA Compendium of Chemical Hazards: Tuolene*. London: HPA, 2010. Available from: http://www.hpa.org.uk/Topics/ChemicalsAndPoisons/CompendiumOfChemicalHazards.

822. Morfey D, Patel A. Airway trauma. *Anaesthesia and Intensive Care Medicine* 2008, 9(7): 312–14.

823. Palmieri TL, Warner P, Mlcak RP, Sheridan R, Kagan RJ, Herndon DN, et al. Inhalation injury in children: a 10 year experience at Shriners Hospitals for Children. *Journal of Burn Care and Research* 2009, 30(1): 206–8.

824. Duffy BJ, McLaughlin PM, Eichelberger MR. Assessment, triage, and early management of burns in children. *Clinical Pediatric Emergency Medicine* 2006, 7(2): 82–93.

825. Upshaw JE, Smith CD, Tagge EP, Evans J. Thermal injury in children. *Journal of the South Carolina Medical Association* 2004, 100(12): 342–6.

826. Gauglitz GG, Herndon DN, Jeschke MG. Emergency treatment of severely burned pediatric patients: current therapeutic strategies. *Pediatric Health* 2008, 2(6): 761–75.

827. Yarrow J, Moiemen N, Gulhane S. Early management of burns in children. *Paediatrics and Child Health* 2009, 19(11): 509–16.

828. Ritenour AE, Morton MJ, McManus JG, Barillo DJ, Cancio LC. Lightning injury: a review. *Burns: Journal of the International Society for Burn Injuries* 2008, 34(5): 585–94.

829. Dollery W. Cardiac monitoring not needed in household electrical injury if the patient is asymptomatic and has a normal ECG. *BestBets*, 2003. Available from: http://www.bestbets.org/bets/bet.php?id=9.

830. Bailey B, Gaudreault P, Thivierge RL. Cardiac monitoring of high-risk patients after an electrical injury: a prospective multicentre study. *Emergency Medicine Journal* 2007, 24(5): 348–52.

831. Adukauskiene D, Vizgirdaite V, Mazeikiene S. Electrical injuries. [In Lithuanian]. *Medicina (Kaunas)* 2007, 43(3): 259–66. Abstract in English available from: http://www.ncbi.nlm.nih.gov/pubmed/17413256.

832. Spies C, Trohman RG. Narrative review: electrocution and life-threatening electrical injuries. *Annals of Internal Medicine* 2006, 145(7): 531–7.

833. Health and Safety Executive. Electrical injuries. Available from: http://www.hse.gov.uk/electricity/injuries.htm, 2010.

834. Vierhapper MF, Lumenta DB, Beck H, Keck M, Kamolz LP, Frey M. Electrical injury: a long-term analysis with review of regional differences. *Annals of Plastic Surgery* 2011, 66(1): 43–6: doi 10.1097/SAP.0b013e3181f3e60f.

835. Brenner RA, Taneja GS, Haynie DL, Trumble AC, Qian C, Klinger RM, et al. Association between swimming lessons and drowning in childhood: a case-control study. *Archives of Pediatrics & Adolescent Medicine* 2009, 163(3): 203–10.

836. Durchholz C, Peters J, Staudt F, Pontz B. Childhood drowning: a retrospective analysis. *Notarzt* 2004, 20(5): 168–72.

837. Ross FI, Elliott EJ, Lam LT, Cass DT. Children under 5 years presenting to paediatricians with near-drowning. *Journal of Paediatrics and Child Health* 2003, 39(6): 446–50.

838. Bierens JJLM, Knape JTA, Gelissen HPMM. Drowning. *Current Opinion in Critical Care* 2002, 8(6): 578–86.

839. Kemp A, Sibert JR. Drowning and near drowning in children in the United Kingdom: lessons for prevention. *British Medical Journal* 1992, 304(6835): 1143–6.

840. Cummings P, Quan L. Trends in unintentional drowning: the role of alcohol and medical care. *Journal of the American Medical Association* 1999, 281(23): 2198–202.

841. Franklin RC, Scarr JP, Pearn JH. Reducing drowning deaths: the continued challenge of immersion fatalities in Australia. *Medical Journal of Australia* 2010, 192(3): 123–6.

842. Youn CS, Choi SP, Yim HW, Park KN. Out-of-hospital cardiac arrest due to drowning: an Utstein Style report of 10 years of experience from St Mary's Hospital. *Resuscitation* 2009, 80(7): 778–83.

843. Barbieri S, Feltracco P, Delantone M, Spagna A, Michieletto E, Bortolato A, et al. Helicopter rescue and prehospital care for drowning children: two summer season case studies. *Minerva Anestesiologica* 2008, 74(12): 703–7.

844. Hyder AA, Borse NN, Blum L, Khan R, El Arifeen S, Baqui AH. Childhood drowning in low- and middle-income countries: urgent need for intervention trials. *Journal of Paediatrics and Child Health* 2008, 44(4): 221–7.

845. Salomez F, Vincent J-L. Drowning: a review of epidemiology, pathophysiology, treatment and prevention. *Resuscitation* 2004, 63(3): 261–8.

846. Peden MM, McGee K. The epidemiology of drowning worldwide. *International Journal of Injury Control and Safety Promotion* 2003, 10(4): 195–9.

847. Franklin RC, Scarr JP, Pearn JH. Reducing drowning deaths: the continued challenge of immersion fatalities in Australia. *Medical Journal of Australia* 2011, 192(3): 123–6.

848. al-Talafieh A, al-Majali R, al-Dehayat G. Clinical, laboratory and X-ray findings of drowning and near-drowning in the Gulf of Aqaba. *Eastern Mediterranean Health Journal* 1999, 5(4): 706–9.

849. Papa L, Hoelle R, Idris A. Systematic review of definitions for drowning incidents. *Resuscitation* 2005, 65(3): 255–64.

850. Diplock S, Jamrozik K. Legislative and regulatory measures for preventing alcohol-related drownings and near-drownings. *Australian & New Zealand Journal of Public Health* 2006, 30(4): 314–17.

851. Driscoll TR, Harrison JA, Steenkamp M. Review of the role of alcohol in drowning associated with recreational aquatic activity. *Injury Prevention* 2004, 10(2): 107–13.

852. Eksborg S, Rajs J. Causes and manners of death among users of heroin, methadone, amphetamine, and cannabis in relation to postmortem chemical tests for illegal drugs. *Substance Use and Misuse* 2008, 43(10): 1326–39.

853. Lossius R, Nakken KO. Epilepsy and sudden death. *Tidsskrift for Den norske legeforening* 2002, 122(11): 1114–17.

854. Office for National Statistics. *Deaths Registered in England and Wales in 2010, By Cause*. Available from: http://www.ons.gov.uk, 2010.

855. Watson RS, Cummings P, Quan L, Bratton S, Weiss NS. Cervical spine injuries among submersion victims. *Journal of Trauma* 2001, 51(4): 658–62.

856. Hwang V, Shofer FS, Durbin DR, Baren M. Prevalence of traumatic injuries in drowning and near drowning in children and adolescents. *Archives of Pediatrics & Adolescent Medicine* 2003, 157(1): 50–3.

857. Faddy S. Drowning and near-drowning: the physiology and pathology. *Australian Journal of Medical Science* 2001, 22(1): 4–13.

858. Layon AJ, Modell JH. Drowning: update 2009. *Anaesthesiology* 2009, 110(6): 1390–401.

859. Ouanes-Besbes L, Dachraoui F, Ouanes I, Abroug F. Drowning: pathophysiology and treatment. *Reanimation* 2009, 18(8): 702–7.

860. Claesson A, Svensson L, Silfverstolpe J, Herlitz J. Characteristics and outcome among patients suffering out-of-hospital cardiac arrest due to drowning. *Resuscitation* 2008, 76(3): 381–7.

861. Edwards ND, Timmins AC, Randalls B, Morgan GA, Simcock AD. Survival in adults after cardiac arrest due to drowning. *Intensive Care Medicine* 1990, 16(5): 336–7.

862. Lee LK, Mao C, Thompson KM. Demographic factors and their association with outcomes in pediatric submersion injury. *Academic Emergency Medicine* 2006, 13(3): 308–13.

863. Modell JH, Graves SA, Ketover A. Clinical course of 91 consecutive neardrowning victims. *Chest* 1976, 70(2): 231–8.

864. Modell JH, Idris AH, Pineda JA, Silverstein JH. Survival after prolonged submersion in freshwater in Florida. *Chest* 2004, 125(5): 1948–51.

865. Nussbaum E, Maggi JC. Pentobarbital therapy does not improve neurologic outcome in nearly drowned, flaccid-comatose children. *Pediatrics* 1988, 81(5): 630–4.

866. Suominen P, Baillie C, Korpela R, Rautanen S, Ranta S, Olkkola KT. Impact of age, submersion time and water temperature on outcome in near-drowning. *Resuscitation* 2002, 52(3): 247–54.

867. Wollenek G, Honarwar N, Golej J, Marx M. Cold water submersion and cardiac arrest in treatment of severe hypothermia with cardiopulmonary bypass. *Resuscitation* 2002, 52(3): 255–63.

868. Wyatt JP, Tomlinson GS, Busuttil A. Resuscitation of drowning victims in south-east Scotland. *Resuscitation* 1999, 41(2): 101–4.

869. Woollard M, Hinshaw K, Simpson H, Wieteska S, editors. *Pre-hospital Obstetric Emergency Training*. Oxford: Wiley-Blackwell, 2009.

870. Centre for Maternal and Child Enquiries. Saving mothers' lives: reviewing maternal deaths to make motherhood safer: 2006–2008. *BJOG: An International Journal of Obstetrics & Gynaecology* 2011, 118(suppl. 1).

871. Bourjeily G, Paidas M, Khalil H, Rosene-Montella K, Rodger M. Pulmonary embolism in pregnancy. *The Lancet* 2010, 375(9713): 500–12.

872. Woollard M, Hinshaw K, Simpson H, Wieteska S. Emergencies in early pregnancy and complications following gynaecological surgery. In *Pre-hospital Obstetric Emergency Training*. Oxford: Wiley-Blackwell, 2009: 53–61.

873. Woollard M, Hinshaw K, Simpson H, Wieteska S. Management of non-obstetric emergencies. In *Pre-hospital Obstetric Emergency Training*. Oxford: Wiley-Blackwell, 2009: 136–65.

874. Woollard M, Hinshaw K, Simpson H, Wieteska S. Anatomical and physiological changes in pregnancy. In *Pre-hospital Obstetric Emergency Training*. Oxford: Wiley-Blackwell, 2009: 18–27.

875. Woollard M, Hinshaw K, Simpson H, Wieteska S. Structured approach to the obstetric patient. In *Pre-hospital Obstetric Emergency Training*. Oxford: Wiley-Blackwell, 2009: 38–52.

876. Woollard M, Hinshaw K, Simpson H, Wieteska S. Emergencies after delivery. In *Pre-hospital Obstetric Emergency Training*. Oxford: Wiley-Blackwell, 2009: 111–24.

877. Woollard M, Simpson H, Hinshaw K, Wieteska S. Obstetric services. In *Pre-hospital Obstetric Emergency Training*. Oxford: Wiley-Blackwell, 2009: 1–6.

878. National Institute for Health and Clinical Excellence. *Hypertension in Pregnancy: The management of hypertensive disorders during pregnancy* (CG107). London: NICE, 2010. Available from: http://www.nice. org.uk/nicemedia/live/13098/50418/50418.pdf.

879. Woollard M, Hinshaw K, Simpson H, Wieteska S. Normal delivery. In *Pre-hospital Obstetric Emergency Training*. Oxford: Wiley-Blackwell, 2009: 28–37.

880. Woollard M, Hinshaw K, Simpson H, Wieteska S. Care of the baby at birth. In *Pre-hospital Obstetric Emergency Training*. Oxford: Wiley-Blackwell, 2009: 125–35.

881. Royal College of Obstetricians and Gynaecologists. *Placenta praevia, Placenta praevia accreta and Vasa praevia: Diagnosis and management* (Green-top Guideline 27). London: RCOG, 2011.

882. Royal College of Obstetricians and Gynaecologists. *The Management of Breech Presentation* (Green-top Guideline 20b). London: RCOG, 2006.

883. Royal College of Obstetricians and Gynaecologists. *Umbilical Cord Prolapse* (Green-top Guideline 50). London: RCOG, 2008.

884. Royal College of Obstetricians and Gynaecologists. *Prevention and Management of Postpartum Haemorrhage* (Green-top guideline 52). London: RCOG, 2009.

885. Mousa HA, Alfirevic Z. Treatment for primary postpartum haemorrhage. *Cochrane Database of Systematic Reviews* 2007, 1: CD003249.

886. Starrs A, Winikoff B. Misoprostol for postpartum hemorrhage: moving from evidence to practice. *International Journal of Gynaecology and Obstetrics* 2012, 116(1): 1–3.

887. National Collaborating Centre for Women's and Children's Health. *Diabetes in Pregnancy* (CG63). London: National Institute for Health and Clinical Excellence, 2008.

888. The British National Formulary, British National Formulary for Children. Available from: http://www. bnf.org/bnf/index.htm, 2012.

889. National electronic Library for Medicines. Available from: http://www.nelm.nhs.uk, 2010.

890. NHS Evidence. *List of Drug Interactions*. Available from: http://www.evidence.nhs.uk/formulary/bnf/current/a 1-interactions/list-of-drug-interactions, 2012.

891. The Medicines and Healthcare products Regulatory Agency. Available from: http://www.mhra.gov.uk, 2012.

892. The Medicines and Healthcare products Regulatory Agency. *Patient Group Directions in the NHS*. Available from: http://www.mhra.gov.uk/Howweregulate/ Medicines/Availabilityprescribingsellingandsupplyingof medicines/ExemptionsfromMedicinesActrestrictions/ PatientGroupDirectionsintheNHS/index.htm, 2012.

893. The Medicines and Healthcare products Regulatory Agency. *Paramedics: Exemptions*. Available from: http://www.mhra.gov.uk/Howweregulate/Medicines/ Availabilityprescribingsellingandsupplyingofmedicines/ ExemptionsfromMedicinesActrestrictions/Paramedics/ index.htm, 2012.

894. NHS Evidence. *Adrenaline*. Available from: http://www.evidence.nhs.uk/formulary/bnf/current/a 1-interactions/list-ofdrug-interactions/ sympathomimetics/adrenaline-epinephrine, 2011.

References

895. NHS Evidence. *Adrenaline*. Available from: http://www.evidence.nhs.uk/formulary/bnfc/current/a1-interactions/list-of-drug-interactions/sympathomimetics/adrenaline-epinephrine, 2011–12.

896. NHS Evidence. *Amiodarone*. Available from: http://www.evidence.nhs.uk/formulary.bnf/current/2-cardiovascular-system/23-anti-arrhythmic-drugs/232-drugs-for-arrhythmias/supraventricular-and-ventricular-arrhythmias, 2011.

897. NHS Evidence. *Amiodarone*. Available from: http://www.evidence.nhs.uk/formulary/bnfc/current/2-cardiovascular-system/23-anti-arrhythmic-drugs/232-drugs-for-arrhythmias, 2011–12.

898. NHS Evidence. *Aspirin*. Available from: http://www.evidence.nhs.uk/formulary/bnf/current/2-cardiovascular-system/29-antiplatelet-drugs/aspirin-antiplatelet, 2011.

899. NHS Evidence. *Atropine*. Available from: http://www.evidence.nhs.uk/formulary/bnf/current/5-anaesthesia/151general-anaesthesia/1513-antimuscarinic-drugs/atropine-sulphate, 2011.

900. NHS Evidence. *Atropine*. Available from: http://www.evidence.nhs.uk/formulary/bnfc/current/15-anaesthesia/151general-anaesthesia/1513-antimuscarinic-drugs/atropine-sulphate, 2011–12.

901. NHS Evidence. *Benzylpenicillin*. Available from: http://www.evidence.nhs.uk/formulary/bnf/current/5-infections/51antibacterial-drugs/511-penicillins/5111-benzylpenicillin-andphenoxymethylpenicillin/benzylpenicillin-sodium, 2011.

902. NHS Evidence. *Benzylpenicillin*. Available from: http://www.evidence.nhs.uk/formulary/bnfc/current/5-infections/51antibacterial-drugs/511-penicillins/ 5111-benzylpenicillin-and phenoxymethylpenicillin/ benzylpenicillin-sodium, 2011–12.

903. NHS Evidence. *Chlorphenamine*. Available from: http://www.evidence.nhs.uk/formulary/bnf/current/a1-interactions/list-of-drug-interactions/antihistamines/antihistamines-sedating/chlorphenamine, 2011.

904. NHS Evidence. *Chlorphenamine*. Available from: http://www.evidence.nhs.uk/formulary/bnfc/curren/a1-interactions/list-of-drug-interactions/antihistamines/antihistamines-sedating/chlorphenamine, 2011–12.

905. NHS Evidence. *Clopidogrel*. Available from: http://www.evidence.nhs.uk/formulary/bnf/current/2-cardiovascularsystem/29-antiplatelet-drugs/clopidogrel, 2011.

906. NHS Evidence. *Dexamethasone*. Available from: http://www.evidence.nhs.uk/formulary/bnf/current/6-endocrine-system/63-corticosteroids/632-glucocorticoid-therapy/dexamethasone, 2011.

907. NHS Evidence. *Dexamethasone*. Available from: http://www.evidence.nhs.uk/formulary/bnfc/current/6-endocrine-system/63-corticosteroids/632-glucocorticoid-therapy/dexamethasone, 2011–12.

908. NHS Evidence. *Diazepam*. Available from: http://www.evidence.nhs.uk/formulary/bnf/current/4-central-nervous-system/41-hypnotics-and-anxiolytics/412-anxiolytics/benzodiazepines/diazepam, 2011.

909. NHS Evidence. *Diazepam*. Available from: http://www.evidence.nhs.uk/formulary/bnfc/current/4-central-nervous-system/48-antiepileptics/482-drugs-used-in-status-epilepticus/diazepam, 2011–12.

910. NHS Evidence. *Furosemide*. Available from: http://www.evidence.nhs.uk/formulary/bnf/current/2-cardiovascular-system/22-diuretics/222-loop-diuretics/furosemide, 2011.

911. NHS Evidence. *Glucagon*. Available from: http://www.evidence.nhs.uk/formulary/bnf/current/6-endocrine-system/61-drugs-used-in-diabetes/614-treatment-of-hypoglycaemia/glucagon, 2011.

912. NHS Evidence. *Glucagon*. Available from: http://www.evidence.nhs.uk/formulary/bnfc/current/6-endocrine-system/61-drugs-used-in-diabetes/614-treatment-of-hypoglycaemia/glucagon, 2011–12.

913. NHS Evidence. *Glucose*. Available from: http://www.evidence.nhs.uk/medicine/glucose, 2011.

914. NHS Evidence. *Glyceryl trinitrate*. Available from: http://www.evidence.nhs.uk/formulary/bnf/current/2-cardiovascularsystem/26-nitrates-calcium-channel-blockers-and-other-antianginal-drugs/261-nitrates/glyceryl-trinitrate, 2011.

915. NHS Evidence. *Heparin*. Available from: http://www.evidence.nhs.uk/formulary/bnf/current/2-cardiovascular-system/28-anticoagulants-and-protamine/281-parenteralanticoagulants/heparin/heparin, 2011.

916. NHS Evidence. *Hydrocortisone*. Available from: http://www.evidence.nhs.uk/formulary/bnf/current/6-endocrine-system/63-corticosteroids/632-glucocorticoid-therapy/hydrocortisone, 2011.

917. NHS Evidence. *Hydrocortisone*. Available from: http://www.evidence.nhs.uk/formulary/bnfc/current/6-endocrine-system/63-corticosteroids/632-glucocorticoid-therapy/hydrocortisone, 2011–12.

918. NHS Evidence. *Ibuprofen*. Available from: http://www.evidence.nhs.uk/formulary/bnf/current/10-musculoskeletal-and-joint-diseases/101-drugs-used-in-rheumatic-diseases-and-gout/1011-non-steroidal-anti-inflammatory-drugs/ibuprofen/ibuprofen, 2011.

919. NHS Evidence. *Ibuprofen*. Available from: http://www.evidence.nhs.uk/formulary/bnfc/current/10-musculoskeletal-and-joint-diseases/101-drugs-used-in-rheumatic-diseases/1011-non-steroidal-anti-inflammatory-drugs/ibuprofen/ibuprofen, 2011–12.

920. NHS Evidence. *Ipratropium bromide*. Available from: http://www.evidence.nhs.uk/formulary/bnf/current/3-respiratory-system /31-bro nchodilators/312-antimuscarinic-bronchodilators/ipratropium-bromide, 2011.

921. NHS Evidence. *Ipratropium bromide*. Available from: http://www.evidence.nhs.uk/formulary/bnfc/current/12-ear-nose-andoropharynx/122-drugs-acting-on-the-nose/1222-topical-nasaldecongestants/antimuscarinic/ipratropium-bromide, 2011–12.

922. NHS Evidence. *Metoclopramide*. Available from: http://www.evidence.nhs.uk/formulary/bnf/current/4-central-nervous-system/46-drugs-used-in-nausea-and-vertigo/domperidone-andmetoclopramide/metoclopramide-hydrochloride, 2011.

923. NHS Evidence. *Morphine*. Available from: http://www.evidence.nhs.uk/medicine/morphine, 2012.

924. NHS Evidence. *Morphine*. Available from: http://www.evidence.nhs.uk/formulary/bnfc/current/4-central-nervoussystem/47-analgesics/472-opioid-analgesics/morphine-salts, 2011–12.

925. NHS Evidence. *Naloxone*. Available from: http://www.evidence.nhs.uk/formulary/bnfc/current/15-anaesthesia/151-general-anaesthesia/1517-antagonists-for-central-and-respiratory-depression/naloxone-hydrochloride, 2011–12.

926. Salvucci AA, Squire B, Burdick M, Luoto M, Brazzel D, Vaezazizi R. Ondansetron is safe and effective for prehospital treatment of nausea and vomiting by paramedics. *Prehospital Emergency Care* 2011, 15(1): 34–8.

927. NHS Evidence. *Ondansetron*. Available from: http://www.evidence.nhs.uk/formulary/bnf/current/4-central-nervous-system/46-drugs-used-in-nausea-and-vertigo/5ht3-receptor-antagonists/ondansetron/ondansetron, 2011.

928. Warden CR, Moreno R, Daya M. Prospective evaluation of ondansetron for undifferentiated nausea and vomiting in the prehospital setting. *Prehospital Emergency Care* 2008, 12(1): 87–91.

929. NHS Evidence. *Ondansetron*. Available from: http://www.evidence.nhs.uk/formulary/bnf/current/4-central-nervoussystem/46-drugs-used-in-nausea-and-vertigo/5ht3-receptor-antagonists/ondansetron, 2011.

930. NHS Evidence. *Ondansetron*. Available from: http://www.evidence.nhs.uk/formulary/bnfc/current/4-central-nervoussystem/46-drugs-used-in-nausea-and-vertigo/5ht3-receptorantagonists/ondansetron, 2011–12.

931. NHS Evidence. *Paracetamol*. Available from: http://www.evidence.nhs.uk/formulary/bnf/current/4-central-nervous-system/47-analgesics/471-non-opioid-analgesics-and-compound-analgesic-preparations/paracetamol, 2011.

932. NHS Evidence. *Paracetamol*. Available from: http://www.evidence.nhs.uk/formulary/bnfc/current/4-central-nervoussystem/47-analgesics/471-non-opioid-analgesics-and-compound-analgesic-preparations/paracetamol, 2011–12.

933. The Task Force on the management of ST-segment elevation acute myocardial infarction of the European Society of Cardiology, Van de Werf F, Bax J, Betriu A, Blomstrom-Lundqvist C, Crea F, et al. Management of acute myocardial infarction in patients presenting with persistent ST-segment elevation. *European Heart Journal* 2008, 29(23): 2909–45.

934. The British National Formulary. Reteplase. *BNF 63*. Available from: http://www.medicinescomplete.com/mc/bnf/current/60577.htm, 2012.

935. NHS Evidence. *Reteplase*. Available from: http://www.evidence.nhs.uk/medicine/reteplase, 2012.

936. NHS Evidence. *Reteplase*. Available from: http://www.evidence.nhs.uk/formulary/bnf/current/2-cardiovascular-system/210-stable-angina-acute-coronary-syndromes-and-fibrinolysis/2102-fibrinolytic-drugs/reteplase, 2011.

937. NHS Evidence. *Salbutamol*. Available from: http://www.evidence.nhs.uk/formulary/bnf/current/3-respiratory-system/31-bronchodilators/311-adrenoceptor-agonists/3111-selective-beta2-agonists/salbutamol, 2011.

938. NHS Evidence. *Salbutamol*. Available from: http://www.evidence.nhs.uk/formulary/bnfc/current/3-respiratory-system/31-bronchodilators/311-adrenoceptor-agonists/3111-selective-beta2-agonists/salbutamol, 2011–12.

939. NHS Evidence. *Syntometrine*. Available from: http://www.evidence.nhs.uk/formulary/bnf/current/7-obstetrics-gynaecology-and-urinary-tract-disorders/71-drugs-used-in-obstetrics/711-prostaglandins-and-oxytocics/oxytocin, 2011.

940. The British National Formulary. Tenecteplase. *BNF 63*. Available from: http://www.medicinescomplete.com/mc/bnf/current/106045.htm, 2012.

941. NHS Evidence. *Tenecteplase*. Available from: http//www.evidence.nhs.uk/medicine/tenecteplase, 2012.

942. NHS Evidence. *Tetracaine*. Available from: http://www.evidence.nhs.uk/formulary/bnf/current/15-anaesthesia/152-local-anaesthesia/tetracaine/tetracaine, 2011.

943. NHS Evidence. *Tetracaine*. Available from: http://www.evidence.nhs.uk/formulary/bnfc/current/15-anaesthesia/152-local-anaesthesia/tetracaine/tetracaine, 2011–12.

944. CRASH-2 trial collaborators. Effects of tranexamic acid on death, vascular occlusive events, and blood transfusion in trauma patients with significant haemorrhage (CRASH-2): a randomised, placebo-controlled trial. *The Lancet* 2010, 376(9734): 23–32.

945. CRASH-2 trial collaborators. The importance of early treatment with tranexamic acid in bleeding trauma patients: an exploratory analysis of the CRASH-2 randomised controlled trial. *The Lancet* 2011, 377(9771): 1096–101.e2.

946. Yeguiayan J-M, Rosencher N, Vivien B. Early administration of tranexamic acid in trauma patients. *The Lancet* 2011, 378(9785): 27–8.

947. Cap AP, Baer DG, Orman JA, Aden J, Ryan K, Blackbourne LH. Tranexamic acid for trauma patients: a critical review of the literature. *Journal of Trauma and Acute Care Surgery* 2011, 71(1): S9–14: doi 10.1097/TA.0b013e31822114af.

948. NHS Evidence. *Tranexamic acid*. Available from: http://www.evidence.nhs.uk/formulary/bnf/current/2-cardiovascularsystem/211-antifibrinolytic-drugs-and-haemostatics/tranexamic-acid, 2011.

949. Consensus Working Group on Pre-hospital Fluids. Fluid resuscitation in pre-hospital trauma care: a consensus view. *Journal of the Royal Army Medical Corps* 2001, 147(2): 147–52.

950. Cotton BA, Jerome R, Collier BR, Khetarpal S, Holevar M, Tucker B, et al. Guidelines for prehospital fluid resuscitation in the injured patient. *Journal of Trauma* 2009, 67(2): 389–402.

951. Dalton AM. Prehospital intravenous fluid replacement in trauma: an outmoded concept? *Journal of the Royal Society of Medicine* 1995, 88(4): 213P–216P.

952. Gausche M, Tadeo RE, Zane MC, Lewis RJ. Out-of-hospital intravenous access: unnecessary procedures and excessive cost. *Academic Emergency Medicine* 1998, 5(9): 878–82.

953. Henderson RA, Thomson DP, Bahrs BA, Norman MP. Unnecessary intravenous access in the emergency setting. *Prehospital Emergency Care* 1998, 2(4): 312–16.

954. Mitra B, Cameron PA, Mori A, Fitzgerald M. Acute coagulopathy and early deaths post major trauma. *Injury* 2012, 43(1): 22–5.

955. Revell M, Greaves I, Porter K. Endpoints for fluid resuscitation in hemorrhagic shock. *Journal of Trauma and Acute Care Surgery* 2003, 54(5): 563–7.

956. Roberts K, Revell M, Youssef H, Bradbury AW, Adam DJ. Hypotensive resuscitation in patients with ruptured abdominal aortic aneurysm. *European Journal of Vascular & Endovascular Surgery* 2005, 31(4): 339–44.

957. Kaweski SM, Sise MJ, Virgilio RW. The effect of prehospital fluids on survival in trauma patients. *Journal of Trauma* 1990, 30(10): 1215–18; discussion 1218–19.

958. Spahn D, Cerny V, Coats T, Duranteau J, Fernandez-Mondejar F, Gordini G, et al. Management of bleeding following major trauma: a European guideline. *Critical Care* 2007, 11(1): R17.

959. Eckstein M, Chan L, Schneir A, Palmer R. Effect of prehospital advanced life support on outcomes of major trauma patients. *Journal of Trauma* 2000, 48(4): 643–8.

References

960. Honigman B, Rohweder K, Moore EE, Lowenstein SR, Pons PT. Prehospital advanced trauma life support for penetrating cardiac wounds. *Annals of Emergency Medicine* 1990, 19(2): 145–50.

961. National Institute for Clinical Excellence. *Pre-hospital Initiation of Fluid Replacement Therapy in Trauma* (TA74). London: NICE. Available from: http://www.nice.org.ak/TA074guidance, 2004.

962. Bulger EM, May S, Brasel KJ, Schreiber M, Kerby JD, Tisherman SA, et al. Out-of-hospital hypertonic resuscitation following severe traumatic brain injury: a randomized controlled trial. *Journal of the American Medical Association* 2010, 304(13): 1455–64.

963. Chung KK, Wolf SE, Cancio LC, Alvarado R, Jones JA, McCorcle J, et al. Resuscitation of severely burned military casualties: fluid begets more fluid. *Journal of Trauma* 2009, 67(2): 231–7; discussion 237.

964. Cooper DJ, Myles PS, McDermott FT, Murray LJ, Laidlaw J, Cooper G, et al. Prehospital hypertonic saline resuscitation of patients with hypotension and severe traumatic brain injury: a randomized controlled trial. *Journal of the American Medical* Association 2004, 291(11): 1350–7.

965. Holcroft JW, Vassar MJ, Turner JE, Derlet RW, Kramer GC. 3% NaCl and 7.5% NaCl/dextran 70 in the resuscitation of severely injured patients. *Annals of Surgery* 1987, 206(3): 279–88.

966. Maningas PA, Mattox KL, Pepe PE, Jones RL, Feliciano DV, Burch JM. Hypertonic saline-dextran solutions for the prehospital management of traumatic hypotension. *American Journal of Surgery* 1989, 157(5): 528–33; discussion 533–4.

967. Thompson R, Greaves I. Hypertonic saline-hydroxyethyl starch in trauma resuscitation. *Journal of the Royal Army Medical Corps* 2006, 152(1): 6–12.

968. Vassar MJ, Perry CA, Gannaway WL, Holcroft JW. 7.5% sodium chloride/dextran for resuscitation of trauma patients undergoing helicopter transport. *Archives of Surgery* 1991, 126(9): 1065–72.

969. Vassar MJ, Perry CA, Holcroft JW. Prehospital resuscitation of hypotensive trauma patients with 7.5% NaCl versus 7.5% NaCl with added dextran: a controlled trial. *Journal of Trauma* 1993, 34(5): 622–32; discussion 632–3.

970. Greaves I, Porter K, Smith JE. Consensus statement on the early management of crush injury and prevention of crush syndrome. *Journal of the Royal Army Medical Corps* 2003, 149(4): 255–9.

971. Holcomb JB. Fluid resuscitation in modern combat casualty care: lessons learned from Somalia. *Journal of Trauma* 2003, 54(suppl.): S46–51.

972. Treharne LJ, Kay AR. The initial management of acute burns. *Journal of the Royal Army Medical Corps* 2001, 147(2): 198–205.

973. Mattox KL, Maningas PA, Moore EE, Mateer JR, Marx JA, Aprahamian C, et al. Prehospital hypertonic saline/dextran infusion for post-traumatic hypotension: the U.S.A. Multicenter Trial. *Annals of Surgery* 1991, 213(5): 482–91.

974. Smith JE, Hall MJ. Hypertonic saline. *Journal of the Royal Army Medical Corps* 2004, 150(4): 239–43.

975. Pons PT, Moore EE, Cusick JM, Brunko M, Antuna B, Owens L. Prehospital venous access in an urban paramedic system: a prospective on-scene analysis. *Journal of Trauma* 1988, 28(10): 1460–3.

976. Jones SE, Nesper TP, Alcouloumre E. Prehospital intravenous line placement: a prospective study. *Annals of Emergency Medicine* 1989, 18(3): 244–6.

977. Minville V, Pianezza A, Asehnoune K, Cabardis S, Smail N. Prehospital intravenous line placement assessment in the French emergency system: a prospective study. *European Journal of Anaesthesia* 2006, 23(7): 594–7.

978. Sampalis JS, Tamim H, Denis R, Boukas S, Ruest SA, Nikolis A, et al. Ineffectiveness of on-site intravenous lines: is prehospital time the culprit? *Journal of Trauma* 1997, 43(4): 608–15; discussion 615–17.

979. Daniels R. Surviving Sepsis Campaign: indications for fluid administration in patients with sepsis. Personal communication, 2011.

980. Dellinger RP, Levy MM, Cadet JM, Bion J, Parker MM, Jaeschke R, et al. Surviving Sepsis Campaign: international guidelines for management of severe sepsis and septic shock 2008. *Critical Care Medicine* 2008, 36(1): 296–327: doi 10.1097/01.CCM.0000298158.12101.41.

981. The National Counter Terrorism Security Office. *Pathogens and Toxins.* Available from: http://www.nactso.gov.uk/AreaOfRisks/PathogensToxins.aspx, 2012.

982. The National Counter Terrorism Security Office. *Radioactive Materials.* Available from: http://www.nactso.gov.uk/AreaOfRisks/RadioactiveMaterials.aspx, 2012.

983. The National Counter Terrorism Security Office. *Hazardous Materials.* Available from: http://www.nactso.gov.uk/AreaOfRisks/Hazardous.aspx, 2012.

984. The National Counter Terrorism Security Office. *Hazardous Chemicals.* Available from: http://www.nactso.gov.uk/Default.aspx, 2011.

985. NHS Evidence. *Chemical, Biological, Radiological, Nuclear and Explosives.* Available from: http://www.evidence.nhs.uk/search?q=chemical%2C+biologica l%2C+radiological%2C+nuclear+and+explosives+, 2011.

986. Holdsworth D, Bland S, O'Reilly D. CBRN response and the future. *Journal of the Royal Army Medical Corps* 2012, 158(1): 58–63.

987. Heptonstall J, Gent N. *CBRN Incidents: A guide to clinical management and health protection.* London: Health Protection Agency, 2008. Available from: http://www.hpa.org.uk/webc/HPAwebFile/HPAweb_C/1194947377166.

988. Health Protection Agency, Chemical Hazards and Poisons Division. *Chemical Hazards and Poisons Report: Issue 15.* Available from: http://www.hpa.org.uk/webc/HPAwebFile/HPAweb_C/1242717232594, 2009.

989. Health Protection Agency. *Immediate Health Effects of Explosions.* Available from: http://www.hpa.org.uk/web/HPAweb&HPAwebStandard/HPAweb_C/1204542905759, 2012

990. Health Protection Agency. *Compendium of Chemical Hazards.* Available from: http://www.hpa.org.uk/Topics/ChemicalsAndPoisons/CompendiumOfChemicalHazards, 2012.

991. Health Protection Agency, Centre for Radiation, Chemical and Environmental Hazards. Available from: http://www.hpa.org.uk/AboutTheHPA/WhoWeAre/CentreForRadiationChemicalAndEnvironmentalHazards, 2012.

992. Castle N, Bowen J, Spencer N. Does wearing CBRN-PPE adversely affect the ability for clinicians to accurately, safely, and speedily draw up drugs? *Clinical Toxicology* 2010, 48(6): 522–7.

References

993. Department of Health, Emergency Preparedness Divison. *NHS Emergency Planning Guidance: The ambulance service guidance on dealing with radiological incidents and emergencies.* Available from: http://www.dh.gov.uk/prod_consum_dh/groups/dh_digitalassets/@dh/@en/@ps/documents/digitalasset/dh_114466.pdf, 2010.

994. Department of Health. *Patient Group Direction for the Supply of Ciprofloxacin Tablets by Healthcare Professionals to Adults and Children Aged Over 1.2 Years Exposed to a Suspected Biological Agent.* Available from: http://www.dh.gov.uk/prod_consum_dh/groups/dh_digitalassets/documents/digitalasset/dh_097640.pdf, 2009.

995. NHS Evidence. *Ciprofloxacin.* Available from: http://www.evidence.nhs.uk/medicine/ciprofloxacin, 2011.

996. Department of Health. *Patient Group Direction for the Further Supply of Doxycycline Capsules to Adults and Children Over 12 Years Known to Have Been Exposed to a Biological Agent.* Available from: http://www.dh.gov.uk/prod_consum_dh/groups/dh_digitalassets/@dh/@en/documents/digitalasset/dh_118794.pdf, 2006.

997. NHS Evidence. *Doxycycline.* Available from: http://www.evidence.nhs.uk/medicine/doxycycline, 2011.

998. Department of Health. *Patient Group Direction for the Supply of Potassium Iodate Tablets by Authorised Persons to Patients Exposed to Radioactive Iodine.* Available from: http://www.dh.gov.uk/prod_consum_dh/groups/dh_digitalassets/@dh/@en/documents/digitalasset/dh_123349.pdf, 2012.

999. Wahl P, Schreyer N, Yersin B. Injury pattern of the Flash-Ball®, a less-lethal weapon used for law enforcement: report of two cases and review of the literature. *Journal of Emergency Medicine* 2006, 31(3): 325–30.

1000. Strote J, Range Hutson H. Taser use in restraint related deaths. *Prehospital Emergency Care* 2006, 10(4): 447–50.

1001. Robb M, Close B, Furyk J, Aitken P. Review article: emergency department implications of the TASER. *Emergency Medicine Australasia* 2009, 21(4): 250–8.

1002. Pollanen MS, Chiasson DA, Cairns TJ, Young JG. Unexpected death related to restraint for excited delirium: a retrospective study of deaths in police custody and in the community. *Canadian Medical Association Journal* 1998, 158(12): 1603–7.

1003. Payne-James J, Sheridan B, Smith G. Medical implications of the Taser. *British Medical Journal* 2010, 340: c853.

1004. Mangus BE, Shen LY, Helmer SD, Maher J, Smith RS. Taser and Taser associated injuries: a case series. *The American Surgeon* 2008, 74(9): 862–5.

1005. Best Evidence Topic reports. BET 1: the best treatment for eye irritation caused by CS spray. *Emergency Medicine Journal* 2011, 28(10): 898.

1006. Rechtin C, Jones JS. Cardiac monitoring in adults after Taser discharge. *Emergency Medicine Journal* 2009, 26(9): 666–7.

1007. Royal College of Paediatrics and Child Health. *Evidence Statement: Major trauma and the use of tranexamic acid in children.* London: RCPCH, 2012.

Index

Index

angina 85, 98, 128, 308, 343

angina pectoris 116

angio-oedema 110, 131, 132, 176–7

angiotensin converting enzyme (ACE) inhibitors 131, 176

ankle trauma 220

ankylosing spondylitis 224

anonymising data 4, 5, 6

anoxia 38

antepartum haemorrhage 264, 268–70

antero-posterior compression (APC) 229

anthrax 427, 429

antibiotics 265, 291

    allergic reactions 131, 176

    febrile illness in children 106, 107–8

    gastroenteritis in children 185, 188

    meningococcal disease 126, 127

    respiratory illness in children 110, 111, 112

    sickle cell crisis 122

anticoagulants 147, 172, 215, 287, 309, 427

anticonvulsants 19, 182–6, 298

antidepressants 91, 161, 165, 194–5, 298, 321

antidiarrhoeals 188

anti-emetics 8, 12, 188, 318, 321, 329

anti-fibrinolytic 365

antihistamines 112, 293

anti-inflammatories 14, 134, 287, 313

antimuscarine bronchodilators 316

antiplatelet therapy 147

antipsychotics 92

antipyretics 14, 107–8, 125, 287, 313, 337

anti-tachycardia pacing (ATP) 156–60

antivirals 110

anxiety and anxiety disorders 82, 89, 91

    HVS 116, 117

    overdose and poisoning 166–8

    pain management 8, 12

anxiolytics 91

aorta 212, 232

abdominal aneurysms 71, 73

    aneurysms 46, 370

    dissection 98, 99

aortic valve stenosis 152

APGAR score 264, 265–6, 267

apnoea 37, 39, 102, 110, 249

    newborns 264, 266

appendicitis 71

Approved Mental Health Professionals (AMHPs) 90, 92

armed forces 19

arrhythmias see cardiac arrhythmia

asphyxia 66, 94, 119, 200, 248

    newborns 264, 265, 266, 267

aspiration of meconium 60, 266

aspiration of vomit see gastric aspiration

aspirin 161, 166, 194, 279, 281, 282, 287

    ACS 129, 130

    clopidogrel 287, 296

    furosemide 154

    gastritis 72

    GL bleeding 145, 146, 147

    stroke and TIA 175

asthma 8, 14, 133–6, 154, 321, 333, 335

    adrenaline 135, 136, 180, 284–5

    aspirin 287

    children 103, 110, 133, 178–81

    COPD 137

    dyspnoea 82, 83, 84

    HVS 116, 117, 118

    hydrocortisone 310–313

    ibuprofen 14, 314–15

    ipratropium bromide 135, 136, 180, 181, 316

    salbutamol 134, 135, 136, 179 81, 316, 343–6

asylum seekers 19

asystole 75, 76, 100, 119

    ALS 45, 46, 48, 62–3, 65

    ROLE 37, 39

ataxia 114, 120

Atenolal 161

atheromatous plaque 77

atherosclerosis 152

ATMIST format 200

atracurium 282

atrial fibrillation 77, 119, 157

atrial flutter 77, 157

atropine 9, 13, 76, 281, 282, 288–90

    fluid therapy 374–407

    haemorrhage during pregnancy 269

    neck and back trauma 226

atropine (CBRNE) 281, 282, 421–24, 430, 432

atropinisation 422

attention deficit hyperactivity disorder (ADHD) 19

automated external defibrillator (AED) 42, 43, 44, 63, 64

    fluid therapy 374–407

AV block 76

AVPU scale 371

    coma 78, 80

    febrile illness in children 107

    head trauma 218

    headache 87

    medical emergencies 95, 96, 97, 101

    meningococcal disease 125

Index

Index

Index

Index

Index

haemothorax 36, 200, 202, 207

    dyspnoea 82

    thoracic trauma 232

hallucinations 89, 90, 91, 166, 168, 169

haloperidol 282

Hartmann's solution 354–9

Hazardous Area Response Team (HART) 164, 413, 414

head injury and trauma 36, 96, 199, 200, 202, 204–5, 214–18

    children 29, 206, 208, 209–10, 217

    coma 80

    convulsions 142, 144, 182

    DLoC 78, 214–18, 301

    fluid therapy 216, 218, 348, 355, 366, 370

    headache 86

    immersion and drowning 248

    incapacitating agents 434, 435, 436

    massive cranial and cerebral destruction 29, 37, 39

mental disorder 89, 90

    morphine sulphate 321

    neck and back trauma 224, 226

    oxygen 214, 216–18, 332, 335

    tranexamic acid 365

head tilt 34, 42, 54–6, 94, 100, 102, 206

headache 78, 86–8, 106, 122, 148, 166, 215, 334–5

    pre-eclampsia 271–2

Health Professions Council 279

Health Professions Order (2001) 279

Health Protection Agency 428, 430

heart attack 99, 128–30

    see also myocardial infarction

heart failure 75, 76, 99, 103, 152–5, 333

    dyspnoea 82, 83, 84, 85

    fluid therapy 350, 357, 371, 373

    HVS 117, 118

    ICDs 156, 157, 158, 159

heart rate 62, 63, 64, 65, 420

    arrhythmias 75, 76, 77

    asthma 133, 135, 178, 180

    CEWs 434

    convulsions 142, 144

    electrocution 246, 247

    febrile illness in children 107

    fluid therapy 371–407

    gastroenteritis in children 189

    hypothermia 119, 121

    immersion and drowning 249

    medical emergencies 101

    meningococcal disease 125

    newborns 58, 59, 61, 266, 267

    normal for children 101, 207

    pregnancy 253

    pulmonary embolism 170, 171

    thoracic trauma 233

    see also pulse

heat cramps 113

heat exhaustion 114, 334, 335

heat related illness 113–15, 368

heat stress 113

heat stroke 113–15, 334, 335

heel fracture 221

Helicobacter pylori 72

hemicorporectomy 29, 37, 39

heroin (diamorphine) 8, 131, 162, 167, 176, 196, 282, 325

    pain management in children 12, 14

HEMS doctors 235

heparin 281, 282, 309, 341, 342, 361, 363

herpes simplex encephalitis 107

hiatal hernia 145

high energy transfer injury 219, 221, 229, 237

hips 220, 221

histamine 53, 321

HIV 110, 112

hives 131, 176

home-made explosives 418

hormone replacement therapy (HRT) 170

household products 161, 194

Human Rights Act (1998) 90

humerus 220, 221

hydrocortisone 132, 177, 281, 282, 310–13

    Addisonian crisis 93, 96

    fluid therapy 375–407

hydrofluoric acid 239, 242

hydrogen cyanide 416–17, 428

hydrogen sulphide 162

hydrostatic squeeze effect 248

hydroxycobalamin 164

hypercapnia 78, 94, 139, 248, 333

hypercarbia 47, 214

hypercholesterolaemia 71

hyperextension 226, 230

hyperflexion 226, 230

hyperglycaemia 8, 47, 78, 95, 148, 191, 201, 215

    children 191–3

hyperglycaemic ketoacidosis see diabetic ketoacidosis (DKA)

hyperkalaemia 46, 47, 48, 49, 63, 65, 367

hypernatraemia 113

hyperoxia 47

hyperpnoea 116

Index

Index

interpreters 19, 20

interstitial lung disease 82

intestinal obstruction 70, 71

intracranial haemorrhage 86, 265, 271, 296

intracranial haematoma 214

intracranial pressure (ICP) 214, 216

    see also raised intracranial pressure

intramuscular route 8, 12, 14, 280, 281, 374–407

intranasal route 8, 12, 14, 280, 281

intraosseous (I/O) access 14, 103, 188, 280, 281

    ALS 45, 48, 65

    convulsions 182–3

    eclampsia 273

    fluid therapy 367, 368, 371, 374–407

    ICDs 157

    maternal resuscitation 52

intravenous or intravascular (I/V) access 8, 11–12, 14, 103, 279, 280, 281

    ACS 129

    ALS 45–8, 65

    arrhythmias 76, 77

    birth 258, 260

    burns and scalds 240, 243–4

    coma 80

    convulsions 182–3, 186, 298

    eclampsia 273

    fluid therapy 366, 368, 371, 374–407

    gastroenteritis in children 187, 188, 190

    GI bleeding 147

    glycaemic emergencies 192

    ICDs 157, 159

    maternal resuscitation 52, 53

    naloxone 325

    neck and back trauma 226

    overdose and poisoning 162, 195, 196

    pre-eclampsia 272

    pregnancy 237, 253, 255, 269–70

    thoracic trauma 233, 235

    vaginal bleeding 275

intubation 62, 64, 104

intussusception 72

iodine 431

ipratropium 179, 316, 343, 373–407

ipratropium bromide (Atrovent) 281, 282, 316–17

    asthma 135, 136, 180, 181, 318

    COPD 139, 140, 318

iris 161, 194

iron tablets 147, 161, 164, 194, 195

irritable bowel syndrome (IBS) 71

irritant gases 162, 416–17, 435

ischaemia Ps 219

ischaemia reperfusion response 47

ischaemic heart disease 36, 75, 77, 82, 85, 158, 166

isoproterenol 116

jaundice 265

jaw thrust 34, 94, 102, 200, 206, 217

    BLS 42, 54, 55

    newborns 58, 59

jugular venous pressure (JVP) 153, 155

Kawasaki's disease 107

Kendrick splint 220

Kennedy Report 27, 28

kernicterus 265

ketamine 9, 10, 11, 281, 282

ketones 80, 148, 150, 193

kidneys 71, 212, 232, 287, 296

knee 220, 221

Kussmaul breathing 150, 193

laburnum 161, 194

lacerations 412, 434, 435

lamotrigine (Lamictal) 142

large intestine 212

laryngeal airway 3, 34

laryngeal crepitus 200, 202

laryngeal mask 34, 62, 94, 200, 672–407

laryngectomy 331

laryngitis 66

laryngoscope 50, 59, 60

laryngospasm 9, 13, 14, 248, 266

larynx 60, 110, 236, 253

lateral compression 229

latex 131, 176

laurel 161, 194

LBBB 129, 130

learning disabilities 17, 18, 19, 25, 133, 319

left ventricular failure 75, 137, 152, 344

leg ulcers 122

levonorgestrel 282

lidocaine 282

lidocaine gel 282

lightning strikes 245

limbs 199, 201, 202, 204–5, 208–10, 219–22, 332, 335

    crush injury 203, 347, 348, 354–5, 370

    fluid therapy 347, 348, 354–5, 366, 370

    medical emergencies 96

    pulmonary embolism 170–2, 173

liver 145, 147, 271, 354

Index

Index

Index

Index

sodium valproate (Epilim) 142

soft tissue injury 313

solvents 80

sore throat 110, 111–12

Sotalol 161

spacer devices 134, 135, 136, 178–9, 181

Special Operations Response Team (SORT) 164, 413, 414, 420

spinal cord injury (SCI) 36, 223–8, 230

spinal nerves 224

spinal shock 223

spiral fractures 17, 219

spleen 212, 213, 232

splinting 201, 208

    limb trauma 219–21

    pain management 7, 8, 9, 11, 12

sporting injuries 223

ST-segment elevation myocardial infarction (STEMI) 85, 99

    ACS 128, 129, 130

    drugs 296, 309, 341, 361

stab wounds 212, 213, 234

stable angina 98, 128

status epilepticus 93, 109, 141–4, 166, 182–4, 298

    cocaine 165

sternocleidomastoid muscle 100

sternum 56, 60, 100, 101, 232

steroids 96, 140, 227, 309

    asthma 134, 135, 136, 180, 181, 344

    febrile illness in children 106, 108

    respiratory illness in children 110, 111, 112

stomach 145, 212

streptokinase 131, 176

streptococci 111, 112

stress 72, 116, 122

    asthma 133

stridor 66, 83, 84, 94, 100, 112

    allergic reactions 131, 132, 176, 177

    burns 239, 242

    croup 110–11

stroke 77, 78, 86, 174–5, 239, 271

    glycaemic emergencies 191

    overdose 166, 167

    oxygen 175, 334, 335

strychnine poisoning 38

stun gun 431

subacute hypothermia 119, 121

subarachnoid haemorrhage 78, 86

subcutaneous route 8, 12, 280, 281

subdural bleed 86

sub-lingual route 280, 281

submersion 37, 38, 39, 248, 250

substance abuse see alcohol; drug misuse

sucking chest wounds 36, 200, 207

suction 34, 42, 200, 206

    FBAO 50

    immersion and drowning 248, 249

    neck and back trauma 224

    newborns 257, 266

    obstetric and gynaecological emergencies 254

sudden unexpected death in epilepsy (SUDEP) 141

sudden unexpected death in infancy (SUDI) 27–9

sudden unexpected death in infancy, children and adolescents (SUDICA) 27–9

suffocation 18, 21

suicide 17, 90, 92, 161, 196

sulphur dioxide 138

supraglottic airway 34, 42, 46, 52, 54, 62

suprapubic pressure 262

supraventricular tachycardia (SVT) 77, 157, 159

surfactant 265

surgical emphysema 233, 236

    trauma emergencies 200, 202, 207

suspect packages 413

suxamethonium 283

symphysis pubis 229, 262

syncope 79, 132, 142, 147, 170, 177

syntocinon 320

syntometrine 258, 260, 269, 281, 283, 360

    misoprostol 320, 360

T piece 135, 136, 180, 181

tachycardia 75, 77, 95, 101

    ACS 122

    allergic reaction 132, **177**

    convulsions 142

    febrile illness in children 107, 108

    fluid therapy 366, 367

    gastroenteritis in children 187, 189

    GI bleeding 147

    glycaemic emergencies 150

    haemorrhage during pregnancy 268, 269–70

    heat related illness 113, 115

    HVS 116

    ICDs 156, 157–8

    overdose 167, 168

    pulmonary embolism 171, 172

    respiratory illness in children 110

    thoracic trauma 235, 236

    trauma emergencies 201, 207

tachypnoea 100, 116–18

Index

ulna 220

umbilical cord 257–8, 264, 266
- around neck 257
- cutting 258, 261, 262
- prolapsed 259, 261, 263, 264

uncomplicated faint 79

uncomplicated vasovagal syncope 79

unipolar affective disorder 89

unstable angina 128

upper airway obstruction 82, 112, 137

upper gastrointestinal bleeding 145–7

upper respiratory tract infections (URTIs) 105, 107, 108, 110, 111–12, 149

ureteric colic 71

ureters 212

urge to push 256, 259

urinary tract infection (UTI) 71, 74, 106, 107, 149, 188

urinary tract obstruction 71

urogenital injury 229

urticaria 131, 132, 176, 177

uterine atony 260

uterus and ovaries 212, 237–8, 254, 258

vacuum mattress 223, 224, 225, 227

vacuum splints 221

vagal manoeuvres 77

vaginal bleeding 73, 237, 253–4, 275–6, 334, 335, 360
- delivery 258, 260, 263
- haemorrhage during pregnancy 268–70

vagotonic procedures 75

valsalva manoeuvre 77

valvular dysfunction 82, 85

vancomycin 131, 176

vapour rubs 112

vascular injury 229

vasodilators 154, 308

vasovagal attack 142

vecuronium 283

vena cava 212

venom 131, 176

venous thromboembolism (VTE) 170

ventilation 35, 93, 94, 96, 102, 331–6
- abdominal trauma 213
- ALS 45–9, 62, 65
- asthma 284
- BLS 42, 43, 44
- convulsions 183
- COPD 139, 140
- DLoC 78, 81
- dyspnoea 85

FBAO 66, 67
- head trauma 214, 216
- hypothermia 120
- ICDs 157
- immersion and drowning 248, 249
- major pelvic trauma 230
- maternal resuscitation 52
- meningococcal disease 126
- neck and back trauma 225, 226
- newborns 59, 265
- overdose and poisoning 162
- pulmonary embolism 172
- sickle cell crisis 122
- thoracic trauma 232, 233, 234, 235
- trauma emergencies 207, 208
- trauma in pregnancy 237

ventilation breaths 59

ventricular fibrillation (VF) 75, 76, 245, 286, 361
- ALS 45–9, 62–3, 65
- hypothermia 119, 120, 121
- ICDs 156–7, 159

ventricular tachycardia (VT) 75, 75, 157–8, 286
- ALS 45–8, 62–3, 65
- convulsions 142
- hypothermia 120, 121
- ICDs 156–7, 158, 159, 160

Venturi mask 333, 336

Verapamil 164

vertical shear (VS) 229

violence 91

viral infections 106, 107, 110

Visual Analogue Scale Dyspnoea (VAS-D) 85

vital signs 96, 199, 201
- abdominal trauma 213
- ACS 129
- children 105, 106
- convulsions 143, 183
- fluid therapy 375–407
- GI bleeding 147
- glycaemic emergencies 192
- haemorrhage during pregnancy 269
- head trauma 216
- heat related illness 115
- hypothermia 121
- limb trauma 219, 222
- overdose and poisoning 167
- thoracic trauma 233

vitamin K 131, 176

Volumatic 134, 178

vomiting 187, 318, 329–30

Index

Notes

Notes

Notes

Notes

Notes

Notes